Alcohol and Seizures

Basic Mechanisms and Clinical Concepts

Alcohol and Seizures

Basic Mechanisms and Clinical Concepts

Editors

Roger J. Porter, M.D.
Deputy Director
National Institute of Neurological Disorders and Stroke
Bethesda, Maryland

Richard H. Mattson, M.D.
Professor of Neurology
Yale University School of Medicine
Chief of Neurology
Veterans Administration Medical Center
West Haven, Connecticut

Joyce A. Cramer, B.S.
Associate in Research
Department of Neurology
Yale University School of Medicine
New Haven, Connecticut
Project Director
Epilepsy Research
Veterans Administration Medical Center
West Haven, Connecticut

Ivan Diamond, M.D., Ph.D.
Director, Ernest Gallo Clinic and Research Center
Professor and Vice Chairman
Department of Neurology
Professor of Pediatrics and Pharmacology
University of California, San Francisco
San Francisco, California

Technical Editor

Devera G. Schoenberg, M.S.
National Institute of Neurological Disorders and Stroke
Bethesda, Maryland

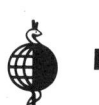

F.A. DAVIS COMPANY • PHILADELPHIA

Copyright © 1990 by F. A. Davis Company

All rights reserved. This book is protected by copyright. No part of it may be reproduced, stored in a retrieval system, or transmitted in any form or by any means, electronic, mechanical, photocopying, recording, or otherwise, without written permission from the publisher.

Printed in the United States of America

Last digit indicates print number: 10 9 8 7 6 5 4 3 2 1

NOTE: As new scientific information becomes available through basic and clinical research, recommended treatments and drug therapies undergo changes. The author(s) and publisher have done everything possible to make this book accurate, up-to-date, and in accord with accepted standards at the time of publication. However, the reader is advised always to check product information (package inserts) for changes and new information regarding dose and contraindications before administering any drug. Caution is especially urged when using new or infrequently ordered drugs.

Library of Congress Cataloging in Publication Data

Alcohol and seizures : basic mechanisms and clinical concepts / editors, Roger J. Porter . . . [et al.].
   p. cm.
   Outgrowth of the International Symposium on Alcohol and Seizures, held Sept. 1988 in Washington, D.C.
   Includes bibliographical references.
   ISBN 0-8036-7008-7
   1. Epilepsy—Complications and sequelae—Congresses.
2. Alcoholism—Complications and sequelae—Congresses.
3. Convulsions—Complications and sequelae—Congresses.   4. Alcohol—Toxicology—Congresses. I. Porter, Roger J., 1942– .
II. International Symposium on Alcohol and Seizures (1988 : Washington, D.C.)
   [DNLM: 1. Alcoholism—complications—congresses. 2. Epilepsy—complications—congresses. 3. Seizures—chemically induced—congresses. 4. Substance Withdrawal Syndrome—therapy—congresses. WM 274 A34973 1989]
RC372.A55   1990
616.8'53—dc20
DNLM/DLC
                                                                                                     90-2712

Authorization to photocopy items for internal or personal use, or the internal or personal use of specific clients, is granted by F. A. Davis Company for users registered with the Copyright Clearance Center (CCC) Transactional Reporting Service, provided that the fee of $.10 per copy is paid directly to CCC, 27 Congress St., Salem, MA 01970. For those organizations that have been granted a photocopy license by CCC, a separate system of payment has been arranged. The fee code for users of the Transactional Reporting Service is: 8036-7008/900 + $.10.

Preface

Two stigmatized disorders, epilepsy and alcoholism, are unfortunately linked by more than chance in some individuals. Although the vast majority of persons with epilepsy are not alcoholic, and while only a small minority of patients with alcoholism suffer epileptic seizures, some patients whose primary problem is epilepsy have seizure exacerbations from alcohol ingestion and some patients with alcoholism have epileptic seizures, usually during withdrawal from the drug. This problem is especially severe in emergency rooms, where seizures related to alcohol—usually in patients who have ingested to excess—present life-threatening implications for a few severely affected patients who develop *status epilepticus*. The sparse literature on alcohol and seizures may be causally related to the combined stigma of the subjects. To better understand the relationship between alcohol and seizures, heretofore a neglected topic, a group of well-known epileptologists and alcohol researchers met in Washington, D.C., for the International Symposium on Alcohol and Seizures in September, 1988. The symposium addressed basic science and clinical issues on the association between alcohol use, seizures, and epilepsy. While the present volume is an outgrowth of this gathering, it is separate from the conference proceedings; it is a comprehensive description of up-to-date clinical investigations and current dilemmas in our understanding of alcohol-related seizures obtained from the foremost authorities worldwide.

Following an introduction to epilepsy and seizures and a description of the magnitude of the problem of alcohol and seizures, the basic scientist illuminates current understanding of the fundamental alterations responsible for alcohol-related seizures. The most basic biochemical changes of ion channels, receptors, neurotransmitters, and cell membranes are considered at length in a series of chapters, followed by discussions of kindling and genetic models. These contributions represent the variety of innovative approaches to understanding how alcohol causes seizures, electrical discharges, and chemical imbalances at all levels of function. The clinical portion of the volume first considers fundamentals of the clinical relationship between alcohol and seizures, then examines the electroencephalogram, etiologies, forms of alcohol seizure patterns, and the relationship to persons with epilepsy. Finally, a series of chapters regarding the appropriateness of antiepileptic drug treatment concludes the clinical sections.

Many physicians, especially in North America, will be surprised that the therapy for alcohol-related seizures varies from place to place around the world. An example is the seemingly novel use of carbamazepine, which is well-documented in Sweden but virtually unknown in the United States. On the other hand, the use of intravenous phenytoin in studies in the United States does not appear to be particularly useful in spite of its popularity. Much work is still needed in evaluating the various therapies for alcohol-related seizures. Even more controversial is the most recent idea that seizures may be caused by alcohol itself rather than by its withdrawal. Little experimental evidence exists to support the epidemiologic data presented in favor of this concept, and a spirited rebuttal is included in the summary chapter. Nevertheless, this provocative thesis causes us to pause to reconsider our time-honored precepts regarding alcohol and its relation to seizures.

We provide a rich diversity of views for the reader to consider and we hope that the efforts of our outstanding contributors will be a service to both investigators and medical practitioners.

Roger J. Porter
Richard H. Mattson
Joyce A. Cramer
Ivan Diamond

Contributors

Brian Alldredge, Pharm.D.
Assistant Clinical Professor of Pharmacy
Division of Clinical Pharmacy
University of California, San Francisco
San Francisco, California

Christer Alling, M.D., Ph.D.
Professor of Psychiatry and Biochemistry
Department of Psychiatry and Biochemistry
University of Lund
Lund, Sweden

Thomas R. Browne, M.D.
Professor and Vice Chairman
Department of Neurology
Associate Professor
Department of Pharmacology and Experimental Therapeutics
Boston University School of Medicine
Boston Veterans Administration Medical Center
Boston, Massachusetts

Peter Carlen, M.D.
Senior Research Scientist
Addiction Research Foundation
Playfair Neuroscience Unit
Toronto, Ontario
Canada

Celia L. Carpenter, B.A.
University of Pittsburgh
School of Medicine
Pittsburgh, Pennsylvania

Arthur W. K. Chan, Ph.D.
Research Institute on Alcoholism
New York State Division of Alcoholism and Alcohol Abuse
Buffalo, New York

John Crabbe, Ph.D.
Research Career Scientist
Department of Veterans Affairs Medical Center
Departments of Medical Psychology and Pharmacology
School of Medicine
Oregon Health Sciences University
Portland, Oregon

Joyce A. Cramer, B.S.
Associate in Research
Department of Neurology
Yale University School of Medicine
New Haven, Connecticut
Project Director
Epilepsy Research
Veterans Administration Medical Center
West Haven, Connecticut

Robert H. Dailey, M.D.
Associate Chief, Department of Emergency Medicine
Merritt Hospital
Clinical Professor of Medicine
University of California, San Francisco
Oakland, California

Robert J. DeLorenzo, M.D., Ph.D., M.P.H.
Professor and Chairman
Department of Neurology
Professor of Pharmacology, Biochemistry and Molecular Biophysics
Director, Molecular Neurobiology and Neuroscience Research Laboratory
Neurologist-in-Chief, Medical College of Virginia Hospitals
Medical College of Virginia
Virginia Commonwealth University
Richmond, Virginia

Orrin Devinsky, M.D.
Director, Epileptology and Clinical Neurophysiology
Hospital for Joint Diseases
Associate Professor of Neurology
New York University School of Medicine
New York, New York

Ivan Diamond, M.D., Ph.D.
Director, Ernest Gallo Clinic and Research Center
Professor and Vice Chairman
Department of Neurology
Professor of Pediatrics and Pharmacology
University of California, San Francisco
San Francisco General Hospital
San Francisco, California

Michael P. Earnest, M.D.
Director of Neurology
Denver General Hospital
Professor of Neurology and Preventive Medicine
University of Colorado School of Medicine
Denver, Colorado

M. Linda Fay
Epilepsy Research
Veterans Administration Medical Center
West Haven, Connecticut

Gerald D. Frye, Ph.D.
Associate Professor
Department of Medical Pharmacology and Toxicology

College of Medicine
Texas A&M University
College Station, Texas

Adrienne S. Gordon
Ernest Gallo Clinic and Research Center
University of California, San Francisco
San Francisco General Hospital
San Francisco, California

David A. Greenberg, M.D., Ph.D.
Associate Professor of Neurology
Department of Neurology
University of California, San Francisco
San Francisco General Hospital
San Francisco, California

W. Allen Hauser, M.D.
Professor of Neurology and Public Health (Epidemiology)
Sergievsky Center
College of Physicians and Surgeons
Columbia University
New York, New York

Matti E. Hillbom, M.D., Ph.D.
Department of Neurology
University of Helsinki
Helsinki, Finland

R. J. E. A. Höppener, M.D.
Mariner 2
The Netherlands

Margaret P. Jacobs
Department of Neurology
Epilepsy Research Center
University of Minnesota
Minneapolis, Minnesota

C. Kwon Kim, Ph.D.
Department of Psychology
University of British Columbia
Vancouver, British Columbia
Canada

Ann Kosobud, Ph.D.
Research Instructor
Department of Physiology and Biophysics
Hahnemann University
Philadelphia, Pennsylvania

Ilo Leppik, M.D.
Professor of Neurology
Comprehensive Epilepsy Program
University of Minnesota
Staff Neurologist
St. Paul Ramsey Medical Center

Director of Pharmacologic Research
MINCEP Epilepsy Care
Minneapolis, Minnesota

J. M. Littleton, M.D., Ph.D.
Professor of Pharmacology
Department of Pharmacology
Kings College
London, England

Ruth B. Loewenson, Ph.D.
Associate Professor of Neurology
Department of Neurology
University of Minnesota
Minneapolis, Minnesota

Michael J. Mana, Ph.D.
Department of Psychology
University of British Columbia
Vancouver, British Columbia
Canada

Shelley S. Marks, B.A.
University of Health Sciences
Chicago Medical School
North Chicago, Illinois

Susanna A. Mathé, M.D.
Department of Neurology
Medical College of Virginia
Virginia Commonwealth University
Richmond, Virginia

Elena M. Mattson
Epilepsy Research
Veterans Administration Medical Center
West Haven, Connecticut

Richard H. Mattson, M.D.
Professor of Neurology
Yale University School of Medicine
New Haven, Connecticut
Chief of Neurology
Veterans Administration Medical Center
West Haven, Connecticut

Charlotte B. McCutchen, M.D.
Associate Professor of Neurology
Department of Neurology
Georgetown University School of Medicine
Chief of Neurophysiology Section
Veterans Administration Medical Center
Washington, D.C.

Robert O. Messing, M.D.
Assistant Professor
Department of Neurology
Ernest Gallo Clinic and Research Center

University of California, San Francisco
San Francisco General Hospital
San Francisco, California

Martha Micks, M.S.
Department of Neurology
University of Minnesota
Minneapolis, Minnesota

Daria Mochly-Rosen
Ernest Gallo Clinic and Research Center
University of California, San Francisco
San Francisco General Hospital
San Francisco, California

A. Leslie Morrow, Ph.D.
Section on Molecular Pharmacology
Clinical Neuroscience Branch
National Institute of Mental Health
Bethesda, Maryland

Stephen K. C. Ng, M.D., Dr.P.H.
Assistant Professor of Public Health and Pediatrics
Sergievsky Center
College of Physicians and Surgeons
Columbia University
New York, New York

Steven M. Paul, M.D.
Section on Molecular Pharmacology
Chief, Clinical Neuroscience Branch
National Institute of Mental Health
Bethesda, Maryland

John P. J. Pinel, Ph.D.
Professor of Psychology
Department of Psychology
University of British Columbia
Vancouver, British Columbia
Canada

Roger J. Porter, M.D.
Deputy Director
National Institute of Neurological Disorders and Stroke
Bethesda, Maryland

J. N. Reynolds, Ph.D.
Addiction Research Foundation
Playfair Neuroscience Unit
Toronto, Ontario
Canada

I. Rougier-Naquet, M.D.
Addiction Research Foundation
Playfair Neuroscience Unit
Toronto, Ontario
Canada

Richard D. Scheyer, M.D.
Post Doctoral Fellow
Department of Neurology
Yale University School of Medicine
New Haven, Connecticut

Roger P. Simon, M.D.
Professor of Neurology
Department of Neurology
University of California, San Francisco
San Francisco, California

Bengt Sternebring, M.D.
Professor
Department of Psychiatry
General Hospital of Malmö
Malmö, Sweden

John K. Sturman, M.D.
Epilepsy Research
Veterans Administration Medical Center
West Haven, Connecticut

Peter D. Suzdak, Ph.D.
Section on Molecular Pharmacology
Clinical Neuroscience Branch
National Institute of Mental Health
Bethesda, Maryland

Martha Taylor, B.S.
Department of Neurology
University of Minnesota
Minneapolis, Minnesota

David M. Treiman, M.D.
Associate Professor of Neurology
Department of Neurology
University of California at Los Angeles
Los Angeles, California
Epilepsy Center
Veterans Administration Medical Center
West Los Angeles, California

Maurice Victor, M.D.
Distinguished Physician
Veterans Administration Medical Center
White River Junction, Vermont
Professor of Neurology
Dartmouth Medical School
Hanover, New Hampshire

David G. Vossler, M.D.
Division of EEG and Clinical Neurophysiology
University of Washington School of Medicine
Seattle, Washington

Jan D. Wallace, M.D.
Yale University School of Medicine
New Haven, Connecticut

Gary P. Young, M.D.
Chief, Emergency Medicine Section
Veterans Administration Medical Center
Portland, Oregon
Assistant Professor of Emergency Medicine and Internal Medicine
Oregon Health Sciences University
Portland, Oregon

Contents

Preface v

PART I
Clinical Overview 1

Chapter 1
Epilepsy and Seizures 3

    Roger J. Porter, M.D.

Chapter 2
Epidemiology of Alcohol Use and of Epilepsy: The Magnitude of the Problem 12

    W. Allen Hauser, M.D.

PART II
Basic Mechanisms of Alcohol-Related Seizures 23

Chapter 3
Models for the Investigation of Alcohol Withdrawal Seizures 25

    Ivan Diamond, M.D., Ph.D.

Chapter 4
Regulation of Neuronal Excitability: Molecular Foundations for the Study of Alcohol Withdrawal 29

    Robert J. DeLorenzo, M.D., Ph.D., M.P.H.

Chapter 5
The Effects of Alcohol on Lipids in Neuronal Membranes 44

    Christer Alling, M.D., Ph.D.

Chapter 6
Calcium Channel Activity in Alcohol Dependency and Withdrawal Seizures 51

    J. M. Littleton, M.D., Ph.D.

Chapter 7
Calcium Channel Changes During Alcohol Withdrawal 60

David A. Greenberg, M.D., Ph.D.; Robert O. Messing, M.D.; Shelley S. Marks, B.A.; and Celia L. Carpenter, B.A.

Chapter 8
Alterations of Neuronal Calcium and Potassium Currents During Alcohol Administration and Withdrawal 68

Peter Carlen, M.D.; I. Rougier-Naquet, M.D.; and J. N. Reynolds, Ph.D.

Chapter 9
Reduced Adenosine Receptor Activation in Alcoholism: Implications for Alcohol Withdrawal Seizures 79

Ivan Diamond, M.D., Ph.D.; Daria Mochly-Rosen; and Adrienne S. Gordon

Chapter 10
Gamma-Aminobutyric Acid (GABA) Changes in Alcohol Withdrawal 87

Gerald D. Frye, Ph.D.

Chapter 11
Ethanol and the GABA/Benzodiazepine Receptor Complex 102

A. Leslie Morrow, Ph.D.; Peter D. Suzdak, Ph.D.; and Steven M. Paul, M.D.

Chapter 12
Development of Tolerance to Ethanol's Anticonvulsant Effect on Kindled Seizures 115

John P. J. Pinel, Ph.D.; Michael J. Mana, Ph.D.; and C. Kwon Kim, Ph.D.

Chapter 13
Alcohol Withdrawal Seizures: Genetic Animal Models 126

John Crabbe, Ph.D., and Ann Kosobud, Ph.D.

PART III
Classification and Diagnosis of Syndromes 141

Chapter 14
Alcohol-Related Seizures 143

Richard H. Mattson, M.D.

Chapter 15
Alcohol Withdrawal Seizures: An Overview 148

Maurice Victor, M.D.

Chapter 16
Alcohol-Related Seizures: A Diversity of Mechanisms? 162

    Stephen K. C. Ng, M.D., Dr.P.H.

Chapter 17
The Electroencephalogram in Patients with Alcohol-Related
Seizures 179

    David G. Vossler, M.D., and Thomas R. Browne, M.D.

Chapter 18
Etiologies of Acute Alcohol-Related Seizures 197

    Michael P. Earnest, M.D.

Chapter 19
Alcohol Withdrawal Seizures and Binge Versus Chronic Drinking . . 206

    Matti E. Hillbom, M.D., Ph.D.

Chapter 20
Alcohol and *Status Epilepticus* 216

    Ilo E. Leppik, M.D.; Margaret P. Jacobs; Ruth B. Loewenson, Ph.D.; W.
    Allen Hauser, M.D.; Martha Micks, M.S.; and Martha Taylor, B.S.

Chapter 21
The Effect of Social Alcohol Use on Seizures in Patients with
Epilepsy 222

    R. J. E. A. Höppener, M.D.

Chapter 22
The Effect of Various Patterns of Alcohol Use on Seizures in
Patients with Epilepsy 233

    Richard H. Mattson, M.D.; M. Linda Fay; John K. Sturman, M.D.; Joyce
    A. Cramer, B.S.; Jan D. Wallace, M.D.; and Elena M. Mattson

Chapter 23
The Effect of Alcohol Use on Anti-Epileptic Drugs 241

    Joyce A. Cramer, B.S., Richard D. Scheyer, M.D.

PART IV
Prevention and Treatment of Alcohol-Related Seizures . . . 251

Chapter 24
Alcohol and Seizures: Principles of Treatment 253

    Orrin Devinsky, M.D., and Roger J. Porter, M.D.

Chapter 25
Treatment of Alcohol Withdrawal Seizures with Benzodiazepines:
Neurochemical Basis 265

    Arthur W. K. Chan, Ph.D.

Chapter 26
Treatment of Alcohol Withdrawal Seizures with Benzodiazepines:
Clinical Applications 283

    David M. Treiman, M.D.

Chapter 27
Treatment of Alcohol Withdrawal Seizures with Phenytoin 290

    Brian K. Alldredge, Pharm.D., and Roger P. Simon, M.D.

Chapter 28
Treatment of Alcohol Withdrawal Seizures with Intravenous
Phenobarbital 298

    Gary P. Young, M.D., and Robert H. Dailey, M.D.

Chapter 29
Treatment of Alcohol Withdrawal with Paraldehyde 304

    Susanna A. Mathé, M.D.; Robert J. DeLorenzo, M.D., Ph.D., M.P.H.

Chapter 30
Treatment of Alcohol Withdrawal Seizures with Carbamazepine
and Valproate 315

    Bengt Sternebring, M.D.

Chapter 31
Treatment of Alcohol Withdrawal Seizures with Other Drugs 321

    Charlotte B. McCutchen, M.D.

Chapter 32
Summary: Questions Answered and Unanswered 329

    Maurice Victor, M.D.

Index 333

PART I

Clinical Overview

Roger J. Porter, M.D.

CHAPTER 1

Epilepsy and Seizures

This chapter provides a basic introduction to epilepsy as a disorder so that seizures associated with alcohol may be placed in appropriate perspective. It also offers the nonneurologist sufficient information about the form and variety of epilepsy and epileptic seizures to allow an understanding of rational diagnosis and treatment. Epilepsy encompasses much more than alcohol-related seizures; the following discussion, therefore, is broader in scope than other chapters in this volume.

Approximately one percent of the population of the United States has epilepsy, the second most common neurologic disorder after stroke. Epilepsy is a heterogeneous symptom complex—a chronic disorder characterized by recurrent seizures. Seizures are finite episodes of brain dysfunction resulting from abnormal discharge of cerebral neurons. The causes of seizures are many and include the gamut of neurologic diseases; metabolic and toxic disorders, infection, neoplasm, and head injury can all result in seizures. In a few subgroups, heredity has proven to be a major factor. The term epilepsy is not usually applied to conditions involving acute seizures, such as meningitis, unless the patient later develops chronic seizures. Occasionally, seizures are caused by an acute underlying toxic or metabolic disorder, in which case therapy should be directed toward that abnormality, for example, hypocalcemia. In most cases of epilepsy, the choice of medication depends on the empirical seizure classification.[11]

Because an epileptic seizure is a definable event—one that is measurable, recordable, and classifiable—one might ask whether an empirical process such as seizure classification is useful for treating epilepsy. In fact, therapy for epilepsy should be based on the seizure type, and a description (usually by history, but occasionally by videotape) is the best clue to the correct therapeutic approach. The seizure diagnosis also yields clues to the etiology of the epilepsy and, to some extent, indicates whether a clearly defined cause will emerge. In treating some patients with epilepsy (those with a brain tumor, for example), the search for the cause and the initiation of therapy based on that cause become paramount. In others, this search is futile, and aggressive studies are not indicated; the major goal in treating such patients is controlling seizures rather than discovering their cause.[10]

The concept unifying treatment of a particular patient is not determining the seizure type but accurately identifying the epileptic syndrome the patient suffers. The classification of epileptic syndromes (the epilepsies) is based not only on seizure type, but also on etiology, age, and other relevant factors. Classifying the syndrome rather than the seizure provides a much clearer view, in many cases, of the prognosis of the disorder, the likelihood of complete control, and the duration of therapy. The level of understanding required of the physician is not trivial, and mastering the classification of seizures is much easier than understanding the classification of epileptic syndromes. The patient will certainly benefit, however, if the physician is able to identify both the seizure type and the syndrome causing the seizures. Unfortunately, the classification of epileptic syndromes is more controversial and less well defined than the classification of seizures. Also, because identification of the seizure type is usually the first step in determining the nature of the epilepsy, emphasis in this chapter is on seizure type recognition rather than on epileptic syndrome determination. The conceptual difference between seizure classification and epilepsy classification has been more extensively reviewed elsewhere.[9]

CLASSIFICATION OF EPILEPTIC SEIZURES

The classification of epileptic seizures as of 1981 is both highly useful and easily applicable to patients with epilepsy.[3] Its success is undoubtedly related to the prolonged refinement of the classification and to the data-oriented nature of its construction. The classification was first organized in its present form in 1969, largely through the exceptional effort of Gastaut, who achieved compromise without sacrificing substance.

Modifications were later superimposed on this seminal document; these modifications came from workshops in the United States and Europe, in which videotaped seizures—the data from which a seizure classification must be constructed—were repeatedly viewed by an international panel of experts. The result, a refinement of the 1969 version, has many improvements and more accurately reflects the nature and heterogeneity of epileptic seizures (Table 1-1).[10]

When classifying epileptic seizures, the physician must first categorize the patient's attacks as either partial or generalized. Partial seizures are those in which a localized onset can be discerned. Such a determination can be made on the basis of many factors, but the major criteria are the clinical nature of the seizures and of the electroencephalogram (EEG) findings, and whether they suggest a localized onset of the seizures. Generalized seizures, a more heterogeneous group, display no evidence of a localized onset in that neither their clinical manifestations nor the abnormal discharges identified by EEG provide a clue to the locus of onset. Therapy for partial seizures is often radically different from therapy for generalized seizures; distinguishing between the two types is thus of great clinical importance.[10]

Table 1-1. INTERNATIONAL CLASSIFICATION OF EPILEPTIC SEIZURES*·†

I. PARTIAL SEIZURES (seizures beginning locally)
  A. Simple partial seizures (consciousness not impaired)
    1. With motor symptoms
    2. With somatosensory or special sensory symptoms
    3. With autonomic symptoms
    4. With psychic symptoms
  B. Complex partial seizures (with impairment of consciousness)
    1. Beginning as simple partial seizures and progressing to impairment of consciousness
      a. With no other features
      b. With features as in A.1-4
      c. With automatisms
    2. With impairment of consciousness at onset
      a. With no other features
      b. With features as in A.1-4
      c. With automatisms
  C. Partial seizures secondarily generalized
II. GENERALIZED SEIZURES (bilaterally symmetrical and without local onset)
  A. 1. Absence seizures
     2. Atypical absence seizures
  B. Myoclonic seizures
  C. Clonic seizures
  D. Tonic seizures
  E. Tonic-clonic seizures
  F. Atonic seizures
III. UNCLASSIFIED EPILEPTIC SEIZURES (inadequate or incomplete data)

*Adapted from Commission,[2] p 493.
†This classification was approved by the International League Against Epilepsy in September 1981.

Partial Seizures

Partial seizures are subdivided into three groups: simple partial seizures, in which consciousness is preserved; complex partial seizures, in which consciousness is altered; and partial seizures (of either type) that progress to generalized tonic-clonic attacks. Consciousness in this context is defined as responsiveness. If the patient has some decrement in his or her ability to respond to exogenous stimuli, then responsiveness, and therefore consciousness, is considered to be altered or lost. Obviously, the degree of difficulty of the task presented affects the application of this definition to a particular patient. Exceptional patients with discrete lesions may be unresponsive but aware (for example, with aphasia); in these patients, whose recall of ictal events is normal, consciousness is considered intact. Although responsiveness is only one aspect of consciousness, this definition allows clinical utilization of the classification of epileptic seizures, because the ability to respond during a seizure can usually be measured.[10]

Seizures may progress, usually in an orderly manner, from one type to another. Although exceptions are possible, the vast majority of partial seizures can be classified as one of six possible progressions (Table 1-2). The concept of progression allows an understanding of *secondary generalization*, that is, the progression of a partial seizure to a generalized tonic-clonic attack. If one views epileptic seizures as a continuum of the spread of the abnormal discharge, then the mildest symptom might be a barely detectable aura (warning) and the most severe symptom a generalized tonic-clonic seizure.

Table 1-2. POSSIBLE PROGRESSION OF PARTIAL SEIZURES*

Seizure Progression	Seizure Name
SP	Simple partial seizures
SP → CP	Complex partial seizures (with SP onset)
CP	Complex partial seizures
SP → GTCS	Partial seizures secondarily generalized—GTCS
CP → GTCS	Partial seizures secondarily generalized—GTCS
SP → CP → GTCS	Partial seizures secondarily generalized—GTCS

*Adapted from Porter,[9] p 18.

The complex partial seizure falls between the two; the involved portion of the brain is sufficient to alter consciousness but insufficient to cause tonic and clonic movement. Consistent with this view of epilepsy, which is readily validated in the clinic when taking a patient's history, is the thesis that the generalized tonic-clonic seizure is the maximal epileptic expression possible in the adult human brain.[12] The characteristics of the generalized tonic-clonic seizure have been well described.[5]

SIMPLE PARTIAL SEIZURES

Simple partial seizures occur with relatively discrete and localized discharges. The patient's ability to comprehend (and later describe) the event reflects the preservation of consciousness. A wide variety of symptoms is possible. Typically, a simple partial seizure begins with a paroxysmal clonic jerking of the arm, gradually slowing in frequency over 30 to 60 seconds, with brief residual weakness. Auras are also simple partial seizures. An aura has traditionally been described as the onset of a seizure; the patient is able to describe the aura because consciousness is maintained. As the seizure discharge spreads, the aura may be followed by a complex partial seizure or a generalized tonic-clonic seizure or both. An aura often occurs in isolation; it is then merely a form of a simple partial seizure.[9]

COMPLEX PARTIAL SEIZURES

Unlike simple partial seizures, complex partial seizures are associated with a decrement in consciousness (responsiveness). Although the seizure begins in a localized area and the attack may be preceded by a simple partial seizure, the spread of the discharge is sufficiently wide (usually bilateral) to alter the patient's ability to respond to exogenous stimuli. Automatic behavior, that is, complicated behavior that requires integration of higher cortical structures and of which the patient has no recollection, is typical, occurring in 96 percent of complex partial seizures in one series.[14] A simplified classification of automatisms is helpful in defining their nature.[9]

De novo *automatisms from internal stimuli* (including "release" phenomena), for example, chewing, lip smacking, swallowing, scratching, rubbing, picking, fumbling, running, and disrobing.

De novo *automatisms from external stimuli*, for example, responding to pin prick, drinking from a cup, chewing gum placed in the mouth, and pushing in response to restraint.

Perseverative automatisms (the continuation of any complex act initiated before loss of consciousness), for example, chewing food, using a fork or spoon, drinking, and walking.

Generalized Seizures

Generalized seizures are epileptic attacks for which no locus of onset can be determined. The group as a whole is heterogeneous; generalized seizures are not related to one another as closely as the various kinds of partial seizures are related.

ABSENCE SEIZURES

The absence seizure is the archetypal generalized seizure. Typically, absence attacks begin in childhood or early adolescence and are characterized by unresponsiveness and a variety of associated phenomena,[7] most notably automatic behavior. Automatisms, however, are often observed in several seizure types and do not distinguish absence attacks from complex partial seizures. Certain distinguishing features are usually helpful: absence attacks are short, usually less than 10 seconds and rarely longer than 45 seconds; the onset is paroxysmal and without warning; and the cessation is likewise sudden and without postictal depression or malaise. Automatisms are common in long attacks; clonic motion, usually of the eyelids, is common in short seizures. A case involving absence seizures has a good prognosis if the patient has normal or above average intelligence and if neurologic examination findings are normal.[13]

MYOCLONIAS

The myoclonias are a heterogeneous group of seizures; moreover, clonic motion is a frequently observed characteristic of other seizure types. The terms most often used to describe the phenomena (myoclonus, myoclonic, clonus, clonic) have been discussed elsewhere,[9] and a volume has been written about epileptic myoclonus.[1] Classifications of myoclonus continue to evolve.[4,6] A review of myoclonia and epilepsy is beyond the scope of this chapter, but emphasis should be placed on the clinical observation that clonic jerking is a surprisingly stereotyped movement; it is not a random flailing about.

CLONIC SEIZURES

Clonic seizures are generalized convulsive seizures that lack a tonic phase and are usually a fragment of a generalized tonic-clonic seizure. In addition, certain patients with epileptic attacks characterized by repetitive myoclonic jerks must be considered to have "clonic seizures." These attacks frequently progress to generalized tonic-clonic seizures.

ATONIC SEIZURES

Atonic seizures are often severely incapacitating attacks in which precipitous loss of tone, usually postural, causes the patient to experience a sudden nodding of the head or to fall to the floor. Although less sudden losses of tone have been described, patients suffering atonic seizures are usually at risk for injury, especially to the face and head, and may require protective helmets.

GENERALIZED TONIC-CLONIC SEIZURE

A generalized tonic-clonic seizure (GTCS) may occur without an antecedent partial or other seizure. Under such circumstances, the attack is termed a *primary* GTCS. The GTCS is the most commonly observed seizure type in alcohol withdrawal. Less clear is whether most of these attacks are primarily or secondarily generalized. Because alcohol withdrawal seizures (AWS) result from a toxic-metabolic disorder, one would expect such seizures to be primarily generalized, that is, without evidence of localized onset. Unfortunately, many alcoholic patients have sustained head injuries and developed post-traumatic partial epilepsy. AWS are often a mixture of GTCSs, partial seizures, and partial seizures progressing to GTCSs. It is interesting that recordings of primary attacks are not common; secondarily generalized tonic-clonic seizures appear to be recorded more often, especially in centers where patients with severe chronic epilepsy are treated and where monitoring equipment is used. Aside from the onset, primary GTCSs are not clinically distinguishable from GTCSs occurring via secondary generalization.

A GTCS is not a random movement of the body and limbs; it is surprisingly stereotyped, although isolated fragments do occur. The typical attack has been well described by Gastaut and Broughton;[5] Tables 1–3 and 1–4 summarize its characteristics. In addition to stereotypical movements, autonomic changes are prominent. Heart rate and blood pressure may double, and bladder pressure may increase up to sixfold. Pupillary mydriasis and glandular hypersecretion of the skin and salivary glands occur. Cyanosis of the skin is correlated with the accompanying apnea.[5]

The EEG accompaniments of a GTCS are usually a desynchronization lasting 1 to 3 seconds, followed by 10 seconds of 10-Hz spikes; as the clonic phase predominates, the spikes are mixed with slow waves, and finally become a polyspike-

Table 1–3. TONIC PHASE OF GENERALIZED TONIC-CLONIC SEIZURES*

1. Usually lasts from 10–20 sec.
2. Begins with brief flexion:
   a. Muscles contract
   b. The eyelids open; eyes look up
   c. The arms are elevated, abducted, and externally rotated; elbows are semiflexed
   d. The legs are less involved, but may be flexed.
3. Extension phase is more prolonged:
   a. Involves first the back and neck
   b. A tonic cry may occur, lasting 2–12 sec
   c. The arms extend
   d. The legs are extended, adducted, and externally rotated.
4. The tremor begins:
   a. The tremor is a repetitive relaxation of the tonic contraction
   b. Starts at 8/sec, gradually coarsens to 4/sec
   c. Leads to the clonic phase.

*Adapted from Gastaut and Broughton,[5] p 28.

Table 1–4. CLONIC PHASE OF GENERALIZED TONIC-CLONIC SEIZURES*

1. Usually lasts about 30 sec.
2. Begins when the muscular relaxations completely interrupt the tonic contraction.
3. Brief, violent flexor spasms of the whole body occur.
4. Often the tongue is bitten.

*Adapted from Gastaut and Broughton,[5] p 29.

and-wave pattern. The EEG tracing is flat or nearly flat after a severe GTCS, but normal brain wave rhythms gradually resume.

CLASSIFICATION OF EPILEPTIC SYNDROMES

Potentially even more useful than the classification of epileptic seizures is the classification of epileptic syndromes. A first attempt was published in 1970, but it was never widely accepted and certain terms were misunderstood and misused, as noted by Wolf.[15] A new classification has been proposed that is controversial and has been rejected by some epileptologists. It represents, however, a start at meaningfully defining the syndromes that cause epileptic seizures. The classification uses 2 fundamental criteria to define the major classes.[2]

First, epileptic syndromes are divided much the same way as epileptic seizures, that is, according to the nature of the attacks suffered by the patient. Epilepsies that have a localized onset (partial seizures) are termed localization-related epilepsies. Those without evidence of a localized onset (generalized seizures) are termed generalized epilepsies.

Both localization-related and generalized epilepsies are then subdivided into syndromes of known cause (symptomatic or "secondary" epilepsies) and idiopathic (primary or "cryptogenic") syndromes. This division is slightly less important than the localization-related/generalized division, which has the advantage that most partial seizures are classified as localization-related, and most generalized seizures are considered a form of generalized epilepsy.

Epileptic syndromes that cannot be easily categorized as either localization-related or generalized are categorized separately. The classification also includes a category of "special syndromes."

The epilepsy syndrome classification has ambiguities that are lessened by the appropriate inclusion of an extensive list of definitions. The classification makes the enormous contribution of clarifying the difference between seizures and epilepsy, and represents an important first step toward classifying syndromes rather than merely classifying seizures on the ward. Because the classification of epileptic syndromes is still evolving and because of its limited relevance to AWS, it will not be discussed further here.

CHRONIC ANTI-EPILEPTIC DRUG THERAPY

Fundamentals of Drug Therapy

Although the major concern of the physician treating AWS is therapy for acute, uncontrolled attacks over a relatively brief period, knowledge of the fundamentals of anti-epileptic drug therapy may be useful for two reasons. First, an understanding of anti-epileptic pharmacology enhances the physician's ability to prescribe effectively. Second, some patients may be candidates for long-term drug therapy.

Seizure classification is important for the pharmacotherapy of epilepsy because seizure type largely determines the appropriate medication. For example, partial seizures and GTCSs are usually treated with phenytoin or carbamazepine, although phenobarbital and primidone also have some effectiveness. Absence seizures respond to ethosuximide or valproic acid; the myoclonias, to valproic acid and occasionally clonazepam.[8] Epilepsy should virtually always be a positive diagnosis; when the diagnosis is uncertain, a therapeutic trial of anti-epileptic drugs is rarely successful. When psychogenic seizures are incorrectly diagnosed as epilepsy, for example, administration of anti-epileptic drugs may result in a temporary placebo effect, temporary worsening of the condition, or intolerance to the medication. Eventually, confusion reigns as more drugs at higher doses are tried. The chief pitfalls in the diagnosis of epilepsy include not recognizing psychogenic seizures, acute anxiety attacks, dissociative states, and syncope. The differential diagnosis of these difficult problems has been reviewed elsewhere.[9]

Drugs Useful for Partial Seizures and GTCSs

In general, drugs useful for treating partial seizures and GTCS—whether primary or secondary—are effective in preventing maximal electroshock (MES) seizures in animals. Of the major drugs available for treating these seizure types, four are most commonly prescribed: phenytoin, carbamazepine, phenobarbital, and primidone. The first two are considered the drugs of choice by most epileptologists.[10] Effective plasma levels are outlined in Table 1–5.

An ED_{50} of 9 mg/kg of phenytoin (Fig. 1–1) is highly effective against MES in rodents. Phenytoin is well absorbed orally, although the absorption rate depends on the formulation used. With intramuscular (IM) injection, absorption is unpredictable. When used intravenously (IV), it is considered a drug of choice for treating

Table 1–5. EFFECTIVE PLASMA LEVELS OF 6 ANTI-EPILEPTIC DRUGS†

Drug	Effective Level (µg/ml)	High Effective Level* (µg/ml)	Toxic Level (µg/ml)
Carbamazepine	4–10	7	8
Primidone	5–15	10	12
Phenytoin	10–20	18	20
Phenobarbital	10–40	35	40
Ethosuximide	50–100	80	100
Valproic acid	50–100	80	100

*Level that should be achieved, if possible, in patients with refractory seizures, assuming that the blood samples are drawn before administration of the morning medication. Higher levels are often possible, without causing toxicity, when the drugs are used alone, that is, as monotherapy.

†Adapted from Porter,[9] p 69.

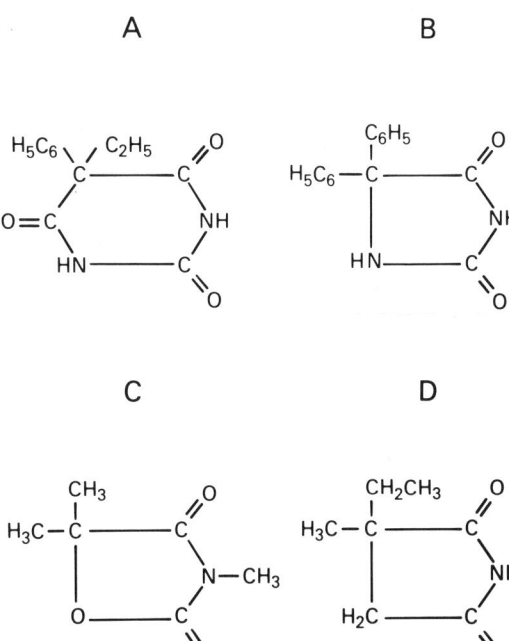

Figure 1–1. Heterocyclic ring structure of some antiepileptic compounds: (A) phenobarbital (B) phenytoin (C) trimethadione (D) ethosuximide.

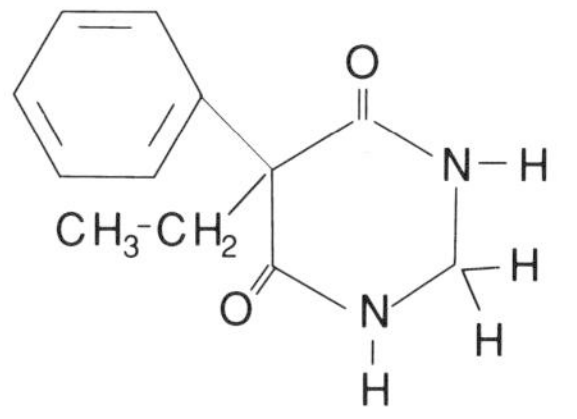

Figure 1–2. The structure of primidone.

status epilepticus. It is highly bound to plasma proteins and is metabolized primarily by parahydroxylation to a clinically inactive metabolite. The dose-dependent kinetics of phenytoin are unique among anti-epileptic drugs. Especially at higher doses (and levels), the maximum capacity of the liver to metabolize phenytoin is attained and the half-life may greatly increase from its usual value of 12 to 36 hours. The most common dose-related side-effects are diplopia and ataxia; idiosyncratic reactions other than skin rash are uncommon. Several minor congeners of phenytoin are marketed, including mephenytoin, ethotoin, and the straight-chain analog, phenacemide.[8]

Carbamazepine, which many researchers consider the drug of choice for this seizure group, is also very effective against MES. The ED$_{50}$ is 9 mg/kg. It is a tricyclic compound, closely related to imipramine (see Fig. 30–1). Absorption is complete, and plasma-protein binding is not clinically important. The drug is metabolized, in part, to a stable epoxide that has anticonvulsant activity. The chronic half-life of carbamazepine is typically 10 to 15 hours. Dose-related side-effects are similar to those of phenytoin; the major idiosyncratic effect is aplastic anemia. This admittedly severe reaction is much less common than has been previously suggested.[8]

Phenobarbital (Fig. 1–1), like other barbiturates and benzodiazepines, is in less favor clinically because of its sedative nature. Aside from the bromides, phenobarbital is the oldest of the currently available anti-epileptic drugs. The ED$_{50}$ of the drug against MES is 22 mg/kg; its antipentylenetetrazol (PTZ) ED$_{50}$ is 13 mg/kg. Absorption is complete, plasma-protein binding is unimportant, and the metabolites are clinically inactive. The half-life may be several days. Dose-related side-effects include sedation, diplopia, and ataxia. Idiosyncratic reactions are usually limited to skin rash. Minor congeners are barbital, metharbital, and mephobarbital.[8]

Primidone is 2-desoxyphenobarbital (Fig. 1–2) and is metabolized to two clinically active compounds, phenobarbital and phenylethylmalonamide; the latter has only weak anti-epileptic action. The ED$_{50}$ of primidone against MES is 11 mg/kg; against PTZ, 59 mg/kg. Absorption is complete; plasma-protein binding is unimportant. The half-life is short—only 8 to 12 hours—but gradually accumulating phenobarbital levels are usually two to three times higher than primidone levels. Toxic side-effects are similar, and often directly related to, phenobarbital.[8]

Drugs Useful for Generalized Seizures

The heterogeneity of the generalized seizures precludes a discussion of therapeutic agents useful for the entire group. In general, ethosuximide is useful against only absence seizures, whereas valproic acid is effective against absence seizures, certain myoclonias, and GTCS.[8] Effective plasma levels are outlined in Table 1–5.

Ethosuximide is the last anti-epileptic compound to be marketed whose origin is the familiar heterocyclic ring structure (Fig. 1–1). Ethosuximide has an ED_{50} of 130 mg/kg against PTZ, but is ineffective against MES in rodents. Absorption is complete, plasma-protein binding is not significant, and metabolites are inactive. The half-life is long, averaging 40 hours. Dose-related side-effects are usually gastrointestinal. Because of its low toxic potential, ethosuximide is generally the drug of choice for absence seizures. Two less important congeners are phensuximide and methsuximide.[8]

Valproate sodium (valproic acid) is one of several carboxylic acids with anti-epileptic activity (see Fig. 30–1). In rodents, its ED_{50} against PTZ is 149 mg/kg; the ED_{50} against MES is 272 mg/kg. Absorption is complete; plasma-protein binding is 90% and may be clinically important. Metabolism is complex and varied; a prominent active metabolite has not been uncovered. Drug interactions, especially with phenobarbital, may be prominent. Dose-related side-effects are usually gastrointestinal; idiosyncratic hepatotoxicity is of some concern.[8] Valproic acid is the drug of choice for patients with absence seizures complicated by concomitant GTCSs. The drug is also very effective against primary GTCSs.

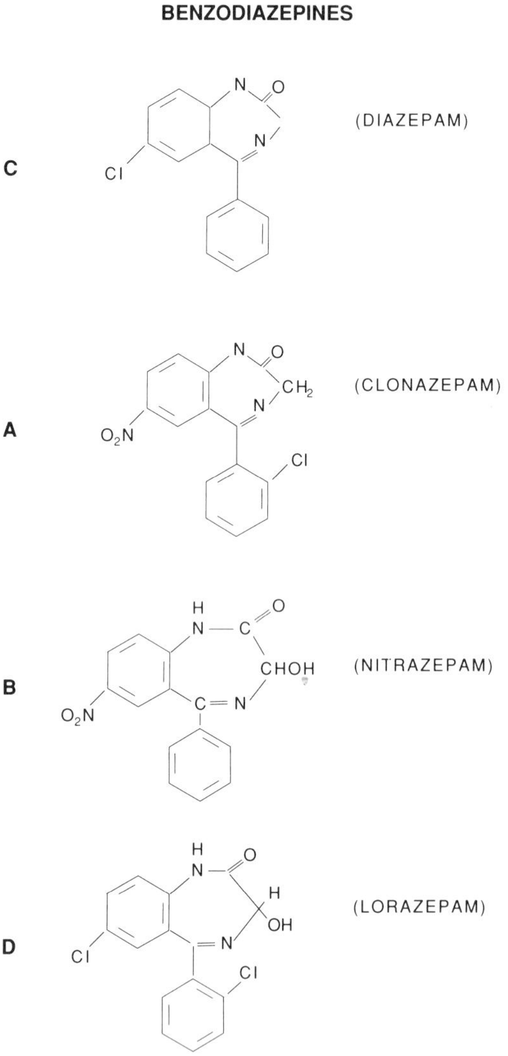

Figure 1–3. The structure of some benzodiazepines used in antiepileptic treatment: (A) clonazepam (B) nitrazepam (C) diazepam (D) lorazepam.

Other Anti-epileptic Drugs

Other anti-epileptic drugs, whose therapeutic usefulness for treating chronic epilepsy is much less than those described, are nonetheless marketed worldwide. Trimethadione (Fig. 1–1) and other oxazolidinediones such as paramethadione and dimethadione are somewhat effective against absence seizures, as are benzodiazepines such as clonazepam and nitrazepam (Fig. 1–3). Other benzodiazepines, notably diazepam and lorazepam (Fig. 1–3), are among the drugs of choice for treating *status epilepticus*. Acetazolamide may have a role in treating catamenial epilepsy, and bromides may be useful in treating porphyria. Steroids and adrenocorticotropic hormone may be effective against infantile spasms.

SUMMARY

Alcohol-related seizures are an isolated but important part of the spectrum of epileptic seizures and syndromes. A full understanding of epilepsy and its pharmacologic treatment will allow the physician more effectively to treat seizures related to alcohol.

References

1. Charleton, MH: Myoclonic Seizures. Exerpta Medica, Amsterdam, 1975, p 167.
2. Commission on Classification and Terminology of the International League Against Epilepsy: Proposal for classification of epilepsies and epileptic syndromes. Epilepsia 26:268, 1985.
3. Commission on Classification and Terminology of the International League Against Epilepsy: Proposal for revised clinical and electroencephalographic classification of epileptic seizures. Epilepsia 22:489, 1981.
4. Gastaut, H: Semeiologie des myoclonies et nosologie analytique des syndromes myocloniques. In Bonduelle, M and Gastaut, H (eds): Les Myoclonies. Masson, Paris, 1968, p 1.
5. Gastaut, H and Broughton, R: Epileptic Seizures: Clinical and Electrographic Features, Diagnosis and Treatment. Charles C Thomas, Springfield, Illinois, 1972, p 286.
6. Marsden, CD, Hallett, M, and Fahn, S: The nosology and pathophysiology of myoclonus. In Marsden, CD and Fahn, S (eds): Neurology 2: Movement Disorders. Butterworth & Co, London, 1982, p 196.
7. Penry, JK, Porter, RJ, and Dreifuss, FE: Simultaneous recording of absence seizures with video tape and electroencephalography. Brain 98:427, 1975.
8. Porter, RJ: Antiepileptic drugs. In Encyclopedia of Neuroscience. Birkhauser, Boston, 1987, p 56.
9. Porter, RJ: Epilepsy: One Hundred Elementary Principles. WB Saunders, London, 1984, p 162.
10. Porter, RJ: Recognizing and classifying epileptic seizures and epileptic syndromes. Neurol Clin 3:495, 1986.
11. Porter, RJ and Pitlick, WH: Antiepileptic drugs. In Katzung, BG (ed): Basic and Clinical Pharmacology, ed 3. Lange Medical Publications, Los Altos, 1987, p 262.
12. Porter, RJ and Sato, S: Secondary generalization of epileptic seizures. In Akimoto, H, et al (eds): Advances in Epileptology: XIIIth Epilepsy International Symposium. Raven Press, New York, 1982, p 47.
13. Sato, S, et al: Valproic acid versus ethosuximide in the treatment of absence seizures. Neurology 32:157, 1982.
14. Theodore, WH, Porter, RJ, and Penry, JK: Complex partial seizures: Clinical characteristics and differential diagnosis. Neurology 33:1115, 1983.
15. Wolf, P: The classification of seizures and the epilepsies. In Porter, RJ and Morselli, PL (eds): The Epilepsies. Butterworth & Co, London, 1985, p 106.

W. Allen Hauser, M.D.

CHAPTER 2

Epidemiology of Alcohol Use and of Epilepsy: The Magnitude of the Problem

The use of agents that alter mind and neurologic function seems to be a constant feature of human society, and alcohol seems to have been the agent of choice throughout time. The use and abuse of alcohol are documented in translations of records recovered from Egyptian pyramids dating back 8000 years.[4] These writings describe wars lost or won because of alcohol abuse, attempts to regulate the distribution of alcohol, and therapies for alcoholism.

The occurrence of seizures has been linked to alcohol use or abuse in medical literature for centuries, starting with the Hippocratic writings. The nature of the assumed relationship, however, has not been constant.[36] Considering the variety of factors to which epilepsy has been attributed over the centuries, it would be remarkable if alcohol use or abuse was not mentioned. Drunkenness has always been considered a cause of epilepsy, but other mechanisms have also been suggested to explain the relationship. These suggestions include alcohol use or abuse in wet nurses, chronic drunkenness in parents, a common genetic predisposition for both drunkenness and epilepsy, and a common trait linking criminality, insanity, alcoholism, and epilepsy.[22] Recently, it has been suggested that persons with epilepsy are more likely to become alcohol abusers, a suggestion not inconsistent with many of the previously mentioned hypotheses.

Although many clinicians now reject folklore developed over centuries about the association between seizures, epilepsy, and alcohol use and abuse, our understanding of the relationship between alcohol use and epilepsy has not advanced significantly over time. Few of our current perceptions are founded upon or confirmed by experimental studies, and because of moral and ethical considerations, experiments involving human subjects cannot currently be undertaken. The few experimental studies involving human subjects that have been reported confuse as much as clarify the relationship between alcohol use and abuse and seizures.

MEASURES OF ALCOHOL USE, ABUSE, AND ALCOHOLISM

A number of methods have been used to estimate the frequency of alcohol use and "alcoholism," both nationally and internationally. Although the most accurate methods of identifying the frequency of alcoholism involve community surveys, these methods are expensive and have thus been undertaken infrequently. Other indirect measures of alcohol use, derived from morbidity and mortality data (hospital admission rates for alcoholism or mortality from cirrhosis), ecologic data (such as per capita consumption of alcohol),[26] or data from opportunistic but frequently biased samples (such as interviews of patients admitted to the hospital) have provided broad estimates of the frequency of alcoholism. Ecologic comparisons have demonstrated positive correlations between mortality from cirrhosis and estimated per capita alcohol consumption.[19]

There is much interest in the frequency of alcohol abuse or "alcoholism," but these concepts are seldom well defined. In part, this is because different measures may be important for evaluating different outcomes. Estimates of the frequency of alcoholism have been variously determined through estimates of the population engaged in heavy drinking, using measures (often complex) of quantity, frequency, and duration;[23] determination of the frequency of alcohol dependency using scales constructed from responses to questions believed to identify alcohol-dependent states; and scales measuring the frequency of adverse social consequences related to drinking, such as loss of jobs, or marital or legal difficulties related to alcohol use.[18] For the last two categories, a scale is usually constructed with the endpoint defined as exceeding a specific number of adverse events over a particular unit of time (not always defined). These three measures (alcohol use, dependency, adverse social consequences) define overlapping but not identical populations.[27] Contrary to intuitive reasoning, alcohol dependency, for example, is not invariably associated with heavy drinking.

Recent population surveys have utilized the Diagnostic Interview Schedule (DIS) to identify persons suffering alcoholism. This questionnaire identifies persons meeting the criteria described in the *Diagnostic and Statistical Manual of Mental Disorders, Third Edition (DSM III)* for alcohol abuse or dependence.[14,40]* This strategy may be problematic: The *DSM III* criteria are sensitive, but not necessarily specific, for the diagnosis of alcohol-related problems.

In evaluating the literature on the frequency of alcohol use or abuse using the measures described, the period of time for which drinking habits or adverse outcomes are being reported should be considered. Partly because of the current tendency to consider alcoholism a lifelong affliction, many surveys report the "lifetime" prevalence of alcohol abuse or dependency, that is, the proportion of the population with any history of heavy drinking or with any history of social problems due to alcoholism. Other studies report the current frequency of alcohol use or abuse (usually a period prevalence ranging from several months to 1 to 3

***Alcohol abuse** is defined in DSM III as a pattern of pathological use of alcohol for at least 1 month *causing* impairment in social or occupational functioning. **Pathological Use** includes: need for daily use of alcohol for adequate functioning; inability to cut down or stop drinking; repeated efforts to control or reduce excessive drinking by "going on the wagon" (periods of temporary abstinence) or restricting drinking to certain times of the day; binges (remaining intoxicated throughout the day for at least 2 days); occasional consumption of a fifth of spirits (or its equivalent in wine or beer); amnesia about events occurring while intoxicated (blackouts); continuation of drinking despite a serious physical disorder that the person knows is exacerbated by alcohol use; drinking of nonbeverage alcohol. **Impairment due to alcohol** includes: violence while intoxicated, absence from work, loss of job, legal difficulties (*e.g.*, arrest for intoxicated behavior, traffic accidents while intoxicated), arguments or difficulties with family or friends because of excessive alcohol use.

Alcohol dependence is defined as *either* a pattern of pathological alcohol use *or* impairment in social or occupational functioning *and either* **tolerance**: need for markedly increased amounts of alcohol to achieve the desired effect, or markedly diminished effect with regular use of the same amount; *or* **withdrawal**: coarse tremor of hands, tongue, and eyelids and at least one of the following: nausea and vomiting; malaise or weakness; autonomic hyperactivity, for example, tachycardia, sweating, or elevated blood pressure; anxiety; depressed mood or irritability; orthostatic hypotension occurring within several hours of cessation or reduction in heavy, prolonged alcohol use and not due to any other physical or mental disorder.[1]

years), and still others report cumulative incidence.

Surveys using random samples have been repeated in the same populations in an attempt to describe time trends in the prevalence of alcohol use. Few studies explore whether patterns of alcohol use or abuse are stable in individual cases over time, and no studies in the United States address the incidence of alcohol abuse using amount, abuse, or dependency criteria.

It seems likely that the neurologic complications of alcohol use (e.g., dementia, seizures, peripheral neuropathy) are related to cumulative dose. Thus none of the standard measures of alcohol use or abuse is truly useful for evaluating the risk of neurologic complications. Only with knowledge of the volume of alcohol a person uses, the duration of use, and the temporal consistency of his or her drinking patterns can the relationship between alcohol use and neurologic complication be determined. Current measures do not provide this information. Although the relationship between the tendency to develop alcohol dependency and the ultimate appearance of neurologic complications may be intriguing, most scales measuring dependency include identified medical difficulties such as "withdrawal seizures." These inclusions negate the usefulness of dependency measures for evaluating the risk of medical complications in general and neurologic complications, including seizures, in particular.

One point of caution in the following discussion: The population of heavy drinkers as identified by amount and frequency questions overlaps with, but is not synonymous with, the population of problem drinkers. Thus, factors that may be dose-related to total alcohol use, such as cirrhosis and the occurrence of seizures, may occur in a group of persons different from those with driving while intoxicated (DWI) convictions, divorce, or job difficulties attributable to alcohol abuse. Neither of these groups is congruous with the population characterized by extended and heavy alcohol use, and for the second group, cause and effect may be difficult to distinguish.

OVERALL FREQUENCY OF HEAVY DRINKING AND ALCOHOL ABUSE

Definitions

For purposes of this discussion, a drink is defined as the equivalent of one ounce of 100-proof whisky. High-volume drinkers are defined by the consumption of more than 1.5 drinks/day. High-maximum drinkers consume more than five drinks or, in recent studies, more than eight drinks at one sitting at least once in the time interval being measured. In the present discussion, heavy drinking is in most cases synonymous with high-volume–high-maximum drinking as far as can be defined from quoted studies. Alcohol abuse refers to the occurrence of social difficulties associated with or due to alcohol use. Generally, four to six independent features must be identified for a person to be considered an abuser of alcohol, although cut-points vary even when similar questionnaires are used. Alcohol dependency is defined as the occurrence of symptoms generally associated with withdrawal, such as shakiness, withdrawal seizures, aberrant patterns of drinking (such as morning drinking), or medical difficulties attributable to alcohol (such as cirrhosis). Again, most surveys have required multiple symptoms to be present for a person to be considered affected. The survey criteria used for the last 40 years are more stringent than the DSM III criteria, which require only one such event for a diagnosis.

Incidence (density) may be defined as the number of newly occurring cases of a disorder within a defined population in a circumscribed period of time. For alcoholism, incidence has been measured in terms of new cases/100,000/year. Prevalence is the proportion of the population afflicted with a disorder at a specific time. *Lifetime* prevalence is the likelihood of being or having been affected with a disorder currently or in the past. Cumulative incidence refers to the risk of suffering from a disorder before reaching a specific age (not necessarily concurrently), based on age-specific incidence rates. For alcohol abuse or dependency, these latter measures usually are reported as a percent.

The earliest epidemiologic studies of alcohol use and abuse were ecologic. Per capita alcohol consumption was shown to be correlated with mortality from cirrhosis.[19] These data suggested differences in the geographic distribution of alcohol use and abuse, and also allowed speculation about the relationship between lifestyle and likelihood of alcohol abuse. The deficiencies of the ecologic approach are obvious, and researchers in the past two decades have used survey methods to better define high-risk groups.

All surveys both in the United States and internationally, indicate that at any specified time a substantial proportion of the population can be considered to engage in *heavy drinking*, no matter how it is defined. Most surveys indicate that the prevalence of frequent heavy drinking among persons over age 10 ranges from 10 to 20 percent. All studies show a higher frequency of heavy alcohol use among men than women: a recent national survey indicates that 20 percent of men can be classified as heavy drinkers compared with 5 percent of women.[3] In this survey, social problems attributable to drinking were identified in 5 percent of men and 2 percent of women. National as well as regional surveys in the 1970s and 1980s suggest that fewer women currently are abstainers than in the preceding decades.[2,8,17,23] However, it does not seem that the rates of heavy drinking or of alcohol abuse or dependency have changed over this same time interval.

Age

Surveys of high school and college students consistently indicate that about 10 percent of teenagers currently engage in heavy drinking.[39,41] Most population-based studies show that the prevalence of heavy alcohol use peaks in the third decade, at which time 30 to 50 percent of men and 10 to 20 percent of women are defined as *heavy drinkers*.[8] After that age, the proportion of the population that drinks heavily decreases. By the seventh decade, 5 to 10 percent of the population are heavy drinkers.

Race

Contrary to the impressions of many clinicians treating inner-city residents, the proportion of abstainers among blacks is higher than among whites, and blacks appear to start drinking at a later age.[31,33,38] When measures of frequency and quantity are used, the proportions of heavy drinkers in the black and Hispanic male populations are similar to those noted in white male populations. However, black women seem to be more likely to drink heavily than white women.

Evaluation of drinking patterns among high school and college students suggests that fewer black than white children and young adults drink, and that fewer can be considered heavy drinkers.[41] When age-specific drinking patterns are evaluated, it appears that a higher proportion of blacks than whites in the fourth and fifth decades can be considered heavy drinkers. Because these conclusions are based on cross-sectional data, it is not clear if blacks start drinking heavily later in life, but continue to drink heavily as they age, or if the patterns reflect a higher frequency of new drinkers. It appears that blacks are more likely than whites to suffer social consequences of drinking—or at least to have a higher rate of arrests, altercations, or DWI convictions associated with alcohol use. Thus, on scales using history of loss of jobs, arrests, or family discord associated with alcohol use or abuse, rates of alcoholism may appear to be higher in blacks, Hispanics, or native Americans. Furthermore, these frequencies may reflect trends in the community from which the data were collected and do not necessarily reflect a specific predilection of minorities to be problem drinkers.

Geographic Patterns of Alcohol Use

In the United States, questions about use (and abuse) of alcohol have been included in several national and regional surveys. Although regional surveys seem to show greater variation and, in general, higher rates of alcohol use or abuse, trends seem consistent across studies.

Drinking in general and heavy drinking specifically are more prevalent in the New England states, the Middle Atlantic area, and the Pacific Coast area.[34] Surveys conducted in the 1960s suggested that people living in urban areas were more likely to be heavy drinkers than people living in rural areas, but subsequent surveys refuted this claim.[8]

Socioeconomic Factors

Lower socioeconomic classes have consistently been shown to have a higher proportion of abstainers, particularly among women.[38] Inconsistent differences have been found in the proportion of heavy drinkers across social classes. Heavy drinkers are over represented among unattached (single, separated, or divorced) men and women. There is a higher proportion of abstainers among persons with less than a high school education; among other educational subgroups, however, researchers have found inconsistent differences in the proportion of heavy drinkers.

Time Trends

National surveys suggest convergence in drinking patterns over time.[17,38] Studies indicate that in the late 1970s a higher proportion of women considered themselves drinkers, and the urban/rural differences are less than in the 1960s. Studies in Iowa extending across periods of drinking-law liberalization suggest that a higher proportion of the population now drink, although the proportion considered to drink heavily has remained the same.[8,28] Similar findings have been reported for adolescents.[39]

Studies that have provided information on both the lifetime and current proportion of people with alcoholism suggest that somewhat less than half the people reporting a lifetime prevalence of alcohol abuse could also be considered abusers at the time of the interview. This finding suggests some lack of permanency of the disorder.[32] The lifetime prevalence of alcohol abuse declines with age. This unexpected pattern suggests that there have been major changes over this century in patterns of alcohol use or abuse with specific cohort effects; that persons who have abused alcohol at some time in their lives die at a much earlier age than those who have not; or that there is an age-related recall bias in data collection. Despite this fall in lifetime prevalence, there appears to be a rather constant proportion of the population (5–6 percent of adults) who at any one time meet criteria for alcoholism.

There are few studies involving repeat interviews of the same persons. About 25 percent of a group of 456 junior high school students (all boys), interviewed as controls for a delinquency study, were reinterviewed at ages 25, 31, and 47.[37] About 25 percent of this group reported multiple symptoms of problem drinking during the time period. In any one age group, about 10 percent of the total cohort were considered alcohol abusers. There seems to have been considerable individual movement into and out of the category of alcohol abuse, however.

I am unaware of incidence studies of alcoholism reported from the United States. In a longitudinal study of drinking patterns of men and boys in Lundby, Sweden, the annual incidence rate for alcohol abuse measured according to DSM III criteria was 30/100,000,[30] and the cumulative incidence was 19.3 percent through age 80. Rates were highest in the 10- to 19-year-old age group, falling with aging. Rates were highest among men classified as working class at the time of the first interview, and among men with only elementary school educations. This study did not address remission or permanency of the condition.

When the reported use frequencies of alcohol among various populations are translated into total alcohol consumption, only about 50 percent of alcohol sales can be accounted for.[8] Surveys tend to exclude teenagers and may not identify adults who drink infrequently or sporadically.

Nonetheless, some researchers have questioned the reliability of drinking estimates provided by population surveys.

INCIDENCE AND PREVALENCE OF EPILEPSY AND SEIZURES

Seizures are among the more frequent symptoms of neurologic dysfunction to affect humans. Even among predominantly white middle-class people in the United States—a group not generally believed to be at high risk for seizures or epilepsy—fully 10 percent of the population can be expected to experience at least one seizure by age 80.[12] This figure may be considerably higher among persons believed to be at high risk for seizures or epilepsy, such as inner-city blacks. For this group, the cumulative incidence for seizures or epilepsy may be more than double the white middle-class rate.[11]

Incidence of Epilepsy

In undertaking etiologic studies of epilepsy, it is important to identify cases as soon as possible after onset. This inclusiveness allows a more complete assessment of potential causes by permitting the study of cases in which the patient dies or goes into early remission. It also enables a better assessment of prognosis. Because of costs and complexities, there are few incidence studies of epilepsy worldwide. Only one series reports the incidence of epilepsy in all age groups in the United States. This series originates from the population-based records-linkage system of the Mayo Clinic in Rochester, Minnesota.[13] The most recent reported incidence of epilepsy is approximately 40/100,000 person-years. In this community, the incidence of epilepsy is high in the first year of life, falls to a stable rate in adulthood, and increases again among persons over age 60.

In most population-based studies of the incidence of epilepsy, about 65 percent of cases have no readily identifiable neurologic antecedent (such as cerebral palsy, stroke, head injury, or infections of the central nervous system), and in slightly over 50 percent of cases, epilepsy is manifest by partial seizures with or without secondary generalization. Rates are slightly higher among men than among women. Extrapolations from prevalence surveys in Harlem, New York suggest that the age-specific incidence rate for epilepsy for inner-city black children may be similar to rates in Rochester. However, the rates for black adults are considerably higher than rates in predominantly white populations.[11]

Prevalence of Epilepsy

Identifying prevalence is useful for determining resource needs in a community. Prevalence is a mix of incidence, mortality, remission, and in-and-out migration in the community; it may also be affected by patterns of medical practice or patient attitudes. Thus, the meaning of prevalence is much more difficult to decipher than the meaning of incidence, and prevalence data are considerably less valuable for etiologic studies.

However, because prevalence may be estimated through one-time population surveys, such studies are much less expensive than incidence studies. For this reason the prevalence of epilepsy is more frequently reported than its incidence in both the United States and other countries. There is great geographic (and socioeconomic) diversity among populations for which prevalence has been estimated, and comparing rates among populations may help explain the genesis of epilepsy. However, these comparisons must be approached cautiously. Variation in prevalence rates probably reflects variation in definitions of epilepsy and in study methodology rather than true differences in the prevalence of epilepsy across diverse populations.

Recent studies of the prevalence of active epilepsy in the United States that include all age groups and that have used comparable definitions provide estimates ranging from 6.7 to 13/1000 population.[9,11,12,24] Prevalence rates, like incidence rates, tend to be slightly higher among men than among women. Rates tend to be higher among older persons and among inner-city residents and minorities, although differences in methodology may explain much of the variation. Both a rural community survey in Mississippi,[9] which included blacks and whites, and a survey of predominantly black and Hispanic inner-city people, revealed higher rates among blacks.[24]

INCIDENCE AND PREVALENCE OF SEIZURES IN PATIENTS WITH CHRONIC ALCOHOLISM

Seizures in Case Series of Patients with Alcoholism

Many clinicians assume that imbibing alcoholic beverages tends to exacerbate seizures in patients with epilepsy.[18] Clinical studies seem to correlate alcohol abuse with a tendency to have poor seizure control in patients with epilepsy.[21] Numerous mechanisms have been suggested to account for a hypothesized increased frequency of seizures in patients with epilepsy who drink alcoholic beverages. Hypotheses include a stimulant effect of the alcohol; a withdrawal effect associated with decreasing blood levels; enhancement of anticonvulsant metabolism through hepatic enzyme induction; alteration of the absorption of anticonvulsant drugs; and noncompliance in patients with epilepsy who drink. Thus, in surveys of alcohol users and abusers using hospital services, one might reasonably expect to find a disproportionate number of persons with a history of epilepsy.

Information about the frequency of seizures or epilepsy among patients with presumed alcoholism has been derived from surveys of persons admitted to hospitals, detoxification units, and psychiatric wards. No surveys have been conducted that relate quantity or frequency measures of alcohol use or measures of social disability or alcohol dependence or DSM III alcohol abuse/dependency criteria to concurrent or past seizures. Because seizure occurrence in association with withdrawal from alcohol is included as an item demonstrating alcohol dependency, any correlation between seizure frequency and alcohol dependency is circular.

In many studies, seizure categorization is less than optimal. Even when an association of seizures with alcoholism is reported, distinctions are rarely made between current and past seizures or between provoked and unprovoked seizures. Studies of admissions to detoxification centers, hospitals, or psychiatric units that mention the frequency with which seizures complicate current admissions seldom distinguish between incidence (newly occurring) seizures and seizures occurring in persons who have previously experienced seizures. It must be remembered that the cumulative risk for any seizure by age 40 is about 4 percent and for epilepsy (recurrent unprovoked seizures), 2 percent. Thus, baseline risks must be taken into account in estimating overall alteration of comorbidity for epilepsy and alcoholism.

Between 4 and 7 percent of alcoholics have convulsive seizures.[20] In a review of all alcohol-related admissions to hospitals in the Feltre region of Italy, 6.6 percent were attributable to seizures.[6] Only 7 percent of the cases involving seizures in this series also involved prior epilepsy (4/1000 of all alcohol-related admissions). This rate is somewhat lower than the expected point prevalence rate of 8/1000 for a group with a mean age of 40.

Alcohol is a substantial risk factor for new onset seizures whether or not withdrawal is involved (see Chapter 16). Although researchers in the United States have seldom considered chronic alcohol abuse as a potential antecedent of epilepsy, this is not true of European researchers. In a Danish study of incidence cases of epilepsy in adults, a history of alcohol abuse was the only identified antecedent in over 20 percent of the cases.[5] Even though the frequency of alcohol use in Denmark may be higher than that in other countries, this proportion seems to have occurred by chance. In the study of seizures in alcoholic patients in Feltre, newly occurring first unprovoked seizures occurred in 1.4 percent of patients admitted for alcohol-related problems, a rate substantially above the expected incidence rate for first unprovoked seizures.[6] Because in most Western countries adults with first seizures tend to be admitted to the hospital to facilitate initial evaluation, this rate is, in all likelihood, considerably inflated.

As with most reports of seizures occurring in the context of staged withdrawal or other medical interventions for alcoholism, first seizures are seldom distinguished from recurrent seizures. Also, most patients admitted to alcohol detoxification centers are sedated with diazepam or chlordiazepoxide, and in many centers anticonvulsant medications are frequently administered as well. The role of anticonvulsants in the management of planned withdrawal is, in fact, the genesis of most recent reports on the frequency of seizures in such situations. Seizures occur in 1 to 7 percent of all patients admitted to detoxification centers.[16,29,35] The rate may be even higher because many patients have had seizures before admission that are not counted. Of course, the seizure may be the reason for admission to the detoxification unit. It appears that first seizures in patients in detoxification centers are rare: as low as 2 or 3 per 1000 admissions. This incidence rate is still five to ten times that expected in the age group usually admitted to such centers, but also suggests that a substantial proportion of patients in such centers have had previous seizures. It is clear that prior seizures (not otherwise defined) are a risk factor for the occurrence of seizures at the time of hospitalization for detoxification, as is concurrent abuse of benzodiazepines or other psychotropic medications.

The incidence of first acute seizure attributed to drug withdrawal (predominantly ethanol) in Rochester, Minnesota was approximately 5 per 100,000 person-years. Rates were almost three times higher among men than among women. The incidence increased almost sixfold from 1935 to 1979 (from 1.3 per 100,000–8 per 100,000 person-years). This increase was noted in both men and women. The male:female ratio of incidence was constant over time, however. It is not clear whether drug and alcohol abuse were more frequent in the later years of the study or if clinicians were reluctant to code alcohol-related events in the early years. We have no information about the prevalence or time trends of alcohol use in this community. Longitudinal studies of persons experiencing a first seizure presumed to be associated with withdrawal suggest that one in three will have seizure recurrence within the next three years.[10] This rate is similar to the recurrence rate reported for idiopathic epilepsy.

Alcohol Use in Case Series of Patients with Epilepsy

Several investigators have reported the frequency of alcohol use in patients with seizures. In a review of 472 adults admitted for seizures to the neurology ward of Denver Municipal Hospital, 42 percent (195) had a history of alcohol abuse.[7] Approximately 60 percent of the patients with alcohol histories had seizures presumed to be related to withdrawal, but 24 percent had seizures categorized as of unknown cause. Only 2 percent had a history of epilepsy, a figure close to the expected cumulative incidence of epilepsy. These data suggest that patients with epilepsy are not overrepresented among patients who are alcohol abusers.

Hillbom,[15] in a review of emergency room contacts for seizures, reported an immediate history of alcohol intoxication in 49 percent of seizure patients. More than half the seizures were attributed to alcohol withdrawal but 15 percent were thought to have no specific etiology and thus would seem to represent first unprovoked seizures. In a random survey of patients admitted to Harlem Hospital, New York, 47 percent of whom were defined as suffering from alcoholism, all patients admitted for seizures were identified as alcoholics.[25] In the series of seizure patients evaluated at the Division of Neurology at Feltre Hospital, in which 6.6 percent of alcohol-related admissions were for seizures, only about one fifth of the seizures were associated with withdrawal from alcohol.[6] Prior epilepsy was identified in 6.5 percent of alcoholic patients. This rate is higher than would be expected given usual cumulative incidence rates for epilepsy. It is impossible to estimate a risk for seizures for alcoholics in general.

Lennox conducted a survey of the frequency and nature of alcohol use in patients with epilepsy and obtained similar information about a control group of nonepileptic persons consisting of medical students, nursing students, and hospitalized patients.[22] The proportion of persons who never used alcohol was higher in the epilepsy group than in the control group (69 percent vs. 47 percent, respectively), although the difference was totally accounted for by a higher proportion of alcohol users among the men in the control group. Although the proportion of persons who drank a "large" amount of alcohol was slightly lower in the epilepsy group than in the control group (7 percent vs. 10 percent), among epilepsy patients who did drink, the proportion who drank a large amount was slightly higher (22 percent vs. 19 percent). Lennox realized the inadequacies of his controls, but believed his data were consistent with the assumption that patients with epilepsy did not use more alcohol than persons not suffering epilepsy. Lennox made two additional observations about the use of alcohol among persons with epilepsy: those who drank frequently also tended to drink a large amount, and the proportion of men who used alcohol increased with advancing age.

A few other researchers have systematically studied the frequency of alcohol use among patients with epilepsy (see Chapter 14). One might reasonably expect a lower proportion of persons with epilepsy to drink because of the usual admonition against such activity by their physicians.

SUMMARY

A substantial proportion of the adult population (roughly 10 percent) drinks heavily. A substantial proportion of the population (roughly 10 percent) suffers from seizures and at least 4.5 percent will have a diagnosis of epilepsy by the age of 80. The chance coexistence of these conditions would not be unusual. Nonetheless, persons suffering seizures and epilepsy seem over-represented among people with history of alcohol abuse, while patients with a history of epilepsy seem under-represented in patient series dealing with the problem of alcoholism. Although the relationship between alcoholism and epilepsy on a constitutional basis must be questioned, alcohol must be considered a major risk-factor for the occurrence of seizures and epilepsy.

References

1. American Psychiatric Association: Diagnostic and Statistical Manual of Mental Disorders, ed 3. APA, Washington, DC, 1980, pp 133, 169.
2. Cahalan, D and Cisin, IH: American drinking practices: Findings of drinking by population subgroups. J Stud Alcohol 29:130, 1968.
3. Clark, W and Midanik, L: Alcohol use and alcohol problems among U.S. adults: Results of the 1979 national survey. In Alcohol Consumption and Related Problems: Alcohol and Health Monograph I. US Dept. of Health and Human Services Publication No (ADM) 82-1190. US Government Printing Office, Washington, DC, 1982.
4. Crothers, TD: Inebriety: A Clinical Treatise of the Etiology, Symptomatology, Neurosis, Psychosis and Treatment and the Medical-Legal Relations. Harvey Publishing, Cincinnati, 1911.
5. Dam, AM, et al: Late-onset epilepsy: Etiologies, types of seizures, and value of clinical investigation, EEG, and computerized tomography scan. Epilepsia 26:227, 1985.
6. Devetag, F, et al: Alcoholic epilepsy: Review of a series and proposed classification and etiopathogenesis. Ital J Neurol Sci 3:275, 1983.
7. Earnest, MP and Yarnell, PR: Seizure admissions to a city hospital: The role of alcohol. Epilepsia 17:387, 1976.
8. Fitzgerald, JL and Mulford, HA: Prevalence and extent of drinking in Iowa: 1979. J Stud Alcohol 42:38, 1981.
9. Haerer, AF, Anderson, DW, and Schoenberg, BS: Prevalence of clinical features of epilepsy in a biracial United States population. Epilepsia 27:66, 1986.
10. Hauser, WA, et al: Clinical findings, seizure recurrence, and sibling risk in alcohol-withdrawal seizure patients. Epilepsia 23:439, 1982.
11. Hauser, WA, et al: Prevalence of epilepsy in a black inner-city community—a telephone survey. Neurology (Suppl 1)36:108, 1986.
12. Hauser, WA, Annegers, JF, and Kurland, LT: The incidence of epilepsy in Rochester, Minnesota 1935–79. Epilepsia 25:666, 1984.
13. Hauser, WA and Kurland, LT: The epidemiology of epilepsy in Rochester, Minn. 1935–67. Epilepsia 16:1, 1975.
14. Helzer, JE, et al: Alcoholism: A cross-national comparison of population surveys with the diagnostic interview schedule. In Rose, RM and

Barrett, J (eds): Alcoholism: Origins and Outcome. Raven Press, New York, 1988, p 31.
15. Hillbom, ME: Occurrence of cerebral seizures provoked by alcohol abuse. Epilepsia 21:459, 1980.
16. Hillbom, ME and Hjelm-Jaeger, M: Should alcohol withdrawal seizures be treated with antiepileptic drugs? Acta Neurol Scand 69:39, 1984.
17. Hilton, ME: Drinking patterns and drinking problems in 1984: Results from a general population survey. Alcoholism: Clinical and Experimental Research 11:167, 1987.
18. Hoppener, RJ, Kuyer, A, and van der Lugt, PJM: Epilepsy and alcohol: The influence of social alcohol intake on seizures and treatment in epilepsy. Epilepsia 24:459, 1983.
19. Jellinek, EM: Estimating the prevalence of alcoholism modified values in the Jellinek Formula and an alternative approach. Quarterly Journal of Studies on Alcohol 20:261, 1959.
20. Lafon, R, et al: L'epilepsie tardive de l'alcoolisme chronique. Rev Neurol 34:624, 1956.
21. Lambie, DG, Stanway, L, and Johnson, RH: Factors which influence the effectiveness of treatment of epilepsy. Aust NZ J Med 16:779, 1986.
22. Lennox, WG: Alcohol and epilepsy. Quarterly Journal of Studies on Alcohol 2:1, 1941.
23. Little, RE, Schultz, FA, and Mandell, W: Describing alcohol consumption: A comparison of three methods and a new approach. J Stud Alcohol 38:554, 1977.
24. Locke, GE, et al: Prevalence of epilepsy in an urban minority population: Los Angeles. Epilepsia 27:618, 1986.
25. McCusker, J, Cherubin, CE, and Zimberg, S: Prevalence of alcoholism in general municipal population. NY State J Med 751, 1971.
26. Miller, GH and Agnew, N: The Ledermann model of alcohol consumption: Description, implications and assessment. Quarterly Journal of Studies on Alcohol 35:877, 1974.
27. Mulford, HA: Stages in the alcoholic process: Toward a cumulative nonsequential index. J Stud Alcohol 38:563, 1977.
28. Mulford, HA and Fitzgerald, JL: Changes in alcohol sales and drinking problems in Iowa: 1961–1979. J Stud Alcohol 44:138, 1983.
29. Newsom, JA: Withdrawal seizures in an in-patient alcoholism program. In Galanter, M (ed): Currents in Alcoholism, Vol VI, Treatment and Rehabilitation and Epidemiology. Grune & Stratton, New York, 1979, p 11.
30. Ojesjo, L: Risks for alcoholism by age and class among males: The Lundby cohort. In Goodwin, DW, Van Dusen, KT, and Mednick, SA (eds): Longitudinal Research in Alcoholism. Kluwer-Nijhoff Publishing, Boston, 1984, p 9.
31. Report of the Secretary's Task Force on Black and Minority Health, Vol VII, Chemical Dependency and Diabetes. US Dept. of Health and Human Services, Washington, DC, 1986.
32. Robins, LN, et al: Alcohol disorders in the community: A report from the epidemiologic catchment area. In Rose, RM and Barrett, J (eds): Alcoholism: Origins and Outcome. Raven Press, New York, 1988, p 15.
33. Robins, LN, Murphy, GE, and Breckenridge, MD: Drinking behavior of young urban Negro men. J Stud Alcohol 29:657, 1968.
34. Room, R: Measurement and distribution of drinking patterns and problems in general populations. In Gross, MM, et al (eds): Alcohol-Related Disabilities. Offset Publication No. 32. World Health Organization, Geneva, 1977, p 61.
35. Sampliner, R and Iber, FL: Diphenylhydantoin control of alcohol withdrawal seizures: Results of a controlled study. JAMA 230:1430, 1974.
36. Temkin, O: The Falling Sickness, ed 2. Johns Hopkins Press, Baltimore, 1971.
37. Vaillant, GE and Milofsky, ES: Natural history of male alcoholism: Paths to recovery. In Goodwin, DW, Van Dusen, KT, and Mednick, SA (eds): Longitudinal Research in Alcoholism. Kluwer-Nijhoff Publishing, Boston, 1984, p 53.
38. Wechsler, H, Demone, HW, and Gottlieb, N: Drinking patterns of Greater Boston adults. J Stud Alcohol 39:1158, 1978.
39. Wechsler, H and McFadden, M: Sex differences in adolescent alcohol and drug use: A disappearing phenomenon. Quarterly Journal of Studies on Alcohol 37:1291, 1976.
40. Weissman, MM, Myers, JK, and Harding, PS: Prevalence and psychiatric heterogeneity of alcoholism in a United States urban community. J Stud Alcohol 41:672, 1980.
41. Welte, JW and Barnes, GM: Alcohol use among adolescent minority groups. J Stud Alcohol 48:329, 1987.

PART II

Basic Mechanisms of Alcohol-Related Seizures

CHAPTER 3

Ivan Diamond, M.D., Ph.D.

Models for the Investigation of Alcohol Withdrawal Seizures

The neurologic and behavioral signs of ethanol intoxication, chronic alcohol abuse, and the alcohol withdrawal syndrome are easily recognized and well known. However, the biochemical and neurophysiologic basis of alcohol withdrawal seizures is not clearly understood and as a result, current therapy is often inadequate. Fortunately, experimental models are beginning to generate new concepts about the interaction of alcohol with the nervous system. In this chapter, some fundamental considerations about ethanol metabolism and the acute and chronic effects of ethanol on neurologic function are summarized and related to subsequent chapters. A more detailed discussion has been presented elsewhere.[1]

EFFECTS OF ALCOHOL ON THE CENTRAL NERVOUS SYSTEM

Ethanol is absorbed rapidly from the gastrointestinal tract into the circulation and widely distributed to all organs and tissue fluids, including the central nervous system (CNS). Ethanol readily equilibrates across the blood-brain barrier so that soon after a person drinks, the concentration of ethanol in the brain approximates that in the blood. There is virtually no ethanol metabolism in the CNS and the effects of ethanol are correlated with blood alcohol levels. Thus, in naive subjects, acute ethanol intoxication occurs at blood alcohol concentrations of 50 to 150 mg/100 ml (11–33 mM) while at 300 to 500 mg/100 ml (65–109 mM), the signs of CNS depression predominate. In nonalcoholic persons, stupor, coma, and death due to respiratory depression can occur at concentrations of 500 to 600 mg/ml (109–130 mM).

Acute Tolerance

Although there is a well-recognized correlation of blood alcohol levels with the neurologic and behavioral effects of ethanol, tolerance to alcohol can develop during a single drinking experience. Thus, after being judged intoxicated at 200 mg/100 ml after 1.5 hours of ethanol consumption, a subject can appear sober 4.5 hours later even though he or she now has a much higher blood alcohol level (275 mg/100 ml).[3] The adaptive change in the brain that accounts for acute tolerance to ethanol is not well understood but probably involves biochemical and physiologic mechanisms that compensate for the acute effects of ethanol on neurologic function.

Chronic Tolerance

The extent of CNS adaptation to ethanol in actively drinking chronic alcoholics is impressive and not often appreciated. Actively drinking alcoholics can appear sober within 6 hours of ethanol consumption despite blood alcohol levels ranging from 120 to 540 mg/100 ml (26–117 mM).[4] Thus, tolerance to ethanol can be so effective that concentrations of ethanol known to be lethal in naive subjects do not cause intoxication in chronic alcoholics. Indeed, a blood alcohol level as high as 1510 mg/100 ml (328 mM) has been reported in an agitated patient who was alert, slightly confused, and oriented to person and place.[2]

Alcohol Withdrawal Syndrome

If alcoholics stop drinking for more than 6–8 hours, they develop a characteristic alcohol withdrawal syndrome (AWS), with symptoms and signs opposite in direction to the effects of ethanol. Thus, it seems likely that adaptive mechanisms in the brain that compensate for the effects of ethanol also account for the development of AWS.

EXPERIMENTAL MODELS

Cellular Models

Recent evidence indicates that ethanol interacts with biologic membranes and changes the functional activity of membrane-bound proteins. In Chapter 4, DeLorenzo considers how ion channels and membrane neurotransmitter receptor systems are likely to be involved in the pathogenesis of AWS and how several anticonvulsants alter neuronal excitability by affecting these mechanisms.

We also know that membrane structure and composition are major targets for the effects of ethanol in the CNS. In Chapter 5, Alling summarizes the acute and chronic effects of ethanol on the biologic properties and lipid composition of membranes in the brain and relates these events to ethanol-induced changes in neuroreceptor systems and the activity of membrane-bound enzymes. He also describes how chronic exposure to ethanol causes the accumulation of an abnormal acidic phospholipid, phosphatidylethanol, and refers to other findings about the accumulation of specific ethanol fatty acid ethyl esters. These new observations are important because collection of abnormal products in neural membranes could play a primary role in the pathogenesis of alcohol-induced organ damage.

Independent studies in several laboratories indicate that calcium channels in neural membranes are also important targets for the acute and chronic effects of ethanol. Littleton, Greenberg and associates, and Carlen, Rougier-Naquet, and Reynolds (Chapters 6–8) describe ethanol-induced changes in calcium channel function. It is now clear from these biochemical and physiologic studies that chronic ethanol consumption induces a substantial increase in calcium channel concentration and activity in neural preparations. Increased calcium channel activity stimulates neuronal excitability, catecholamine release, and turnover of inositol phospholipids. These changes appear to have important implications for the pathogenesis of AWS because treatment with calcium channel blockers can prevent the convulsions that develop during alcohol withdrawal. It is still not clear how chronic exposure to ethanol alters cellular regulatory events to increase the number of calcium channels in neural membranes. Once these molecular mechanisms are understood, it should be possible to design therapeutic agents selectively to prevent the development of AWS.

Several specific neuroreceptor systems have emerged recently as major targets for the acute and chronic effects of ethanol in the brain. Diamond, Moehly-Rosen, and Gordon (Chapter 9) have shown in cultured neural cells that acute exposure to ethanol stimulates adenosine A_2 receptor-dependent cAMP production. By contrast, chronic exposure to ethanol reduces adenosine receptor-stimulated cAMP levels when measured in the absence of alcohol.

This desensitization of adenosine receptor-dependent cAMP signal transduction appears to be a form of cellular "dependence" on ethanol. Similar findings were also obtained when freshly isolated lymphocytes from actively drinking alcoholics were examined. Lymphocytes from alcoholics showed a 75 percent reduction in adenosine-stimulated cAMP levels. Because adenosine is an endogenous anticonvulsant, impaired adenosine-dependent cAMP production in alcoholics could play a role in generating AWS. This finding raises the possibility that treatment with adenosine A_2 receptor agonists might prevent convulsions during alcohol withdrawal.

Many investigators have implicated the GABA/benzodiazepine receptor complex in ethanol's acute and chronic effects in the brain. Treatment with benzodiazepines has been very effective in relieving the symptoms of alcohol withdrawal. In Chapter 11, Morrow, Suzdak, and Paul discuss their studies with the benzodiazepine inverse agonist Ro 15-4513, which blocks ethanol potentiation of GABA-receptor-dependent chloride uptake and prevents ethanol intoxication in animals. Moreover, chronic administration of ethanol to animals decreases GABA-receptor–chloride-channel function. Because these effects are reversed following alcohol withdrawal, it is possible that "subsensitivity" of the GABA-receptor–chloride-channel complex plays a role in AWS. Based on a review of the literature, Frye (Chapter 10) also concludes that a compensatory reduction in GABA activity is probably involved in physical dependence on alcohol.

Animal Models

In order to investigate the pathophysiologic significance of molecular changes caused by chronic exposure to alcohol, it is useful to have well-defined models of AWS. Crabbe and Kosobud (Chapter 13) describe the power and advantages of genetics to investigate this question. They have created genetic animal models of AWS by selecting mice bred for resistance or sensitivity to developing convulsions during ethanol withdrawal. However, the differences between these inbred mouse lines are not due to differences in ethanol metabolism. Crabbe and Kosobud found that genetic control of AWS is distinct from genetic regulation of other responses to ethanol, and appears to be related to a genetic predisposition to dependence on depressant drugs. This important animal model should be very useful in relating molecular events to physical dependence, AWS, and the development of specific anticonvulsants. In this regard, Pinel, Mana, and Kim (Chapter 12) have observed tolerance to ethanol's anticonvulsant effect in a different experimental animal model, kindled seizures in rats. Ethanol is an anticonvulsant and it is possible that AWS are related to the development of tolerance to ethanol's anticonvulsant effect. Pinel, Mana, and Kim have used ethanol to help develop an "effect-dependent" model of drug tolerance. Their experiments indicate that tolerance to the anticonvulsant effect of ethanol is not simply due to prolonged exposure to ethanol. Instead, it is an adaptation to the effect of ethanol in preventing the seizure. This model has interesting implications and suggests that tolerance to ethanol and other anticonvulsants develops much more readily in subjects who experience the anticonvulsant effect of the drug than in those who do not.

SUMMARY

Investigations using cellular and animal models have greatly increased our understanding of the pathophysiology of AWS. As a result of studying the interaction of ethanol with biologic membranes, investigators have begun to identify the molecular events that play a role in the development of ethanol intoxication, tolerance, and physical dependence. At the same time, cellular and animal models have been established that make it possible to test hypotheses and develop new strategies for therapy. It is gratifying to see how advances in basic research are beginning to generate new ideas about preventing and treating alcohol dependence and withdrawal seizures.

References

1. Diamond, I and Charness, ME: Alcohol toxicity. In Asbury, AK, McKhann, GM, and McDonald, WI (eds): Diseases of the Nervous System. WB Saunders, Philadelphia, 1986, p 1324.
2. Johnson, RA, Noll, EC, and Rodney, WM: Survival after a serum ethanol concentration of 1.5%. Lancet ii:1394, 1982.
3. Mirsky, A, et al: Adaptation of the central nervous system to varying concentrations of alcohol in the blood. J Stud Alcohol 2:35, 1941.
4. Urso, T, Gavaler, JS, and Van Thiel, D: Blood ethanol levels in sober alcohol users seen in an emergency room. Life Sci 28:1053, 1981.

Robert J. DeLorenzo, M.D., Ph.D., M.P.H.

CHAPTER 4

Regulation of Neuronal Excitability: Molecular Foundations for the Study of Alcohol Withdrawal

A complete discussion of all aspects of the mechanisms of neuronal excitability is beyond the scope of this chapter, and neuronal excitability has been the subject of several excellent monographs and articles.[9,17,23,47] This limited review highlights some of the important advances that have been made in molecular neurobiology that have direct bearing on neuronal excitability and alcohol withdrawal. The role of excitatory transmitters, calcium, and membrane receptors in regulating ion channels and neuronal excitability is emphasized. The importance of calcium as a major second messenger system in modulating neuronal excitability is discussed in detail, because several advances have recently been made in this area.

Understanding the basic regulation of neuronal excitability is a major research focus and studies indicate that numerous biochemical processes regulate neuronal excitability. However, a direct correlation between a molecular event or second messenger effect and changes in excitability is often difficult to prove and clearly document. Recent research has indicated that several models of excitability may help us understand the molecular regulation of membrane excitability. Advances in neuroscience and the more sophisticated technology of molecular neurobiology have made these developments possible. I will discuss several specific research areas, including the role of excitatory amino acids (EAAs), calcium second-messenger systems, membrane receptors, and sustained repetitive firing in regulating neuronal excitability. This review demonstrates the direct bearing of molecular research on control of the physiologic processes of neuronal activity. These details provide the substrate for more specific discussion of the molecular mechanism underlying the increased excitability that occurs in alcohol withdrawal syndromes (AWS).

EAA RECEPTORS

L-glutamate was proposed as an excitatory neurotransmitter over 30 years ago.[53] However, only recently has the study of EAAs included investigation of their role in epilepsy, neuronal excitability, and learning.[53,61] The two main excitatory neurotransmitters currently known are glutamate and aspartate.[8] Many pathways in the brain utilize these neurotransmitters, including hippocampal afferents and major cortical output tracts that are widely activated during convulsions.

EAAs bind to specific membrane receptors.[37,62] Currently, four major types of EAA receptors have been characterized in detail. An example is the binding of an EAA analog N-methyl-D-aspartate (NMDA). The NMDA receptor has now been well studied. Three types of non-NMDA receptors that bind other analogs of EAAs but have different properties from the NMDA receptor have also been identified. The non-NMDA receptors bind EAAS such as kainic acid, quisqualate, and 2-amino-4-phosphonobutyrate (2-APB), but do not bind NMDA.

Excitatory transmission regulated by EAA receptors is distinct from classical, fast-acting synaptic transmission. EAAs regulate specific ion channels that allow calcium and sodium to enter the cell when the channel is activated by occupation of the EAA receptor.[37,62] These specific channels are opened or gated by the EAA, and the currents activated by EAA receptors are rapid and long lasting. The postsynaptic localization of these receptors, as well as their presence over the cell body, has been implicated in explaining how EAAs alter neuronal excitability, causing depolarization and long-lasting neuronal changes. Thus, this type of calcium entry is independent of depolarization and can be activated by specific EAAs. Important convulsants, such as kainic acid, alter neuronal excitability by binding to these receptor sites and activating calcium and sodium channels. Compounds that bind to the EAA receptors but do not activate the channel to inhibit EAA have effects on these receptors. Several of these compounds have been shown to have potent anticonvulsant actions and have been demonstrated to be very effective in maximal electric shock (MES)-induced seizures in animals.[62]

Because of their potential importance to epileptogenesis, EAA receptors and the calcium channels they regulate have been the focus of extensive research.[42,61] These receptor sites are responsible for mediating some of the effects of kainic acid in producing convulsant discharge in the brain. NMDA receptors have been implicated in long-term potentiation and in long-term alterations of neuronal excitability. The EAA analog, 2-APH, is a potent anticonvulsant in various seizure models. These and other investigations provide strong evidence that EAA receptors and their regulation of calcium channels are important mechanisms in modulating neuronal excitability and, potentially, in anticonvulsant drug actions. Studies should be directed at investigating the effect of chronic alcohol consumption on this system.

CALCIUM REGULATION OF NEURONAL FUNCTION

Calcium plays a major role in modulating normal activity and function of the nervous system.[51,52,54] One of its most widely recognized roles is modulating synaptic neurotransmission. Several now classic studies have demonstrated the importance of calcium in stimulus secretion coupling.[29] Calcium also plays a critical role as a second messenger in neuronal and nonneuronal tissues.

Our laboratory has investigated the role of calcium in regulating neuronal excitability and producing anticonvulsant effects. Several lines of evidence indicate its importance in these areas.[13] Because of the importance of calcium as a second messenger, it is reasonable to assume that alterations in the normal function of calcium-regulated processes may underlie some of the abnormalities of neuronal excitability occurring in seizure disorders and withdrawal states. Accumulating evidence suggests that abnormalities in major calcium-regulated enzymatic processes or ion channels may underlie alterations in neuronal excitability and result in seizure activity.[13,57,58]

The major role of calcium in regulating neuronal excitability and synaptic function makes this an important area for investigating mechanisms of neuronal excitability. The role of calcium in anticonvulsant drug action and regulating seizure excitability has been recently reviewed.[13,58] Several advances in neuroscience research techniques have permitted a more mechanistic view of how calcium regulates neuronal excitability. This research will be discussed in relation to anticonvulsant drug effects. Anticonvulsants have been shown to determine the entry of calcium into cells through both voltage- and transmitter-regulated calcium channels. Thus, the relation of calcium channels to neuronal excitability has direct bearing on the mechanism of action of anticonvulsant drugs. Also, anticonvulsants inhibit important calcium-mediated enzyme systems that play essential roles in cell function and neuronal excitability. These mechanisms may also be significant for certain anticonvulsant effects.

Calcium Channels and Neuronal Excitability

The entry of calcium into a cell triggers many biochemical and biophysical actions.[20,54] This major second-messenger effect of calcium has been clearly linked to the regulation of neuronal excitability and cell metabolism.[51,54] Thus, controlling calcium entry into the cell is the first key step in regulating calcium's role as a second messenger. Alterations in calcium channel function have a major impact on neuronal excitability.

Depolarization-dependent action potentials are typically mediated by a large sodium current into the cell. Calcium simultaneously enters the cell during depolarization. Researchers now more clearly understand the importance of this calcium entry during the action-potential generation. Accumulation of increased concentrations of calcium within a neuron is related to sustained repetitive firing of neurons, which can occur *in vitro* or during epileptic activity. Calcium entry is also regulated by specific EAA receptors. This recently characterized type of calcium channel opens or closes in response to binding of EAAs to specific calcium-channel-linked receptors. The ability of these channels to produce tonic, long-lasting excitability changes in hippocampal and other cortical neurons has implications for long-term potentiation, memory, and excitability.

In understanding the role of calcium in neuronal excitability and anticonvulsant drug action, it is important to consider both voltage-regulated and EAA-modulated calcium channels. Only in the last 5 years has the heterogeneity of calcium channels been appreciated. The regulation of calcium channels in a fashion similar to the regulation of the chloride channel by the benzodiazepines, barbiturates, and convulsant drugs may play an important role in modifying neuronal excitability.

Voltage-Gated Calcium Channels

Voltage-regulated or -gated calcium channels are implicated in regulating neuronal excitability. As an action potential arrives at a nerve terminal, depolarization of the nerve terminal membrane causes entry of calcium through voltage-gated calcium channels, with subsequent release of neurotransmitters. This classic paradigm for calcium-mediated neurotransmitter release was the first indication of the importance of calcium in neuronal excitability. Initially, however, little was understood about the specific mechanisms of calcium channels in the brain.

Early understanding of the neuropharmacology of calcium channels came from studies involving nonneuronal tissue. Calcium entry in smooth muscle and cardiac cells was well characterized by pharmacologists during the 1970s. Dihydropyridine calcium-channel blockers and related molecules were shown to be effective in blocking calcium channels in peripheral tissue.[3,27,58] These compounds were classified as *organic calcium channel blockers*. This development represented a major advance in pharmacology. Numerous analogs were developed and specific binding sites for the dihydropyridines and other analogs were identified and characterized. This advance led to the first molecular characterization of calcium channels and to an understanding of their regulation by specific receptor sites.

A major controversy developed when it was observed that the organic calcium-channel blockers, effective in inhibiting calcium entry into nonneuronal tissue, seemed to be ineffective in blocking voltage-gated calcium entry into neurons.[44] Numerous investigators demonstrated that calcium entry as a result of neuronal activity was not significantly inhibited by therapeutic or relevant concentrations of the organic calcium-channel blockers.[58] Because there was at that time no clear evidence that more than one type of calcium channel existed, this dichotomy was not well understood and was attributed to unusual properties of the neuronal membrane and to specific differences in drug penetration into the nervous system. Recent studies using benzodiazepines and phenothiazines[11,14,19,34] demonstrated that these compounds can in fact significantly block voltage-gated calcium channels in neurons. These results suggested that calcium channels in the brain were distinct from calcium channels in peripheral tissue.

With the development of patch- and voltage-clamp technology, more sophisticated characterization of calcium channels was possible. It is now clear that overall there are at least three, and possibly more, types of calcium channels in neurons.[44,48,60] One type of voltage-gated calcium channel is insensitive to dihydropyridines and a second type is sensitive to them. A third type has been postulated to exist in brain membrane. Although terminology has not developed for these different channels, initial classification by Tsien[48] is currently in use and differentiates these channels as T, N, and L channels.

The heterogeneity of calcium channels provided a major insight into different mechanisms of regulating calcium excitability in the nervous system. These observations also explain the fact that the major voltage-gated calcium channels in the brain that are insensitive to dihydropyridines are a different class of channel than those found in peripheral tissues. However, in certain regions of the nervous system and at certain sites on the cell body, there are calcium channels that are sensitive to dihydropyridines and similar to calcium channels in nonneuronal tissue. Recent observations have indicated that different types of calcium channels are distributed in characteristic patterns over the surface of a neuron. Some channels may be localized at the synapse and others may be present at higher density at the cell body. The heterogeneity and individual function of specific types of calcium channels are important areas for further investigation, for example, in the development of specific drugs to regulate each type of channel.

Several anticonvulsant compounds block or alter calcium entry through voltage-gated calcium channels. Ferrendelli and Daniels-McQueen and Ferrendelli and Kinocherf[21,22] have described the ability of phenytoin, phenobarbital, and carbamazepine, but not ethosuximide, to block voltage-dependent calcium entry into isolated nerve terminal preparations. Subsequent studies have demonstrated that benzodiazepines as well as phenytoin and barbiturates can regulate calcium entry into isolated neurons. The effective concentrations of anticonvulsants in blocking calcium entry are in the low micromolar range. The concentrations are approximately one order of magnitude higher than the levels of these drugs achieved therapeutically in spinal fluid. Although these concentrations may be relevant to anticonvulsant actions, more likely they relate to toxic side-effects.

Modulating the Calcium Signal in Controlling Neuronal Excitability

The widespread second messenger effects of calcium on neuronal and other cell function have intrigued scientists for many years. However, only in the last 10 years have significant advances been made in understanding the molecular mechanisms that mediate calcium effects. The discovery of a calcium-binding protein, calmodulin, was the first major breakthrough.[7,33] Evidence now suggests that many of the effects of calcium on cell function are mediated by calmodulin. The role of calmodulin in modulating nerve transmission and neuronal excitability has been extensively investigated and reviewed.[10,11,12,14,15] Several important calcium-regulated processes are mediated by calmodulin and by a major calmodulin target enzyme system, calmodulin kinase II (CaM kinase II).[2,25,56] Figure 4-1 presents a hypothetical model of the role of calmodulin in synaptic excitability. Evidence from multiple laboratories has now confirmed the original calmodulin hypothesis of neurotransmission and substantiated the role of calmodulin in mediating some of the effects of calcium on neuronal excitability. Anticonvulsant drugs that antagonize calcium-mediated effects, including phenytoin, carbamazepine, and the benzodiazepines, also inhibit calmodulin activation of CaM kinase II.[13,16] Concentrations required to inhibit CaM kinase II are in the low micromolar concentration ranges for anticonvulsant drug effects. This enzyme plays an important role in mediating calcium-dependent protein phosphorylation of membrane and soluble proteins.

CaM kinase II has been implicated by several investigators as a major molecular mechanism mediating some of the second messenger effects of calcium in the cell. Thus, control of this important calcium-mediated event by phenytoin, carbamazepine, and diazepam may be a major action of these anticonvulsant drugs. The

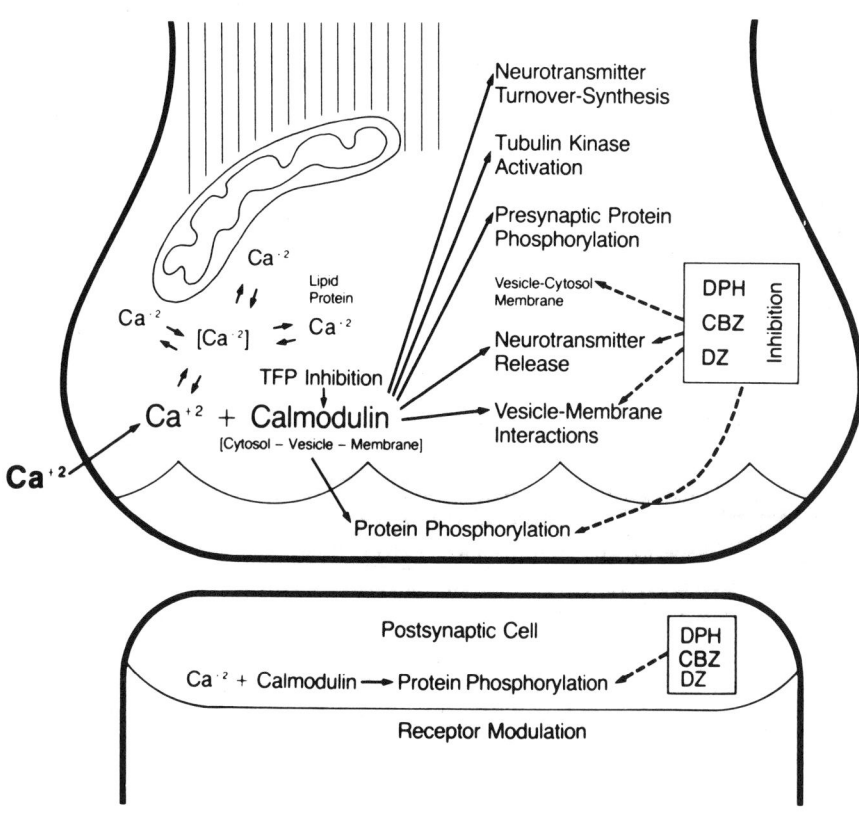

Figure 4-1. Schematic model showing the roles of calcium and calmodulin in regulating synaptic protein phosphorylation, neurotransmitter release and turnover, and vesicle-membrane interactions. Additionally, the inhibitory effects of phenytoin (DPH), carbamazepine (CBZ) and diazepam (DZ) on these calcium-stimulated processes are seen. The inhibitory effects of these anticonvulsants or synaptic membrane protein phosphorylation may also modulate the depolarization-dependent entry of calcium into the nerve terminal.

precise relationship of this particular effect to clinically useful anticonvulsant activity or their related side-effects must still be elucidated.

The importance of CaM kinase II in regulating neuronal excitability is widely recognized. Injection of CaM kinase II into identified invertebrate neurons regulates potassium and calcium currents.[55] In addition, CaM kinase II levels in hippocampal neurons are chronically altered during the long-term alteration of neuronal excitability that occurs in kindling.[24] CaM kinase II activity is inhibited by specific anticonvulsants,[13,16] and the subunits of CaM kinase II are a major protein component of the postsynaptic density that localizes this important enzyme system directly at the synapse.[26,30,31] Further understanding the role of CaM kinase II in the pathophysiology of epilepsy and in controlling neuronal excitability is clearly important.

Another major molecular mechanism regulating the effects of calcium on neuronal excitability and cell function is the major enzyme system, protein kinase C. C-kinase has been implicated in many of the effects of calcium on cell function and also in some of the effects of calcium in regulating specific ion conductances.[51] Although no researchers have directly investigated the effects of anticonvulsant drugs on the C-kinase system, this is an important area for investigation. Modulation of these calcium target enzyme systems by anticonvulsant drugs is a significant area for new drug development.

RECEPTOR REGULATION OF MEMBRANE EXCITABILITY: BENZODIAZEPINE RECEPTORS

Because their use is so ubiquitous, benzodiazepines have been actively investigated in numerous laboratory settings, and their clinical and laboratory effects have been extensively reviewed.[32,49,50,59] Much of the earlier research with these compounds focused on their effects on animal and human behavior. Benzodiazepines are an important class of compounds with anti-anxiety or anxiolytic effects. In addition to these important clinical actions, benzodiazepines also have sedative, muscle relaxant, and anticonvulsant properties. Their anticonvulsant effects are particularly intriguing. These compounds are effective in blocking both pentylenetetrazol (PTZ)-induced seizures in animals and, at higher concentrations, MES-induced seizures. Diazepam is the most commonly prescribed first drug for treating generalized tonic-clonic seizures (GTCSs) and status epilepticus in hospital emergency rooms. Thus, the anticonvulsant properties of the benzodiazepines are not only of academic importance, but have widespread clinical use.

The anxiolytic effects of benzodiazepines made them one of the most frequently prescribed pharmacologic agents in the 1970s, and because of their widespread use, extensive research was undertaken to elucidate their mechanisms of action. The demonstration of a high-affinity specific benzodiazepine receptor site in brain membranes was the first major breakthrough in understanding the molecular action of these compounds. This nanomolar benzodiazepine receptor was carefully identified and characterized in the brain.[6,45,46] It was shown to be highly specific to the brain and absent in other tissues. Subsequently, a second high-affinity benzodiazepine receptor was identified. Because initially it seemed to be more prevalent in peripheral, nonneuronal tissues, this receptor was called the peripheral benzodiazepine binding site.[42] More recently, this "peripheral site" has also been shown to be present in the brain.

The nanomolar benzodiazepine receptor is associated with the chloride channel and gamma-aminobutyric acid (GABA) receptors in the brain.[49,50,59] The elegant research that has been done characterizing this benzodiazepine receptor is a classic demonstration of anticonvulsant receptor-mediated regulation of neuronal excitability. Benzodiazepine binding to the nanomolar receptor site potentiates GABA effects on neuronal inhibition, providing one clear mechanism by which these compounds regulate neuronal excitability. Correlative neuropharmacologic studies have indicated that the anxiolytic and anti-PTZ-induced anticonvulsant ac-

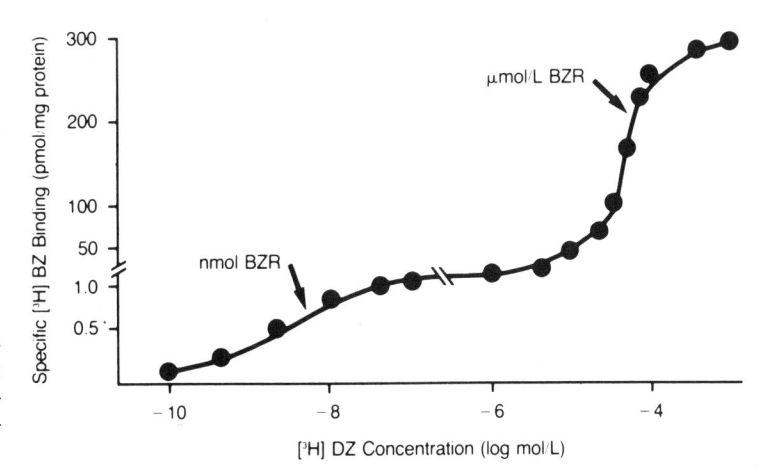

Figure 4–2. Specific [³H] benzodiazepine binding curve; the data illustrate specific saturable binding in the nanomolar and micromolar ranges.

tivities of these compounds are mediated through the high-affinity benzodiazepine nanomolar receptors. However, the effects of benzodiazepines on MES-induced seizures and on generalized convulsions in the emergency room cannot be clearly explained by these nanomolar actions.

Recently, new classes of benzodiazepine binding sites with binding affinities in the high nanomolar and low micromolar range have been elucidated.[4,5] These new types of receptors are stereospecific and bind benzodiazepines in concentrations that are consistent with their anticonvulsant effects on MES-induced seizures, sustained repetitive firing, and GTCSs. Further investigation into the specific mechanisms by which these binding sites regulate membrane excitability is just beginning. The multiple classes of benzodiazepine receptors (Fig. 4–2) are especially important in view of the diverse anticonvulsant properties of these compounds. A discussion of both high- and low-affinity benzodiazepine receptors has important bearing on anticonvulsant drug development and on understanding the molecular mechanisms of action of anticonvulsant compounds.

Nanomolar Benzodiazepine Receptors

In the 1970s, use of radioactively labeled benzodiazepine derivatives allowed the detection of specific nanomolar benzodiazepine receptor sites in brain membranes.[45,46] These sites had a very high affinity for the benzodiazepines, binding in low nanomolar concentration ranges. Binding to these receptors is reversible, saturable, and stereospecific. Nanomolar benzodiazepine receptors have now been identified in the human brain. They are widely distributed and are not present in significant density in peripheral tissues. The potency of benzodiazepine binding to these receptors correlates with their ability to inhibit PTZ-induced seizures, promote muscle relaxation, and produce anxiolytic effects.[4,59] However, these studies also demonstrated that benzodiazepine binding to the nanomolar receptors does not correlate with their ability to inhibit MES-induced seizures in animals.[4]

The specific membrane-binding protein that accounts for the majority of nanomolar benzodiazepine binding has been identified. This protein has a molecular weight of approximately 50,000 daltons on sodium-dodecyl-sulfate (SDS) polyacrylamine gel electrophoresis,[1] and is being purified from animal and human brain. Specific antibodies have been made against the receptor. Such studies characterize the distribution and function of the nanomolar benzodiazepine receptor in regulating neuronal excitability.

High-affinity benzodiazepine binding has also been observed in peripheral, non-neuronal tissue.[43] Here benzodiazepines bind to a different class of benzodiazepine receptor molecules. Both the potency and tissue distribution of this binding are different from the potency and tissue distribution of binding to central receptors. This second class of high-affinity benzodiazepine binding sites was designated "peripheral type receptors,"[43] but it was subsequently shown that the peripheral benzodiazepine receptor is also present in neuronal tissue. Thus, both peripheral and central high-affinity benzodiazepine receptors exist in the brain.

Relationship Between Nanomolar Benzodiazepine Receptors and the GABA Receptor Site

GABA, the major inhibitory neurotransmitter in the brain, has been extensively characterized, and plays a major role in regulating neuronal excitability by controlling chloride permeability.[49,50,59] Specific binding sites for GABA molecules have been identified in neuronal membranes. Although not all GABA receptors are linked to the chloride channel, a large proportion of these receptors are directly involved in regulating chloride channel function.[49,50,59] An overwhelming amount of data indicates that the major inhibitory effect of GABA on the nervous system is mediated through its ability to regulate chloride channel permeability. GABA binding to the GABA receptor potentiates the opening of the chloride channel, allowing chloride ions to flow more easily into the cell. The entry of chloride ions causes cellular hyperpolarization and inhibits neuronal firing, because chloride ions increase the internal electrical negativity of the cell. This action is believed to be the major mechanism by which GABA produces its inhibitory effect on neurons. Functions of GABA on neuronal systems have been closely linked with the effects of the benzodiazepines.[49,50,59] Most evidence now indicates that a significant portion of the nanomolar benzodiazepine receptors in the brain are associated with the GABA binding sites and with the chloride channel in neuronal membranes. The GABA nanomolar benzodiazepine receptor/chloride iontophore macromolecular complex is an important example of the relationship between membrane receptors and neuronal excitability. A model of this receptor-linked channel system is shown in Figure 4–2. The ability of the benzodiazepines to regulate chloride conductances is a major molecular mechanism mediating some of their neuronal stabilizing effects. Benzodiazepine binding to the nanomolar receptor has been postulated to potentiate GABA binding. Increased GABA binding as a result of benzodiazepine activity causes neuronal inhibition and stabilization of neuronal excitability. This action is currently one of the best characterized pharmacologic effects of a neuroleptic compound.

Anticonvulsant Properties of the Nanomolar Benzodiazepine Receptor

The association of the nanomolar benzodiazepine receptor with the GABA receptor and chloride channel provided an important insight into the molecular basis of the anticonvulsant effects of the benzodiazepines. The ability of the benzodiazepines to inhibit PTZ-induced seizures in animals is closely correlated with their ability to bind to the nanomolar receptor site. Thus, evidence strongly suggests that the nanomolar benzodiazepine receptor mediates the anticonvulsant effects of these compounds on this type of seizure. Because of the importance of this finding to anticonvulsant research, other anticonvulsant properties associated with the chloride channel have been thoroughly investigated.[49,59] These studies provide a splendid example of how anticonvulsant drugs can regulate specific channel conductances in neuronal membranes.

Numerous investigations have provided data to indicate the existence of the benzodiazepine/barbiturate/GABA receptor/chloride iontophore complex.[50] The chloride channel is surrounded by a GABA receptor, a nanomolar central benzodiazepine receptor, and a receptor site that binds picrotoxin and related convulsants and barbiturates and related depressants (Fig. 4–3). Several reviews have characterized in detail this channel and its properties related to the benzodiazepines,

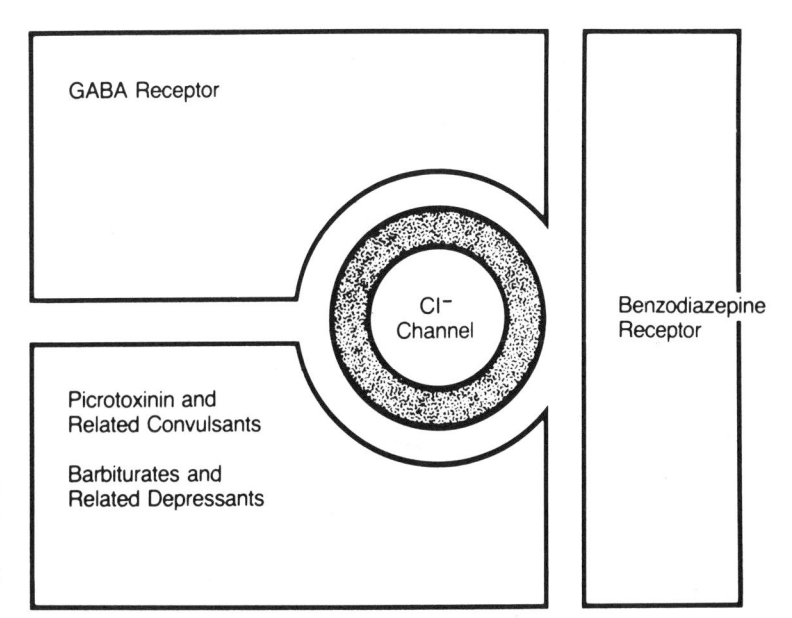

Figure 4–3. Schematic model of the benzodiazepine-barbiturate-GABA receptor chloride iontophore complex. (Adapted from Olsen, RW, et al.[49])

to GABA, and to convulsant and barbiturate molecules.[63] Picrotoxin binds to the proposed site (Fig. 4–3) and modulates benzodiazepine and GABA receptor binding in a way that inhibits chloride channel permeability, thus making the cell more excitable. Barbiturate binding to the proposed site potentiates benzodiazepine receptor binding and, thus, indirectly potentiates the GABA effect of opening the chloride channel and enhancing neuronal inhibition. This complex interaction between GABA, benzodiazepines, picrotoxin and related convulsants, and the barbiturates and related depressants is a prime example of how pharmacologic agents modulate the function of ion channels through specific receptor binding. It is possible that similar types of receptor-mediated channel regulation exist for other ionic channels in the brain. However, at this time no other channel system has been as closely linked at a molecular level to anticonvulsant and convulsant action as the chloride channel. Phenytoin and carbamazepine have been shown to produce a use-dependent inhibition of the sodium channel, and the benzodiazepines, phenytoin, and carbamazepine inhibit voltage-sensitive calcium channels. However, the molecular mechanisms of these effects have not been elucidated.

Novel Benzodiazepine Binding Sites

High-nanomolar and low-micromolar benzodiazepine binding sites have been identified recently in brain membranes.[1,4,5] In addition, another benzodiazepine receptor that binds in the high nanomolar range has been identified in brain cytosol.[5] These novel benzodiazepine binding sites have been shown to be stereospecific (Fig. 4–4) and have potencies for benzodiazepine binding that correlate with the ability of these compounds to inhibit MES-induced seizures. Diazepam binding to micromolar benzodiazepine receptors is displaced by phenytoin. These results indicate that high-nanomolar and low-micromolar-affinity benzodiazepine receptors may represent an important anticonvulsant binding site in brain membranes that mediate some of the effects of benzodiazepines used in high concentration to regulate status epilepticus, GTCSs, and MES-induced seizures.

It has been shown that micromolar benzodiazepine binding to synaptosome membranes regulates depolarization-dependent calcium uptake in nerve terminal preparations.[57,58] Micromolar benzodiazepine receptor binding in neuronal mem-

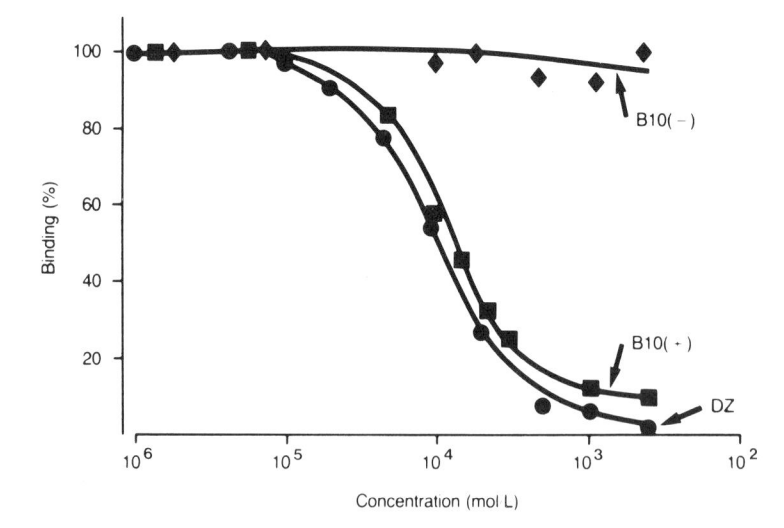

Figure 4–4. Stereospecificity of binding of the micromolar binding site demonstrated by displacement of the pharmacologically active B10(+) compared with the negligible displacement exhibited by the pharmacologically inactive B10(−). (Adapted from Bowling, AC and DeLorenzo, RJ.[4])

brane of identified leech neurons has been shown to regulate specific calcium channels (Fig. 4–5) in isolated neurons.[28] Recently, it has been shown that benzodiazepines in micromolar concentrations regulate calcium and sodium channels in isolated vertebrate neurons in culture.[18] These studies indicate that benzodiazepine binding sites that function in both therapeutic and toxic concentrations may mediate benzodiazepine effects on multiple types of channel systems. Thus, the regulation of the chloride channel by nanomolar benzodiazepine receptors may be analogous to the regulation of other channels, such as calcium, potassium, and sodium channels. These results indicate that benzodiazepines may have their dual anticonvulsant effects by regulating different channels in neuronal membrane.

SUSTAINED REPETITIVE FIRING: MODULATION BY DRUGS AND SECOND MESSENGERS

An understanding of basic mechanisms of excitability should result from studying not only how populations of neurons interact, but also how the electrophysiologic processes in isolated neurons are altered in epileptogenesis. Experiments exploring in detail the basic mechanisms

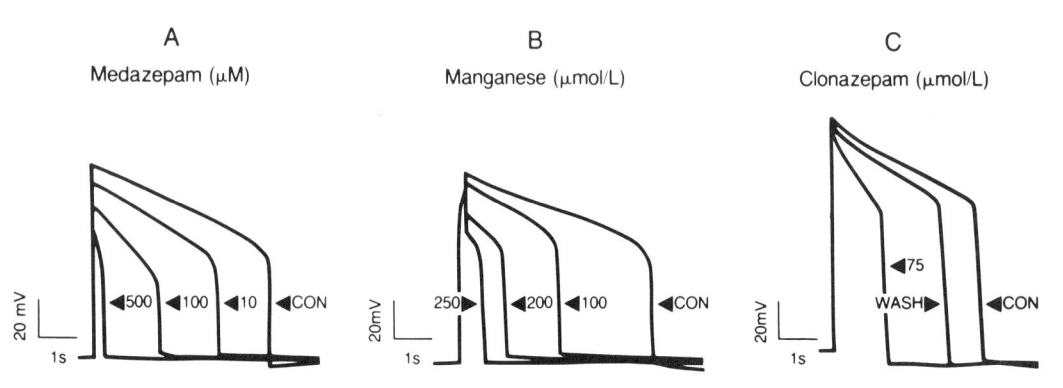

Figure 4–5. Effects of medazepam (A) and manganese (B) on Sr^{2+} potentials in the lateral N cells of the leech ganglia. Both medazepam and manganese inhibited Sr^{2+} on Ca^{2+} potentials. The effects of medazepam were reversible over time (C). The results demonstrate that benzodiazepines can inhibit Ca^{2+} potentials in identified neurons. (Adapted from Johansen, J, et al.[28])

controlling neuronal excitability in isolated vertebrate and invertebrate neurons can be useful in making predictions about electrophysiologic mechanisms that may be present in central neurons and that may alter excitability. A growing body of evidence[28,35,36,39,40,64] indicates that sustained high-frequency repetitive firing (SRF) is an important property of vertebrate and invertebrate neurons that correlates with the excitability state of the neuron. SRF is present in central nervous system neurons and may be involved in anticonvulsant drug action and epileptogenesis. Although no direct evidence has demonstrated the link between SRF and epilepsy, information about SRF obtained from *in vitro* studies on isolated neurons may be related to altered neuronal excitability and anticonvulsant action.

Several anticonvulsant drugs regulate SRF.[36] The correlation of certain types of anticonvulsant activity with actions on SRF indicate that SRF is a good model for studying drugs effective against GTCS- and MES-induced seizures.[36] Anticonvulsants effective against generalized absence seizures are usually not effective against SRF; thus, different mechanisms of action are implicated by this type of electrophysiologic testing. The potential importance of understanding SRF and its relationship to anticonvulsant action has been highlighted by Macdonald and McLean and is an important area for investigating the molecular mechanisms of action of anticonvulsant drugs.

Anticonvulsant Action and SRF

SRF is a nonsynaptic property of neurons. Specific anticonvulsants limit SRF and thus stabilize isolated neurons. Macdonald and McLean[36] have demonstrated that phenytoin, carbamazepine, valproic acid, the benzodiazepines, and phenobarbital all effectively limit SRF. Ethosuximide, however, has no effect on SRF.[38,41] The ability of specific anticonvulsants to limit SRF appears to be a common property and may be an important anticonvulsant mechanism of these compounds.

The relevance of limitation of SRF to anticonvulsant action is further strengthened by several important observations. The therapeutic efficacy of each anticonvulsant drug in controlling seizures in animals and humans is similar to its therapeutic efficacy in controlling SRF in isolated, cultured neurons. These results indicate that therapeutic cerebral spinal fluid (CSF) levels of anticonvulsant drugs correlate with the concentrations most effective against SRF.[36] The effects of anticonvulsants in limiting SRF have been shown in a wide variety of neurons maintained in culture from different regions of the mammalian central nervous system. This evidence suggests that this effect is not unique to specific regions or cell types. Anticonvulsants prevent bursting in the epileptic focus and restrict the spread of epileptic activity from the focus to normal surrounding tissue. Thus, suppression of SRF by anticonvulsants may inhibit excitability by inhibiting the spread of seizure activity. Membrane properties of nonepileptic neurons may be important in understanding drug mechanisms of action and may have a special relationship to the properties of SRF. Thus, SRF is an important model for studying the excitability of isolated neurons.

Benzodiazepine Receptors and SRF

Benzodiazepines are effective in nanomolar concentrations in blocking PTZ-induced seizures in animals and in treating absence seizures (Fig. 4-6). In addition, benzodiazepines in high nanomolar and low micromolar ranges inhibit MES-induced seizures in animals (Fig. 4-7). Furthermore, benzodiazepines are effective in humans in stopping GTCSs and status epilepticus when given in intravenous doses that produce low micromolar serum concentrations. The potency of the benzodiazepines in blocking MES-induced seizures does not correlate in time or concentration (Figs. 4-5 and 4-6) with their ability to inhibit PTZ-induced seizures or bind to the nanomolar central benzodiazepine receptor.[4] Thus, other mechanisms appear to underlie this generalized anti-

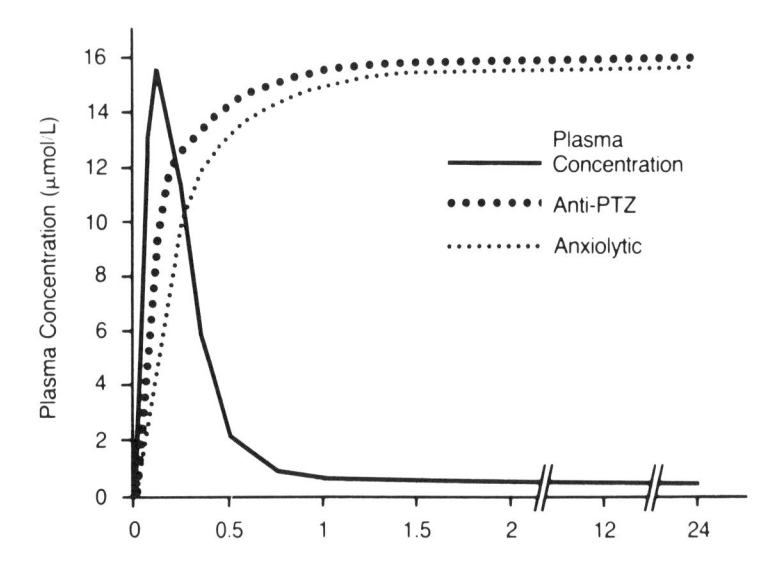

Figure 4–6. Benzodiazepine blood levels and clinical effects. The data demonstrate that following a single (intravenous) dose of diazepam (10 mg) in man, the antipentylenetetrazole (anti-PTZ) and anti-anxiety (anxiolytic) effects last for longer than 24 hours, while peak diazepam levels last for only 30 minutes.

convulsant property of the benzodiazepines in high concentration.

Macdonald and McLean[36] showed that diazepam and clonazepam in high nanomolar and low micromolar concentrations reduced SRF. They demonstrated that these concentrations are above therapeutic free-serum concentrations achieved in ambulatory patients treated with benzodiazepines, but are within the ranges of free-serum concentrations achieved in patients treated for *status epilepticus* or for acute GTCSs. In addition to the discrepancy in concentration ranges, the potency of benzodiazepines in suppressing SRF does not correlate with benzodiazepine binding to the nanomolar central receptor or with their ability to inhibit PTZ-induced seizures. However, there is more evidence for a direct correlation between benzodiazepine potency in inhibiting MES-induced seizures and limiting SRF.

Benzodiazepines uniquely inhibit both GTCSs at higher concentrations and absence seizures at lower concentrations. The ability of benzodiazepines to block

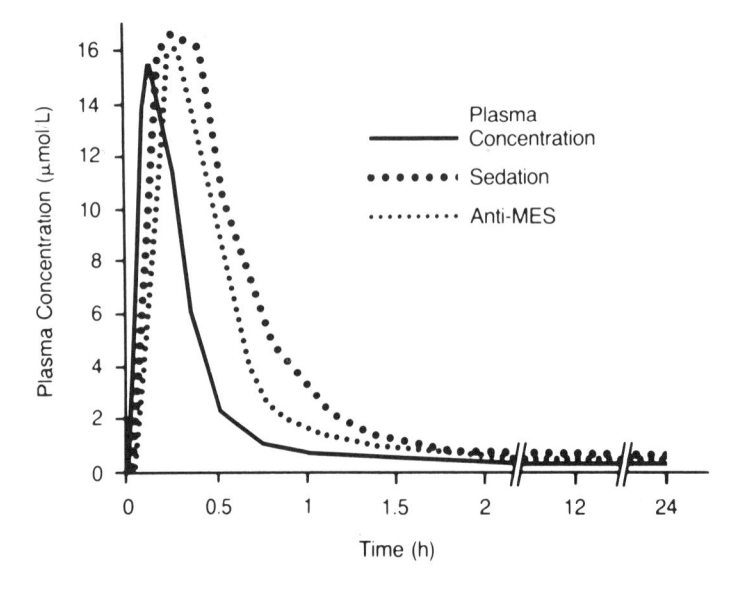

Figure 4–7. Benzodiazepine blood levels and clinical effects. The data demonstrate that following a single dose of intravenous diazepam, anti-maximal electric shock (Anti-MES) and sedation effects correlate in time with the initial peak levels of diazepam.

generalized absence seizures and PTZ-induced seizures in animals at low concentrations is most likely secondary to potentiation of GABA effects produced by binding to the nanomolar central benzodiazepine receptor. However, their inhibition of MES-induced seizures, GTCSs, *status epilepticus*, and SRF appears to be mediated by mechanisms distinct from those related to their effects on the nanomolar benzodiazepine receptor.[4] Macdonald and McLean[36] have suggested that limitation of SRF may underlie some anticonvulsant actions of the benzodiazepines in humans and experimental animals and may be related to unique mechanisms of action of anticonvulsant benzodiazepines. These mechanisms may also mediate some of the effects of these drugs on alcohol withdrawal.

The high-nanomolar and low-micromolar-affinity benzodiazepine binding sites fall in the concentration ranges for benzodiazepine binding that produce effects on MES-induced seizures in animals, effects on GTCSs in humans, and SRF in cultured neurons. These novel benzodiazepine receptors[4,5] have a broad range of benzodiazepine affinities (Fig. 4–2) and are comprised of multiple binding sites. The recently described soluble benzodiazepine-binding protein isolated from mammalian central nervous system[5] has a binding potency that correlates with the high nanomolar concentrations of the benzodiazepines that inhibit SRF. The higher binding constants for the low-micromolar benzodiazepine binding sites could be related to some of the clinical effects of these drugs on seizure activity in animals and humans. However, it is also possible that these lower-affinity binding sites may be involved in mediating some of the toxic side-effects of the benzodiazepines. For example, benzodiazepines block calcium entry into neurons at low micromolar concentrations.[34,57,58] Blocking calcium channels, and perhaps sodium and potassium channels as well,[64] could also account for some of the sedative and neuroleptic effects of the benzodiazepines.

The further characterization of high-nanomolar and low-micromolar-affinity benzodiazepine binding sites is an important area for anticonvulsant research, because it is now clear that some of the most useful anticonvulsant actions of the benzodiazepines are mediated in this concentration range. The isolation of a specific high-nanomolar-affinity binding site in the brain provides the first insight into the molecular mechanism by which benzodiazepines may regulate SRF and MES-induced seizures. Further studies are needed, however, to demonstrate the correlation between binding to these novel receptors and their effects on physiologic actions such as seizures and limitation of SRF.

SUMMARY

Understanding the basic mechanisms underlying neuronal excitability has been a major research effort of neuroscientists for the last three decades. Numerous biochemical second messengers and electrophysiologic processes have been shown to modulate neuronal excitability. However, clear correlations of many of these effects with changes in electrical activity are often difficult to determine. Over the last five years, several major new research areas have identified specific areas of promise that might provide an insight into the regulation of neuronal excitability. Understanding the regulation of ion channels by receptors and neurotransmitter substances is an important research advance that has led to the development of excitability models and may help us understand basic mechanisms of AWS. Although a complete discussion of all aspects of neuronal excitability is not possible here, EAAs, calcium mechanisms, and receptor-regulated excitability have been discussed in relationship both to neuronal excitability and to changes in excitability that occur in alcohol withdrawal. Each of these important areas of research has provided new insights into the molecular mechanisms that regulate neuronal excitability. Some of these insights may provide the foundation to investigate the molecular mechanisms of alcohol withdrawal.

References

1. Battersby, MK, Richards, JG, and Mohler, N: Benzodiazepine receptors: Photoaffinity labelling and localization. Eur J Pharmacol 57:277, 1979.
2. Bennett, MK, Erondu, NE, and Kennedy, MB: Purification and characterization of a calmodulin-dependent protein kinase that is highly concentrated in brain. J Biol Chem 258:12735, 1983.
3. Bolger, GT, et al: Characterization of binding of the calcium channel antagonist [³H]nitrendipine, to guinea pig ileal smooth muscle. J Pharmacol Exp Ther 225:291, 1983.
4. Bowling, AC and DeLorenzo, RJ: Micromolar benzodiazepine receptors: Identification and characterization in the central nervous system. Science 216:1247, 1982.
5. Bowling, AC and DeLorenzo, RJ: Photoaffinity labeling of a novel benzodiazepine binding protein in rat brain. Eur J Pharmacol 57:277, 1979.
6. Braestrup, C and Squires, RF: Pharmacological characterization of benzodiazepine receptors. Eur J Pharmacol 48:263, 1978.
7. Cheung, WY: Calmodulin role in cellular regulation. Science 207:19, 1980.
8. Czuczwar, S, Frey, H, and Loscher, W: N-methyl-D,L-aspartic acid-induced convulsions in mice and their blockade by antiepileptic drugs and other agents. In Nistico, G, et al (eds): Neurotransmitters, Seizures, and Epilepsy, ed 3. Raven Press, New York, 1986, p 235.
9. Delgado-Escueta, AV, Ward, AA, Woodbury, DM, and Porter, RJ, (eds): New Wave of Research in the Epilepsies. In Advances in Neurology, vol 44. Raven Press, New York, 1986, p 3.
10. DeLorenzo, RJ: Calcium-calmodulin protein phosphorylation in neuronal transmission: A molecular approach to neuronal excitability and anticonvulsant drug action. In Delgado-Escueta, AV, et al (eds): Advances in Neurology, Vol 34, Status Epilepticus. Raven Press, New York, 1983, p 325.
11. DeLorenzo, RJ: The calmodulin hypothesis of neurotransmission. Cell Calcium 2:365, 1981.
12. DeLorenzo, RJ: Calmodulin in neurotransmitter release and synaptic function. Fed Proc 41:2275, 1982.
13. DeLorenzo, RJ: A molecular approach to the calcium signal in the brain: Relationship to synaptic modulation and seizure discharge. Adv Neurol 44:435, 1986.
14. DeLorenzo, RJ: Role of calmodulin in neurotransmitter release and synaptic function. Ann NY Acad Sci 356:92, 1980.
15. DeLorenzo, RJ, et al: Stimulation of Ca^{2+}-dependent neurotransmitter release and presynaptic nerve terminal protein phosphorylation by calmodulin and a calmodulin-like protein isolated from synaptic vesicles. Proc Natl Acad Sci USA 76:1838, 1979.
16. DeLorenzo, RJ, Burdette, S, and Holderness, J: Benzodiazepine inhibition of the calcium-calmodulin protein kinase system in brain membrane. Science 213:546, 1981.
17. DeLorenzo, RJ and Dashefsky, L: Anticonvulsants. In Handbook of Neurochemistry, Vol 9, Plenum Publishing, New York, 1985, p 363.
18. DeLorenzo, RJ and Taft, WC: Anticonvulsant receptors: Regulation of depolarization-induced calcium uptake. In Porter, RJ (ed): Advances in Epileptology: XVth Epilepsy International Symposium. Raven Press, New York, 1984, p 37.
19. DeLorenzo, RJ, Taft, WC, and Andrews, WT: Regulation of voltage-sensitive calcium channels in brain by micromolar affinity benzodiazepine receptors. In Katz, B and Rahamimoff, R (eds): Calcium, Neuronal Function and Neurotransmitter Release. Martinus Nijhoff, Boston, 1985, p 375.
20. Douglas, WW: Stimulus-secretion coupling: The concept and clues from chromaffin and other cells. Br J Pharmacol 34:451, 1986.
21. Ferrendelli, JA and Daniels-McQueen, S: Comparative actions of phenytoin and other anticonvulsant drugs on potassium- and veratroidine-stimulated calcium uptake in synaptosomes. J Pharmacol Exp Ther 220:29, 1982.
22. Ferrendelli, JA and Kinocherf, DA: Phenytoin: Effects on calcium flux and cyclic nucleotides. Epilepsia 18:331, 1977.
23. Glaser, GH, Penry, JK, and Woodbury, DW: Antiepileptic Drugs: Mechanisms of Action. Raven Press, New York, 1980.
24. Goldenring, JR, et al: Kindling induces a long-lasting change in the activity of a hippocampal membrane calmodulin-dependent protein kinase system. Brain Res 377:47, 1986.
25. Goldenring, JR, et al: Purification and characterization of a calmodulin-dependent kinase from rat brain cytosol able to phosphorylate tubulin and microtubule-associated proteins. J Biol Chem 258:12632, 1983.
26. Goldenring, JR, McGuire, JS, Jr, and DeLorenzo, RJ: Identification of the major postsynaptic density protein as homologous with the major calmodulin-binding subunit of a calmodulin-dependent protein kinase. J Neurochem 42:1077, 1984.
27. Gould, RJ, Murphy, KM, and Snyder, SH: [³]Nitrendipine-labeled calcium channels discriminate inorganic calcium agonists and antagonists. Proc Natl Acad Sci USA 79:3656, 1982.
28. Johansen, J, et al: Benzodiazepine inhibition of calcium conductance in identified leech neurons. Proc Natl Acad Sci USA 82:3935, 1985.
29. Katz, B and Miledi, R: Further study of the role of calcium in synaptic transmission. J Physiol (Lond) 207:789, 1970.
30. Kelly, PT, McGuinness, TL, and Greengard, P: Evidence that the major postsynaptic density protein is a component of a Ca^{++} calmodulin-dependent protein kinase. Proc Natl Acad Sci USA 81:945, 1984.
31. Kennedy, MR, Bennett, MK, and Erondu, NE: Biochemical and immunochemical evidence that the "major PSD protein" is a subunit of a calmodulin-dependent protein kinase. Proc Natl Acad Sci USA 80:7357, 1983.
32. Killiam, EK and Suria, A: Benzodiazepines. In Glaser, GH, Penry, JK, and Woodbury, DM

(eds): Antiepileptic Drugs: Mechanisms of Action. Raven Press, New York, 1980, p 597.
33. Klee, CB, Crouch, TH, and Richmand, PG: Calmodulin. Ann Rev Biochem 49:489, 1980.
34. Leslie, SW, Friedman, MB, and Coleman, RR: Effects of chlordiazepoxide on depolarization-induced calcium influx into synaptosomes. Biochem Pharmacol 29:2439, 1980.
35. Macdonald, RL and McLean, MJ: Cellular bases of barbiturate and phenytoin anticonvulsant drug action. Epilepsia 23:S7, 1982.
36. Macdonald, RL and McLean, MJ: Anticonvulsant drugs: Mechanisms of action. Adv Neurol 44:713, 1986.
37. Mayer, ML and Westbrook, GL: The physiology of excitatory amino acid receptors. Trends in Neurosciences 10:197, 1987.
38. McLean, MJ and Macdonald, RL: Carbamazepine and 10, 11-epoxycarbamazepine produce use- and voltage-dependent limitation of rapidly firing action potentials of mouse central neurons in cell culture. J Pharmacol Exp Ther 238:727, 1986.
39. McLean, MJ and Macdonald, RL: Multiple actions of phenytoin on mouse spinal cord neurons in cell culture. J Pharmacol Exp Ther 227:779, 1983.
40. McLean, MJ and Macdonald, RL: Limitation of high frequency repetitive firing of cultured mouse neurons by anticonvulsant drugs. Neurology 34:188, 1984.
41. McLean, MJ and Macdonald, RL: Sodium valproate, but not ethosuximide, produces use- and voltage-dependent limitation of high frequency repetitive firing of action potentials of mouse central neurons in cell culture. J Pharmacol Exp Ther 237:1001, 1986.
42. Meldrum, B and Chapman, A: Excitatory amino acid antagonists and anticonvulsant agents: Receptor subtype involvement in different seizure models. In Nistico, G, et al (eds): Neurotransmitters, Seizures, and Epilepsy, ed 3. Raven Press, New York, 1986, p 223.
43. Mestre, M, et al: Electrophysiological and pharmacological evidence that peripheral type benzodiazepine receptors are coupled to calcium channels in the heart. Life Sci 36:391, 1985.
44. Miller, RJ: Multiple calcium channels and neuronal function. Science 235:46, 1987.
45. Mohler, H, Battersby, MK, and Richards, JG: Benzodiazepine receptor protein identified and visualized in brain tissue by a photoaffinity label. Proc Natl Acad Sci USA 77:1666, 1980.
46. Mohler, H and Okada, T: Properties of [^{3}H]-diazepam binding to benzodiazepine receptors in rat cerebral cortex. Life Sci 20:2101, 1977.
47. Nistico, G, et al (eds): Neurotransmitters, Seizures, and Epilepsy, ed 3. Raven Press, New York, 1986.
48. Nowycky, MC, Fox, AP, and Tsien, RW: Three types of neuronal calcium channels with different calcium agonist sensitivity. Nature 316:440, 1985.
49. Olsen, RW, et al: Benzodiazepine/barbiturate/GABA receptor-chloride ionophore complex in a genetic model for generalized epilepsy. Adv Neurol 44:365, 1986.
50. Olsen, RW, et al: Biochemical pharmacology of the GABA/benzodiazepine receptor/ionophore protein. Fed Proc 43:2773, 1984.
51. Rasmussen, H: The calcium messenger system. N Engl J Med 314:1094, 1986.
52. Rasmussen, H and Goodmann, DBP: Relationships between calcium and cyclic nucleotides in cell activation. Physiol Rev 57:421, 1977.
53. Rothman, S and Olney, J: Excitotoxicity and the NMDA receptor. Trends in Neurosciences 10:299, 1987.
54. Rubin, RP: The role of calcium in the release of neurotransmitter substances and hormones. Pharmacol Rev 22:389, 1972.
55. Sakakibara, M, et al: Modulation of calcium-mediated inactivation of ionic currents by Ca^{2+} calmodulin-dependent protein kinase II. Journal of Biophysics 50:319, 1986.
56. Schulman, H and Greengard, P: Stimulation of brain membrane protein phosphorylation by calcium and an endogenous heat-stable protein. Nature 271:478, 1978.
57. Taft, WC and DeLorenzo, RJ: Micromolar-affinity benzodiazepine receptors regulate voltage-sensitive calcium channels in nerve terminal preparations. Proc Natl Acad Sci USA 81:3118, 1984.
58. Taft, WC and DeLorenzo, RJ: Regulation of calcium channels in brain: Implications for the clinical neurosciences. Yale J Biol Med 60:99, 1987.
59. Tallman, JF, et al: Receptors for the age of anxiety: Pharmacology of the benzodiazepines. Science 207:274, 1980.
60. Tsien, R: Calcium currents in heart cells and neurons. In Kaczmarek, L and Levitan, I (eds): Neuromodulation: The Biochemical Control of Neuronal Excitability. Oxford University Press, New York, 1987, p 206.
61. Turski, L, et al: Excitatory neurotransmission within the substantia nigra pars reticulata regulates threshold for seizures produced by pilocarpine in rats. Neurosciences 18:61, 1987.
62. Watkins, J and Olverman, H: Agonists and antagonists for excitatory amino acid receptors. Trends in Neurosciences 10:265, 1987.
63. Woodbury, DM, Penry, JK, and Pippenger, CE: Antiepileptic Drugs, ed 2. Raven Press, New York, 1982.
64. Yang, J, et al: Effects of medazepam on voltage-gated ion currents of cultured chick sensory neurons. Eur J Pharmacol 143:373, 1987.

CHAPTER 5

Christer Alling, M.D., Ph.D.

The Effects of Alcohol on Lipids in Neuronal Membranes

ETHANOL-MEMBRANE INTERACTIONS

Partitioning of Ethanol

The biochemical effects of alcohol on the central nervous system (CNS) start in the neuronal membranes. Neuronal membranes are heterogeneous mixtures of lipids and proteins. Phospholipids make up the skeleton of the membrane bilayer structure and provide, with cholesterol and other lipids, a matrix for membrane proteins. Ethanol, a small, lipid-soluble, and amphiphilic molecule, dissolves in the lipid bilayer and perturbs the cell membrane structure. Nuclear magnetic resonance (NMR) and thermodynamic measurements have demonstrated that ethanol is located near the membrane surface with the hydroxyl group anchored to the polar headgroup of the phospholipids.[51,53] The partitioning of ethanol into membranes involves two processes.[39] The partition coefficient is constant with increasing ethanol concentrations in the interior of the membrane, and the binding coefficient to the polar headgroup increases with increasing ethanol concentrations.

Fluidization

As early as 1901 it was proposed that ethanol's effects, such as intoxication and sedation, were the result of perturbation of neuronal membrane lipids.[49] However, this membrane hypothesis was not corroborated until 1977 when Chin and Goldstein first demonstrated that ethanol at physiologically attainable levels (25–100 mmol/liter) dose-dependently decreases the order in brain membranes.[20] This finding was later confirmed by fluorescence polarization.[22] Measurements with various probes that dissolve at different depths of the membrane have indicated that the disordering effect is greatest in the membrane core.[21,37] The effect seems to be related to the original membrane fluidity: the more fluid the membrane, the greater the effect. These changes in membrane fluidity can be correlated with the sedative effect of ethanol in animals. One important study demonstrated that neuronal membranes from ethanol-sensitive animals ("LS" mice) were more prone to the fluidizing effect of ethanol than membranes from less sensitive animals ("SS" mice).[29]

Biphasic Effects

There is evidence that ethanol has an ordering effect at low concentrations near the membrane surface but a disordering effect at high concentrations in the interior membrane core.[32,34,50] Other studies support the hypothesis that ethanol specifi-

Table 5-1. ACUTE ETHANOL EFFECTS ON NEURORECEPTOR COMPLEXES

Receptor Systems	Effects
Catecholamine receptors	Increase in α-adrenoceptor binding Altered G-protein function Activation of adenylate cyclase
Serotonin receptors	Reduced binding but increased affinity for both S1 and S2 receptors Stimulated phosphoinositide breakdown
Acetylcholine receptors	No effects on QNB binding Changes in muscarinic-stimulated phosphoinositide metabolism
GABA/benzodiazepine receptor/chloride channel	Stimulation of chloride uptake by increased efficiency of GABA binding
Opiate receptors	Preferential inhibition of ligand binding to δ as compared with μ receptors. κ receptors are resistant.
Glutamate receptors	Stimulation of glutamate binding at ethanol concentration below 100 mmol/Liter.

cally interacts with the polar headgroup of phosphatidylcholine.[56,57] Ethanol also has a biphasic behavioral effect, often causing stimulation at low concentrations and depression at high blood levels.[52] Interference may exist between the biphasic effects on membrane lipids, and ethanol may have a similar biphasic effect on GABA receptors.[61,67]

Disruption of Neuronal Receptor Systems

The evidence that specific lipid components within the neuronal membrane show selective sensitivity to ethanol suggests that these membrane-bound proteins, which are dependent on the lipids surrounding them for optimal activity, also differ in their sensitivity to ethanol. Receptors, ionophores, and enzymes therefore do not react uniformly.[11,13,35,60] The neuronal receptor could be affected by ethanol with regard to ligand binding, transduction proteins, adenylate cyclase, and phosphodiesterase, or second messengers (Table 5-1).

CHRONIC EFFECTS AND ADAPTATION

Chronic consumption of alcohol is thought to result in an adaptation within the neuronal membrane. This cellular tolerance implies that a greater amount of ethanol is required to achieve the same effect than is required in the naive organism. The membranes seem to change their chemical structure to resist the perturbation effects of ethanol. This maladaptive state is also characterized by neuronal hyperexcitability during withdrawal from ethanol. This condition is the opposite of that observed during intoxication. Since Hill and Bengham[33] proposed that the lipid composition of some critical membranes is reorganized as a result of adaptation, there have been many experiments to elucidate the molecular abnormalities in the structure of these membranes. There is biophysical evidence for membrane adaptation, that is, both for decreased partitioning of ethanol into the membranes and for a resistance to the disordering effect of ethanol. When neurochemical methods are applied, however, the results are far from conclusive. Most studies have focused on changes in bulk membrane lipids. These alterations include increased cholesterol concentrations and greater saturation among the phospholipid fatty acids. Even more interesting are selective changes among special lipids—boundary lipids—that affect the charge distribution over the membranes or are prerequisites for protein function.

Cholesterol and Fatty Acids

Increased cholesterol content of biomembranes results in a decreased fluidization effect of ethanol.[19] When synaptosomal plasma membranes were prepared from mice, rats, or chickens who chronically had been fed alcohol for some time, elevated concentrations of cholesterol were found.[22,24,48,58] On the other hand, negative findings have also been reported.[9,40,45,65] However, strain differences, age, mode and length of ethanol exposure, and tissue preparation technique do not account for the disparate findings.

The fatty acid composition both of the total phosphoglyceride fraction and of the individual phospholipids has been studied in ethanol-exposed rats. Most of the attention has focused on the phospholipids because of their properties, such as high proportions of polyunsaturated fatty acids and rapid turnover, which make them important as regulators of membrane fluidity. Decreased proportions of polyunsaturated and increased proportions of saturated fatty acids have been reported in synaptosomes.[43,44] Moreover, dietary fatty acid composition seems to influence ethanol sensitivity. Although fatty acid changes are difficult to induce in brain membranes by dietary means,[9] rats receiving a diet enriched with saturated fatty acids were less sensitive to ethanol,[36] whereas rats fed a diet deficient in essential fatty acids had greater motor impairment after an acute dose of ethanol.[37] Ethanol also enhanced the depletion of polyunsaturated fatty acids in the brain when the diet was deficient in these fatty acids.[5] Other studies have found no changes among the polyunsaturated fatty acids.[24,58,66]

Thus, there is currently no simple model of imbalance between saturated and polyunsaturated fatty acids that is explained by or correlated with the compensatory reorganization of neuronal membranes that have adapted to ethanol. Several studies have documented an increased proportion of oleic acid, a monounsaturated fatty acid, following ethanol administration. In rodents, chronic ethanol treatment has been reported to induce increased proportions of oleic acid in synaptosomes, both in the total phospholipid fraction[40] and in phosphatidylcholine.[9] Increased proportions of oleic acid have also been found in peripheral tissues such as heart, liver, and erythrocytes.[40,44,47,55,66] Furthermore, an increase in oleic acid was consistently found in erythrocytes and platelets from human alcoholics.[2] An elevated oleic acid level is obviously one of the most general effects of chronic ethanol exposure on the fatty acid composition in different membranes. Among the different phospholipids, phosphatidylcholine contributes the most oleic acid to the membranes following chronic ethanol exposure. Phosphatidylcholine is located primarily in the outer leaflet of membranes. It has been suggested that ethanol, because of its amphiphilic properties, should be situated mainly in the water–lipid interface, thereby increasing the volume of the polar headgroup region.[25,61] Increased oleic acid in phosphatidylcholine could be a suitable correction to maintain the intermolecular spaces. These findings indicate that the interaction between ethanol and membrane lipids and their fatty acids might be more complex than fluidization.

Acidic Phospholipids

CONCENTRATIONS AFTER CHRONIC ETHANOL EXPOSURE

Investigators have focused on the acidic phospholipids because of their role in charge distribution over the membranes and their ability to bind calcium ions. When calcium ions bind to membranes, the phospholipid headgroups condense and the rigidity of the membrane increases.[63] Ethanol inhibits calcium binding to phosphatidylserine vesicles.[27,54] In 1983, two reports indicated that alcohol exposure in rats[8] and guinea pigs[59] increases brain acidic phospholipids. Subsequent studies demonstrated this phenomenon in rats.[5,59] Furthermore, primary astrocyte cultures exposed to ethanol had an increased ration of acidic:neutral phospholipids.[6] The extent of such changes, conditions for their occurrence, and their specificity remain to be elucidated before their significance is fully understood.

Table 5-2. NEURORECEPTORS AND MEMBRANE PROTEINS SHOWN TO BE DEPENDENT ON PHOSPHATIDYLSERINE FOR PROPER FUNCTION

System	Investigators
Opiate binding	Abood and Takeda, 1976[1]
Muscarinic binding	Aronstam, Abood, and Baumgold, 1977[11]
Glutamate binding	Foster et al, 1982[28]
[^{3}H] flunitrazepam binding	Hammond and Martin, 1987[31]
Na$^+$,K$^+$ ATPase activity	Floreani and Carpenedo, 1987[27]
Acetylcholine release	Vannucchi and Pepeu, 1987[62]

INTERACTION BETWEEN ACIDIC PHOSPHOLIPIDS AND MEMBRANE PROTEINS

Several membrane proteins, especially receptor proteins, require one or more of the following acidic phospholipids in their microenvironment to function properly: phosphatidylserine, phosphatidylinositol, or phosphatidic acid (Table 5-2). One of the best-studied proteins in this regard is Na$^+$,K$^+$-ATPase,[26] whose activity increased following acute ethanol exposure. Repeated doses resulted in a cumulative increase, which paralleled a rise in phosphatidylserine in synaptosomal plasma membranes.[59]

Phosphatidylserine has been reported to normalize electrophysiologic and behavioral parameters associated with aging in rats.[17,18] In another study, phosphatidylserine reduced age-dependent spontaneous EEG bursts in rats.[10] These studies all demonstrate that phosphatidylserine is involved in neurotransmission.[1,28,31] An elevated concentration of acidic phospholipids after ethanol exposure may therefore be a pathophysiologic factor in alcohol-induced hyperexcitability.

MODE OF ETHANOL ADMINISTRATION AND KINDLING

Experimental models for ethanol exposure include a variety of time periods, alcohol concentrations, and mode of administration, such as inhalation, liquid diet, and injection. The severity of intoxication fluctuates tremendously. When different reports were compared, it was noted that repeated episodes of intoxication and subsequent withdrawal induced increases in acid phospholipids, whereas a sustained amount of ethanol administered continuously had no effect on phospholipid levels. Because repeated intoxication/withdrawal episodes increase convulsions in the withdrawal phase,[23] it is tempting to speculate that there is a relation between the increase in acidic phospholipids and their role in charge distribution and neurotransmission. The phenomenon may be similar to the kindling model for hyperexcitability, which suggests that hyperexcitability develops after repeated electrical amygdaloid stimulation.[12]

Abnormal Lipids

An abnormal lipid with acidic characteristics has been found in ethanol-intoxicated rats.[3,8,14] This lipid has been identified as phosphatidylethanol, and was shown to have been formed enzymatically by phospholipase D in the presence of ethanol.[7,30,38] This biochemical reaction can be stimulated by phorbol esters and is mediated by protein kinase C. Because the activity of C-kinase is controlled by a receptor-mediated mechanism, it is possible that phosphatidylethanol is formed as a result of an overactive agonist operating during some stage of ethanol intoxication. Vasopressin, which mobilizes calcium and stimulates phospholipase D, is one such agonist candidate.[15] The eventual physiologic consequences of the formation of phosphatidylethanol in neuronal membranes remain to be proven, but most likely the molecule affects membrane properties. A study of the effects of phosphatidylethanol on the fusion ability of lipid vesicles demonstrated that this abnormal lipid promoted protein-induced fusion but inhibited Ca^{++}-induced fusion, thus differing from other phospholipids.[16]

Another example of a reaction between ethanol and lipids is the formation of fatty acid ethyl esters during ethanol exposure. Ethyl esters were first identified in the heart,[41] but have recently been found in the human brain.[42]

The formation of abnormal lipids in neuronal membranes is unique. The psychotropic agent, ethanol, itself becomes a part of the new molecules, making this phenomenon even more fascinating.

ACKNOWLEDGMENT

Supported by grants from the Medical Research Council (05249), the Bank of Sweden Tercentenary Foundation, and the Swedish Alcohol Research Fund.

References

1. Abood LG and Takeda F: Enhancement of stereospecific opiate binding to neural membranes by phosphatidylserine. Eur J Pharmacol 39:71, 1976.
2. Alling C, et al: Anionic glycerophospholipids in platelets from alcoholics. Drug Alcohol Depend 16:309, 1986.
3. Alling C, et al: Changes in fatty acid composition of major glycerophospholipids in erythrocyte membranes from chronic alcoholics during withdrawal. Scand J Clin Lab Invest 44:283, 1984b.
4. Alling C, et al: Effect of maternal essential fatty acid supply on fatty acid composition of brain, liver, muscles and serum in 21-day-old rats. J Nutr 102:772, 1972.
5. Alling C, et al: Effects of chronic ethanol treatment on lipid composition and prostaglandins in rats fed essential fatty acid deficient diets. Alcoholism: Clinical and Experimental Research 8:238, 1984.
6. Alling C, et al: Lipids and fatty acids in membranes from astroglial cells cultured in ethanol-containing media. Drug Alcohol Depend 18:126, 1987.
7. Alling C, et al: Phosphatidylethanol formation in rat organs after ethanol treatment. Biochim Biophys Acta 793:119, 1984.
8. Alling C, Gustavsson L and Änggård E: An abnormal phospholipid in rat organs after ethanol treatment. FEBS Lett 152:24, 1983.
9. Alling C, Liljequist S, and Engel J: The effect of chronic ethanol administration on lipids and fatty acids in subcellular fractions of rat brain. Med Biol 60:149, 1982.
10. Aporti F, et al: Age-dependent spontaneous EEG bursts in rats: Effects of brain phosphatidylserine. Neurobiol Aging 7:115, 1986.
11. Aronstam RS, Abood LG, and Baumgold J: Role of phospholipids in muscarinic binding by neural membranes. Biochem Pharmacol 26:1689, 1977.
12. Ballenger JC and Post KM: Kindling as a model for alcoholic withdrawal syndromes. Br J Psychiatry 133:1, 1978.
13. Bannisko P and Losowsky MS: Cell receptors and ethanol. Alcoholism: Clinical and Experimental Research 10:505, 1986.
14. Benthin G, et al: Formation of phosphatidylethanol in frozen kidneys from ethanol-treated rats. Biochim Biophys Acta 835:385, 1985.
15. Bocckino SB, Wilson PB, and Exton JH: Ca^{++}-mobilizing hormones elicit phosphatidylethanol accumulation via phospholipase D activation. FEBS Lett 225:201, 1987.
16. Bondeson J and Sundler R: Phosphatidylethanol counteracts calcium-induced membrane fusion but promotes proton-induced fusion. Biochim Biophys Acta 899:258, 1987.
17. Bruni A, et al: Serine phospholipids as endocoids. Prog Clin Biol Res 192:507, 1985.
18. Calderini G, et al: Pharmacological properties of phosphatidylserine in the aging brain: Biochemical aspects and therapeutic potential. In Horrocks LA, Freysz L, and Toffano G (eds): Phospholipid Research and the Nervous System, Biochemical and Molecular Pharmacology, Vol 4, Fidia Research Series. Padova, Liviana Press, 1986, p. 233.
19. Chin JH and Goldstein DB: Cholesterol blocks the disordering effects of ethanol in biomembranes. Lipids 19:929, 1984.
20. Chin JH and Goldstein DB: Drug tolerance in biomembranes: A spin label study of the effects of ethanol. Science 196:684, 1976.
21. Chin JH and Goldstein DB: Membrane-disordering action of ethanol: Variation with membrane cholesterol content and depth of the spin label probe. Mol Pharmacol 19:425, 1981.
22. Chin JH, Parsons LM, and Goldstein DB: Increased cholesterol content of erythrocyte and brain membranes in ethanol-tolerant mice. Biochim Biophys Acta 513:358, 1978.
23. Clemmesen L and Hemmingsen R: Physical dependence on ethanol during multiple intoxication and withdrawal episodes in the rat: Evidence of a potentiation. Acta Pharmacol Toxicol 55:345, 1984.
24. Crews FR, Majchrowicz E, and Meek R: Changes in cortical synaptosomal plasma membrane fluidity and composition in ethanol-dependent rats. Psychopharmacology 81:208, 1983.
25. Cullis PR, Hornby AP, and Hope MJ: Effects of anesthetics on lipid polymorphism. In Fink BR (ed): Molecular Mechanisms of Anesthesia, Vol 2, Progress in Anesthesiology. Raven Press, New York, 1980, p 397.
26. Floreani M, Bonetti AC, and Carpendo F: Increase of Na^+/K^+-ATPase activity in intact rat brain synaptosomes after interaction with phosphatidylserine vesicles. Biochem Biophys Res Commun 101:1337, 1981.
27. Floreani M and Carpenedo F: Phosphatidylserine vesicles increase rat brain synaptosomal adenylate cyclase activity. Biochem Biophys Res Commun 145:631, 1987.
28. Foster AC, et al: Regulation of glutamate receptors: Possible role of phosphatidylserine. Brain Res 242:374, 1982.
29. Goldstein DB, Chin JH, and Lyon RC: Ethanol disordering of spin-labeled mouse brain mem-

branes: Correlation with genetically determined ethanol sensitivity of mice. Proc Natl Acad Sci USA 79:4231, 1982.
30. Gustavsson L and Alling C: Formation of phosphatidylethanol in rat brain by phospholipase D. Biochem Biophys Res Commun 142:958, 1987.
31. Hammond JR and Martin IL: Modulation of [^{3}H]-flunitrazepam binding to rat cerebellar benzodiazepine receptors by phosphatidylserine. Eur J Pharmacol 137:49, 1987.
32. Harris RA and Schroeder F: Ethanol and the physical properties of brain membranes. Mol Pharmacol 20:128, 1981.
33. Hill MW and Bengham AD: General depressant drug dependency: A biophysical hypothesis. Adv Exp Med Biol 59:1, 1975.
34. Hitzemann RJ, et al: Ethanol-induced changes in neuronal membrane order: An NMR study. Biochim Biophys Acta 859:189, 1986.
35. Hunt WA: Alcohol and biological membranes: Neuroreceptors. Guilford Press, New York, 1985, p 103.
36. John GR, Littleton JM, and Jones PA: Membrane lipids and ethanol tolerance in the mouse: The influence of dietary fatty acid composition. Life Sci 27:545, 1980.
37. Jones AW, et al: Tolerance to ethanol in rats bred on essential fatty acid deficient diets. Pharmacol Biochem Behav 19:115, 1983.
38. Kobyashi M and Kanfer JN: Phosphatidylethanol formation via transphosphatidylation by rat brain synaptosomal phospholipase D. J Neurochem 48:1597, 1987.
39. Kreishman GP, Graham-Brittain C, and Hitzemann RJ: Determination of ethanol partition coefficients to the interior and the surface of dipalmityl-phosphatidylcholine liposomes using dentrium nuclear magnetic resonance spectroscopy. Biochem Biophys Res Comm 130:301, 1985.
40. La Droitte P, Lamboeuf Y, and De Saint Blanquat G: Ethanol sensitivity and membrane lipid composition in three strains of mouse. Comp Biochem Physiol 77C:351, 1984.
41. Lange LG, Bergmann SR, and Sobel BE: Identification of fatty acid ethyl esters as products of rabbit myocardial ethanol metabolism. J Biol Chem 256:12968, 1981.
42. Laposata EA, et al: Metabolism of ethanol by human brain to fatty acid ethyl esters. J Biol Chem 262:4653, 1987.
43. Littleton JM and John GR: Synaptosomal membrane lipids of mice during continuous exposure to ethanol. J Pharm Pharmacol 29:579, 1977.
44. Littleton JM, John GR, and Grieve SJ: Alterations in phospholipid composition in ethanol tolerance and dependence. Alcoholism: Clinical and Experimental Research 3:50, 1979.
45. Lyon RC and Goldstein DB: Changes in synaptic membrane order associated with chronic ethanol treatment in mice. Mol Pharmacol 23:86, 1983.
46. Magruder JD, Waide-Jones M, and Reitz RC: Ethanol-induced alterations in rat synaptosomal plasma membrane phospholipids. Mol Pharmacol 27:256, 1985.
47. Marco C, et al: Ethanol sensitivity and fatty acid composition of chick liver mitochondria and microsomal membranes. Biochem Int 11:291, 1985.
48. Marco C, et al: The fatty acid composition of mitochondria, microsomes and myelin from neonatal chick brain. Neuropharmacology 25:1051, 1986.
49. Meyer HH: Zur Theorie der Alkoholnarkose. 3. Mitteilung: Der Einfluss wechslender Temperatur auf Wirkungsstärke und Teilungscoefficient der Narcotica. Archives of Experimental Pathology and Pharmakology 46:338, 1901.
50. Michaelis EK, et al: Ethanol effects on synaptic glutamate receptor function and on membrane lipid organization. Pharmacol Biochem Behav (Suppl 1)18:1, 1983.
51. Miller KW: The nature of the site of general anesthesia. Int Rev Neurobiol 27:1, 1985.
52. Pohorecky LA: Biophasic action of ethanol. Biobehavior Reviews 1:231, 1977.
53. Pope JM, Walker LW, and Dubro D: On the ordering of N-alkane and N-alcohol solutes in phospholipid bilayer model membrane systems. Chem Phys Lipids 35:259, 1984.
54. Ross DH, Garrett KM, and Cardenas HL: Role of calcium in ethanol-membrane interactions: A model for tolerance and dependence. Drug Alcohol Depend 4:183, 1979.
55. Rowach H, et al: Fatty acid composition of rat liver mitochondrial phospholipids during ethanol inhalation. Biochim Biophys Acta 795:125, 1984.
56. Rowe ES: Induction of lateral phase separations in binary lipid mixtures by alcohol. Biochemistry 26:46, 1987.
57. Rowe ES: Thermodynamic reversibility of phase transitions: Specific effects of alcohols on phosphatidylcholines. Biochim Biophys Acta 813:321, 1985.
58. Smith TL and Gerhart MJ: Alterations in brain lipid composition of mice made physically dependent on ethanol. Life Sci 31:1419, 1982.
59. Sun GY and Sun AY: Chronic ethanol administration induced an increase in phosphatidylserine in guinea pig synaptic plasma membranes. Biochem Biophys Res Commun 113:262, 1983.
60. Tabakoff B and Hoffmann PL: Biochemical pharmacology of alcohol. In Meltzer HY (ed): Psychopharmacology: The Third Generation of Progress. Raven Press, New York, 1987, p 1521.
61. Tilcock CPS and Cullis PR: Lipid polymorphism. In Rubin E (ed): Alcohol and the Cell, Annals of the New York Academy of Sciences, Vol 492. The New York Academy of Sciences, New York, 1987, p 88.
62. Vannucchi MG and Pepeu G: Effect of phosphatidylserine on acetylcholine release and content in cortical slices from aging rats. Neurobiol Aging 8:403, 1987.
63. Viret J and Leterrier F: A spin label study of rat membranes: Effects of temperature and divalent cations. Biochim Biophys Acta 436:811, 1976.
64. Vrbaski SR, Grudic-Injac B, and Ristic M: Phospholipid and ganglioside composition in rat brain after chronic intake of ethanol. J Neurochem 42:1235, 1984.

65. Wing DR, et al: Changes in membrane lipid content after chronic ethanol administration with respect to fatty acyl compositions and phospholipid type. Biochem Pharmacol 33:1625, 1984.
66. Wing DR, et al: Effects of chronic ethanol administration on the composition of membrane lipids in the mouse. Biochem Pharmacol 31:3431, 1982.
67. Wixon HN and Hunt WA: Effect of acute and chronic treatment on gamma-aminobutyric acid levels and on aminooxyacetic acid-induced GABA accumulation. Substance and Alcohol Actions Misuse 1:481, 1980.

CHAPTER 6

J. M. Littleton, M.D., Ph.D.

Calcium Channel Activity in Alcohol Dependency and Withdrawal Seizures

Although the neurochemical mechanisms underlying seizures in alcohol withdrawal are unknown, they are important both theoretically and practically. The physical withdrawal syndrome usually occurs as a consequence of neuronal adaptation to a drug causing dependence. Removal of the drug exposes this adaptation so that changes occur that are the opposite of those induced by acute administration of the drug. Thus, in the case of alcohol, central nervous system (CNS) hyperexcitability occurs on withdrawal.[15] Understanding the mechanism of withdrawal seizures, therefore, should also explain drug adaptation in the CNS. Practically, this knowledge should improve treatment of withdrawal detoxification; therapy would involve attacking the mechanism of withdrawal rather than simply masking the hyperexcitability with other sedative/hypnotics, which is the basis of most current therapy.

If the basis of withdrawal seizures is an adaptive response of central neurons to alcohol, then we must first understand the mechanism by which alcohol produces acute intoxification. This knowledge is essential because we presume it is this mechanism that evokes the adaptive response. Much recent evidence suggests that one of the major reasons for the neuronal depressant action of ethanol is a potentiation of the effects of gamma-aminobutyric acid (GABA) on Cl$^-$ flux at the GABA$_A$ receptor.[40] That this effect is probably related to the intoxicating effect of alcohol is shown by experiments utilizing the imidazodiazepine RO 15-4513, which both prevents the effect of ethanol on Cl$^-$ flux and also reduces many of the behavioral effects of acute administration of ethanol.[39] Although not all the evidence is totally convincing,[23] the "alcohol antagonist" properties of RO 15-4513 argue strongly for a role of GABA$_A$ receptors in intoxication.

The consensus at present is not that alcohol influences the GABA$_A$ receptor by a specific drug-protein interaction (although Franks and Lieb[6] stress a specific interaction) but that ethanol influences many membrane-associated proteins involved in neuronal excitability and that the GABA$_A$ receptor is one of the most sensitive. It may be that the cooperative interactions between the polypeptides that make up the GABA$_A$ receptor/Cl$^-$ ionophore-benzodiazepine receptor are altered by the presence of ethanol molecules. At higher concentrations, ethanol probably affects flux of other ions both via receptor- and voltage-operated channels. Thus, inhibitory effects of ethanol on depolarization-induced Na^+ and Ca^{2+} flux have been described.[14] These effects could result either from membrane stabilization via the $GABA_A$ receptor or from a direct effect of ethanol on the appropriate ion channel protein.

Assuming that the acute effects of ethanol on neuronal function are largely inhibitory and are a consequence of potentiation of Cl^- flux at the $GABA_A$ receptor and inhibition of voltage-operated channels (probably an oversimplification), we can now consider what might be an appropriate adaptation of neurons to these effects. The most direct adaptation would be to alter the $GABA_A$ receptor so that the effects of alcohol on Cl^- flux are negated. Changes that are appropriate in this regard have been reported[1] and can be adduced as a mechanism for alcohol tolerance at the neuronal level. However, they are not associated with changes in the effect of GABA on the receptor or with alterations in the number of $GABA_A$ receptors sufficient to explain the neuronal hyperexcitability on withdrawal. In other words this adaptation *decreases* the effect of ethanol but does not oppose it. I have previously called these two types of adaptation *decremental* and *oppositional*, respectively.[26] Although decremental adaptation can explain tolerance, I believe that only oppositional adaptation can explain physical dependence.

If we cannot find evidence for oppositional adaptation in the $GABA_A$ receptor, then presumably we should look "downstream" from this action of alcohol on neuronal excitability for mechanisms that could oppose it. As discussed above, ethanol decreases depolarization-induced cation flux into neurons, probably by indirect and direct mechanisms. An oppositional adaptation based on enhanced cation flux might restore neuronal excitability in the presence of alcohol (tolerance) and cause hyperexcitability on removal of alcohol (physical dependence). Although there is no evidence for increased Na^+ flux after chronic administration of alcohol, there is now considerable evidence for an increase in voltage-operated Ca^{2+} channels associated with the development of ethanol physical dependence. Before this evidence can be discussed, it is necessary to consider the various types of neuronal Ca^{2+} channels and their function in developing and mature neurons.

Electrophysiologic evidence[34] suggests that at least three distinct types of voltage-operated Ca^{2+} channels are present on neurons. The three types have different pharmacologic characteristics as well as different electrical properties. Channels with a *long* opening period have been designated L-type; channels that open *transiently* T-type; and those with an intermediate opening period N-type (*neither* T nor L). Only the L-type channel is susceptible to inhibition by calcium channel antagonist drugs[34] which currently are used to treat cardiovascular disease. The most potent group of calcium channel antagonists on these channels is the 1,4-dihydropyridines (DHPs), and the L-type channel is sometimes described as the DHP-sensitive channel. DHP drugs bind to the channels with a high affinity and exhibit saturable specific binding.[7] Functionally the DHPs can have either antagonist (inhibitory) effects on the channel or agonist (excitatory) effects.[37] Which effect predominates depends on many factors, including membrane voltage, G-proteins and guanosine triphosphate (GTP), and the stereochemistry of the DHP. Therefore, one cannot simply assume that the functional consequences of a DHP antagonist will always reflect inhibition of depolarization-induced Ca^{2+} entry. The situation is further complicated by our imperfect understanding of the functional roles of these different types of Ca^{2+} channels in neurons.

In neurons developed *in vivo* or in culture there may be little distinction between the roles of different types of channel. Thus, in bovine adrenal chromaffin cells in culture (a model for undifferentiated sympathetic neurons that I will introduce later) and in the similar PC12 cells (derived from a rat pheochromocytoma), both N- and L-type channels can readily be shown to be coupled to Ca^{2+} entry, although only in the bovine chromaffin cells can this coupling be shown to be directly related to transmitter release.[21]

It seems that in such primitive cells intracellular Ca^{2+}, which is intimately involved in the growth and differentiation process,[19] may be controlled by these membrane Ca^{2+} channels. This finding has important implications for modulating Ca^{2+} channels as an adaptive response to alcohol, and will be discussed later.

In mature neurons the situation is probably much more complex. During differentiation it becomes increasingly difficult to demonstrate any role for the L-type channel either in depolarization-induced Ca^{2+} entry or in neuronal functions such as neurotransmitter release.[21] This does not mean that the L-type channels disappear. Radioligand binding studies utilizing DHPs suggest that a large number of L-type channel proteins exist in the mature CNS.[7] One explanation may be that L-type channels are concentrated at cellular sites where it is not easy to demonstrate effects on Ca^{2+} entry or transmitter release, for example on dendrites.[32] Concentration at such a site would enable L-type channels to control neuronal sensitivity to incoming stimuli. It is similarly difficult to ascribe functional roles to the other types of Ca^{2+} channels. Although it seems likely that N-type channels are coupled to transmitter release from nerve terminals, it has been suggested that T-type channels on the soma and axon hillock are responsible for the electrical "bursting" activity of some neurons.[32]

Whether L-type Ca^{2+} channels have any functional role at all in the mature CNS has been disputed, largely because calcium channel antagonists seem to be without central effects *in vivo*. The DHPs, for example, are largely without sedative/hypnotic actions and do not have gross electrophysiologic effects on neuronal activity in the normal brain. However, the fact that DHP-sensitive Ca^{2+} channels *can* influence neuronal activity is shown by the actions *in vitro* and *in vivo* of DHP Ca^{2+} channel agonists such as BAY K 8644. This compound has been shown to potentiate both depolarization-induced neurotransmitter release[31] and breakdown of inositol phospholipids[20] in brain slices. At the level of the intact animal, BAY K 8644 causes convulsions.[2] This finding suggests that an increase in DHP-sensitive Ca^{2+} channel activity may indeed lead to CNS hyperexcitability.

Together these studies suggest that an increase in Ca^{2+} channel activity is a logical adaptive mechanism opposing the inhibitory effects of alcohol on neuronal excitability. The Ca^{2+} channel most amenable to study is the DHP-sensitive channel, which can be investigated by studying radioligand binding (to ascertain numbers of channel proteins and their affinity for DHPs) and by studying the functional effects of DHP antagonists and agonists. The major problem with this approach is that the DHP-sensitive channels seem to play a relatively minor role in the mature CNS. This fact makes it difficult to assess the consequences of any increase in the activity of this type of channel. In undifferentiated neurons in culture and in other tissues, however, the roles of DHP-sensitive Ca^{2+} channels are better defined, and it is therefore easier to assess the functional significance of any alcohol-induced alterations in these channels.

ALTERATIONS IN Ca^{2+} CHANNELS INDUCED BY ALCOHOL IN CELL CULTURES

The presence of alcohol inhibits depolarization-induced Ca^{2+} entry in PC12 cells[30] and, presumably by the same mechanism, inhibits depolarization-induced catecholamine release from bovine chromaffin cells.[13] When either cell type is grown in a culture medium containing ethanol, an increase in the number of DHP binding sites on the cells occurs.[12,30] This increase is variable, depending on ethanol concentration and the duration of exposure, but can be well in excess of 100 percent. The greater number of DHP binding sites can be shown by experiments on $^{45}Ca^{2+}$ entry[8] and catecholamine release to represent a functional increase in DHP-sensitive Ca^{2+} channels.[12,30] As I have noted, this increase in Ca^{2+} channels may be an adaptive mechanism to the presence of ethanol. The fact that it occurs in such simple systems implies that it is a fundamental property of excitable cells. I will discuss this possibility later. I will now briefly describe the mechanism by which this change in DHP binding sites takes place and the cellular consequences it produces.

The increase in number of DHP binding sites follows a similar time course in PC12 and bovine chromaffin cell cultures. Significant increases occur within 3 or 4 days[30] and maximum increase is reached after about 6 days of growth in ethanol. DHP binding affinity changes little during this period. This time course is consistent with a genuine "up-regulation" of the DHP-sensitive calcium channel by synthesis of "new" channel proteins. Experiments utilizing cycloheximide (which inhibits protein synthesis at the mRNA translation stage) and lomofungin and anisomycin (which inhibit mRNA synthesis[3]) suggest strongly that initiation of protein synthesis via regulation of the Ca^{2+} channel gene is the cause of the increased number of DHP binding sites. As yet the trigger for the up-regulation by ethanol is unknown, although a reduction in Ca^{2+} entry caused by the presence of the drug seems logical.

Some of the consequences I have mentioned of an up-regulation of DHP-sensitive Ca^{2+} channels—alterations in depolarization-induced Ca^{2+} entry[8] and neurotransmitter release[12,13]—would be expected immediately to follow an increase in the number of channels, and both have been reported. However, several possibly more important long-term changes occur in these cells, probably as a consequence of the increased number of Ca^{2+} channels. These changes include increased synthesis and spontaneous release of catecholamines[12] as well as greater basal and receptor-stimulated turnover of inositol phospholipids.[3] These values do not seem to revert to control levels as fast as the number of Ca^{2+} channels returns to normal (about 16 hours) on removal of ethanol from the culture medium.[12]

Experiments using cell cultures suggest, therefore, that the continued presence of ethanol in the vicinity of excitable cells evokes an adaptive up-regulation in the synthesis of functional L-type Ca^{2+} channels. This increase opposes the inhibitory effect of ethanol on the cells but also confers long-term changes on cell function that cannot be immediately reversed by inhibition of the L-type channel.

ALTERATIONS IN Ca^{2+} CHANNELS INDUCED BY ALCOHOL IN THE INTACT ANIMAL

Ethanol physical dependence can be induced in laboratory animals by a variety of techniques, including administration of alcohol by inhalation.[9] When rats receive alcohol by inhalation, changes in [^{3}H]DHP binding characteristics in the brain and some peripheral tissues begin after 3 or 4 days.[4,11] As in the cell culture systems I have described, the major change is an increase in the number of DHP binding sites, but I have also noted a small decrease in binding affinity during the period when the increase in the number of binding sites is taking place.[10] Once the number of binding sites stabilizes (6-10 days, depending on the tissue studied), the binding affinity returns to normal values.[10] The extent of the change seems greatest in the heart (>100 percent increase) and less in smooth muscle and in the brain ($\approx$50 percent increase), but there is considerable individual variation.[11]

In relation to alcohol withdrawal seizures (AWS), it is necessary to demonstrate that the increase in the number of DHP binding sites in the brain represents a genuine increase in the number of functional Ca^{2+} channels. This hypothesis is difficult to demonstrate because the true function of the DHP-sensitive channels in mature neurons is unknown. We have previously reported several changes in brain preparations where Ca^{2+}-dependent phenomena are enhanced in preparations from ethanol-dependent animals.[17,28] These changes might well be a consequence of increased numbers of DHP-sensitive channels, but this possibility has not been rigorously investigated. Recently, we have studied the effects of DHP Ca^{2+} channel agonists and antagonists on brain slice preparations to ascertain whether ethanol dependence is associated with functional alterations in Ca^{2+} channels. We reasoned that an increase in DHP-sensitive channels might increase the ability of the agonist BAY K 8644 to induce neurotransmitter release, particularly from neuronal cell bodies (where the DHP-sensitive channels may be located). We also investigated the possibility that depolarization-induced inositol lipid breakdown, which is known to be DHP sensitive,[20] might be enhanced in brain preparations from ethanol-dependent rats.

In cortical slice preparations from ethanol-dependent rats there was a greater potentiation of electrically induced [³H]norepinephrine release by BAY K 8644 than in control preparations.[4] We also found a greater stimulation of inositol lipid breakdown induced by K⁺ depolarization and BAY K 8644 in the cortical preparations from ethanol-dependent rats.[4] Both actions of BAY K 8644 were potently inhibited by DHP Ca^{2+} channel antagonists, although these compounds had very little effect on the changes induced by depolarization *per se*.[5] These results strongly suggest that the increase in the number of DHP binding sites represents an increase in functional proteins even if the normal function of DHP binding sites differs from those studied here. In order to address the problem of the cellular site of these DHP binding sites, we compared K⁺-induced release of [³H]dopamine from brain slice preparations obtained from corpus striatum (rich in dopaminergic terminals) and substantia nigra (rich in dopaminergic cell bodies).[35] BAY K 8644 potentiated release to a greater extent in preparations obtained from both brain areas of ethanol-dependent rats than in control preparations. The effect of the Ca^{2+} channel antagonist was to inhibit release of [³H]dopamine in the preparations from substantia nigra (cell bodies) but not in striatal preparations (nerve terminals).[35] Only in the case of nigral preparations from ethanol-dependent animals was this inhibition significant. All these results suggest that there is an increase in the number of functional DHP-sensitive Ca^{2+} channels on central neurons in ethanol-dependent animals. These channels may normally be more numerous on cell bodies but the alcohol-induced increase in their numbers may well occur on both cell bodies and nerve terminals.

Although it is difficult to obtain unequivocal evidence for a functional increase in the number of DHP-sensitive Ca^{2+} channels in the CNS, the function of this increase in peripheral tissues is better established. Thus, in heart and smooth muscle, the number of DHP binding sites correlates closely with DHP-sensitive Ca^{2+} flux and contraction. In both heart and smooth muscle (vas deferens) of the rat, the induction of alcohol physical dependence is associated with an increase in DHP binding sites[11] and with more contractile responses to DHP-sensitive stimuli.[16] Although not strictly relevant to AWS, this finding provides further evidence that the hyperexcitability of excitable tissues is produced by an increase in the number of functional Ca^{2+} channels during the induction of alcohol physical dependence. The role of this change in the phenomena of alcohol tolerance and physical dependence in the intact animal will be considered here.

EFFECTS OF THE DHP Ca^{2+} CHANNEL AGONISTS AND ANTAGONISTS IN THE INTACT ANIMAL

Acute administration of the DHP Ca^{2+} channel agonist BAY K 8644 has a convulsant effect in intact animals.[2] The type of convulsion produced by relatively small doses of BAY K 8644 closely resembles AWS.[27] This fact suggests that an increase in the number of DHP-sensitive channels in the CNS could underlie the seizure activity associated with alcohol withdrawal. BAY K 8644 also inhibits the sedative effects of alcohol at some doses,[5] but this effect is not great.

In contrast to these effects of the Ca^{2+} channel agonist (BAY K 8644) on the behavior of otherwise untreated animals, the effects of DHP antagonists are almost nonexistent. They have very little sedative/hypnotic activity themselves but do potentiate the sedative/hypnotic effect produced by ethanol.[18] This finding suggests that in circumstances of normal neuronal electrical activity, the DHP-sensitive Ca^{2+} channels play little part in determining neuronal excitability. However, when the number of channels is increased, such as in alcohol tolerance and physical dependence, the Ca^{2+} channel antagonists may have important behavioral effects.

One might predict that when ethanol tolerance has been induced, a DHP Ca^{2+} channel agonist such as BAY K 8644 might have a greater convulsive effect, but this possibility has not yet been rigorously investigated. One might also predict that the DHP antagonists should have a greater potentiating effect on ethanol under these conditions because they should reduce the extent of tolerance due to the increased number of DHP-sensitive Ca^{2+} channels. This prediction has not been tested either; in fact both predictions would be difficult to test, based as they are on complex interactions between the DHPs and ethanol.

More simply, if AWS is a consequence of increased central neuronal excitability due to an increased number of DHP-sensitive Ca^{2+} channels, then the DHP antagonists should reduce this excitability. This phenomenon has now been unequivocally shown in rats[25] and mice.[27] It has also been demonstrated that the protective effect of the DHP Ca^{2+} channel antagonists against AWS is stereoselective and is prevented by the DHP Ca^{2+} channel agonist, BAY K 8644.[27] There seems little doubt that the DHP drugs influence AWS by virtue of their interaction with Ca^{2+} channels in the CNS.

Although this aspect (seizures) of the alcohol withdrawal syndrome can be prevented by DHP Ca^{2+} channel antagonists, there may well be other parts of the syndrome that cannot be reversed by acute administration of DHPs. In cell culture experiments, several long-term consequences of Ca^{2+} channel up-regulation were noted that did not revert to normal as fast as the removal of the excess channels.[12] In the intact animal, too, one would predict that some changes in neuronal function induced by the increase in Ca^{2+} channels would be reversible only slowly after blockage of these channels. This prediction in turn suggests that an appropriate approach to treat the withdrawal syndrome would be to prevent the increase in the number of Ca^{2+} channels ever taking place, or at least to attempt to reverse the increase well before withdrawing alcohol. Rather surprisingly, it appears that the DHP Ca^{2+} channel antagonists might also be useful in this respect.

Because chronic administration of DHP Ca^{2+} channel antagonists can be shown to *decrease* the number of DHP binding sites in peripheral tissues,[36] two groups have investigated the effects of repeatedly administering DHPs together with ethanol.[24,42] In one series of experiments, DHP binding sites in the brain were shown to be up-regulated when ethanol alone was given, but this effect was prevented when the DHP Ca^{2+} channel antagonist was also given.[20] Both groups found that concurrent administration of the DHP significantly reduced the development of alcohol tolerance.[24,42] In subsequent experiments, administration of a DHP Ca^{2+} channel antagonist with alcohol was shown to prevent AWS even when the DHP was withdrawn 24 hours before removal of ethanol from the animals.[41] This kind of regimen deserves much more extensive investigation because it may allow the DHPs to be used clinically to inhibit all aspects of the withdrawal syndrome rather than seizures alone.

CONCLUSIONS

The evidence presented is consistent with the view that alcohol physical dependence is associated with an adaptive up-regulation of DHP-sensitive Ca^{2+} channels on excitable cells. On removal of alcohol from a dependent animal, the increase in the number of Ca^{2+} channels on central neurons causes hyperexcitability expressed as the physical withdrawal syndrome. Treatment with DHP Ca^{2+} channel antagonists can prevent this syndrome, particularly the associated seizures.

Although these changes represent a logical adaptive response to the inhibitory effects of alcohol, there are many unresolved problems. The most puzzling aspect is the role of the DHP binding sites in the normal brain and the lack of effects of DHP Ca^{2+} channel antagonists on normal excitability. The relation of these Ca^{2+} channels to intracellular second messengers, such as the products of inositol phospholipid breakdown, may be important. DHP-sensitive channels normally may mediate relatively slow changes in excitability within cells via intracellular mediators, rather than causing immediate changes. In alcohol dependence, however, the dramatic increase in the number of channels may make their density on neuronal membranes sufficiently great to play a more direct role in cell excitability.

The relation between an increased number of DHP-sensitive channels and increased inositol phospholipid breakdown is also an interesting problem. In some cell types, diacylglycerol-induced activation of protein kinase C has been reported to trigger up-regulation of an L-type of Ca^{2+} channel.[38] Thus, the increased inositol lipid breakdown could be the cause of the increased number of channels, or it could be a consequence of the increase. I currently favor the second explanation but the question is far from resolved.

Much of the evidence presented for the association of alcohol physical dependence with this up-regulation involves radioligand binding of DHP Ca^{2+} channel antagonists. I have established a functional basis for this association using the DHP Ca^{2+} channel agonist, BAY K 8644. This approach provides only limited information, since it appears that DHPs can act as either agonists or antagonists, depending on the state of the channel. Their action depends on the presence of GTP, which probably mediates alterations in the channel via a G-protein.[37] In other words, we do not know whether the increase in the number of binding sites represents mainly an increase in the conformation that is activated by DHPs ("agonist conformation") or inactivated by DHPs ("antagonist conformation"). Some of our unpublished evidence involving peripheral tissue favors the former possibility, but only painstaking electrophysiologic research will answer this important question.

Finally, what is the role of the DHP Ca^{2+} channel antagonists in therapy for AWS? A small clinical trial in Austria of a Ca^{2+} channel antagonist (albeit a non-DHP type) suggested its efficacy in alcohol withdrawal,[22] and similar findings have been reported in East Berlin using the DPH nimodipine.[33] There is every reason to suppose that this approach will become useful clinically. There is, however, one serious problem. All the DHPs currently in use have been developed for their selectivity on the cardiovascular system. Cardiovascular side-effects are an inevitable consequence of their use in withdrawal (these side-effects may or may not be useful in themselves, but that is a separate question). The development of DHPs relatively selective for the CNS would represent an advance. This development is possible only if there are differences in the channel proteins in the CNS and cardiovascular system. This is probably the case. The sea-snail toxin ω-conotoxin selectively inhibits neuronal L-type Ca^{2+} channels rather than peripheral channels.[29] The situation is therefore very promising. It should be possible to develop DHP drugs that are effective in controlling seizures (and possibly other aspects of AWS), that have few side-effects, and that neither potentiate the sedative effects of alcohol nor have abuse potential of their own. This development would be a considerable advance on current treatment.

SUMMARY

The acute intoxicating effects of alcohol involve a depression of neuronal activity via potentiation of GABA-mediated Cl^- flux. As a consequence, depolarization-induced entry of Ca^{2+} into central neurons is reduced. A major adaptive response is for neurons to increase the number of a subtype of Ca^{2+} channels on their surface membrane. This subtype may be mainly located on the cell body and is sensitive to inhibition by DHP Ca^{2+} channel antagonists. Removal of alcohol from an organism in this adapted state causes CNS hyperexcitability, expressed as the physical withdrawal syndrome, as a consequence of the increase in the number of Ca^{2+} channels. DHP Ca^{2+} channel antagonists can prevent AWS and offer a novel approach to the therapeutic management of the withdrawal syndrome.

References

1. Allan, AM and Harris, RA: Acute and chronic ethanol treatments alter GABA receptor-oper-

ated chloride channels. Pharmacol Biochem Behav 27:665, 1987.
2. Bolger, TG, Weissman, BA, and Skolnick, P: The behavioural effect of the calcium antagonist BAY K 8644 in the mouse: Antagonism by nifedipine. Naunyn Schmiedebergs Arch Pharmacol 328:373, 1985.
3. Brennan, CH: Unpublished material, 1987.
4. Dolin, SJ, et al: Increased dihydropyridine-sensitive calcium channels in rat brain may underlie ethanol physical dependence. Neuropharmacology 26:275, 1987.
5. Dolin, SJ, Halsey, MJ, and Little, HJ: Effects of BAY K 8644 on general anaesthetic potencies of ethanol and argon. Br J Pharmacol 89:622P, 1986.
6. Franks, NP and Lieb, WR: Volatile general anaesthetics activate a novel neuronal K^+ current. Nature 333:662, 1988.
7. Glossman, H and Ferry, DR: Assay for calcium channels. Methods Enzymol 109:513, 1985.
8. Greenberg, DA, Carpenter, CL, and Messing, RO: Ethanol-induced component of $^{45}Ca^{2+}$ uptake in PC12 cells is sensitive to Ca^{2+} channel modulating drugs. Brain Res, 410:143, 1987.
9. Griffiths, PJ, Littleton, JM, and Ortiz, A: Changes in monoamine concentrations in mouse brain associated with ethanol dependence and withdrawal. Br J Pharmacol 50:489, 1974.
10. Guppy, LJ: Unpublished material, 1987.
11. Guppy, LJ and Littleton, JM: Increased [^{3}H]dihydropyridine binding sites in brain, heart and smooth muscle of ethanol dependent rats. Br J Pharmacol 92:662P, 1987.
12. Harper, JC and Littleton, JM: Putative alcohol dependence in adrenal cell cultures: Relation to calcium channel activity. Br J Pharmacol 92:661P, 1987.
13. Harper, JC, Pagonis, C, and Littleton JM: An adaptive increase in neuronal calcium channels alters catecholamine release in alcohol dependence. Proceedings of 6th International Catecholamine Symposium (in press).
14. Harris, RA and Bruno, P: Membrane disordering by anaesthetic drugs: Relationship to synaptosomal sodium and calcium fluxes. J Neurochem 44:1274, 1985.
15. Himmelsbach, CK: Clinical studies of drug addiction. Arch Intern Med 69:766, 1942.
16. Hudspith, MJ, et al: Dihydropyridine-sensitive calcium channels and inositol phospholipid metabolism in ethanol physical dependence. Ann NY Acad Sci 492:156, 1987.
17. Hudspith MJ, et al: Effect of ethanol in vitro and in vivo on Ca^{2+} activated enzymes of membrane lipid metabolism in rat synaptosomal and brain slice preparations. Alcohol 2:133, 1985.
18. Isaacson RL, et al: Nimodipine's interactions with other drugs: 1: Ethanol. Life Sci 36:2195, 1985.
19. Kater, SB, et al: Calcium regulation of the neuronal growth cone. Trends in Neuroscience 11:315, 1988.
20. Kendall, DA and Nahorski, SR: Dihydropyridine calcium channel activators and antagonists influence depolarisation-induced inositol phospholipid hydrolysis in brain. Eur J Pharmacol 115:31, 1985.
21. Kongsamut, S and Miller, RJ: Nerve growth factor modulates the drug sensitivity of neurotransmitter release from PC12 cells. Proc Natl Acad Sci USA 83:2243, 1986.
22. Koppi, S, et al: Calcium channel blocking agent in the treatment of acute ethanol withdrawal: Caroverine versus meprobamate in a randomized double blind study. Neuropsychobiology 17:49, 1987.
23. Lister, RG and Nutt, DJ: Is RO 15-4513 a specific alcohol antagonist? Trends in Neuroscience 10:223, 1987.
24. Little, HJ and Dolin, SJ: Lack of tolerance to ethanol after concurrent administration of nitrendipine. Br J Pharmacol 92:606P, 1987.
25. Little, HJ, Dolin, SJ, and Halsey, MJ: Calcium channel antagonists decrease the ethanol withdrawal syndrome. Life Sci 39:2059, 1986.
26. Littleton, JM: Tolerance and physical dependence on alcohol at the level of synaptic membranes: A review. J R Soc Med 76:593, 1983.
27. Littleton, JM and Little, HJ: Dihydropyridines and the ethanol withdrawal syndrome: Stereospecificity and the effects of BAY K 8644. Br J Pharmacol 92:663P, 1987.
28. Lynch, M and Littleton, JM: Possible association of alcohol tolerance with increased synaptic calcium sensitivity. Nature 303:175, 1983.
29. McCleskey, EW, et al: ω-Conotoxin: Direct and persistent blockade of specific types of calcium channels in neurons but not muscle. Proc Natl Acad Sci USA 84:4327, 1987.
30. Messing, RO, et al: Ethanol regulates calcium channels in clonal neural cells. Proc Natl Acad Sci USA 83:6213, 1986.
31. Middlemiss, D and Spedding, M: A functional correlate for the dihydropyridine binding site in rat brain. Nature 314:94, 1985.
32. Miller, RJ: Multiple calcium channels and neuronal function. Science 235:46, 1987.
33. Nickel, B and Schmickaly, R: Calcium channel blockers in the treatment of alcohol withdrawal syndromes. Alcohol Alcohol 23:A60, 1988.
34. Nowycky, MC, Fox, AP, and Tsien, RW: Three types of neuronal calcium channel with different calcium agonist sensitivity. Nature 316:440, 1985.
35. Pagonis, C and Littleton, JM: The Ca^{2+} antagonist, PN 200-110, inhibits [^{3}H]dopamine release from nigral but not striatal slices from ethanol dependent rats. Br J Pharmacol 91:416P, 1987.
36. Panza, G, et al: Evidence for down-regulation of [^{3}H]nitrendipine recognition sites in mouse brain after long term treatment with nifedipine or verapamil. Neuropharmacology 24:1113, 1985.
37. Scott, RH and Dolphin, AC: Activation of a G-protein promotes agonist responses to calcium channel ligands. Nature 330:760, 1987.
38. Strong, JA, et al: Stimulation of protein kinase C recruits covert calcium channels in Aplysia bag cell neurons. Nature 325:714, 1987.
39. Suzdak, PD, et al: Ethanol stimulates γ-aminobutyric acid-mediated chloride transport in rat

brain synaptosomes. Proc Natl Acad Sci USA 83:4071, 1986.
40. Suzdak, PD, et al: A selective imidazodiazepine antagonist of ethanol in the rat. Science 234:1243, 1986.
41. Whittington, MA and Little, HJ: Nitrendipine prevents the ethanol withdrawal syndrome when administered chronically with ethanol prior to withdrawal. Br J Pharmacol 94:385P, 1988.
42. Wu, PH, Pham, T, and Naranjo, CA: Nifedipine delays the acquisition of tolerance to ethanol. Eur J Pharmacol 139:233, 1987.

CHAPTER 7

David A. Greenberg, M.D., Ph.D.
Robert O. Messing, M.D.
Shelley S. Marks
Celia L. Carpenter

Calcium Channel Changes During Alcohol Withdrawal

The principal clinical features of ethanol intoxication and withdrawal are related to altered nervous system function. In addition, the nervous system is a major site of pathology following prolonged, excessive ethanol intake.[11] Despite the frequency with which these problems are encountered in clinical practice, the molecular basis for ethanol's adverse effects on the nervous system is poorly understood. The widespread dependence of neurotropic drug action on biologic membranes has focused attention on the cell membrane and its macromolecular components as mediators of ethanol's effects. Whether membrane lipids or proteins are the primary targets for ethanol is debated, but it is generally agreed that both are affected, and both are likely to be important in expressing ethanol's pharmacologic properties. Certain membrane proteins such as neurotransmitter receptors, ion channels, transport proteins, and enzymes are particularly well suited for study because they have well-characterized roles in neuronal function, and in many cases are amenable to pharmacologic manipulation. These characteristics not only facilitate their investigation in the laboratory, but also offer potential therapeutic approaches to reversing ethanol-induced changes.

ETHANOL AND CALCIUM

The pivotal role of Ca^{2+} in regulating the activity of excitable cells[9] has prompted interest in its possible involvement in neuronal responses to ethanol. The concentration of free intracellular Ca^{2+} ($[Ca^{2+}]_i$) is maintained at low levels by the relative impermeability of the cell membrane to Ca^{2+}, and by mechanisms for Ca^{2+} sequestration and extrusion. Electrical or chemical stimulation increases $[Ca^{2+}]_i$ by promoting entry of extracellular Ca^{2+} through membrane ion channels, or by mobilizing Ca^{2+} from intracellular stores via the action of second-messenger inositol phosphates. Elevation of $[Ca^{2+}]_i$ activates intracellular biochemical processes involving protein kinases, proteases, and phospholipases, and regulates neurotransmitter synthesis and release, ion channel number and gating properties, neurotransmitter receptor density, and cytoskeletal elements.

Ethanol has been shown to influence several aspects of cellular Ca^{2+} homeostasis and to modify Ca^{2+}-dependent neuronal responses; in many instances, long-term exposure to ethanol has resulted in apparent adaptation to these acute effects. Studies of the acute effects of ethanol suggest it inhibits adenosine triphosphate

(ATP)-dependent Ca^{2+} sequestration[8,12] and Na^+/Ca^{2+} exchange,[19] while enhancing plasmalemmal Ca^{2+}-ATPase activity.[26] The net result of these perturbations is an increase in $[Ca^{2+}]_i$ that can be demonstrated with fluorescent Ca^{2+} indicator dyes.[4,22] The physiologic consequences of ethanol-induced elevation of $[Ca^{2+}]_i$ may include enhancement of spontaneous neurotransmitter release[3,22,23] and of Ca^{2+}-activated K^+ currents.[2,25] Following chronic exposure to ethanol, its acute effects on Ca^{2+} sequestration,[12] Na^+/Ca^{2+} exchange,[20] and Ca^{2+}-activated K^+ currents[6] are attenuated.

Ethanol also reduces voltage-dependent Ca^{2+} currents in several preparations, and chronic ethanol treatment elicits adaptation to this effect. Ethanol inhibits Ca^{2+} currents in cultured dorsal root ganglion[21] and Aplysia[1] neurons. In the former case, chronic ethanol exposure diminishes the acute effect of ethanol.[7] Ethanol also inhibits the rapid phase of K^+-stimulated Ca^{2+} uptake into rat brain synaptosomes.[13,14] Chronic administration of ethanol in vivo abolishes this acute in vitro effect.[14] Because inhibition of Ca^{2+} flux by membrane-perturbing drugs, including ethanol, appears to correlate poorly with disordering of bulk membrane lipids,[13] it has been suggested that ethanol may interact with the Ca^{2+} channel or its lipid microenvironment in a relatively selective fashion.

In many in vitro studies, the ethanol concentrations employed are greater than those required to produce clinical symptoms in nonalcoholic human subjects. There are several possible explanations for this discrepancy. In vitro biochemical assays are often conducted under conditions designed to yield changes of large magnitude, whereas quantitatively minor changes may be responsible for cognitive and behavioral impairment related to ethanol. In vitro studies may also underestimate physiologic effects that are amplified in vivo through complex neuronal systems. In addition, particular clinical features of ethanol intoxication, such as cerebellar ataxia or death from respiratory depression, may reflect involvement of specific groups of preferentially sensitive neurons, rather than the overall extent of neuronal dysfunction. Finally, higher ethanol concentrations may be chosen to reflect more closely the blood levels that occur in alcoholic patients in whom tolerance has developed.

CELL CULTURE APPROACH

Depending on the question studied, one or another experimental system may be most suitable for ethanol research. Whole animals are ideal for investigating behavioral or nutritional aspects of ethanol consumption, or the effects of ethanol on integrated physiologic systems. However, the complexity of intact organisms can confound efforts to identify precise molecular mechanisms of ethanol action. Fractionated cell preparations make neuronal membranes directly accessible for study, but the heterogeneity of the original preparation is retained, and fractionation may cause parts of neurons, endogenous regulatory factors, or receptor-effector coupling to be lost.

An alternative approach involves studying neural cells in culture, which allows experiments to be conducted on intact, living cells under closely controlled conditions. Primary cultures of dissociated neurons have numerous applications, but include diverse cell types, contain relatively few cells, and can be maintained for only brief periods of time. In contrast, continuous clonal cell lines of nervous system origin yield large, homogeneous populations of cells such as are commonly required for biochemical studies. Several neural cells lines express phenotypic neuronal properties and are stable in culture for prolonged periods, so that both acute and long-term effects of ethanol on selected neuronal functions can be investigated. The major disadvantage of continuous cell lines is that they consist of transformed cells, which are likely to differ from "normal" cells in several respects. However, if the cellular function or constituent under study is well defined and its properties in a given cell line correspond to those in untransformed cells, the superior yield and uniformity of cultured cell lines can generate information not otherwise available using existing methods.

PC12, the cell line we have used, is a clonal cell line of neural crest origin, originally derived from a rat pheochromocytoma. PC12 cells in culture express a wide variety of neuronal properties, including voltage-dependent and receptor-gated ion channels; mechanisms for the synthesis, storage, release, and reuptake of neurotransmitter catecholamines, acetylcholine, and gamma-amino butyric acid (GABA); and physiologic responses to acetylcholine, substance P, and adenosine. PC12 cells respond to nerve growth factor (NGF) with extension of neurites; elaboration of neuronal growth cones; cessation of cell division; enhanced expression of Na$^+$ channels and of muscarinic cholinergic and delta opiate receptors; and increased levels of choline acetyltransferase, acetylcholine, glutamic acid decarboxylase mRNA, neuropeptide Y-like immunoreactivity, cyclic adenosine monophosphate (cAMP), neurofilament proteins, and synapsin I. Finally, PC12 cells can form functional synapses in culture. For these reasons, PC12 has been widely used as a model neural system.

ACUTE EFFECT OF ETHANOL

Ion flux through voltage-dependent Ca^{2+} channels can be studied by measuring K$^+$-stimulated ^{45}Ca^{2+} uptake into PC12 cells. Ca^{2+} flux elicited in this manner appears to correspond to L-type (long-lasting) Ca^{2+} channels identified in electrophysiologic preparations, since it is inhibited by cationic Ca^{2+} channel blockers and organic Ca^{2+} channel antagonists and enhanced by Ca^{2+} channel agonists. Therefore, we used this method to investigate the acute effect of ethanol on voltage-dependent Ca^{2+} channels.

PC12 cells were grown at 37°C in Dulbecco's modified Eagle's medium containing 10 percent horse serum, 5 percent fetal calf serum, 50 units of penicillin/ml, 50 μg of streptomycin/ml, and 2 mM glutamine, under a humidified atmosphere of 90 percent air and 10 percent CO$_2$. Nerve growth factor was not employed. Control and ethanol-containing media were re-

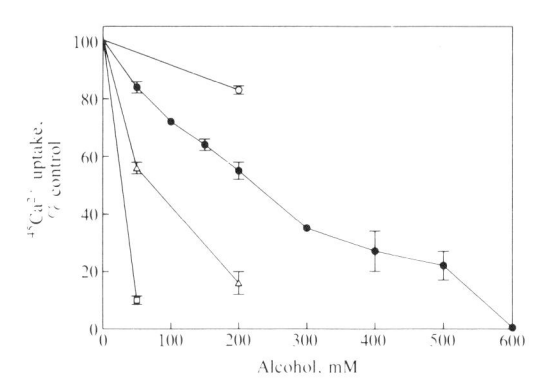

Figure 7–1. Acute inhibition of voltage-dependent ^{45}Ca^{2+} uptake in PC12 cells by ethanol and other alcohols. Data shown are mean values ± SEM from 3–5 different cultures exposed for 25 minutes to ethanol (●), methanol (○), propanol (△), or butanol (□). (From Messing, et al,[18] with permission.)

placed every 24 hours, at which time the concentration of ethanol remaining in cultures was 95 percent of that added initially. Voltage-dependent (K$^+$-depolarization-evoked) ^{45}Ca^{2+} uptake was defined as the difference between uptake in 50 mM K$^+$ (depolarizing) and 5 mM K$^+$ (nondepolarizing) buffers. Inhibition of uptake by ethanol was concentration dependent, with 16 percent inhibition at 50 mM ethanol and 50 percent inhibition at 211 mM ethanol (Fig. 7–1).[18] The ability of n-alkanols to reduce uptake was directly related to their carbon chain length, and other osmotically active agents failed to reproduce the effect of ethanol. It is therefore most likely that ethanol acts on Ca^{2+} channels by partitioning into hydrophobic compartments of the cell membrane, and not simply through an osmotic effect. The measured reduction in net ^{45}Ca^{2+} accumulation by PC12 cells exposed to ethanol was clearly due to a decrease in ^{45}Ca^{2+} influx, because ^{45}Ca^{2+} efflux was not significantly affected by 200 mM ethanol.

LONG-TERM EFFECT OF ETHANOL

A striking feature of the pharmacology of ethanol is the emergence of reduced behavioral sensitivity with prolonged exposure. One view is that such adaptation results from compensatory changes in neuronal activity that permit normal neuronal function in the drug's continued presence. Accordingly, cells might respond to acute inhibition of Ca^{2+} flux by ethanol with decreased sensitivity to this acute effect or, alternatively, by an enhanced capacity for Ca^{2+} uptake that counteracts the acute inhibitory effect. We attempted to distinguish between these possibilities by measuring K$^+$-stimulated ^{45}Ca^{2+} uptake in cells grown with or without 200 mM ethanol for prolonged periods. After 6 days of exposure to 200 mM ethanol, there was no change in the potency with which ethanol inhibited Ca^{2+} uptake acutely (IC$_{50}$ = 194 mM in both cases). However, the same ethanol exposure schedule increased K$^+$-stimulated ^{45}Ca^{2+} uptake, measured in the absence of ethanol, by 75 percent (Fig. 7–2).[18]

Ca^{2+} current is the product of the unitary channel conductance, the probability of channel opening in response to depolarization, and the number of functional channels. Therefore, chronic exposure to ethanol could enhance Ca^{2+} flux in PC12 cells by increasing any of these factors. The availability of radioligand probes for L-type Ca^{2+} channels present in PC12 cells prompted us to investigate whether an increase in the number of channels might underlie the long-term enhancement of Ca^{2+} flux by ethanol. Initially, we used the dihydropyridine (DHP) Ca^{2+} channel antagonist, [^{3}H]nitrendipine, to label channels in membranes from PC12 cells grown for 6 days with or without 200 mM ethanol.[18] Scatchard plots of these data (Fig. 7–3) were linear, indicating that [^{3}H]nitrendipine bound to a homogeneous population of receptor sites under both conditions of growth. Plots describing binding to ethanol-treated cultures were parallel to those generated from control cultures, indicating that ethanol exposure resulted in no change in the affinity (K$_D$ = 120–140 pM) with which [^{3}H]nitrendipine binds to Ca^{2+} channel receptor sites. However, long-term culture with ethanol resulted in an approximately

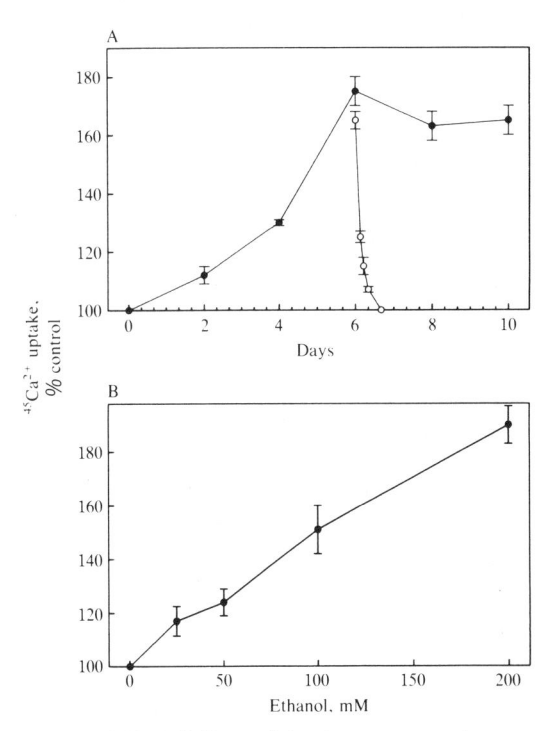

Figure 7–2. (A) Reversible, long-term enhancement of voltage-dependent ^{45}Ca^{2+} uptake in PC12 cells by exposure to 200 mM ethanol for various periods or (B) to various concentrations of ethanol for 6 days. Some cells were withdrawn from ethanol following long-term exposure (A,○). Data shown are mean values ± SEM from 3–9 different cultures. (From Messing, et al,[18] with permission.)

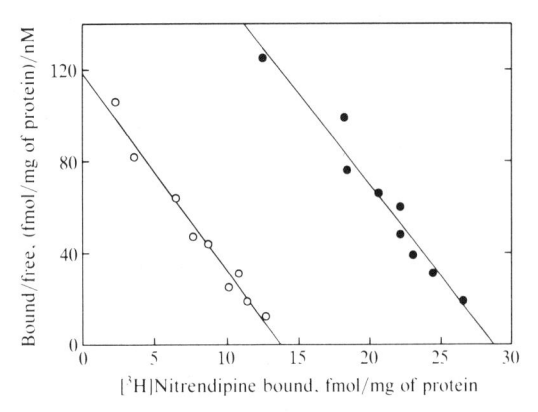

Figure 7–3. Scatchard plots of [^{3}H]nitrendipine binding to PC12 membranes prepared from cells grown for 6 days in the absence of ethanol (○) or in the presence of 200 mM ethanol (●). Data shown are from a representative experiment. (From Messing, et al,[18] with permission.)

two-fold increase in the number of binding sites, from 12.4 to 23.8 fmol/mg protein.[18] This finding suggests that chronic ethanol treatment may enhance voltage-dependent Ca^{2+} flux by causing an increase in the number of Ca^{2+} channels expressed by the cell.

Ca^{2+} channel receptors detected by radioligand binding studies on disrupted membrane preparations might not correspond to functional receptors on the cell surface. For example, some such binding sites might be located intracellularly, or in sequestered domains of the cell membrane where they are unavailable for sensing changes in membrane potential or for transporting Ca^{2+} across the membrane. To determine if the increase in the number of Ca^{2+} channel antagonist binding sites induced by chronic ethanol exposure involves physiologically accessible receptors, we examined the effects of growing cells for 6 days in 200 mM ethanol on the binding of another DHP Ca^{2+} channel antagonist, (+)-[^{3}H]PN 200-110, to intact PC12 cells. As was the case for [^{3}H]nitrendipine binding to PC12 membranes, binding of (+)-[^{3}H]PN 200-110 to intact PC12 cells was altered by ethanol treatment. In both control and ethanol-treated cells, K_D values were in the range of 65 to 85 pM, but ethanol exposure resulted in an approximate doubling of the number of binding sites, from 2.26 to 4.15 fmol/10^6 cells. This magnitude of increase is similar to that observed for [^{3}H]nitrendipine binding to disrupted membranes. Therefore, the additional Ca^{2+} channel receptors induced by culturing cells in ethanol appear to represent physiologically relevant sites.

PROPERTIES OF ETHANOL-INDUCED CALCIUM CHANNELS

At least three varieties of voltage-dependent Ca^{2+} channels can be distinguished by electrophysiologic and pharmacologic criteria. N-type channels, which are insensitive to conventional Ca^{2+} channel antagonist drugs, appear to account for the major portion of K^+-stimulated $^{45}Ca^{2+}$ uptake into brain synaptosomes. These channels have also been implicated in Ca^{2+}-evoked neurotransmitter release. Because most studies of acute and chronic effects of ethanol on Ca^{2+} channels have utilized brain synaptosomes, the bulk of data concerning ethanol's effects on Ca^{2+} channels probably applies to N-type channels. In contrast, Ca^{2+} channels expressed by PC12 cells are classified as L-type, as defined by their sensitivity to Ca^{2+} channel agonist and antagonist drugs. We were interested in whether the additional Ca^{2+} channels expressed following ethanol exposure were also L-type, because this characteristic would suggest a possible use for Ca^{2+} channel antagonist drugs in treating alcohol withdrawal syndromes (AWS).

In one set of experiments, we compared the voltage dependence of $^{45}Ca^{2+}$ uptake into PC12 cells in ethanol-treated and control cells. Treated cells were exposed to 200 mM ethanol for 6 days, and $^{45}Ca^{2+}$ uptake was measured at increasing concentrations of extracellular K^+, corresponding to increasing degrees of membrane depolarization. There was no appreciable difference between the K^+-dependence of uptake under the two conditions, as demonstrated by the similar concentrations of K^+ required for half-maximal (25–30 mM) and maximal (50–60 mM) stimulation.[10]

Subtypes of voltage-dependent Ca^{2+} channels also exhibit differential sensitivity to ionic Ca^{2+} channel blockers. Therefore, we examined the effects of several such ions on K^+-stimulated $^{45}Ca^{2+}$ uptake in control PC12 cells and cells treated for 6 days with 200 mM ethanol. Ethanol exposure had no effect on the relative potencies of blocking ions, which under both conditions had the following order: La^{3+}, $Cd^{2+} > Co^{2+}$, Ni^{2+}, $Mn^{2+} > Mg^{2+}$.[10]

The most definitive pharmacologic criterion for establishing that Ca^{2+} channels are L-type is sensitivity to Ca^{2+} channel agonist and antagonist drugs, especially DHPs. To determine if Ca^{2+} channels induced by chronic ethanol exposure are drug sensitive or drug resistant, we compared the ability of several such drugs to modify K^+-stimulated $^{45}Ca^{2+}$ uptake into control and ethanol (200 mM, 6 days)-treated cells. All antagonist drugs tested completely inhibited uptake, and were at least as potent in ethanol-treated cells as in control cells. Half-maximal inhibitory concentrations (nM) in treated and untreated cells were: nifedipine (2 and 4), flunarizine (485 and 590), verapamil (441 and 912), and diltiazem (900 and 1919). In addition, the Ca^{2+} channel agonist, BAY K 8644, stimulated $^{45}Ca^{2+}$ uptake with similar potency (half-maximally-effective concentrations of 19 and 14 nM) and to a similar maximal extent (209 percent and 248 percent) in ethanol-treated and control cells.[10] This finding establishes that Ca^{2+} channels in PC12 cells chronically exposed to ethanol, like channels in control cells, are L-type.

ETHANOL WITHDRAWAL

To determine whether the ethanol-induced increase in $^{45}Ca^{2+}$ uptake was reversible, uptake was measured in cells cultured for 6 days with 200 mM ethanol, and then for additional periods without ethanol. Under these conditions, $^{45}Ca^{2+}$ uptake declined to control levels within 16 hours of ethanol withdrawal (Fig. 7–2).[18] The duration of this in vitro withdrawal period is of interest because it corresponds to the interval after cessation of drinking during which alcoholic patients are most likely to experience AWS. Although the mechanisms responsible for generating such seizures are unknown, one possibility is that unmasking enhanced Ca^{2+} influx by withdrawal of ethanol may enhance neurotransmitter release at central synapses involved in epileptogenesis.[16,17]

CALCIUM CHANNEL BLOCKADE AND THE MECHANISM OF ETHANOL'S CHRONIC EFFECT

Because acute exposure to ethanol inhibits voltage-dependent Ca^{2+} flux in PC12 cells and chronic ethanol treatment increases Ca^{2+} flux, one could suppose that the chronic effect is an adaptation that reflects the ability of the cell to sense and correct the acute inhibition. However, long-term changes in the number of Ca^{2+} channels could also be elicited by a signal other than acute reduction of Ca^{2+} flux by ethanol. To test this hypothesis, cells were exposed to Ca^{2+} channel antagonist drugs for the same period (6 days) and at the same relative (acute IC_{50}) concentration employed in long-term experiments involving ethanol. If acute inhibition of uptake was the cause of the long-term increase in the number of channels, then prolonged treatment with Ca^{2+} channel antagonists should also increase Ca^{2+} channel radioligand binding. The drug concentrations used were 200 mM ethanol, 4 nM nifedipine, and 900 nM verapamil or 1900 mM diltiazem. Binding of (+)-[^{3}H]PN 200-110 was measured in PC12 membranes that had been thoroughly washed to remove any drug that remained bound to its receptor.

Results of these studies showed no significant increase in (+)-[^{3}H]PN 200-110 binding due to chronic exposure to Ca^{2+} channel antagonists. Ethanol increased the number of binding sites by 89% over that measured in control cultures, but nifedipine and verapamil did not increase binding, and diltiazem increased binding by only 8%. Thus, acute inhibition of Ca^{2+} flux is not an adequate stimulus for a long-term increase in the number of channels, and the acute and chronic effects of ethanol on Ca^{2+} flux in PC12 cells do not appear to be causally related.

STUDIES ON BRAINS OF ALCOHOLIC PATIENTS

Although we have found an increase in the number of Ca^{2+} channel binding sites in PC12 cultures chronically treated with ethanol,[18] and others have obtained similar results in both PC12 cells and rat brain synaptosomes,[5,24] it is uncertain whether a similar phenomenon occurs in relation to alcoholism in human subjects. The changes we observed were reversible within 16 hours, indicating that if analogous changes take place in the brains of human alcoholics, they might disappear with resolution of the alcohol withdrawal period. Alternatively, excessive drinking over many years might lead to more persistent alterations in the number or function of Ca^{2+} channels, which could in turn contribute to the pathogenesis of alcohol-related neurologic disorders.

To address these issues, we conducted studies of (+)-[³H]PN 200-110 binding to brain samples obtained at autopsy from alcoholic and nonalcoholic patients. Human frontal cerebral cortex was frozen at autopsy and maintained at −70°C until experiments were performed. Five patients without central nervous system (CNS) disease or a history of alcoholism, six alcoholics, and seven patients with Alzheimer's disease were studied. Tissue was thawed, white matter was removed, and gray matter was assayed for (+)-[³H]PN 200-110 binding.

There was no significant difference in mean age nor in the time between death and autopsy between the control and alcoholic populations investigated. The alcoholics, however, were significantly younger (55 ± 6 years) than the Alzheimer's (74 ± 4 years) patients. Neither (+)-[³H]PN 200-110 binding affinity nor the number of binding sites was significantly different in alcoholic as compared with control patient samples, although affinity was marginally lower in the Alzheimer's group compared with controls.

None of the alcoholic patients we studied was withdrawing from alcohol at the time of death. It is therefore possible that changes in the number of Ca^{2+} channels akin to those we observed *in vitro* occurred while these patients were drinking, but had resolved before they died. Obvious practical limitations preclude obtaining human brain tissue immediately at the onset of alcohol withdrawal, which might be the only way to detect such changes. In any event, our findings argue against the hypothesis that permanent changes in brain Ca^{2+} channels result from chronic alcoholism.

SUMMARY

Evidence suggests that membrane ion channels may mediate some of the effects of ethanol on the nervous system. Our experimental findings indicate that long-term exposure of cultured neural cells to ethanol enhances $^{45}Ca^{2+}$ influx through voltage-dependent Ca^{2+} channels in a reversible fashion. Accordingly, persistent augmentation of Ca^{2+} flux during ethanol withdrawal might contribute to the state of neuronal hyperexcitability associated with AWS, including withdrawal seizures. Therefore, it is of considerable interest that some investigators have found Ca^{2+} channel antagonist drugs to be capable of attenuating AWS in laboratory animals.[15] The application of this finding to human patients awaits appropriately controlled clinical testing.

ACKNOWLEDGMENTS

This research was supported in part by USPHS research grants AA07032 (D.A.G.) and NS01151 (R.O.M.), research grants from the Alcoholic Beverage Medical Research Foundation (D.A.G. and R.O.M.), and an Alfred P. Sloan Research Fellowship in Neuroscience (D.A.G.).

References

1. Camacho-Nasi, P and Treistman, SN: Ethanol-induced reduction of neuronal calcium currents in Aplysia: An examination of possible mechanisms. Cell Mol Neurobiol 7:191, 1987.
2. Carlen, PL, Gurevich, N, and Durand, D: Ethanol in low doses augments calcium-mediated mechanisms measured intracellularly in hippocampal neurons. Science 215:306, 1982.
3. Carmichael, FJ and Israel, Y: Effects of ethanol on neurotransmitter release by rat brain cortical slices. J Pharmacol Exp Ther 193:824, 1975.
4. Daniell, LC, Brass, EP, and Harris, RA: Effect of ethanol on intracellular ionized calcium concentrations in synaptosomes and hepatocytes. Mol Pharmacol 32:831, 1987.
5. Dolin, S, et al: Increased dihydropyridine-sensitive calcium channels in rat brain may underlie ethanol physical dependence. Neuropharmacology 26:275, 1987.
6. Durand, D and Carlen, PL: Decreased neuronal inhibition in vitro after long-term administration of ethanol. Science 224:1359, 1984.
7. Eskuri, S and Pozos, R: Development of ethanol tolerance in sensory neurons in culture. Alcoholism: Clinical and Experimental Research 9:197, 1985.
8. Garrett, KM and Ross, DH: Effects of in vivo ethanol administration on Ca^{2+}/Mg^{2+} ATPase and ATP-dependent Ca^{2+} uptake activity in synaptosomal membranes. Neurochem Res 8:1013, 1983.
9. Greenberg, DA: Calcium channels and calcium channel antagonists. Ann Neurol 21:317, 1987.

10. Greenberg, DA, Carpenter, CL, and Messing, RO: Ethanol-induced component of $^{45}Ca^{2+}$ uptake in PC12 cells is sensitive to Ca^{2+} channel modulating drugs. Brain Res 410:143, 1987.
11. Greenberg, DA and Messing, RO: Alcohol and the nervous system. In Aminoff, MJ (ed): Neurology and General Medicine. Churchill Livingstone, New York, 1989, p 533.
12. Harris, RA: Ethanol and pentobarbital inhibit intrasynaptosomal sequestration of calcium. Biochem Pharmacol 30:3209, 1981.
13. Harris, RA and Bruno, P: Membrane disordering by anesthetic drugs: Relationship to synaptosomal sodium and calcium fluxes. J Neurochem 44:1274, 1985.
14. Leslie, SW, et al: Inhibition of fast- and slow-phase depolarization-dependent synaptosomal calcium uptake by ethanol. J Pharmacol Exp Ther 225:571, 1983.
15. Little, HJ, Dolin, SJ, and Halsey MJ: Calcium channel antagonists decrease the ethanol withdrawal syndrome. Life Sci 39:2059, 1986.
16. Lynch, MA, Archer, ER, and Littleton, JM: Increased sensitivity of transmitter release to calcium in ethanol tolerance. Biochem Pharmacol 35:1207, 1986.
17. Lynch, MA and Littleton, JM: Possible association of alcohol tolerance with increased synaptic Ca^{2+} sensitivity. Nature 303:175, 1983.
18. Messing, RO, et al: Ethanol regulates Ca^{2+} channels in clonal neural cells. Proc Natl Acad Sci USA 83:6213, 1986.
19. Michaelis, ML, Michaelis, EK, and Tehan, T: Alcohol effects on synaptic membrane calcium ion fluxes. Pharmacol Biochem Behav 18:19, 1983.
20. Michaelis, ML, et al: Effects of chronic alcohol administration on synaptic membrane Na^+-Ca^{2+} exchange activity. Brain Res 414:239, 1987.
21. Oakes, SG and Pozos, RS: Electrophysiologic effects of acute ethanol exposure. II: Alterations in the calcium component of action potentials from sensory neurons in dissociated culture. Developmental Brain Research 5:251, 1982.
22. Rabe, CS and Weight, FF: Effects of ethanol on neurotransmitter release and intracellular free calcium in PC12 cells. J Pharmacol Exp Ther 244:417, 1988.
23. Seeman, P and Lee, T: The dopamine-releasing actions of neuroleptics and ethanol. J Pharmacol Exp Ther 190:131, 1974.
24. Skattebol, A and Rabin, RA: Effects of ethanol on $^{45}Ca^{2+}$ uptake in synaptosomes and in PC12 cells. Biochem Pharmacol 36:2227, 1987.
25. Yamamoto, H-A and Harris, RA: Calcium-dependent ^{86}Rb efflux and ethanol intoxication: Studies of human red blood cells and rodent brain synaptosomes. Eur J Pharmacol 88:357, 1983.
26. Yamamoto, H-A and Harris, RA: Effects of ethanol and barbiturates on Ca^{2+}-ATPase activity of erythrocyte and brain membranes. Biochem Pharmacol 32:2787, 1983.

Peter Carlen, M.D.
I. Rougier-Naquet, M.D.
J. N. Reynolds, Ph.D

CHAPTER 8

Alterations of Neuronal Calcium and Potassium Currents During Alcohol Administration and Withdrawal

Until now, alcohol-related seizures had not been studied electrophysiologically at the cellular level. In recent years, however, considerable interest has been shown in the ionic mechanisms associated with the acute and chronic administration of alcohol and other sedative/hypnotics.[4,8] Still, relatively little information is available concerning the electrophysiologic changes associated with ethanol withdrawal. Our group examined the acute and chronic effects of ethanol in *in vitro* rat hippocampal neurons. The hippocampus is a well-recognized area of epileptogenesis, and its organized structure makes it a model system useful in characterizing the electrophysiologic manifestations of several types of epilepsy.

We will review the ionic mechanisms of ethanol withdrawal as measured by intracellular current and voltage-clamp recordings in hippocampal neurons. Then we will describe the acute cellular electrophysiologic effects of ethanol and compare them with the phenomena resulting from chronic ethanol administration and withdrawal. Finally, we will compare these data with data on the acute and withdrawal effects of other sedative/hypnotic drugs.

Our working hypothesis is that in hippocampal neurons, acutely applied sedative doses of ethanol increases free cytosolic Ca^{2+} levels, resulting in augmented Ca^{2+}-activated K^+ conductance (gK_{Ca}) and diminished voltage-dependent inward Ca^{2+} currents. Decreasing inward depolarizing Ca^{2+} currents and increasing outward hyperpolarizing gK reduce neuronal excitability (Fig. 8–1). Chronic ethanol administration causes an underlying neuronal hyperexcitability that may be due to compensatory changes in voltage-dependent inward Ca^{2+} currents and gK_{Ca}. When ethanol is withdrawn, the decreased gK_{Ca} effect is "unmasked," voltage-dependent Ca^{2+} currents increase, and neuronal hyperexcitability ensues. This effect could be enhanced if the coupling between transiently increased intracellular Ca^{2+} and gK is also diminished during the early withdrawal phase.

METHODS OF RECORDING ELECTROPHYSIOLOGIC DATA FROM BRAIN SLICES

Because additional information is available elsewhere,[2,5] we will highlight only

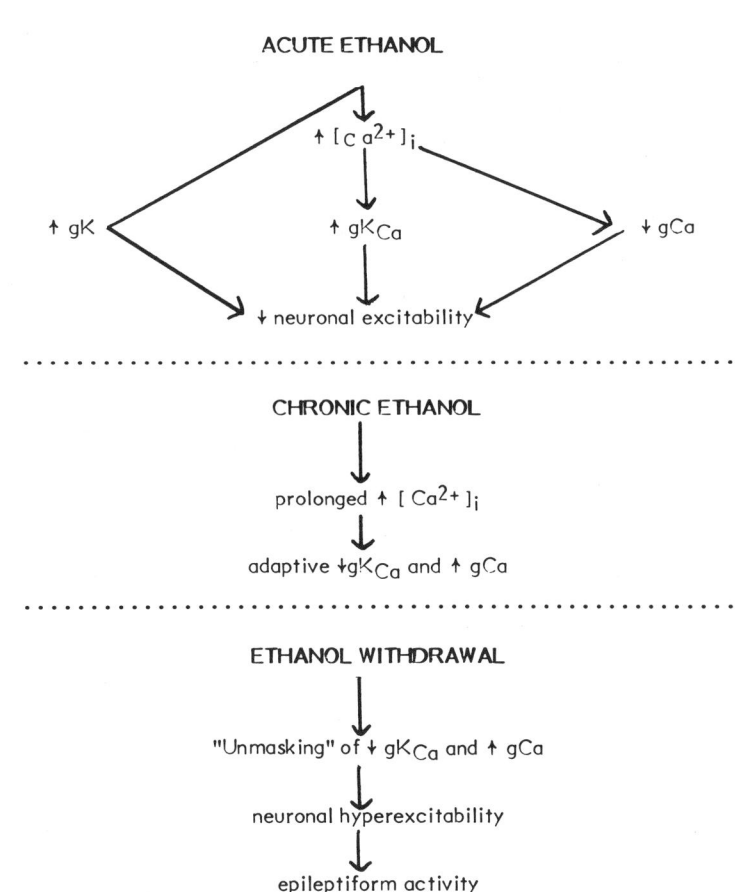

Figure 8-1. Hypothesis of mechanisms of acute, chronic, and withdrawal effects of ethanol on central mammalian neurons.

```
                        ACUTE ETHANOL
                              │
                              ▼
                         ↑ [Ca²⁺]ᵢ
                       ╱     │     ╲
                      ▼      ▼      ▼
                    ↑ gK   ↑ gK_Ca  ↓ gCa
                       ╲     │     ╱
                        ▼    ▼    ▼
                      ↓ neuronal excitability

                       CHRONIC ETHANOL
                              │
                              ▼
                    prolonged ↑ [Ca²⁺]ᵢ
                              │
                              ▼
                  adaptive ↓gK_Ca and ↑ gCa

                      ETHANOL WITHDRAWAL
                              │
                              ▼
              "Unmasking" of ↓ gK_Ca and ↑ gCa
                              │
                              ▼
                    neuronal hyperexcitability
                              │
                              ▼
                      epileptiform activity
```

important details of our electrophysiologic recording methods.

Preparation of Hippocampal Slices

Adult rats (usually male Wistar), weighing 150 to 200 g, were anesthetized with halothane and then decapitated. Brains were quickly removed and placed into ice-cold artificial cerebrospinal fluid (ACSF). Transverse slices (400 μm) of the hippocampus were cut (Fig. 8-2D) with a tissue chopper (earlier experiments) or with a vibratome, and maintained at 30°C in ACSF containing (in mM): Na⁺, 150; K⁺, 4.25; Ca²⁺, 2; Mg²⁺, 2; Cl⁻, 131; HCO₃, 26; H₂PO₄, 1.25; SO₄⁻², 2; dextrose 10, and at pH 7.4 when equilibrated with 95 percent O₂/5 percent CO₂. For voltage-clamp recordings, the slices were perfused with an ACSF containing K⁺ and Na⁺ channel blockers as follows (in mM): tetrodotoxin (TTX) 0.5 or 1×10^{-3}; tetraethylammonium (TEA) 10; 4-aminopyridine 5; CsCl₃. Also, the Na⁺ was reduced to 140 mM, Cl⁻ was substituted for SO₄⁻² and H₂PO₄, and Ca²⁺ was increased to 4 mM.

Electrophysiologic Recordings

For recordings, slices were transferred to an interface-type recording chamber where oxygenated ACSF perfused the slice at a rate of 0.8 to 1 ml/minute. Intracellular recordings were made with glass microelectrodes filled with 3M KCl (resistances of 60–120 megohms) or 3M K acetate (resistances of 80–150 megohms) for current-clamp recordings, and 3M CsCl (resistances of 50–90 megohms) for voltage-clamp recordings. Orthodromic excitatory postsynaptic potentials (EPSPs) and inhibitory postsynaptic potentials (IPSPs)

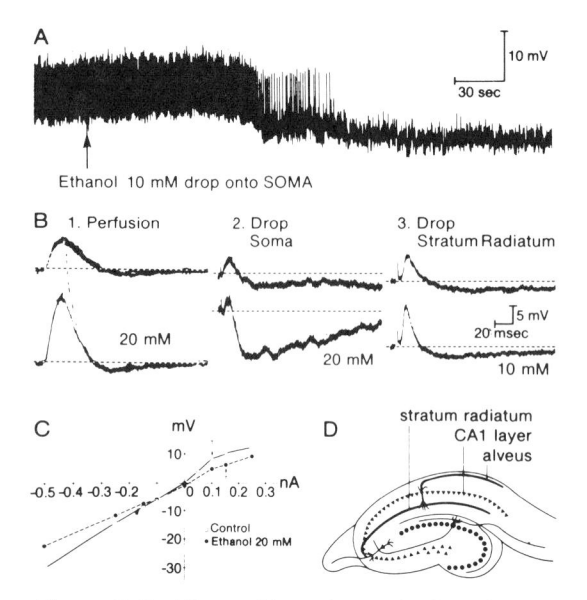

Figure 8–2. Effects of low doses of ethanol measured intracellularly in CA1 cells of a hippocampal slice preparation. (A) Spontaneous activity and resting membrane potential obtained with a potassium acetate electrode were monitored on a DC chart recorder. Approximately 1.5 min after focal application of a drop containing 10 mM ethanol onto the somatic region of the CA1 cell, the cell hyperpolarized; this was followed by cessation of the spontaneous spiking. Spike heights were attenuated by the chart recorder. (B) An EPSP-IPSP sequence elicited by stratum radiatum stimulation. (1) Bath perfusion of 20 mM ethanol caused increased EPSP and IPSP. The stimulation for both records was 18 µA. The EPSP sometimes reached threshold causing the neuron to fire (lower trace). (2) Drop application of ethanol (20 mM) onto the somatic area greatly enhanced IPSP 5 min after ethanol application. (3) Ethanol (10 mM) focally applied to the stratum radiatum increased the EPSP 2 min after ethanol application. Stimulation currents for (2) and (3) were 22 and 100 µA, respectively. (C) Injected current plotted against the peak voltage response. Cell input resistance (R$_{in}$) was decreased after ethanol exposure; R$_{in}$ was measured in all cells with 100-msec constant-current pulses injected by an active bridge amplifier. With no injected current, the ethanol plot crosses the y-axis at −1 mV, reflecting the degree of resting membrane hyperpolarization seen 5 min after ethanol exposure in this cell.

Control R$_{in}$ was 60 megohms, reduced with ethanol perfusion to 44 megohms. (D) Diagram of the hippocampal slice preparation. The stratum radiatum contains excitatory afferents to the apical dendrites of CA1 cells. (From Carlen, et al,[5] p 307, with permission.)

were generated by low-intensity stimulation of Schaffer collaterals or perforant pathways to elicit responses in CA1 or dentate granule (DG) neurons respectively, using monopolar tungsten stimulating electrodes. Long-lasting postspike train afterhyperpolarizations (AHPs) were elicited by injecting depolarizing current pulses through the recording electrode into the neuron (0.1–0.6 nA, 100 ms) of sufficient intensity to activate a train of 3 to 5 action potentials. Only AHPs following the same number of spikes were compared.

Voltate-clamp recordings were obtained using an Axoclamp IIa amplifier. The gain was maximal and compatible with stability (2.5–4), and the sampling rate was 5 to 6 K Hz. Capacity compensation was continuously monitored on an oscilloscope.

RESULTS

Acute Ethanol Administration

Twenty mM ethanol, which is a moderately intoxicating concentration near the "legal limit" in many jurisdictions, inhibited hippocampal CA1 and DG neurons.[5,23] We had measured similar effects in CA1 neurons at concentrations ranging from 5 to 100 mM, although most experiments were done with 20 mM. The acute electrophysiologic actions of ethanol are detailed below.

Membrane hyperpolarization of 0.5 to 10 mV (Fig. 8–2A) occurred within 2–3 minutes of ethanol application in about 80% of neurons tested. This hyperpolarization was associated with decreased input resistance (Fig. 8–2C) in about 75% of CA1 neurons but not in DG neurons. This effect occurred in the presence of TTX, and in low-Ca^{2+}, high-Mg^{2+} perfusate, both of which block nerve-evoked synaptic transmission.

In both neuronal types, EPSPs and IPSPs (Fig. 8–2B) increased in the presence of ethanol, suggesting enhanced nerve-evoked presynaptic transmitter release by ethanol, a well-known effect at the neuromuscular junction with higher anesthetic doses.

The long-lasting postspike train AHP is

Figure 8–3. Augmentation of AHPs by ethanol. (A) (1) Postspike train AHP is shown in control medium following a 0.35-nA, 100-msec constant-current pulse. Spikes were retouched and full heights (not shown) were 80 mV. (2) TTX (2×10^{-5} M) was applied in large drops to the stratum radiatum, pyramidale, and oriens, blocking fast Na^+ spikes. A higher depolarizing current injection (3.5 nA) elicited a Ca^{2+} spike followed by an AHP that was probably mediated by increased K^+ conductance. (3) 3 min after drop application of 10 mM ethanol to the soma, the AHP (at 3.5 nA) was increased, but the Ca^{2+} spike was slightly decreased. Bridge balance was not corrected after ethanol application. (B) Increases in depth and length of AHP after drop application of 10 mM ethanol to the soma in control solution. The current pulse for control and ethanol measurements was 0.75 nA, and each pulse caused four spikes. A chart recorder was used for (B) and (C), and depolarizing responses to 100-msec current pulses were cut off because of high gain. (C) In the presence of TTX, the AHP following the Ca^{2+} spike increased in depth and was markedly prolonged after drop application of 20 mM ethanol to the soma. A 1.0 nA constant-current depolarizing pulse was used. (From Carlen, et al,[5] p. 308, with permission.)

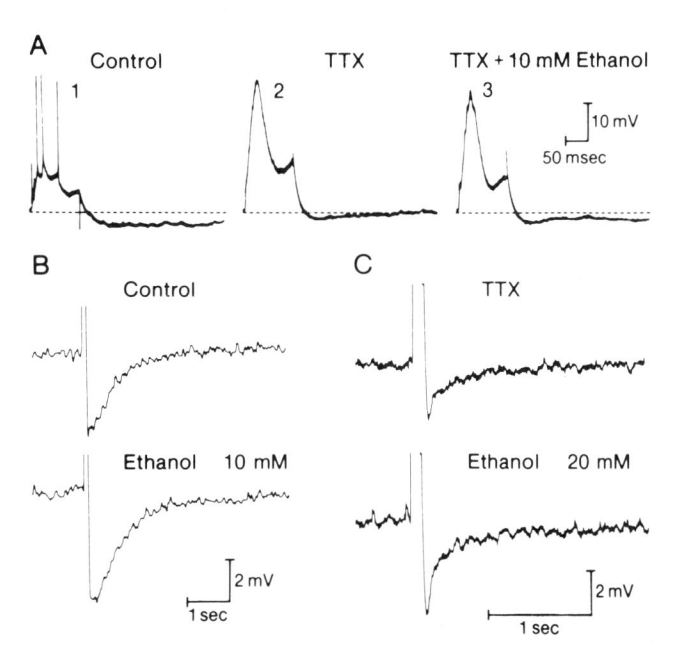

an ubiquitous, powerful, intrinsic inhibitory neuronal mechanism, thought to be caused by a spike-evoked, voltage-dependent inward flux of Ca^{2+} ions that activate a gK.[15,16] The AHPs were consistently increased in both amplitude and duration by acute ethanol application (Fig. 8–3).

In the presence of TTX, Ca^{2+} spikes were elicited in CA1 neurons. They were unaffected or slightly depressed by ethanol (Fig. 8–3A). Focally applied gamma-aminobutyric acid (GABA) responses in CA1, DG, and layer V parietal cortex neurons were not enhanced by ethanol.

These data led us to speculate that acute ethanol actions could be mediated by increased intracellular Ca^{2+} levels. Because the ethanol-mediated hyperpolarization occurred in the presence of low or zero extracellular Ca^{2+} and high Mg^{2+} or Mn^{2+} concentrations, and Ca^{2+} spikes were not enhanced,[5] the increased intracellular Ca^{2+} concentration could come from intracellular stores (e.g., mitochondria or endoplasmic reticulum) through release of Ca^{2+} or by blocking of a Ca^{2+} extrusion mechanism. These data do not exclude the possibility that ethanol has a direct effect on gK. Because there was little if any shunt associated with the hyperpolarization in DG neurons, a neurogenic pump might be involved in this case.

To further characterize ethanol's effects on neuronal Ca^{2+} currents, single-electrode voltage-clamp recordings of the relatively electrotonically compact DG neurons were performed. These experiments were done using K^+ and Na^+ channel blockers and lower temperature both to minimize non-Ca^{2+} conductances and to improve the quality of the space clamp. It is known that in many neuronal preparations Ca^{2+} currents are partly inactivated by intracellular Ca^{2+}.[14] Hence, we predicted that ethanol, if it does raise intracellular Ca^{2+}, could decrease Ca^{2+} currents. We found three different types of voltage-dependent Ca^{2+} currents in voltage-clamped DG neurons: a transient low-threshold (TLT) current (e.g. Fig. 8–8, upper left trace), a large transient high-threshold (THT) current (Fig. 8–4) activated only from a hyperpolarized holding potential (V_H) and probably localized in

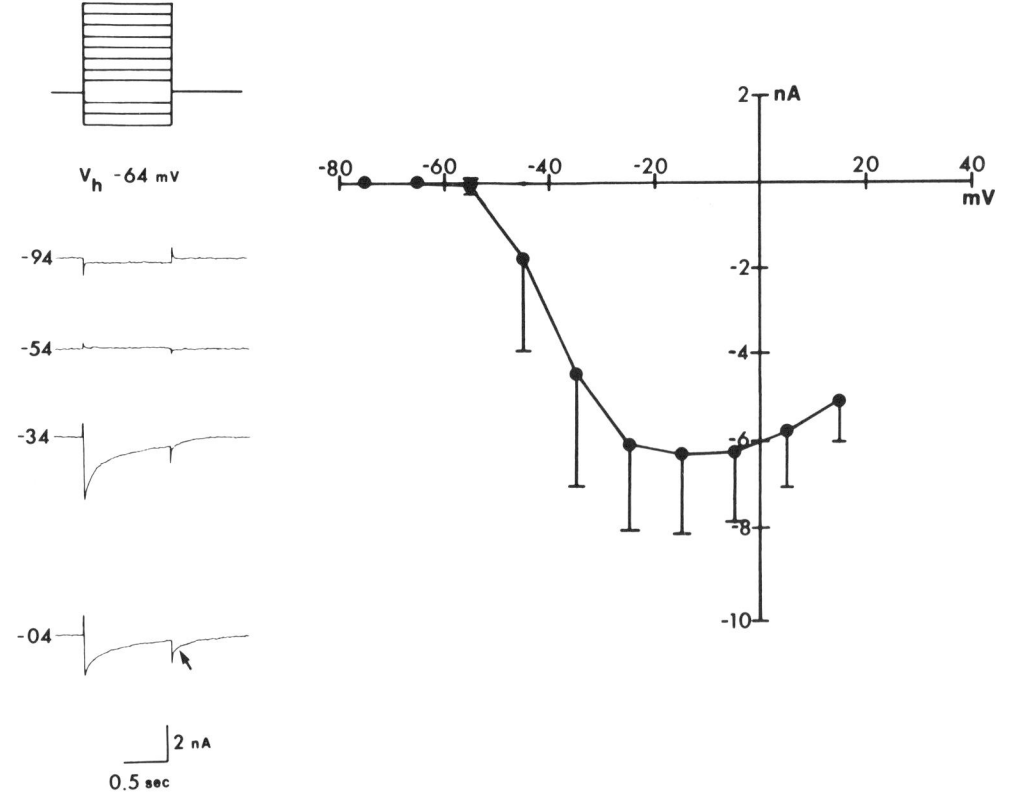

Figure 8–4. Rapidly inactivating high threshold (THT) Ca^{2+} current in dentate gyrus granule neurons. An example of current responses to hyperpolarizing and depolarizing voltage steps in a granule neuron using a CsCl electrode is shown on the left. The holding potential (V$_h$) was −64 mV, and the command potential is shown at the left of each current response. The arrow indicates the inward tail current which follows the THT current. A cumulative plot of the peak inward current (leak-corrected) against command potential is plotted on the right for 15 dentate gyrus granule neurons (mean ± SD) recorded using CsCl electrodes. Note that the peak of the inward current occurs at command potentials of around −15 mV.

the dendrites, and a sustained high-threshold (SHT) current probably localized in the perisomatic region and most easily activated from a depolarized V$_H$ (Fig. 8–5).[7,23] The SHT current is blocked by dihydropyridine (DHP) calcium antagonists (e.g., nimodipine).

Following perfusion of 20 mM ethanol, there was a slight to moderate decrease in the amplitude of the TLT current in 3 of 9 neurons. Otherwise, the TLT current was unaffected by ethanol. In 15 of 17 neurons, the THT current was depressed by ethanol; in 6 of these 17 cells, there was a concomitant decrease in the following tail current. In 13 of 14 neurons, the SHT was diminished. The holding current was slightly increased by ethanol for the hyperpolarized V$_H$ in 6 neurons, and for the depolarized V$_H$ in 4 neurons. The leak conductance was usually unchanged by acute ethanol administration. GABA-mediated Cl$^-$ conductance was not increased by ethanol in 3 voltage-clamped neurons.

Chronic Ethanol Administration

As a model for chronic alcohol-induced brain damage and dysfunction, rats were fed a liquid diet containing ethanol for 5 months. The diet was then discontinued for 3 weeks.[13] Hippocampal slices were prepared from these animals and from pair-fed controls. Of the many electrophysiologic parameters measured, the only significant differences in the ethanol-treated group compared with the control

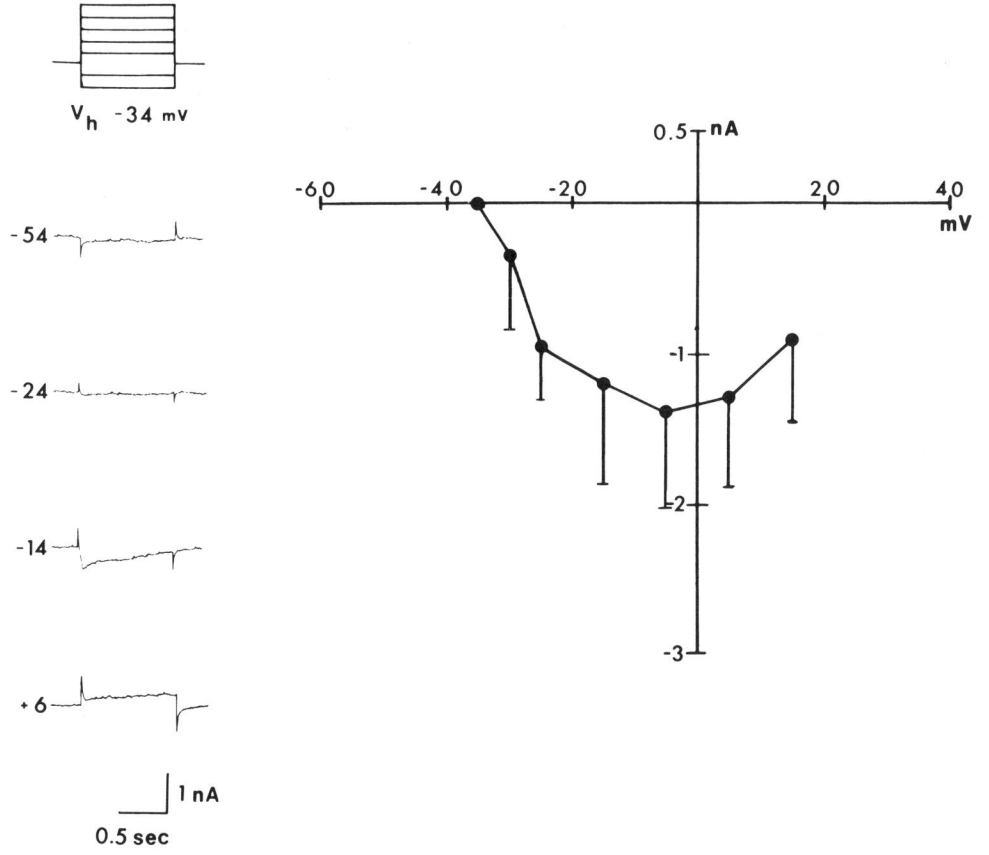

Figure 8–5. Slowly inactivating high threshold (SHT) Ca^{2+} current in dentate gyrus granule neurons. On the left side, an example of current responses to hyperpolarizing and depolarizing voltage steps in a granule neuron recorded using a CsCl electrode is shown. The holding potential (V_h) was -34 mV, and the command potential is shown at the left of each current response. On the right side, a cumulative plot of the peak inward current (leak-corrected) against command potential for 16 dentate gyrus granule neurons (mean ± SD) using CsCl electrodes is shown. Note that the peak of the inward current occurs at command potentials of around -5 mV.

group were diminished IPSPs and AHPs in both DG and CA1 neurons.

Ethanol Withdrawal

Two types of ethanol-withdrawal experiments were performed: *in vivo* administration of ethanol and *in vitro* exposure to ethanol of hippocampal slices from a drug-naive animal.[26] Both experiments demonstrated neuronal hyperexcitability consequent to ethanol withdrawal.

IN VIVO ETHANOL ADMINISTRATION

Ethanol was administered by gastric intubation to 12 Wistar rats every 8 hours for 3 days, with an initial dose of 8 g/kg and subsequent doses determined by their pre-dose level of intoxication (ambulatory, 3g/kg; nonambulatory but conscious, 1.5 g/kg; unconscious, no ethanol). A second group of 12 animals received a sucrose solution by gastric intubation. The ethanol-treated animals all demonstrated an exaggerated startle response and tremulousness within 3 days. Twelve hours after the last dose, hippocampal slices were prepared and extra- and intracellular recordings were performed in the CA1 region. The perfusate contained no ethanol.

In slices from ethanol-treated animals, extracellular recordings showed increased

SPONTANEOUS ACTIVITY FROM ETHANOL TREATED ANIMALS

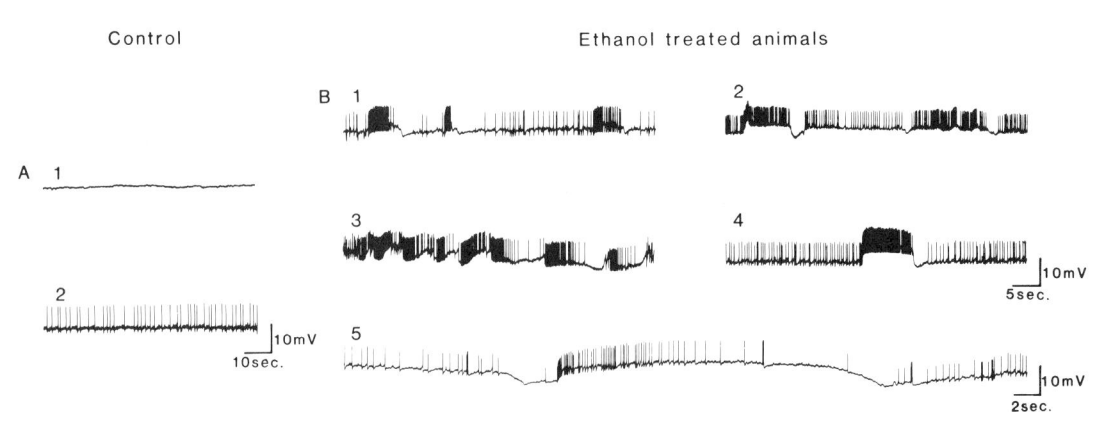

Figure 8–6. Spontaneous activity from ethanol-treated animals. (A) Type of spontaneous activity noted in control slices. Usually there was no firing (A1), but occasional spikes were noted (A2). (B) Various forms of neuronal hyperactivity noted in slices from ethanol-treated animals.

excitability with multiple evoked population spikes and some spontaneous bursts of population spikes. Slices from sucrose-treated animals showed no such activity. Intracellular recordings from neurons of animals withdrawn from ethanol showed significantly increased spontaneous spiking activity (Fig. 8–6). Paroxysmal depolarization shifts of 8 to 20 mV were noted in 19 of 33 neurons. None of this type of activity was noted in neurons from the sucrose-treated animals. The ethanol-with-

1. Afterhyperpolarization
2. Accommodation

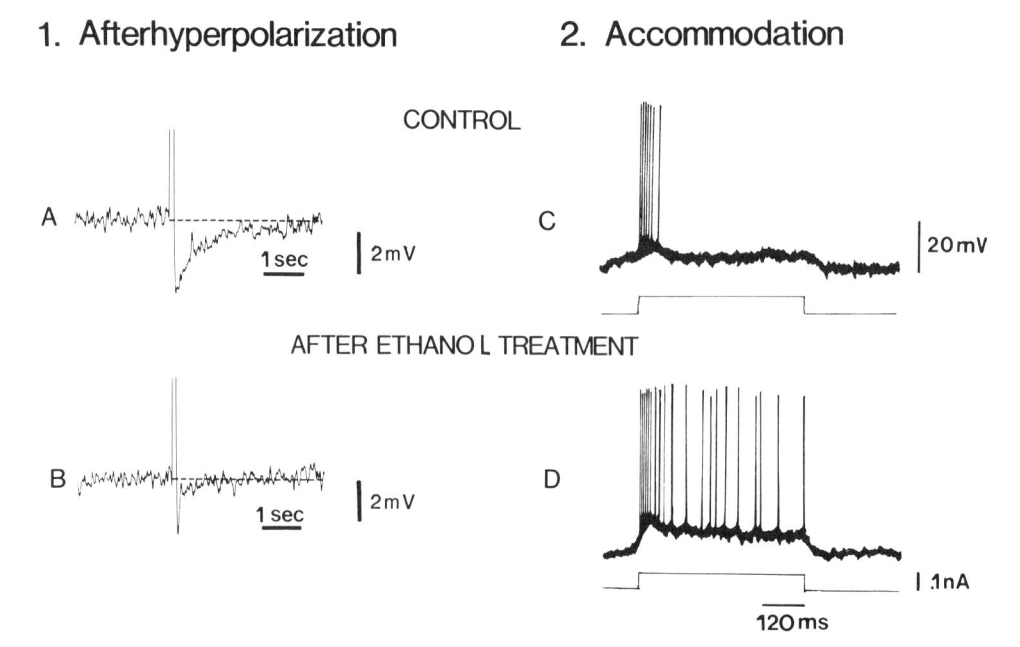

CONTROL

AFTER ETHANOL TREATMENT

Figure 8–7. AHPs (1) and spike frequency accommodation (adaptation) (2) are diminished in neurons from a rat intubated with ethanol for 3 days. In these neurons, current injection of 0.1nA and 100 ms evoked 4 spikes follow by an AHP (A and B). Accommodation was measured during a 0.1nA, 600 ms pulse.

Figure 8–8. Ethanol withdrawal enhances the THT current in a dentate granule neuron from a drug-naive animal which was bathed in 100 mM ethanol for 6 hr prior to recording. The holding potential (V_h) was −72mV and at the bottom of each vertical panel is the depolarizing voltage step command. Note in the left panel that only the TLT current is visible when the neuron was still bathed in 100 mM ethanol. After 15 min of perfusion in ethanol-free solution (withdrawal, 15 min), a THT current apparently overshadows the TLT current. Ethanol withdrawal had reduced the threshold for the THT current and also widened and deepened the THT current triggered from +30 and +60 mV voltage steps. These Ca^{2+} current enhancing effects of ethanol withdrawal were reversed within 10 min of re-adding 100 mM ethanol to the perfusate (bottom panel).

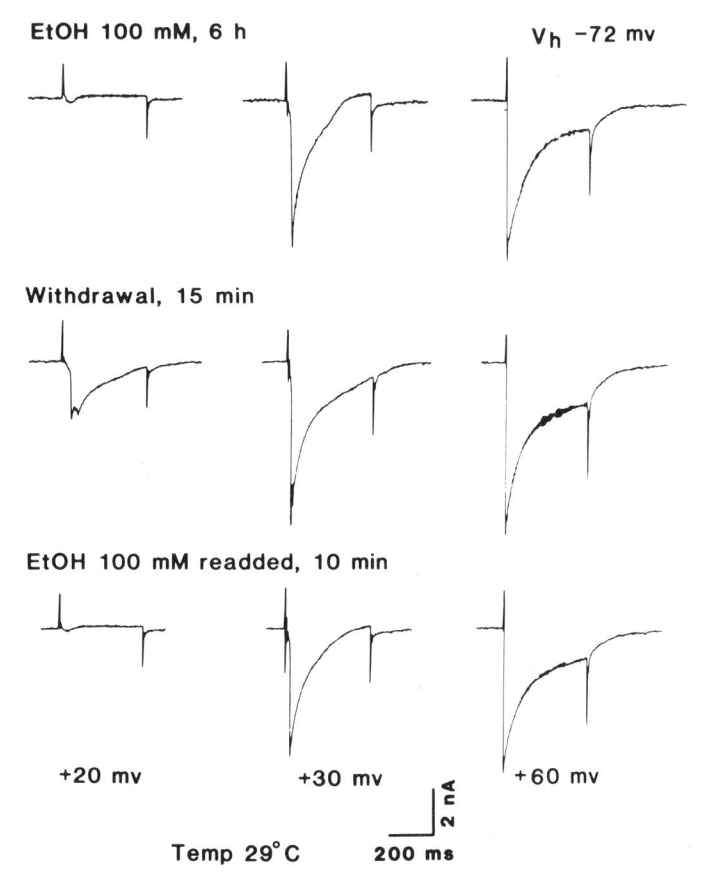

drawn neurons also had smaller postspike train AHPs, decreased spike frequency adaptation to a 600-ms depolarizing constant current pulse (Fig. 8–7), and decreased IPSPs without any significant change in the EPSPs.

IN VITRO ETHANOL ADMINISTRATION

Hippocampal slices from drug-naive rats were incubated in 100 mM ethanol for 2 to 3 hours. When the perfusate was changed to an ethanol-free solution, findings of neuronal hyperexcitability similar to those described above developed within 10 to 15 minutes. Findings included increased evoked and spontaneous population spikes, increased spontaneous spiking with membrane depolarization and sometimes bursting behavior, smaller AHPs and IPSPs, and decreased spike frequency adaptation. Using the same *in vitro* experimental paradigm, slices were bathed for 2 or more hours in 100 mM ethanol, and subsequently used for voltage-clamp recordings of Ca^{2+} currents in DG neurons. These recordings were performed at 29 to 35°C in 11 neurons that had undergone *in vitro* ethanol withdrawal. The threshold for the THT current decreased in 7 of 11 neurons and the amplitude or width of the THT current increased in every neuron (Fig. 8–8). The SHT current also increased upon alcohol withdrawal in 4 of 5 neurons. Re-adding 100 mM ethanol in 4 neurons caused depression of the Ca^{2+} currents that were enhanced upon ethanol withdrawal.

DISCUSSION

These data suggest that K^+ and Ca^{2+} conductances may play major roles in the acute and chronic neuronal effects of ethanol.[8] Acute ethanol application enhanced IPSPs and AHPs. IPSPs are mediated in part by increased gK.[27] AHPs are mediated entirely by increased gK.[15,16] Although the ethanol-induced hyperpolarization could be due to increased gK, this possibility is less likely in DG neurons, where no associated decrease in input resistance (R_{in}) (or increased conductance) was noted. The increase in EPSPs and IPSPs could also be due to increased presynaptic transmitter release. Increased intracellular Ca^{2+} or increased sensitivity to ambient intracellular Ca^{2+} could explain in part the ethanol-induced augmentation of gK-dependent events and the possibly increased presynaptic transmitter release. Although ethanol has been postulated to work through GABAergic mechanisms,[21] we were unable to demonstrate any ethanol enhancement of the neuronal response to focally applied GABA. In CA1 neurons, the GABA response is complicated, involving increases in gK and gCl.[2]

Elevated levels of intracellular Ca^{2+} were first postulated[5] and then shown to result from acute ethanol administration,[9,25] possibly from inhibition of the Na^+/Ca^{2+} membrane exchange mechanism.[19] Elevated levels of intracellular Ca^{2+} also inactivated voltage-dependent Ca^{2+} current in many different neurons.[14,17] Low concentrations (20 mM) of ethanol also diminished voltage-dependent Ca^{2+} currents in hippocampal DG neurons. Other sedative/hypnotics enhanced gK in pharmacologically relevant doses.[4,8] Pentobarbital (1–100 μM) acted similarly to ethanol by increasing AHPs and IPSPs, hyperpolarizing the neuron, and decreasing Ca^{2+} spikes.[24] Midazolam (5 nM), a water-soluble benzodiazepine, had the same actions as ethanol and pentobarbital in CA1 neurons, except that it required extracellular Ca^{2+} to cause a hyperpolarization, and it caused enhanced Ca^{2+} spikes.[6]

In the animal model where hippocampal slices were prepared following 5 months of ethanol administration and 3 weeks withdrawal,[13] it was assumed that the acute hyperexcitable withdrawal phase was completed and a more stable state of alcohol-induced brain damage was present. AHPs and IPSPs were diminished in this model.[13] One possible explanation for the AHP data is that intracellular Ca^{2+} levels chronically elevated by prolonged ethanol exposure could diminish (inactivate) the inward Ca^{2+} flux associated with the train of spikes preceding the AHP. Another possibility is that coupling between increased intracellular free Ca^{2+} and the AHP was diminished. It is generally thought that the increased gK associated with the IPSP in these neurons is probably not Ca^{2+} dependent.[28] Finally, chronic ethanol treatment could interfere directly with gK mechanisms rather than indirectly via Ca^{2+}.

The *in vivo* and *in vitro* ethanol withdrawal-induced neuronal hyperexcitability raised other interesting issues. First, the epileptiform activity in hippocampal slices removed from ethanol-treated animals provided a relevant model for studying alcohol withdrawal seizures (AWS) and demonstrated that the electrophysiologic correlates of epilepsy were present and maintained in a small piece of central nervous system (CNS) tissue. Even more convenient is the model of ethanol withdrawal epilepsy induced *in vitro*. We have not yet examined what concentrations of ethanol are necessary or sufficient to create withdrawal epilepsy in slices removed from drug-naive animals. Second, unlike the acute effects of ethanol, the effects of ethanol withdrawal appears to include decreased gK and enhanced Ca^{2+} currents. The smaller AHPs and IPSPs were compatible with decreased gK. The decreased spike frequency accommodation was also related to diminished gK. THT and SHT Ca^{2+} currents were augmented upon alcohol withdrawal. Furthermore, DHP-sensitive Ca^{2+} channel activity is increased in ethanol-exposed rats exhibiting physical dependence and hyperexcitability.[12] In contrast, [^{3}H]nitrendipine binding was reduced in neocortical membranes of animals fed lower doses of ethanol and not exhibiting overt signs of drug withdrawal.[1]

One might also attribute the ethanol-withdrawal-induced neuronal hyperactivity and increased Ca^{2+} currents to altered intracellular homeostasis. Michaelis and associates[18] showed that the Na^+/Ca^{2+} membrane antiporter was significantly increased in the fraction enriched in functional synaptic complexes after 3 weeks of ethanol diet. If this antiporter became even more active during acute ethanol withdrawal, then intracellular Ca^{2+} levels could drop, resulting in decreased Ca^{2+}-dependent inactivation of these neuronal Ca^{2+} currents. Both decreased gK and increased Ca^{2+} currents depolarized the neuron and caused hyperexcitability. Decreased IPSPs are associated with epileptiform activity in both in vitro and in vivo models of epilepsy.[27] The underlying biochemical mechanisms for these ionic conductance changes in alcohol withdrawal are yet to be identified.

Although sedative and anti-epileptic drug withdrawal epilepsy are clinically well-recognized events, there is a remarkable paucity of biochemical and electrophysiologic data concerning the pathogenesis of these common problems. We have demonstrated similar epileptiform activity in hippocampal slices removed from rats fed high doses (50 mg/kg/day) of the anticonvulsant clonazepam for 4 weeks.[11] In a parallel series of experiments using EEG electrodes in rats, Naquet and associates[20] demonstrated that within 1 week of initiating clonazepam feeding, abnormal EEG activity was apparent. Eight of 20 rats later showed sporadic epileptiform discharges. When the benzodiazepine blocker CGS 8216 was given intraperitoneally (25 mg/kg) to 7 animals fed clonazepam for 4 weeks, overt epileptiform activity quickly became apparent both in the EEG and behaviorally. After 4 weeks, the clonazepam feedings were abruptly discontinued. Within 12 hours of withdrawal, epileptiform activity was apparent in the EEG of all animals. This abnormal activity persisted up to 2 weeks. Finally, when a hippocampal slice from a drug-naive rat was bathed in a 20 nM clonazepam solution for over 2 hours and then exposed to drug-free perfusate, epileptiform activity became apparent. This activity was also associated with decreased gK (i.e., fewer AHPs),[10] and is consistent with our in vitro AWS model.

Brailowsky and associates[3] showed that chronic (6 hours–14 days) localized application of GABA, the inhibitory neurotransmitter, into the somatosensory cortex of rats caused, upon withdrawal, the development of focal epileptogenic activity localized to the infused site. These data suggest that many inhibitory substances or influences, when applied chronically, can cause a neuronal hyperexcitable state upon withdrawal. In order to elucidate the pathophysiology of alcohol withdrawal epilepsy, more research is necessary, particularly on the time and dose of alcohol required, regional susceptibility in the CNS, neurochemical (including second messenger) processes affected by alcohol withdrawal, the role of excitotoxic amino acids, neuropeptide, and neurotransmitter interactions, membrane biophysical changes, and the details of the relevant ionic events.

SUMMARY

To better understand the effects of ethanol withdrawal, we first studied the acute effects of ethanol. Electrophysiologic experiments were performed on adult rat hippocampal slices. Ethanol, perfused in concentrations ranging from 5 to 100 mM (mainly 20 mM), caused in dentate granule (DG) and CA1 neurons a hyperpolarization and an augmented postspike train long-lasting AHP thought to be due to a Ca^{2+}-activated gK. The ethanol-induced hyperpolarization persisted in a low-Ca^{2+}, high-Mg^{2+} perfusate. Ethanol also increased IPSPs, but Ca^{2+} spikes were unaffected or depressed. Single-electrode voltage-clamp recordings of Ca^{2+} currents in DG neurons at 23°C showed that 20 mM ethanol depressed these currents. These data suggest that acute ethanol administration could increase intracellular Ca^{2+} concentration.

Ethanol withdrawal was studied using two experimental paradigms. Adult rats received oral doses of ethanol for 3 days and were allowed to withdraw for 12 hours. In a separate set of experiments, hippocampal slices from drug-naive animals were exposed to 100 mM ethanol in vitro for over 2 hours, and ethanol was withdrawn during electrophysiologic recording. In both cases, extracellular recordings from the CA1 region showed epileptiform phenomena including evoked and spontaneous multiple population spikes. Intracellular recordings from CA1 neurons showed decreased AHPs and IPSPs, and impaired spike frequency adaptation. Increased spontaneous spiking and membrane depolarizations were also noted during ethanol withdrawal. When voltage-clamped Ca^{2+} currents were examined in DG neurons exposed to 100 mM ethanol for more than 2 hours *in vitro* at 29 to 33°C, it was found that ethanol withdrawal was accompanied by enhanced amplitude and decreased threshold of voltage-dependent Ca^{2+} currents. These results are compatible with evidence of decreased neuronal gK and increased Ca^{2+} currents during the hyperexcitable state associated with ethanol withdrawal.

ACKNOWLEDGMENTS

Supported by the Alcoholic Beverages Medical Research Foundation and the MRC. Manuscript prepared by Yvonne Bedford.

References

1. Bergamaschi, A, Govoni, S, and Trabucchi, M: Alcohol and calcium interactions at the CNS level: An in vivo study. Pharmacol Res Comm 19:975, 1987.
2. Blaxter, TJ, et al: Hyperpolarizing response to γ-aminobutyric acid in rat hippocampal pyramidal cells is mediated by a calcium-dependent potassium conductance. J Physiol 373:181, 1986.
3. Brailowsky, S, et al: The GABA-withdrawal syndrome: A new model of focal epileptogenesis. Brain Res 442:175, 1988.
4. Carlen, PL, et al: Enhanced neuronal K^+ conductance: Possible common mechanism for CNS depressant drugs. Can J Physiol Pharmacol 63:831, 1985.
5. Carlen, PL, Gurevich, N, and Durand, D: Ethanol in low doses augments calcium-mediated mechanisms measured intracellularly in hippocampal neurons. Science 215:306, 1982.
6. Carlen, PL, Gurevich, N, and Polc, P: Low-dose benzodiazepine neuronal inhibition: Enhanced Ca^{++}-mediated K^+ conductance. Brain Res 271:358, 1983.
7. Carlen, PL, Niesen, CE, and Blaxter, T: Calcium currents in voltage-clamped dentate granule neurons in vitro. Can J Physiol Pharmacol 65:vii, 1987.
8. Carlen, PL, and Wu, PH: Calcium and sedative-hypnotic drug actions. Internat Rev Neurobiol 29:161, 1988.
9. Davidson, M, Wilce, P, and Shanley I: Ethanol increases synaptosomal free calcium concentration. Neurosci Lett 89:165, 1988.
10. Davies, MF, Sasaki, SE, and Carlen, PL: Benzodiazepine-induced epileptiform activity in vitro. Brain Res 437:237, 1988.
11. Davies, MF, Sasaki, SE, and Carlen, PL: Hyperexcitability of hippocampal CA1 neurons in brain slices of rats chronically administered clonazepam. J Pharmacol Exp Ther (in press).
12. Dolin, A, et al: Increased dihydropyridine-sensitive calcium channels in rat brain may underlie ethanol physical dependence. Neuropharmacology 26:275, 1987.
13. Durand, D and Carlen, PL: Decreased neuronal inhibition in vitro after long-term ethanol administration. Science 224:1359, 1984.
14. Eckert, R and Chad, JE: Inactivation of Ca channels. Prog Biophys Mol Biol 44:215, 1984.
15. Gustafsson, B and Wigstrom, H: Evidence for two types of after hyperpolarizations in CA1 pyramidal cells in the hippocampus. Brain Res 206:462, 1981.
16. Hotson, JR and Prince, DA: A calcium-activated hyperpolarization follows repetitive firing in hippocampal neurons. J Neurophysiol 43:409, 1980.
17. Krnjevic, K and Lisiewicz, A: Injections of calcium ions into spinal motoneurones. J Physiol (London) 225:363, 1972.
18. Michaelis, ML, et al: Effects of chronic alcohol administration on synaptic membrane Na^+-Ca^{2+} exchange activity. Brain Res 414:239, 1987.
19. Michaelis, ML, Kitos, TE, and Tehran, T: Differential effects of ethanol on two synaptic membrane Ca^{2+} transport systems. Alcohol 2:129, 1985.
20. Naquet, IA, et al: EEG abnormalities including epileptiform activity in rats induced by chronic high dose clonazepam administration, withdrawal or benzodiazepine blocker administration. XX Canadian Congress of Neurological Sciences, 1985.
21. Nestoros, JN: Ethanol specifically potentiates GABA-mediated neurotransmission in feline cerebral cortex. Science 209:708, 1980.
22. Niesen, CE, Baskys, A, and Carlen, PL: Reversed ethanol effects on potassium conductances in aged hippocampal dentate granule neurons. Brain Res 445:137, 1988.
23. Niesen, CE, Blaster, TJ, and Carlen, PL: Electrophysiological, pharmacological and spatial separation of three calcium currents in rat dentate granule neurons. Soc Neurosci 13:103, 1987.
24. O'Beirne, M, Gurevich, N, and Carlen, PL: Pentobarbital inhibits hippocampal neurons by increasing potassium conductance. Can J Physiol Pharmacol 65:36, 1987.
25. Pozos, RS and Oakes, SG: The effects of ethanol on electrophysiology of calcium channels. In Galanter, M (ed): Recent Developments in Alcoholism, Vol 5. Plenum Press, New York, 1987, p 327.
26. Rougier-Naquet, IA, et al: Hyperexcitability of hippocampal CA1 neurons in slices from rats undergoing ethanol withdrawal or in slices following 2 hours exposure to ethanol. Soc Neurosci 12:52, 1986.
27. Taylor, CP: How do seizures begin: Clues from hippocampal slices. TINS 11:375, 1988.
28. Thalmann, RH and Ayala, GF: A late increase in potassium conductance follows synaptic stimulation of granule neurons of the dentate gyrus. Neurosci Lett 29:243, 1982.

CHAPTER 9

Ivan Diamond, M.D., Ph.D.
Daria Mochly-Rosen, Ph.D.
Adrienne S. Gordon, Ph.D.

Reduced Adenosine Receptor Activation in Alcoholism: Implications for Alcohol Withdrawal Seizures

Alcoholics who are physically dependent on alcohol experience a severe withdrawal syndrome when they stop drinking.[13] One of the most prominent features of this syndrome is the development of grand mal convulsions 24 to 48 hours after alcohol withdrawal. Although alcohol withdrawal seizures (AWS) are well known to physicians, the pathophysiology of this limited convulsive disorder is not well understood. Recent evidence suggests that the neuromodulator adenosine appears to mediate many effects of ethanol in the brain.[9–11,29] Moreover, adenosine is an endogenous anticonvulsant that causes inhibition of neuronal and motor activity.[1,2,4,14–17,23,26–28,36,37,40] There are several types of adenosine receptors,[8,17,40] and Phillis and Barroco[26] have presented evidence that the inhibitory effects of adenosine may be mediated primarily through the A_2 adenosine receptor. In this chapter we suggest that desensitization of A_2 adenosine-receptor-dependent cyclic adenosine monophosphate (cAMP) production in alcoholics could play a role in generating AWS.

ETHANOL AND NEURAL CELLS IN CULTURE

Studies with neural cells in culture have provided many new insights into the regulation of neuronal excitability under precisely controlled conditions. Moreover, the use of intact cells makes it possible to avoid cellular disruption and loss of important cofactors and metabolites, problems that limit studies with most brain preparations. Richelson's laboratory was among the first to use neural cells in culture to examine the effects of ethanol on the cAMP signal transduction system.[42] In this system, activated neurotransmitter receptors are coupled to stimulation of adenylyl cyclase via G_s a GTP-binding protein. It is now clear that relatively low concentrations of ethanol added to intact cells stimulate receptor-dependent cAMP production.[19,20,25,42]

ADENOSINE-RECEPTOR-DEPENDENT cAMP PRODUCTION IN NEURAL CELLS

Most cells in culture, including NG108-15 neuroblastoma x glioma hybrid cells, express only the A_2 receptor and not the A_1 receptor. Figure 9–1 shows that A_2-adenosine-receptor-dependent cAMP production in NG108-15 cells is stimulated by acute exposure to ethanol. cAMP levels increase in proportion to concentration and chain length of the alcohol.[19] Thus, the effect of ethanol on receptor-stimulated cAMP production is not an artifact

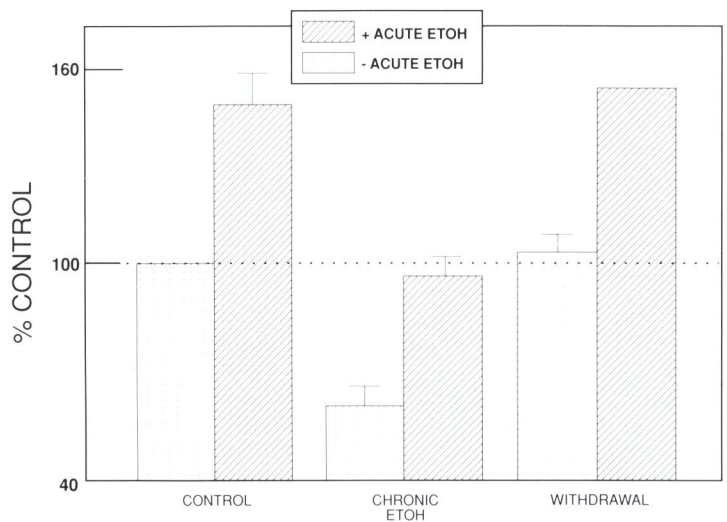

Figure 9–1. Ethanol-induced changes in adenosine receptor-dependent cAMP levels in NG108-15 cells. Cells were grown without (CONTROL) or with 200 mM ethanol (CHRONIC ETOH) for 48 hr (n = 9). All cells were treated with phenylisopropyladenosine (PIA) to activate adenosine receptors and assayed in triplicate for cAMP levels in the absence (open bars) or presence (shaded bars) of 200 mM ethanol. In a separate experiment, cells were grown with 100 mM ethanol for 48 hr and kept without ethanol for an additional 48 hr (WITHDRAWAL). cAMP levels were assayed in the absence (n = 5) or presence (n = 2) of 100 mM ethanol. Each bar represents the mean ± SEM.

of changes in osmolarity, but is more directly related to the solubility of the alcohol in the lipid membrane. In addition, acetaldehyde has no effect on cAMP levels, consistent with the observation that neuronal cells have only negligible amounts of alcohol dehydrogenase,[3] and that the acute toxic effect of ethanol in the nervous system appears to be caused by alcohol and not by its metabolic products.

Goldstein and Goldstein[18] proposed that physical dependence develops as a cell or organism makes homeostatic adjustments that compensate for the primary effects of a drug. Therefore, it may be anticipated that NG108-15 cells chronically exposed to ethanol would adapt to the continued presence of the alcohol by reducing endogenous cAMP signal transduction. Figure 9–1 also shows that NG108-15 cells adapt to chronic exposure to ethanol by decreasing adenosine-receptor-dependent cAMP levels. This adaptive decrease appears to be an example of cellular "dependence," because intracellular cAMP levels are equal to control levels only in the continued presence of ethanol, and are abnormally low if ethanol is removed from the cultures. Because adenosine receptors are inhibitory, decreased adenosine receptor responses after ethanol withdrawal would lead to increased excitability. Thus, ethanol-induced changes in cAMP levels appear to parallel such clinical events as acute intoxication, physical dependence, and AWS. After discontinuing drinking, patients are at greatest risk of developing seizures during the first 2 days of alcohol withdrawal. In this regard, it is interesting that recovery of normal adenosine receptor cAMP levels occurs 48 hours after ethanol is removed from the culture (Fig. 9–1).

ETHANOL-INDUCED HETEROLOGOUS DESENSITIZATION

Richelson[35] reported that chronic exposure to ethanol depresses prostaglandin E_1, (PGE_1) PGE_1-mediated cAMP formation in NIE-115 cells. We found that NG108-15 cells also have reduced PGE_1-stimulated cAMP production. This reduction is similar to the decrease in adenosine-receptor-dependent cAMP levels (Table 9–1).[25] Therefore, it appears that chronic exposure of NG108-15 cells to ethanol causes heterologous desensitization of receptors that activate adenylyl cyclase.[25] Others have reached similar conclusions using different experimental preparations.[39,47]

Receptor activation leading to increased cAMP production requires at least three membrane components:[44] receptors for hormones and neurotransmitters; G_s, the GTP-binding protein that couples recep-

Table 9–1. EFFECTS OF CHRONIC ETHANOL (100 mM) ON α_s*

	Decrease	
cAMP production		
Adenosine-receptor-dependent	27 ± 6	(n = 4)
PGE$_1$-Receptor-dependent	25.6 ± 5.7	(n = 3)
α_s function (cyc⁻ reconstitution)	29 ± 1	(n = 3)
α_s protein (Western blot analysis)	38.5 ± 6	(n = 4)
α_s mRNA (Northern blot analysis)	30 ± 2	(n = 5)

*NG108-15 cells were treated with 100 mM ethanol for 48 hr. Adenosine-receptor-dependent cAMP levels were determined in intact control and ethanol-treated cells using phenylisopropyladenosine as described. cAMP assays and Western and Northern blot analyses were carried out on the same cells. n indicates the number of independent experiments on cell cultures grown at different times. The amount of α_s mRNA was also determined by slot blot analysis using 0.625, 1.25, 2.5, and 5.0 µg of total RNA. The results are from 4 separate RNA preparations analyzed on 4 Northern blots and 1 slot blot. Western, Northern, and slot blots were analyzed by scanning autoradiograms with a Hoeffer GS 300 densitometer connected to a Hewlett Packard 3390A integrator. Each band was analyzed by scanning 4 separate segments and the areas from each scan were added to compensate for variations in band width across the lane. Results are expressed as percent decrease (mean ± SEM) of ethanol-treated cells as compared with controls.

tor activation to adenylyl cyclase stimulation; and adenylyl cyclase, the enzyme that synthesizes cAMP. Alterations in G$_s$ could account for the reduced stimulation of cAMP production by both adenosine and PGE$_1$ in cells adapted to ethanol. Therefore, we investigated whether chronic ethanol treatment altered the amount or function of α_s, the GTP-binding subunit of G$_s$.

To assay α_s function, we used a mutant S49 lymphoma cell line, cyc⁻, which lacks α_s. Because of the deficiency in α_s protein, membranes from cyc⁻ cells cannot increase cAMP production when challenged with a β-adrenergic agonist. However, if the mutant cell membranes are reconstituted with α_s extracted from membranes of another source, adenylate cyclase activity is stimulated by β-adrenergic receptor activation. This reconstitution system, therefore, can be used as a biologic assay for α_s function. NG108-15 cells were incubated with 100 mM ethanol for 48 hours to cause heterologous desensitization of adenosine- and PGE$_1$-receptor-dependent cAMP production (Table 9–1).[25] Next, α_s was extracted from control and ethanol-adapted NG108-15 cells and used to reconstitute receptor-stimulated adenylyl cyclase activity in membranes from the S49 cyc⁻ cells. Consistent with the decrease in adenosine and PGE$_1$-mediated cAMP production in intact cells (Table 9–1), chronic ethanol caused a 29 percent reduction in the ability of membrane extracts of NG108-15 cells to complement the α_s deficiency of cyc⁻ membranes (Fig. 9–2).

Decreased cAMP production in the reconstitution assay with cyc⁻ membranes could be due to a decrease in α_s protein in the ethanol-dependent cells. Using anti-α_s antibodies in a Western blot analysis, we measured membrane-bound α_s in control and ethanol-treated NG108-15 cells. We found that chronic exposure to ethanol resulted in a 38.5 percent decrease in α_s protein (Table 9–1).[25]

To investigate the mechanism underlying the ethanol-induced decrease in α_s protein, we compared the amount of α_s-specific mRNA in ethanol-treated and control NG108-15 cells, using a cDNA probe for α_s mRNA.[25] Northern blot analysis of total cellular RNA showed a 30% reduction in α_s mRNA in the ethanol-treated cells (Table 9–1). In contrast, the amount of β-tubulin mRNA was slightly increased in the same experiments and the amount of α_i mRNA, the GTP-binding subunits of the inhibitory G-protein that

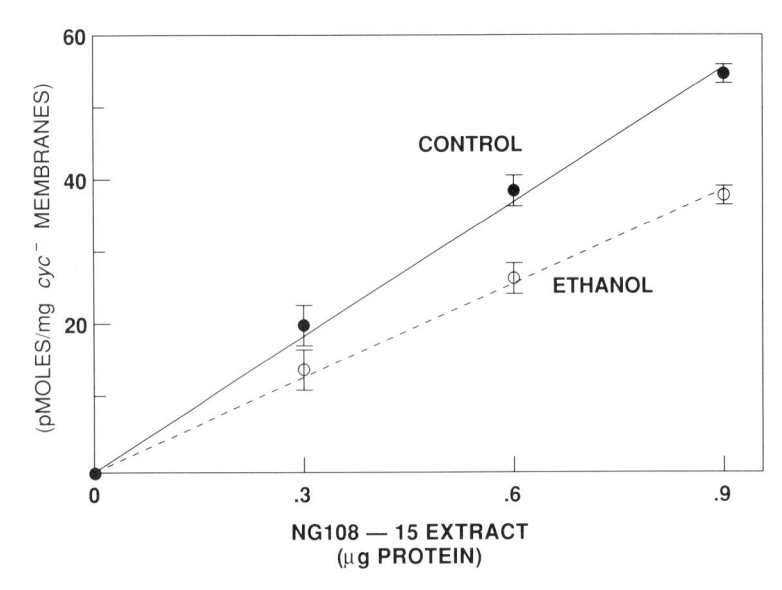

Figure 9–2. Activity of α_s in NG108-15 membranes measured by reconstitution of α_s-deficient cyc⁻ membranes. Increasing amounts of Lubrol PX extracts from NG108-15 membranes isolated from control (closed circles) and ethanol-treated cells (open circles) were incubated with cyc⁻ membranes, and receptor-stimulated adenylyl cyclase activity was measured. From Mochly-Rosen, et al,[25] 1988.

couples activation of certain receptors to adenylyl cyclase inhibition, was not altered (unpublished observations). It appeared, therefore, that the absolute amount of α_s limited cAMP production in NG108-15 cells and the ethanol-induced heterologous desensitization was due to reduced α_s mRNA.[25]

STUDIES IN ALCOHOLICS

Our results in cell culture indicate that chronic exposure to ethanol produces an adaptive decrease in receptor-dependent cAMP signal transduction. Desensitization of adenosine-receptor-stimulated cAMP levels might be pathophysiologically significant in chronic alcholism and AWS. Because human lymphocytes have the same A_2 adenosine receptors as NG108-15 cells, we could directly test whether cells from alcoholics have altered adenosine-receptor-dependent cAMP levels. We undertook a controlled age- and sex-matched study of cAMP levels in lymphocytes of chronic alcoholics, normal subjects, and patients with nonalcoholic liver disease.[12] The alcoholic patients had a lifetime ethanol consumption of nearly 2 tons (Table 9–2). Each of the alcoholic patients had normal weight for height and all subjects appeared well nourished. Half the alcoholics had normal findings on neurologic examination; the other half had mild memory deficits, mild peripheral neuropathy, and mild cerebellar gait ataxia. Extensive clinical laboratory measurements were performed on all three types of subject. There was no laboratory

Table 9–2. PROFILE OF PATIENTS*

Patients	Age (years)	Sex (M;F)	ETOH (kg)
Controls (10)	49.6 ± 3.6	9;1	145 ± 77
Alcoholics (10)	48.6 ± 3.6	9;1	1914 ± 319
Patient with nonalcoholic liver disease (10)	45.3 ± 3.6	5;5	45 ± 23

*Volunteer, actively drinking alcoholics were matched for age and sex with control subjects. Patients with nonalcoholic disease could not be sex-matched. Lifetime alcohol consumption was calculated as described by Diamond, et al.[12]

Table 9–3. cAMP LEVELS IN LYMPHOCYTES*

	Basal	PIA
	\(pmol/10^6 cells)	
Controls	9.55 ± 1.65	15.81 ± 2.52
Alcoholics	2.30 ± 0.34	3.72 ± 0.53
	(p = .0004)	(p = .0005)
Patients with nonalcoholic liver disease	8.33 ± 1.29	14.04 ± 1.93
	(p = .0005)	(p = .0005)

*Lymphocytes were isolated and assayed for cAMP in the absence (basal) and in the presence of 80 mM phenylisopropyladenosine, as described by Diamond, et al.[12]

evidence of malnutrition in the alcoholic subjects. Hemoglobin levels and mean corpuscular volumes in these subjects were normal, indicating adequate iron and folic acid ingestion. Transketolase activity was also normal, suggesting a diet containing adequate thiamine, and markers for malnutrition such as serum albumin levels and lymphocyte counts were also normal. Alcoholics and patients with liver disease exhibited abnormalities of some liver enzymes, but there were no statistically significant differences between the alcoholic and matched liver-disease group. Laboratory values for alcoholic patients were similar to values for normal controls except that alcoholic patients had significantly elevated serum glutamic-oxaloacetic transaminase and globulin levels.

REDUCED cAMP LEVELS IN LYMPHOCYTES FROM ALCOHOLICS

The most striking difference between alcoholics and normal subjects or patients with nonalcoholic liver disease was in lymphocyte cAMP levels (Table 9–3). Thus, lymphocytes from alcoholics showed a four-fold reduction in basal and adenosine-receptor-stimulated cAMP levels compared with cells from nonalcoholic subjects (Fig. 9–3). Moreover, the lymphocytes from alcoholics showed marked resistance to acute ethanol stimulation of receptor-dependent cAMP production and this difference in stimulated cAMP levels appeared to distinguish alcoholic from nonalcoholic patients (Fig. 9–4). This manifestation of "tolerance" at a cel-

Figure 9–3. Basal and stimulated cAMP levels in lymphocytes from alcoholics (open bars) and control subjects (closed bars). Each bar represents the mean ± SEM (n = 10 for basal and PIA; n = 9 for PIA plus ethanol). From Diamond, et al,[12] 1987.

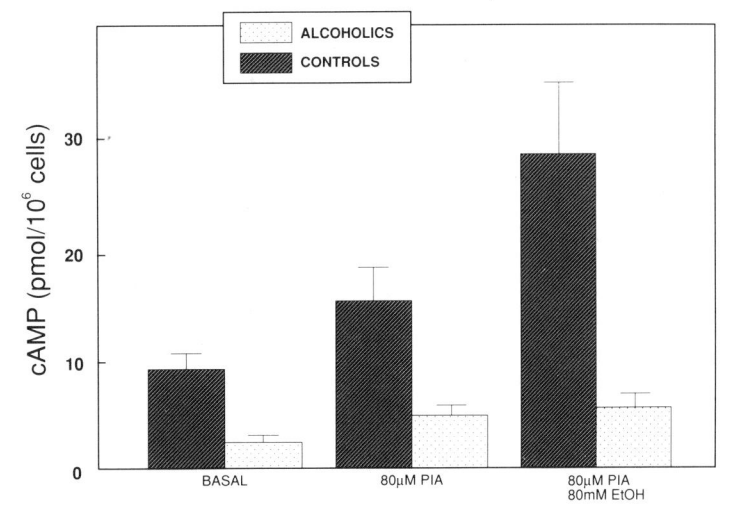

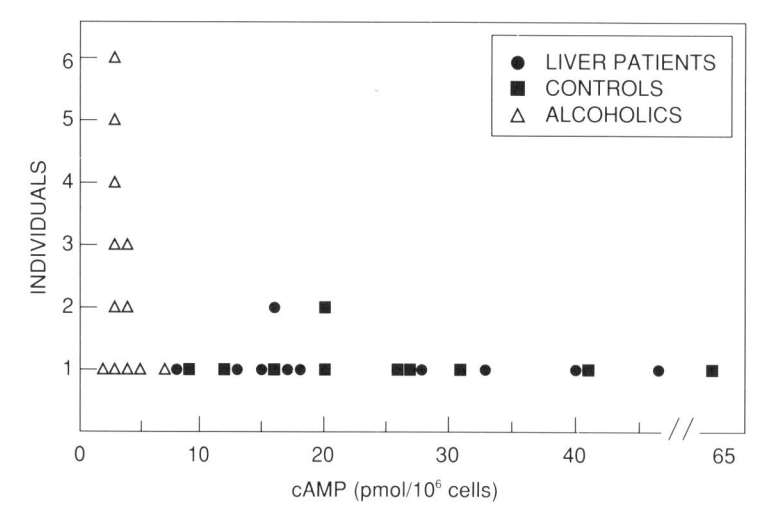

Figure 9–4. Ethanol stimulation of adenosine receptor-dependent cAMP levels in freshly isolated lymphocytes from alcoholics, patients with nonalcoholic liver disease and control subjects. Each point indicates cAMP levels from an individual patient after stimulation for 60 minutes by 80 uM PIA and 80 mM ethanol.

lular level may parallel clinical tolerance to ethanol in chronic alcoholics.[13] We have also found similar results in a blinded study in which basal and adenosine-receptor-stimulated cAMP levels were measured in lymphocytes from every 10th patient admitted to San Francisco General Hospital.[43] Alcoholics were identified after the assays were completed. Patients had diverse medical disorders and were taking a variety of medications. Despite the likelihood of under-reporting of alcoholism in the "nonalcoholic" group, lymphocytes from alcoholics had lower levels of cAMP and were resistant to the acute effects of ethanol compared with cells from nonalcoholics. Consistent with these findings, Tabakoff and associates[45] reported that platelet membranes from alcoholics show a significant reduction in PGE_1-stimulated cAMP levels.

Our results indicate that lymphocytes from alcoholics are distinguishable from lymphocytes from nonalcoholic subjects. Cells from alcoholics exhibit reduced basal cAMP levels, reduced adenosine-receptor-stimulated cAMP levels, and increased resistance to ethanol stimulation of adenosine-receptor-dependent cAMP accumulation. Therefore, basal and receptor-stimulated cAMP levels in lymphocytes may be valuable biologic markers for alcohol abuse.

ETHANOL AND cAMP SIGNAL TRANSDUCTION: IMPLICATIONS FOR AWS

Signal transduction, where activation of a receptor on the outside of a cell by a neurotransmitter or hormone results in production of an intracellular second messenger, appears to be particularly sensitive to acute and chronic exposure to ethanol.[5-7,12,19-22,24,25,30-35,38,39,41-43,45-47] Using a model system of neural cells in culture, we identified adenosine-receptor-dependent cAMP production as a major target of ethanol action. Acute addition of ethanol stimulated adenosine-dependent cAMP production, whereas chronic exposure to ethanol caused a heterologous desensitization of this signaling mechanism when measured in the absence of alcohol. We predicted that the decrease in receptor-dependent cAMP levels that we observed in neural cells in culture after chronic exposure to ethanol might occur in alcoholics. We confirmed this hypothesis in a controlled clinical study with freshly isolated lymphocytes.

Our results indicate that adenosine-receptor-dependent cAMP signal transduction is altered by acute and chronic exposure to ethanol in patients as well as in neural cells in culture. This finding may be of pathophysiologic significance in AWS. Because adenosine is an endogenous anticonvulsant, it may be anticipated that an ethanol-induced desensitization of adenosine receptor activation during alcohol withdrawal would constitute a reduction in endogenous anticonvulsant activity. This occurrence could promote AWS. It remains to be determined whether therapy directed at increasing brain A_2 adenosine receptor activity will be effective in preventing or treating AWS.

SUMMARY

Adenosine is an inhibitory neuromodulator with anticonvulsant properties. Recent evidence suggests that adenosine may mediate the effects of ethanol in the brain. We have found that ethanol acutely stimulates adenosine-receptor-dependent cAMP levels by 35 percent to 50 percent in NG108-15 cells, a cloned neural cell line. However, chronic ethanol exposure caused a 35 percent to 48 percent reduction in adenosine-stimulated cAMP levels when assayed without ethanol. cAMP returned to control levels when ethanol was added back to these cells. This is a form of "cellular dependence" on ethanol. These cellular changes appeared to parallel the clinical events of acute ethanol intoxication and physical dependence. We have also found that reduced cAMP production in ethanol-dependent cells is associated with a 29 percent decrease in functional activity of the α subunit of G_s, the GTP-binding protein that couples receptor activation to adenylyl cyclase stimulation. This action is caused by a 39 percent decrease in the amount of α_s protein and a 30 percent decrease in α_s mRNA. These results indicate that chronic exposure to ethanol alters the regulation of adenosine-dependent cAMP signal transduction in neural cells. An alteration in cAMP signal transduction could have pathophysiologic significance in alcoholics. Freshly isolated lymphocytes from alcoholics showed a 75 percent reduction in adenosine-receptor-dependent cAMP production compared with cells from patients with nonalcoholic liver disease and cells from control subjects. In the central nervous system, desensitization of adenosine receptor activation during alcohol withdrawal would constitute a reduction in endogenous anticonvulsant activity. This occurrence could play a role in generating AWS.

ACKNOWLEDGMENTS

This work was supported by grants from NIAAA and the Alcoholic Beverage Medical Research Foundation.

References

1. Ault, B and Wang, CM: Adenosine inhibits epileptiform activity arising in hippocampal area CA3. Br J Pharmacol 87:695, 1986.
2. Barraco, RA, et al: Anticonvulsant effects of adenosine analogues on amygdaloid-kindled seizures in rats. Neurosci Lett 46:317, 1984.
3. Beisswenger, TB, Holmquist, B, and Vallee, BL: $_x$-ADH is the sole alcohol dehydrogenase isozyme of mammalian brains: Implications and inferences. Proc Natl Acad Sci USA 82:8369, 1985.
4. Bowker, HM and Chapman, AG: Adenosine analogues: The temperature-dependence of the anticonvulsant effect and inhibition of ^{3}H-D-aspartate release. Biochem Pharmacol 35:2949, 1986.
5. Charnes, ME, Gordon, AS, and Diamond, I: Ethanol modulation of opiate receptors in cultured neural cells. Science 222: 1246, 1983.
6. Charness, ME, Querimit, LA, and Diamond, I: Ethanol increases the expression of functional delta-opioid receptors in neuroblastoma x glioma NG108-15 hybrid cells. J Biol Chem 261:3164, 1986.
7. Charness, ME, Querimit, LA, and Henteleff, M: Ethanol differentially regulates G proteins in neural cells. Biochem Biophys Res Comm 155:138, 1988.
8. Chin, JH and DeLorenzo, RJ: A new class of adenosine receptors in brain. Characterization by 2-chloro[^{3}H]adenosine binding. Biochem Pharmacol 35:847, 1986.
9. Dar, MS, et al: Behavioral interactions of ethanol and methylxanthines. Psychopharmacology 91:1, 1987.
10. Dar, MS, Mustafa, SJ, and Wooles, WR: Possible role of adenosine in the CNS effects of ethanol. Life Sci 33:1363, 1983.
11. Dar, MS and Wooles, WR: Effect of chronically administered methylxanthines on ethanol-induced motor incoordination in mice. Life Sci 39:1429, 1986.
12. Diamond, I, et al: Basal and adenosine receptor-stimulated levels of cAMP are reduced in lymphocytes from alcoholic patients. Proc Natl Acad Sci USA 84:1413, 1987.

13. Diamond, I and Charness, ME: Alcohol toxicity. In Asbury, AK, McKhann, GM, and McDonald, WI (eds): Diseases of the Nervous System. WB Saunders, Philadelphia, 1986, p 1324.
14. Dragunow, M: Endogenous anticonvulsant substances. Neurosci Biobehav Rev 10:229, 1986.
15. Dragunow, M and Goddard, GV: Adenosine modulation of amygdala kindling. Exp Neurol 84:654, 1984.
16. Dragunow, M, Goddard, GV, and Laverty, R: Is adenosine an endogenous anticonvulsant? Epilepsia 26:480, 1985.
17. Dunwiddie, TV: The physiological role of adenosine in the central nervous system. Int Rev Neurobiol 27:63, 1985.
18. Goldstein, DB and Goldstein, A: Possible role of enzyme inhibition and repression in drug tolerance and addiction. Biochem Pharmacol 8:48, 1961.
19. Gordon, AS, et al: Adaptation to ethanol in cultured neural cells and human lymphocytes from alcoholics. Ann NY Acad Sci 492:367, 1987.
20. Gordon, AS, Collier, K, and Diamond, I: Ethanol regulation of adenosine receptor-stimulated cAMP levels in a clonal neural cell line: An in vitro model of cellular tolerance to ethanol. Proc Natl Acad Sci USA 83:2105, 1986.
21. Harper, JF and Brooker, G: Alcohol potentiation of isoproterenol-stimulated cyclic AMP accumulation in rat parotid. J Cyclic Nucleotide Res 6:51, 1980.
22. Hynie, S, Lanefelt, F, and Fredholm, BB: Effects of ethanol on human lymphocyte levels of cyclic AMP in vitro: Potentiation of the response to isoproterenol, prostaglandin E_2 or adenosine stimulation. Acta Pharmacologica et Toxicologica 47:58, 1980.
23. Lee, KS, Schubert, P, and Henemann, U: The anticonvulsive action of adenosine: A postsynaptic, dendritic action by a possible endogenous anticonvulsant. Brain Res 321:160, 1984.
24. Luthin, GR and Tabakoff, B: Activation of adenylate cyclase by alcohols requires the nucleotide-binding protein. J Pharmacol Exp Ther 228:579, 1984.
25. Mochly-Rosen, D, et al: Chronic ethanol causes heterologous desensitization of receptors by reducing α_s messenger RNA. Nature 333:848, 1988.
26. Phillis, JW and Barraco, RA: Adenosine, adenylate cyclase, and transmitter release. Adv Cyclic Nucleotide Protein Phosphorylation Res 19:243, 1985.
27. Phillis, JW and Wu, PH: Adenosine mediates sedative action of various centrally active drugs. Med Hypotheses 9:361, 1982.
28. Popoli, P, Benedetti, M, and Scotti de Carolis, A: Anticonvulsant activity of carbamazepine and N6 L-phenylisopropyladenosine in rabbits: Relationship to adenosine receptors in the central nervous system. Pharmacol Biochem Behav 29:533, 1988.
29. Proctor, WR and Dunwiddie, TV: Behavioral sensitivity to purinergic drugs parallels ethanol sensitivity in selectively bred mice. Science 224:519, 1984.
30. Rabin, RA, et al: Effects of ethanol administration and withdrawal on neurotransmitter receptor systems in C57 mice. J Pharmacol Exp Ther 213:491, 1980.
31. Rabin, RA: Effect of ethanol on inhibition of striatal adenylate cyclase activity. Biochem Pharmacol 34:4329, 1985.
32. Rabin, RA, Bode, DC, and Molinoff, PB: Relationship between ethanol-induced alterations in fluorescence anisotropy and adenylate cyclase activity. Biochem Pharmacol 35:2331, 1986.
33. Rabin, RA and Molinoff, PB: Activation of adenylate cyclase by ethanol in mouse striatal tissue. J Pharmacol Exp Ther 216:129, 1981.
34. Rabin, RA and Molinoff, PB: Multiple sites of action of ethanol on adenylate cyclase. J Pharmacol Exp Ther 227:551, 1983.
35. Richelson, E, et al: Effects of chronic exposure to ethanol on the prostaglandin E_1 receptor-mediated response and binding in a murine neuroblastoma clone (NIE-115). J Pharmacol Exp Ther 239:687, 1986.
36. Rosen, JB and Berman, RF: Differential effects of adenosine analogs on amygdala, hippocampus, and caudate nucleus kindled seizures. Epilepsia 28:658, 1987.
37. Sagratella, S, et al: Modulatory action of purinergic drugs on high potassium-indced epileptiform bursting in rat hippocampal slices. Pharmacol Res Commun 19:819, 1987.
38. Saito, T, et al: Ethanol's effects on cortical adenylate cyclase activity. J Neurosci 48:1817, 1987.
39. Saito, T, Lee, JM, and Tabakoff, B: Ethanol's effects on cortical adenylate cyclase activity. J Neurochem 44:1037, 1985.
40. Snyder, SH: Adenosine as a neuromodulator. Annu Rev Neurosci 8:103, 1985.
41. Stenstrom, S, et al: Acute effects of ethanol and other short-chain alcohols on the guanylate cyclase system of murine neuroblastoma cells (Clone NIE-115). J Pharmacol Exp Ther 236:458, 1986.
42. Stenstrom, S and Richelson, E: Acute effect of ethanol on prostaglandin E_1-mediated cyclic AMP formation by a murine neuroblastoma clone. J Pharmacol Exp Ther 221:334, 1982.
43. Stewart, SA, et al: Unpublished material.
44. Stryer, L and Bourne, HR: G proteins: A family of signal transducers. Annual Review of Cell Biology 2:391, 1986.
45. Tabakoff, B, et al: Differences in platelet enzyme activity between alcoholics and non-alcoholics. N Engl J Med 318:134, 1988.
46. Tabakoff, B and Hoffman, PL: Development of functional dependence on ethanol in dopaminergic systems. J Pharmacol Exp Ther 208:216, 1979.
47. Valverius, P, Hoffman, PL, and Tabakoff, B: Effect of ethanol on mouse cerebral cortical β-adrenergic receptors. Mol Pharmacol 32:217, 1987.

CHAPTER 10

Gerald D. Frye, Ph.D.

Gamma-Aminobutyric Acid Changes in Alcohol Withdrawal

The neurobiologic prominence and apparent significance of gamma-aminobutyric acid (GABA) as an "inhibitory" neurotransmitter in the mammalian central nervous system (CNS) continue to fuel speculation that GABA-mediated neurochemical communication is a likely target for disease processes involved in psychiatric and neurologic disorders including alcohol abuse and alcoholism.[50] There is continued interest in the potential role that GABAergic transmission plays in the neuropharmacology of ethanol, both in the reinforcing properties of ethanol that underlie psychologic dependence and in the pharmacologic consequences of intoxication, functional tolerance, and physical dependence.[34] This chapter interprets recent clinical and experimental findings on the role of GABAergic neurotransmission in these adaptive processes. Particular attention has been paid to the relationship between the expression of seizure susceptibility during the ethanol withdrawal syndrome and changes in GABAergic mechanisms. This chapter addresses the recent literature from the perspective that an adaptive reduction of GABAergic inhibition could be partly responsible for the ethanol withdrawal syndrome. The excellent review by Hunt[41] is frequently consulted for earlier literature on the effects of ethanol on GABAergic transmission.

BASIS FOR GABAergic CHANGES DURING ALCOHOL WITHDRAWAL

GABAmimetics and Withdrawal Suppression

The hypothesis that reduced inhibitory GABAergic tone in the CNS might be responsible for hyperexcitability during the ethanol withdrawal syndrome is based primarily on two observations. First, many clinical and animal studies show that drugs known to augment GABAergic neurotransmission can suppress the ethanol withdrawal syndrome. For example, sodium valproate, gamma-vinyl GABA or diaminobutyric acid, which increase the availability of endogenous GABA, and agents like muscimol, barbiturates, and benzodiazepines, which interact more directly with GABA receptors, effectively block withdrawal signs such as seizures (Fig. 10–1).[41] Conversely, drugs that block either GABA synthesis or GABA receptors can induce behavioral events such as seizures that resemble ethanol withdrawal reactions.[24,41] Thus, pharmacologic modulation of GABAergic inhibition to offset or enhance the effects of ethanol withdrawal indirectly supports the view that physical dependence or the withdrawal syndrome may involve a deficit of GABAergic inhibitory tone.

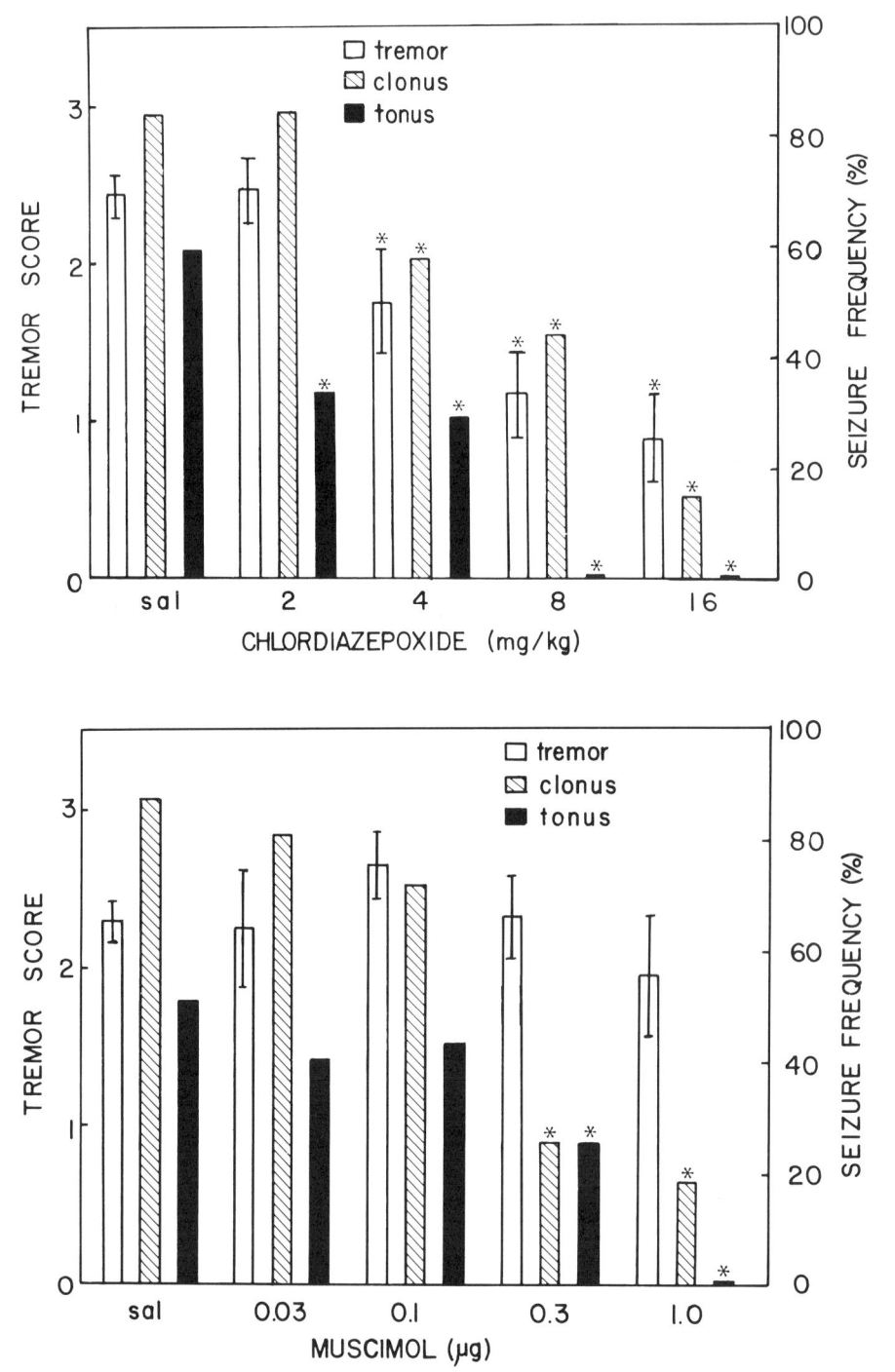

Figure 10–1. Chlordiazepoxide (CDZ) (A) and muscimol (MUS) (B) suppress ethanol withdrawal, audiogenic seizures in a dose-related manner buy only CDZ blocks forelimb tremors. After feeding ethanol-containing liquid diet for 12 days, rats were withdrawn from ethanol. Thirty minutes before testing, either CDZ or saline were injected intraperitoneally. Muscimol or saline were injected intracisternally 5 minutes before testing. Susceptibility to audiogenically induced clonic (clonus) or clonic-tonic (tonus) seizures and the severity of forelimb tremors were evaluated 6.5–8.5 hours after withdrawal. (From Frye, GD, McCown, TJ, and Breese, GR,[29] with permission.)
*$p < 0.05$ when compared with saline-treated group

GABAergic Enhancement by Ethanol

A second finding consistent with a role for compensatory GABAergic hypoactivity in physical dependence is that ethanol directly stimulates GABAergic neurotransmission. Although ethanol does not directly activate a specific receptor in the classic sense,[76] some electrophysiologic and biochemical results suggest that ethanol can either increase the efficiency of endogenous or exogenously applied GABA[1,2,41,59,74,85] or perhaps even directly activate GABAergic receptor mechanisms via an allosteric interaction.[74,85] Sedative/hypnotic drugs, such as the barbiturates and benzodiazepines, also increase GABA receptor-transducer efficiency by acting on allosteric regulatory sites distinct from binding sites recognizing GABA. Interaction of ethanol with the GABA receptor may be functionally relevant to the pharmacologic consequences of ethanol treatment; many measures of acute intoxication can be increased or decreased by direct-acting GABA agonists or antagonists, respectively (Fig. 10–2).[2,11,15,25,41,48,49]

Ethanol and GABAergic Adaptation

Sustained stimulation of GABA receptors caused by the GABAmimetic effects of ethanol intoxication could induce adaptation in the form of GABA receptor hypoactivity. One example of GABAergic adaptation may be the "run down" or "desensitization" of GABA receptors within seconds of sustained exposure to high agonist concentrations.[43] Theoretically, "adaptive" changes in response to a continuing pharmacologic stimulus would be most likely to occur in the immediate vicinity of the site where a drug acts.[30,37] If ethanol increases the relative efficiency of GABAergic neurotransmission, this action could be the force driving adaptive or homeostatic mechanisms to reduce GABAergic tone.

Consistent with this view are recent findings that incubation of embryonic rat or chick forebrain neurons with GABA (1 mM) reduced [^{3}H]muscimol binding,[51,81] suggesting an adaptive reduction in GABA transduction capacity. In addition, cessation of a sustained intracortical infusion of GABA (0.1–1 mg/hr) in rats and photosensitive baboons caused transient epileptiform activity in cortical EEG re-

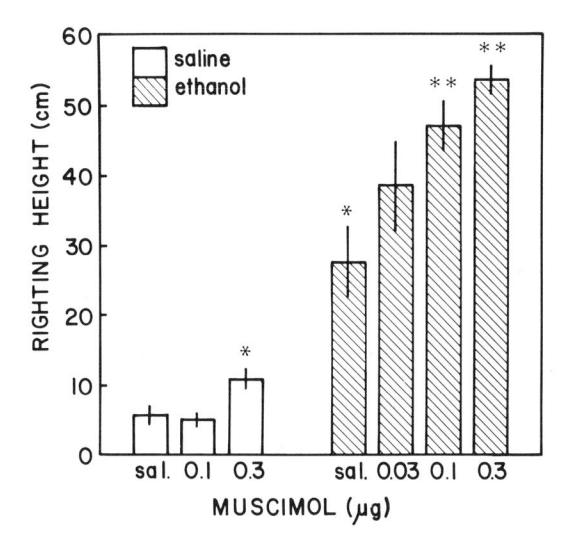

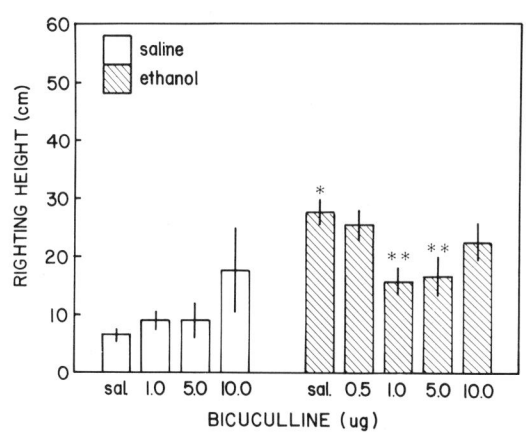

Figure 10–2. Muscimol (MUS) (A) increases and bicuculline (BIC) (B) reduces ethanol-induced impairment of the aerial righting reflex. Ethanol (2.25g/kg, ip) or saline treatment was followed 50 minutes later by intracisternal injection of MUS, BIC or saline (sal). the height of aerial righting was measured 10 minutes later by determining the minimal height from which inverted rats were able to land upright on a foam rubber pad. (From Frye, GD, and Breese, GR,[25] with permission.)
*$p < 0.5$ when compared to saline + saline treatment
*$p < 0.5$ when compared to saline + ethanol treatment

cordings.[1,7] These data suggest that abrupt termination of a sustained GABA stimulus might result in a withdrawal-like syndrome.

Whether acute ethanol treatment exerts a sustained GABAmimetic effect could be irrelevant to understanding how physical dependence and the withdrawal syndrome develop. It is possible that ethanol-induced depression caused by a non-GABAergic mechanism might still be offset by reducing GABAergic inhibition throughout the CNS. However, a CNS impaired by GABAmimetic effects of ethanol could also evoke a change in a different redundant physiologic system to offset the effects of ethanol, as has been suggested for opiates.[53] In this case, an adaptive reduction in GABAergic inhibition might play a role in offsetting ethanol-induced CNS depression only if the redundant mechanism happened to involve GABA. I will now address these issues based on the experimental evidence available.

PRESYNAPTIC GABAergic ACTIVITY IN ETHANOL DEPENDENCE

GABA Synthesis

If physical dependence on ethanol results from an adaptive reduction in GABAergic inhibition, this effect could be expressed as a change in presynaptic mechanisms regulating GABA synthesis, release, and reuptake. An obvious site where ethanol might modify GABA homeostasis is the level of primary synthetic and catabolic enzymes. Most investigations have focused on glutamic acid decarboxylase (GAD), a cytoplasmic enzyme that is found primarily in neurons and that is rate limiting for GABA synthesis. GABA transaminase (GABA-T), which catalyzes the first step in GABA inactivation, has also been studied, though it is not always closely associated with GABA-receptive neurons.[22] In general, neither pharmacologically relevant in vitro ethanol concentrations (3–100 mM) nor acute or chronic ethanol treatment in vivo, nor ethanol withdrawal consistently change the activities of either GAD or GABA-T.[41,44]

GABA Release and Reuptake

Acute administration of ethanol might enhance inhibition by increasing the amount of GABA released into the synapse or by slowing clearance from the synaptic cleft by reuptake mechanisms. In unrestrained rats, [^{14}C]GABA released into push-pull perfusates of several brain areas was not changed by the presence of ethanol in the perfusate.[65] However, in vitro ethanol (55 mM) increased potassium-stimulated release of endogenous GABA from slices of cerebral cortex.[56] Other in vitro studies examining the release of exogenous radiolabeled GABA from preloaded brain tissue preparations have not shown significant enhancement of basal or stimulated release by moderate ethanol concentrations (<100 mM), although at higher ethanol levels (>200 mM) GABA release was impaired.[38,39,41,63,72]

Chronic effects of ethanol on GABA release have not been rigorously studied. In the absence of ethanol, neither basal nor potassium-evoked GABA release from brain tissue of ethanol-dependent animals appear to be altered. Inhibition of basal GABA release by 500 mM ethanol is reduced in preparations from young ethanol-dependent animals, suggesting that tolerance to the inhibitory effects of excessive ethanol concentrations can occur,[72] although one must question the relevance of this finding to the intact animal.

The effects of ethanol on GABA reuptake processes have also received relatively little study. These processes appear to resist direct effects of ethanol. However, there is no change in reuptake kinetics in the ethanol-dependent animal.[41]

Although initial studies suggest that moderate, acute, and chronic ethanol exposure do not significantly alter GABA release and reuptake processes, this area needs further investigation. For example, it is possible that the ability of ethanol to increase endogenous GABA release,[56] but not preloaded exogenous [^{3}H]GABA release,[38,39,41,63,72] may be explained by the actions of ethanol on two different pools of GABA. GABAergic neurotransmission appears to depend primarily on the pool of newly synthesized GABA, which would not be labeled by preloading.[50] Also, there is increasing evidence that presynaptic GABA autoreceptors may regulate GABA release.[61,87] Direct effects of ethanol on GABA autoreceptors might alter presynaptic GABAergic homeostasis.

Steady-State GABA Concentrations

Other attempts to identify the relative effects of ethanol exposure on GABAergic neurotransmission *in vivo* involved measuring changes in the amount of GABA found in brain tissue under steady-state conditions. A nonselective survey of this literature does not reveal a particular pattern, because increases, decreases, and lack of change in GABA content have been reported with roughly equal frequency after both acute and chronic ethanol treatments.[17,25,41,57,67,68,70] Variables such as the magnitude and timing of ethanol treatments,[41] failure to prevent postmortem-induced increases in GABA content,[3] and the lack of appropriate dietary controls[19,41] may explain the wide range of findings. The relatively large glial GABA pool in brain tissue can also distort interpretation of steady-state GABA data and obscure subtle changes in steady-state GABA concentrations. However, one would not expect these factors to completely mask a large change in GABA content in response to ethanol or its withdrawal. A recent study that avoided some of these concerns by measuring the effects of acute and chronic ethanol treatment on stabilized GABA concentrations in synaptosomes isolated from various rat brain regions revealed no significant changes[26] (Fig. 10-3). Taken together, these findings do not support a major effect of ethanol on steady-state GABA concentrations in brain tissue.

GABA Turnover

Estimation of GABA turnover based on its rate of accumulation in brain tissue after metabolic inhibition with GABA-T inhibitors, such as aminooxyacetic acid

Figure 10-3. Acute and chronic ethanol treatment does not change GABA concentrations in synaptosomes from hippocampus. Rats receiving a single intraperitoneal dose of saline or ethanol (0.5-4.0 g/kg) were killed 30 minutes later when motor impairment was maximal. Other animals were fed liquid diets for 12 days to establish physical dependence. One group was fed dextrose (DEX) equicaloric with ethanol. Another was fed ethanol (ETOH) and killed while intoxicated. The third group was fed ethanol and withdrawn (WD) from ethanol for 12 hours before sacrifice. Synaptosomes were prepared from 6 brain regions of each animal. Acute and chronic ethanol treatment also failed to change GABA concentrations (nmol/mg protein) of synaptosomes isolated from cortex (saline = 15.96 ± 0.78), tectum (saline = 42.33 ± 3.91), striatum (saline = 20.08 ± 2.47), brainstem (saline = 24.96 ± 2.49), or cerebellum (saline = 6.95 ± 0.59). Values represent the mean ± S.E.M. for 6-8 measurements. (Adapted from Frye, G, and Fincher, A.[23])

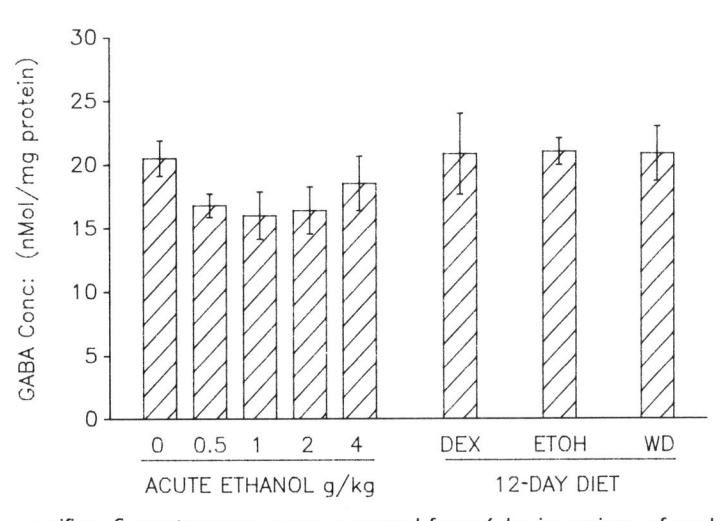

and gabaculine, is thought to provide a more direct and sensitive index of endogenous GABA dynamics related to neurotransmission and to better reflect drug-induced perturbations. Turnover studies suggest that a single injection of ethanol causing mild moderate intoxication reduces GABA accumulation in the cerebellum, cerebral cortex, striatum, and hypothalamus, but this effect is not observed at higher doses of ethanol.[16,73,89] The effects of continuous ethanol treatment are less clear. When blood ethanol concentrations remained elevated, one study found no change in GABA turnover,[89] but others revealed reduced GABA accumulation in the cerebellum, septum, olfatory tubercle, hippocampus, striatum, and cerebral cortex.[70,73] The extent of changes in GABA accumulation after a short period of ethanol withdrawal is also unclear; some researchers have reported no change,[70] others a partial reduction in some brain areas.[16,89] These findings might be consistent with a role for reduced GABA formation in the development of physical dependence and in the expression of the ethanol withdrawal syndrome, because animals that showed no evidence of tolerance or dependence on ethanol[70] did not show changes in GABA turnover. Any effects of ethanol on GABA appear to be reversible within the first 24 hours of withdrawal from ethanol treatment.[70,89]

It is possible that using GABA-T inhibitors in turnover studies could artifically modify the effects of ethanol in a particular brain area. One might expect accumulating GABA to diffuse via interstitial spaces. This action might change GABA-regulated neuronal activity throughout the brain. One report describes an attempt to localize transaminase inhibition by measuring GABA accumulation after a 5 µg microinjection of gamma-vinyl-GABA in the substantia nigra. The rate of GABA accumulation did not change after either acute or chronic ethanol treatment or ethanol withdrawal.[26]

Studies on ethanol's effects on GABA neurotransmitter levels in humans have been limited primarily to measurements of GABA content in the plasma or cerebrospinal fluid (CSF). A single ethanol treatment yielding a blood level of 1.3 mg/ml in healthy men increased plasma GABA levels.[4] Other studies in alcoholics failed to reveal any consistent changes in CSF concentrations of GABA in ethanol-dependent persons during the withdrawal syndrome.[41]

Presynaptic Interactions

In summary, acute and chronic ethanol treatment do not consistently change steady-state GABA concentrations measured in either samples of CSF, whole brain tissues, or brain tissue fractions enriched in nerve terminals. Turnover studies measuring GABA accumulation in whole brain tissue after peripheral treatment with GABA-T inhibitors suggest that acute ethanol treatment may slightly inhibit presynaptic GABA dynamics. This inhibition may persist in some brain areas during chronic ethanol treatment through the early stages of the withdrawal syndrome. After withdrawal, values consistently return to control levels. It is important, however, to note that changes in GABA utilization are not found in all brain areas and that when present the changes are relatively small. One would expect changes in all brain regions if ethanol was exerting direct biochemical effects on GABA homeostatic mechanisms. Whether small reductions in GABA turnover are responsible for the ethanol withdrawal syndrome cannot be determined from these data.

POSTSYNAPTIC GABAergic ACTIVITY IN ETHANOL DEPENDENCE

Apparent GABAergic hypoactivity during ethanol withdrawal could result from an adaptive or compensatory reduction in the number of postsynaptic GABA receptors available or in the receptor-transducer efficiency of GABA receptors. Several types of biochemical and electrophysiologic investigations have tested whether changes in GABA receptors or their transducer roles are induced by ethanol exposure.

Ethanol and GABA Receptor Ligand Binding

Initial studies of GABA receptors using radioligand binding techniques and [³H]GABA suggested that acute ethanol treatment increased the apparent number of binding sites for the ligand. Prolonged exposure and ethanol withdrawal appeared to reduce the number of GABA binding sites and/or their affinity for the ligand.[2,41,84] Although the finding is consistent with the idea that acute administration of ethanol enhances GABAergic transmission and leads to an adaptive GABAergic hypoactivity, increasing knowledge of GABA receptor subtypes and their regulation has forced a reevaluation. It is now clear that nonselective ligands like [³H]GABA can bind to at least two types of GABA binding sites, GABA$_A$ and GABA$_B$, which are pharmacologically and physiologically distinct. GABA$_A$ sites are activated by muscimol, blocked by bicuculline, and gated to a chloride channel[6] (Fig. 10-4). GABA$_A$ receptors also have selective binding sites for other exogenous ligands such as the benzodiazepines, barbiturates, and picrotoxin. These may represent recognition sites for endogenous allosteric modulators. GABA$_B$ receptors recognize a different conformation of the GABA molecule, represented by baclofen but not muscimol. GABA$_B$ sites are blocked by baclofen but not bicuculline, and appear to be linked to a potassium rather than a chloride conductance.[6,64] Both GABA$_A$ and GABA$_B$ receptors generally exert inhibitory cellular actions.[6] To date, I am unaware of any studies describing the influence of ethanol on GABA$_B$ ligand binding.

Interpretation of the effects of ethanol on the GABA$_A$ receptor and associated sites for benzodiazepines, barbiturates, and picrotoxin-like ligands is very complex. Essentially, ethanol *in vitro* does not appear to influence the binding of ligands to GABA$_A$ or benzodiazepine sites and fails to alter the modulatory actions of barbiturates to increase the binding of these ligands to the GABA$_A$ receptor com-

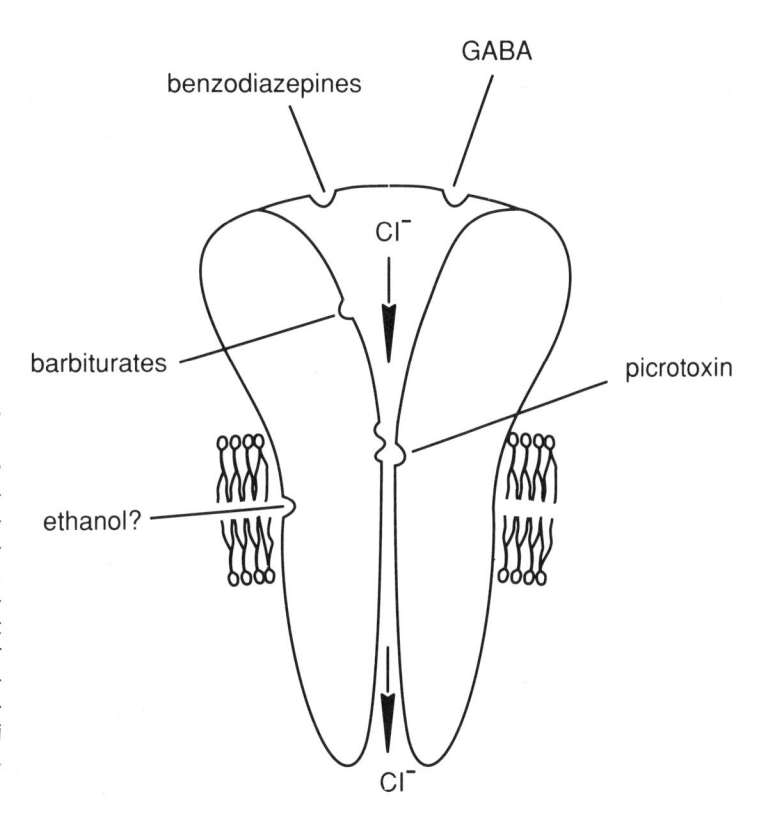

Figure 10-4. Schematic of the GABA$_A$-gated chloride channel. The GABA$_A$-gated chloride channel includes distinct recognition sites for GABA, benzodiazepines, barbiturates and picrotoxin-like convulsants. Ethanol does not directly compete for these binding sites but may interact with the receptor complex at a membrane interface to influence channel activity. (Adapted from Eldefrawi and Eldefrawi, FASEB J 1:262, 1987.)

plex.[35] Binding of [^{35}S]TBPS, a picrotoxin site ligand, is inhibited by ethanol (>200 mM) *in vitro*, which is far in excess of relevant ethanol concentrations *in vivo*.[47,71,82] Acute *in vivo* ethanol treatment may increase the availability of GABA$_A$ recognition sites, perhaps by influencing an endogenous allosteric modulator of the GABA receptor; however, this remains a controversial issue.[35,41,84] Chronic ethanol treatment and withdrawal appear to reduce the number of GABA$_A$ recognition sites available while having no effect on the central benzodiazepine binding site.[41,84] Physical dependence on ethanol apparently does not change [^{35}S]TBPS binding to the picrotoxin recognition site;[47,82] however, binding to the peripheral benzodiazepine receptor that is not associated with the GABA$_A$ site is increased under this condition.[75,78]

Radioligand binding studies do not effectively characterize the actions of drugs such as ethanol on the status of the functional GABA$_A$ receptor that regulates transmembrane chloride currents. For example, desensitized GABA$_A$ receptors have among the highest affinities for GABA$_A$ ligands and exhibit little or no transducer efficiency.[90] Thus, the ability of chronic ethanol treatment to change GABA binding characteristics does not necessarily indicate functionally relevant changes in the transducer role of GABA receptors on neurons.

Ethanol and GABA-Gated Chloride Uptake

There has been much interest recently in the apparent ability of ethanol to increase the efficiency of GABA as an agonist at GABA$_A$ receptors. Ethanol increases GABA$_A$ agonist-induced chloride flux both in subcellular particles known as "synaptoneurosomes"[62] or "microsacs"[1] and in intact cultured spinal neurons,[85] and may directly activate GABA$_A$-gated chloride flux even in the absence of GABA.[62,85] These actions of ethanol are shared by barbiturates like pentobarbital, while benzodiazepines such as diazepam only increase the efficiency of GABA at the GABA$_A$ receptor but do not appear to act directly in GABA's absence. Ethanol may also activate other chloride conductances besides those gated by GABA.[12,27,86]

Recent examination of the chronic effects of ethanol in synaptoneurosomes suggests that the ability of ethanol to stimulate GABA$_A$-induced chloride flux is lost in preparations from physically dependent animals.[1,62] The response returns to normal when recovery from the ethanol withdrawal syndrome is largely complete. Surprisingly, direct stimulation of chloride flux by ethanol in the absence of exogenous GABA$_A$ agonists appears to be unaltered by chronic ethanol treatment.[62] The efficacy but not the potency of muscimol alone to stimulate chloride flux is reduced 25 percent in synaptoneurosomes prepared from cerebral cortex of dependent rate.[62] These measures are unaltered in samples isolated from cerebellar tissue of dependent mice.[1] Down-regulation of GABA$_A$ receptor-transducer efficiency also appears to result from chronic benzodiazepine treatment.[60]

Failure of ethanol to stimulate muscimol-induced ^{36}Cl$^-$ flux may represent a form of functional tolerance that offsets acute ethanol effects on this measure. In fact, as little as 5 minutes of *in vivo* ethanol exposure (4 g/kg, ip) appears to be sufficient completely to prevent the *in vitro* effect of ethanol, suggesting that this mechanism could underlie some type of acute functional tolerance.[1] A reduction in the magnitude of muscimol-evoked ^{36}Cl$^-$ flux after chronic ethanol treatment would seem more consistent with a compensatory change leading to rebound cellular hyperexcitability thought to be associated with physical dependence and the withdrawal syndrome. Lack of subsensitivity to muscimol in mouse cerebellum and its presence in rat cerebral cortex probably do not reflect a species difference, because both species express severe signs of ethanol withdrawal. There may be innate differences between the regulation of GABA$_A$ receptors in cerebral cortex and spinal cord and their regulation in the cerebellum, because only receptors in cerebral cortex and spinal cord exhibit increased ^{36}Cl$^-$ flux in the presence of ethanol alone. The degree of adaptive change in GABA$_A$ receptor efficacy could also depend on the relative magnitude of ethanol-induced depression of neural activity within the particular brain region. If so, greater change might be expected in the cerebral cortex, which appears more sensitive to ethanol than the cerebellum.

Electrophysiologic Recording of Ethanol and GABA Interaction

Various electrophysiologic recording techniques have also been used to examine the proposed interaction of ethanol with GABA. At present, there is no clear consensus about whether ethanol alters the regulation of neuronal excitability by GABA. Several studies using extracellular and intracellular recording techniques have suggested that iontophoretically applied or systemically administered ethanol can significantly enhance synaptic inhibition thought to be mediated by endogenous GABA; ethanol also has been reported to enhance the inhibitory effects of exogenously applied GABA.[10,12,36,41,45,49,88] Other investigations using these techniques as well as patch-clamp recording methods have not supported an ethanol-mediated increase in efficiency of $GABA_A$ receptor–transducer activity.[10,40,52,69,79] In contrast to the relatively consistent effects of ethanol and related sedative/hypnotics on biochemical $^{36}Cl^-$ flux described above, only barbiturates and benzodiazepines appear consistently to increase electrophysiologic measures of GABAergic neurotransmission.[5]

Electrophysiologic evaluation of the chronic effects of ethanol on GABAergic transmission has only recently begun. Preliminary results so far do not indicate a significant change in GABA-mediated hyperpolarizations in functionally tolerant and physically dependent animals. Postsynaptic potentials recorded intracellularly in CA1 pyramidal cells in ethanol-bathed, hippocampal slices from ethanol-dependent rats did not change as the ethanol concentration was lowered to simulate ethanol withdrawal.[14] Moreover, neither the efficacy nor the potency of baclofen, the $GABA_B$ agonist, to inhibit excitatory postsynaptic potentials (EPSPs) recorded from the CA1 region of hippocampal slices was changed in tissues from ethanol-dependent animals relative to ethanol-naive controls.[91] Clearly, additional studies about the reversible chronic effects of ethanol on neuronal responses to GABA are needed.

Ethanol-Induced Loss of GABAergic Inhibition

The results of studies of prolonged exposure to ethanol for several months suggest that there may be permanent reductions in inhibitory input to the dentate gyrus and hippocampal circuits.[18] Such changes appear to result, in part, from loss of small GABA-immunoreactive hippocampal neurons.[46] Such changes would seem an unlikely basis for the phenomenon of physical dependence and the withdrawal syndrome which rapidly dissipate in the absence of ethanol intoxication. However, repeated alcohol detoxification in humans has recently been correlated with an increased incidence of severe withdrawal signs, including seizures, perhaps as a result of a kindling-like phenomenon.[9] Electrical kindling of rat hippocampus leading to generalized clonic-tonic convulsions is also associated with loss of GABA-immunoreactive cells in the CA1 region.[42] Whether permanent loss of synaptic inhibition could result from adaptive pressures on GABAergic neurons and contribute to the development of the controversial disorder called "alcoholic epilepsy"[13] is speculative.

Postsynaptic Interactions

In summary, there is convincing evidence that ethanol enhances postsynaptic $GABA_A$ receptor responses. Studies of GABA-evoked $^{36}Cl^-$ flux consistently show that acute administration of ethanol increases activation of the GABA receptor; an effect that is rapidly lost during continued intoxication. Approximately one half of the researchers who have used electrophysiologic recording methods also report a GABAmimetic action of acute ethanol. The failure of other electrophysiologic studies to confirm this action and its rapid loss in biochemical preparations suggest that GABA receptor augmentation may not be the primary mechanism causing ethanol intoxication. Conclusions about the role of functional GABA receptor hypoactivity in ethanol dependence are premature due to the limited data available.

GABAergic NEUROPHARMACOLOGY OF ETHANOL DEPENDENCE

Differential Suppression of Withdrawal Signs

As previously described, suppression of various ethanol withdrawal signs by administering direct and indirect GABA agonists is consistent with the hypothesis that GABAergic hypoactivity plays a functional role in the ethanol withdrawal syndrome.[41] These data must be considered circumstantial rather than conclusive, however, because they do not directly demonstrate a GABAergic deficit in the ethanol-dependent animal. The fact that indirect-acting GABAmimetics that rely on accumulation of endogenous GABA suppress some aspects of the ethanol withdrawal syndrome suggests that sufficient presynaptic GABAergic reserve must exist in this condition to overcome any adaptive hypoactivity. Similarly, suppression of withdrawal signs by direct-acting agonists indicates that sufficient receptor reserve is still available. It is important to note that direct-acting GABA$_A$ agonists like muscimol, 4,5,6,7-tetrahydroisoxazolo-[5,4-c]pyridin-3-ol (THIP) as well as GABA do not block all ethanol withdrawal signs (See Fig. 10–1). Intracisternal injections of these agents in ethanol-dependent rats during ethanol withdrawal completely suppress susceptibility to sound-induced seizures at doses that have no effect on forelimb tremors, while ethanol and chlordiazepoxide at similar doses completely reverse both responses.[29] The GABA$_B$ agonist baclofen also fails to suppress withdrawal tremors in ethanol-dependent Rhesus monkeys.[80] However, progabide, a drug that can activate both GABA$_A$ and GABA$_B$ receptors, reduces forelimb tremors in rats at doses slightly larger than those blocking audiogenic seizures,[20] suggesting that simultaneous activation of both types of GABA receptors may be important in the mechanisms regulating tremor.

If GABA receptors are hypoactive after continuous ethanol exposure, a cross-tolerance to CNS depressant effects of direct-acting GABA agonists might also be expected. In this regard, the motor-impairing actions of THIP and muscimol were reduced in mice treated chronically with ethanol when compared to ethanol-naive controls.[54,77] However, the potency of muscimol to enhance anesthetic actions of ethanol was equally great in ethanol-tolerant and -naive rats.[55] Several reports suggest that the potency of indirect-acting GABAmimetics to stimulate dopamine turnover is blunted in ethanol-tolerant animals.[41] Thus, there is evidence of cross-tolerance between ethanol and GABAmimetics, but its presence may depend on the particular physiologic response that is being measured.

Neuroanatomic Correlates of GABAmimetic Action

A few attempts have been made to identify specific GABAergic synapses within neural circuits that might be involved in the expression of specific ethanol withdrawal responses. For example, activation of GABAergic receptors in the inferior

Figure 10–5. Blockade of ethanol-withdrawal-induced audiogenic seizures by microinjection of muscimol or baclofen (A) into or by electrolytic lesions (B) of the inferior colliculus. Rats were fed ethanol-containing liquid diets for 12 days to establish physical dependence. One week before the start of ethanol treatment, animals either were surgically implanted with indwelling cannula directed to the inferior colliculus or had electrolytic lesions placed in the medial geniculate body (MGB), inferior colliculus (IC), or sham operations. Seven hours after withdrawal of ethanol diets, rats in (A) were microinjected bilaterally (0.5 μl) with saline, muscimol, or baclofen. Susceptibility to audiogenicity seizures were evaluated 7.5 hours after withdrawal. (From Frye, GD, McCown, TJ, Breese, GR, et al,[24] with permission.)
*$p < 0.05$ when compared with saline-microinjected group or sham group as appropriate.

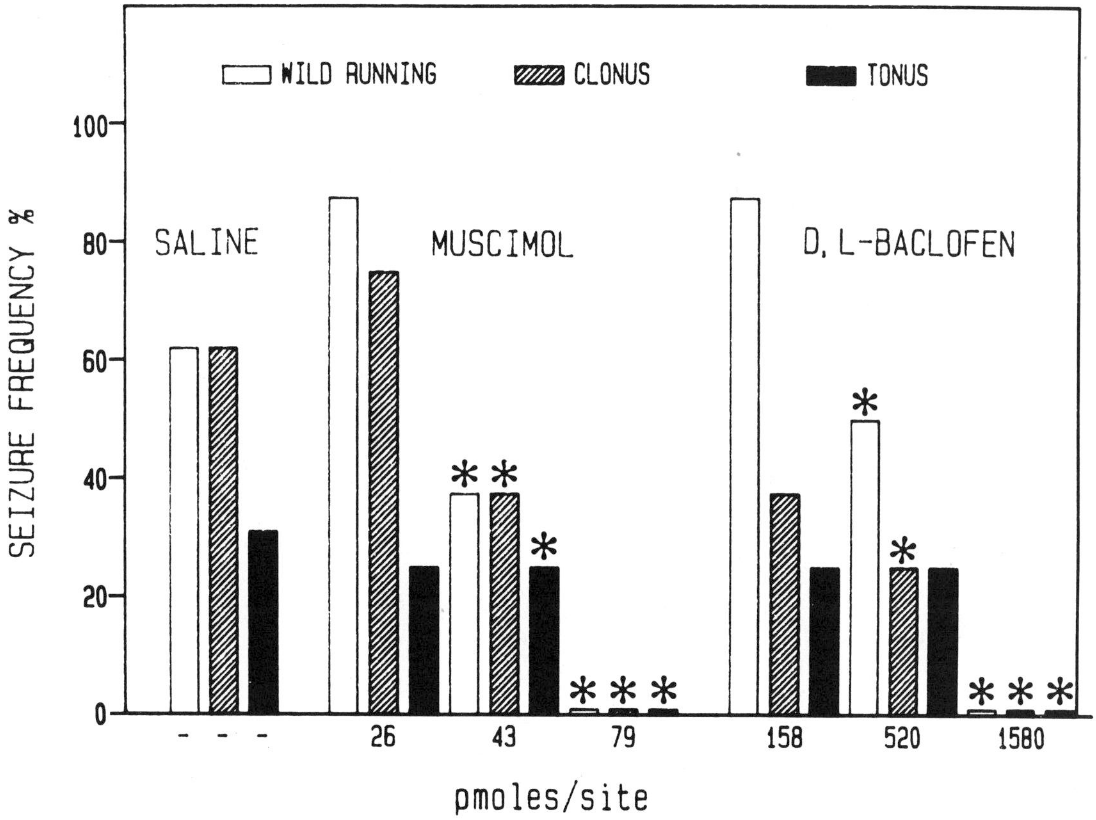
WILD RUNNING
CLONUS
TONUS
SALINE
MUSCIMOL
D, L-BACLOFEN
SEIZURE FREQUENCY %
100
80
60
40
20
0
- - -
26
43
79
158
520
1580
pmoles/site

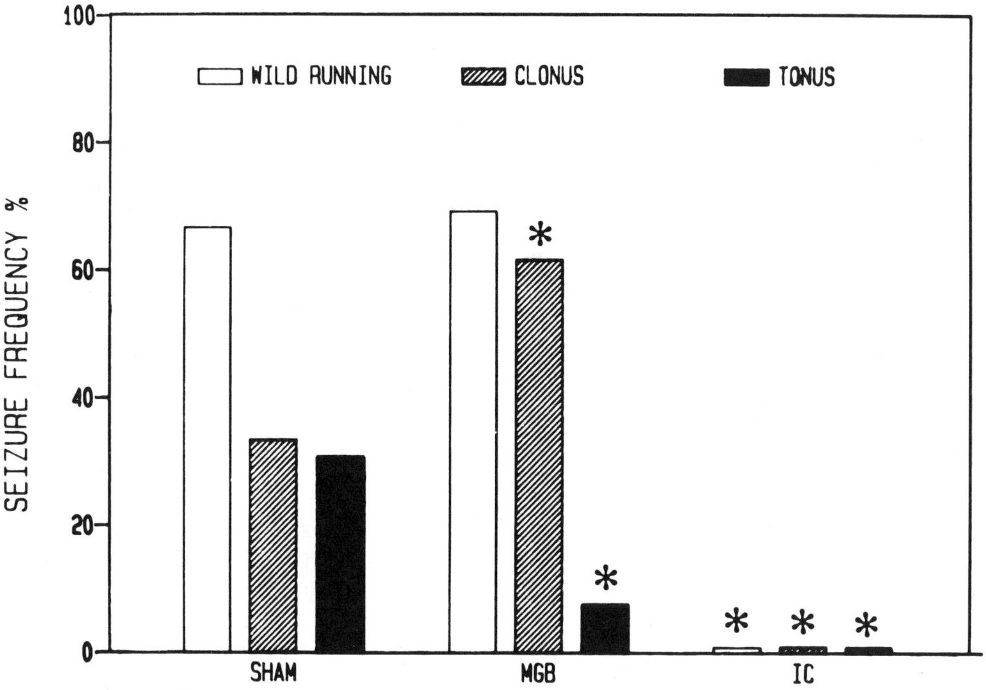
WILD RUNNING
CLONUS
TONUS
SEIZURE FREQUENCY %
100
80
60
40
20
0
SHAM
MGB
IC

colliculus with microinjections of either GABA_A or GABA_B agonists can completely suppress the susceptibility of ethanol-dependent rats to sound-induced seizures[24,28] (Fig. 10–5). Partial suppression of sound-induced withdrawal reactions is also observed after muscimol microinjection into the substantia nigra[27] and medial septal area.[28] Interestingly, GABAergic inhibition in the inferior colliculus and the substantia nigra also contribute to the genesis and modulation of sound-induced seizures in the epilepsy-prone rat.[21]

When the inferior colliculus of ethanol-naive rats is microinfused with bicuculline methiodide (BMI), picrotoxin, or Ro5-3663, which block the GABA_A receptor recognition site, GABA-gated chloride channel, or a benzodiazepine binding site, respectively, seizures are evoked that closely resemble sound-induced responses during ethanol withdrawal.[24,28] Infusion of BMI into the substantia nigra also induces seizures, but these responses are qualitatively distinct from both those evoked by inferior colliculus stimulation and those occurring in response to sound during ethanol withdrawal.[29] It is interesting that the inferior colliculus must be intact for ethanol-dependent rats to express sound-induced seizures. However, interruption of afferent auditory input to the auditory cortex does not appear to be the primary basis for this antagonism of audiogenic seizures, because lesions of the medial geniculate body do not block seizures.[28]

It is not clear whether development of postsynaptic GABAergic hypoactivity in the inferior colliculus during ethanol-induced physical dependence is responsible for susceptibility to audiogenic seizures. There is no increase in the sensitivity of the inferior colliculus to the convulsant effects of bilateral microinjections of the GABA_A antagonists, BMI, or picrotoxin in rats undergoing severe ethanol withdrawal relative to ethanol-naive controls.[23] However, baclofen microinjections into the inferior colliculus appear to be 10 times less potent in suppressing ethanol withdrawal-related audiogenic seizures[24] than in preventing running seizures induced by electrical stimulation of the inferior colliculus in ethanol-naive rats.[58] By contrast, muscimol appears equipotent in both tests. This fact suggests reduced efficiency of GABA_B receptors.

In contrast to the inferior colliculus, the substantia nigra appears to exhibit clear GABA_A subsensitivity after chronic ethanol treatment. The efficiency of intranigral microinjections of muscimol that dampen photic-stimulated field potentials recorded from several subcortical brain areas of ethanol-naive rats is significantly reduced in ethanol-dependent animals.[32] However, microinjections of muscimol into the substantia nigra still were sufficient to suppress the spontaneous EEG spiking observed during ethanol withdrawal in that structure. Intranigral muscimol injection also blocked spiking in the inferior colliculus but not spiking in the visual cortex.[31]

Overview of GABAergic Neuropharmacology

In summary, pharmacologic studies indicate that the expression of some ethanol withdrawal signs, but not others, can be suppressed by activating GABA receptors. For example, ethanol withdrawal seizures can be inhibited but tremor is resistant. Also, chronic ethanol treatment causes subsensitivity to GABA agonists under some conditions, but not under others. A relationship between the development of GABA receptor subsensitivity and the onset of ethanol functional tolerance or dependence has yet to be identified.

SUMMARY

Experimental evidence provides qualified support for the hypothesis that compensatory GABAergic hypoactivity plays a role in the development of functional tolerance to and physical dependence on ethanol. Under some circumstances, drugs thought to act at GABAergic synapses show cross-tolerance with ethanol and can substitute for ethanol to suppress some signs of the ethanol withdrawal syndrome. In particular, the findings that ethanol *in vitro* increases $GABA_A$ agonist-induced chloride flux but that this action is rapidly lost after ethanol treatment *in vivo* suggests that this change might be important in acute functional tolerance to ethanol. However, it is also clear that not all measures of ethanol tolerance or dependence are sensitive to GABAergic drugs. This fact might indicate that compensatory GABAergic hypoactivity is not a primary causative factor in the expression of these forms of ethanol-induced functional tolerance and physical dependence. Thus, the conclusion that there is no uniform underlying mechanism responsible for tolerance to ethanol[66] probably is valid for physical dependence as well. Eventually these results may prove positive from a clinical perspective because they may make it possible to develop drugs that selectively alleviate certain serious aspects of the withdrawal syndrome during detoxification without placing the patient at further risk of developing dependence on other nonspecific CNS depressants introduced during therapy for acute withdrawal.

References

1. Allan, A, and Harris, R: Acute and chronic ethanol treatments alter GABA receptor-operated chloride channels. Pharmacol Biochem Behav 27:665, 1987.
2. Allan, A, and Harris, R: Involvement of neuronal chloride channels in ethanol intoxication, tolerance and dependence. In Galanter, M (ed): Recent Developments in Alcoholism. Plenum Press, New York, 1987, p 313.
3. Balcom, R, Lenox, R, and Meyerhoff, J: Regional gamma-aminobutyric acid levels in rat brain determined after microwave fixation. J Neurochem 24:609, 1975.
4. Bannister, R, et al: Acute ethanol ingestion raises plasma gamma-aminobutyric acid levels in healthy men. Alcohol Alcoholism 23:45, 1988.
5. Barker, J and Owne, D: Electrophysiological pharmacology of GABA and diazepam in cultured CNS neurons. In Olsen, RW and Venter, JC (eds): Benzodiazepine/GABA Reception and Chloride Channels: Structural and Functional Properties. Alan R Liss, New York, 1986, p 135.
6. Bowery, N: Classification of GABA receptors. In Enna, SJ (ed): The GABA Receptors. Humana Press, New York, 1983, p 177.
7. Brailowsky, S, et al: Epileptogenic gamma-aminobutyric acid-withdrawal syndrome after chronic, intracortical infusion in baboons. Neurosci Lett 74:75, 1987.
8. Brailowsky, S, et al: The GABA-withdrawal syndrome: A new model of focal epileptogenesis. Brain Res 442:175, 1988.
9. Brown, M, et al: Alcohol detoxification and withdrawal seizures: Clinical support for a kindling hypothesis. Biol Psychiatry 23:507, 1988.
10. Carlen, P, et al: Enhanced neuronal K+ conductance: A possible common mechanism for sedative-hypnotic drug action. Can J Physiol Pharmacol 63:831, 1985.
11. Castellano, C and Pavone, F: Effects of ethanol on passive avoidance behavior in the mouse: Involvement of GABAergic mechanisms. Pharmacol Biochem Behav 29:321, 1988.
12. Celentano, J, Gibbs, T, and Farb, D: Ethanol potentiates GABA- and glycine-induced chloride currents in chick spinal cord neurons. Brain Res 455:377, 1988.
13. Chan, AWK: Alcoholism and epilepsy. Epilepsia 26:323, 1985.
14. Chestnut, T: The effect of ethanol withdrawal on GABA function in the in vitro hippocampus. Neuroscience Abstract 13: 510, 1987.
15. Daoust, M, et al: GABA transmission, but not benzodiazepine receptor stimulation, modulates ethanol intake by rats. Alcohol 4:469, 1987.
16. Dar, M and Wooles, W: GABA mediation of the central effects of acute and chronic ethanol in mice. Pharmacol Biochem Behav 22:77, 1985.
17. Dar, M, and Wooles, W: Striatal and hypothalamic neurotransmitter changes during ethanol withdrawal in mice. Alcohol 1:453, 1984.
18. Durand, D and Carlen, P: Decreased neuronal inhibition in vitro after long-term administration of ethanol. Science 224:1359, 1984.
19. Edmonds, H, Jr, et al: Neurochemical, electroencephalographic and behavioral correlates of ethanol withdrawal in the rat. Neurobehavioral Toxicology Teratology 4:33, 1982.
20. Fadda, F, et al: Suppression by progabide of ethanol withdrawal syndrome in rats. Eur J Pharmacol 109:321, 1985.
21. Faingold, C, et al: Inferior colliculus neuronal response abnormalities in genetically epilepsy-prone rats: Evidence for a deficit of inhibition. Life Sci 39:869, 1986.
22. Fonnum, F: Biochemistry, anatomy, and pharmacology of GABA neurons. In Meltzer, H (ed): Psychopharmacology: The Third Generation of Progress. Raven Press, New York, 1987, p 173.
23. Frye, G: Effect of chronic ethanol withdrawal on seizure responses to inferior colliculus microinjections of bicuculline methyliodide, picrotoxinin and kainic acid. Neuroscience Abstracts 13:510, 1987.
24. Frye, G, et al: GABAergic modulation of inferior colliculus excitability: Role in ethanol withdrawal audiogenic seizures. J Pharmacol Exp Ther 237:478, 1986; Erratum and additional information. J Pharmacol Exp Ther 238:1143, 1986.
25. Frye, G, and Breese, G: GABAergic modulation of ethanol-induced motor impairment. J Pharmacol Exp Ther 223:750, 1982.
26. Frye, G, and Fincher, A: Effect of ethanol on gamma-vinyl GABA-induced GABA accumulation in the substantia nigra and on synapto-

somal GABA content in six rat brain regions. Brain Res 449:71, 1988a.
27. Frye, G, and Fincher, A: Guinea pig ileum contractile responses to ethanol and GABA$_A$ agonist, 3-aminopropane sulfonic acid. Alcoholism Clinical Experimental Research 12:319, 1988b.
28. Frye, G, McCown, T, and Breese, G: Characterization of susceptibility to audiogenic seizures in ethanol-dependent rats after microinjection of gamma-aminobutyric acid (GABA) agonists into the inferior colliculus, substantial nigra or medial septum. J Pharmacol Exp Ther 227:663, 1983.
29. Frye, G, McCown, T, and Breese, G: Differential sensitivity of ethanol withdrawal signs in the rat to gamma-aminobutyric acid (GABA) mimetics: Blockade of audiogenic seizures but not forelimb tremors. J Pharmacol Exp Ther 226:720, 1983.
30. Goldstein, D: Pharmacology of Alcohol. Oxford University Press, New York, 1983, p 100.
31. Gonzalez, L, and Czachura, J: GABA modulation of electrical seizure discharge during ethanol withdrawal. Neuroscience Abstracts 13:511, 1987.
32. Gonzalez, L, and Czachura, J: Reduced electrophysiological responses to intranigral muscimol observed after chronic ethanol exposure. Alcoholism: Clinical Experimental Research 12:323, 1988.
33. Gonzalez, L, and Hettinger, M: Intranigral muscimol suppresses ethanol withdrawal seizures. Brain Res 298:163, 1984.
34. Gordis, E (ed): Sixth Special Report to the US Congress on Alcohol and Health. US Government Printing Office, Washington, DC, 1987.
35. Greenberg, D, et al: Ethanol and the gamma-aminobutyric acid-benzodiazepine receptor complex. J Neurochemistry 42:1062, 1984.
36. Groul, D: Ethanol alters synaptic activity in cultured spinal cord neurons. Brain Res 243:25, 1982.
37. Haefely, W: Biological basis of drug-induced tolerance, rebound, and dependence: Contribution of recent research on benzodiazepines. Pharmacopsychiatry 19:353, 1986.
38. Howerton, T and Collins, A: Ethanol-induced inhibition of GABA release from LS and SS mouse brain slices. Alcohol 1:471, 1984.
39. Howerton, T, Marks, M, and Collins, A: Norepinephrine, gamma-aminobutyric acid and choline reuptake kinetics and the effect of ethanol in long-sleep and short-sleep mice. Substance and Alcohol Actions/Misuse 3:89, 1982.
40. Huck, S, Gratzl, R, and Griessmayer, F: Ethanol has no effect on GABA-induced membrane currents in cells cultured from dissociated embryonic rat hippocampus. Neuroscience Abstract 13:65, 1987.
41. Hunt, W: The effect of ethanol on GABAergic transmission. Neurosci Biobehav Rev 7:87, 1983.
42. Kamphuis, W, et al: Decrease in number of hippocampal gamma-aminobutyric acid (GABA) immunoreactive cells in the rat kindling model of epilepsy. Exp Brain Res 64:491, 1986.
43. Krnjevic, K: Desensitization of GABA receptors. In Costa, E et al (eds): GABA and Benzodiazepine Receptors. Raven Press, New York, 1981, p 111.
44. Kuriyama, K, et al: Alcohol, acetaldehyde and salsolinol-induced alterations in function and metabolism of cerebral GABAergic and cholinergic neurons: Possible involvements in alcohol dependence and withdrawal. Prog Clin Biol Res 241:271, 1987.
45. Lee, R, Shimizu, N, and Woodward, D: Interactions of ethanol with glutamate and GABA evoked responses of cerebellar purkinje neurons. Neuroscience Abstracts 13:1132, 1987.
46. Lescaudron, L, et al: Effects of long-term ethanol consumption on GABAergic neurons in the mouse hippocampus: A quantitative immunocytochemical study. Drug Alcohol Depend 18:377, 1986.
47. Liljequist, S, Culp, S, and Tabakoff, B: Effect of ethanol on the binding of ^{35}S-T-butylbicyclophosphorothionate to mouse brain membranes. Life Sci 38:1931, 1986.
48. Liljequist, S and Engel, J: Effects of GABA and benzodiazepine receptor antagonists on the anti-conflict actions of diazepam or ethanol. Pharmacol Biochem Behav 21:521, 1984.
49. Liljequist, S and Engel, J: Effects of GABAergic agonists and antagonists on various ethanol-induced behavioral changes. Psychopharmacology 78:71, 1982.
50. Lloyd, K and Morselli, P: Psychopharmacology of GABAergic drugs. In Meltzer, HY (ed): Psychopharmacology: The Third Generation of Progress. Raven Press, New York, 1987, p 183.
51. Maloteaux, J, et al: GABA induces down-regulation of the benzodiazepine-GABA receptor complex in rat cultured neurons. Eur J Pharmacol 144:173, 1987.
52. Mancillas, J, Siggins, G, and Bloom, F: Systemic ethanol: Selective enhancement of responses to acetylcholine and somatostatin in hippocampus. Science 231:161, 1986.
53. Martin, W: Pharmacological redundancy as an adaptive mechanism in the central nervous system. Fed Proc 29:13, 1970.
54. Martz, A, Deitrich, R, and Harris, R: Behavioral evidence for the involvement of gamma-aminobutyric acid in the actions of ethanol. Eur J Pharmacol 89:53, 1983.
55. Mattucci-Schiavone, L and Ferko, A: Effect of muscimol on ethanol-induced central nervous system depression. Pharmacol Biochem Behav 27:745, 1987.
56. McBride, W, et al: Effects of ethanol on monoamine and amino acid release from cerebral cortical slices of the alcohol-preferring P line of rats. Alcoholism: Clinical Experimental Research 10:205, 1986.
57. McCown, T, Frye, G, and Breese, G: Evidence for site specific ethanol actions in the CNS. Alcohol and Drug Research 6:423, 1986.
58. McCown, T, Givens, B, and Breese, G: Amino acid influences on seizures elicited within the inferior colliculus. J Pharmacol Exp Ther 243:603, 1987.

59. Mereu, G and Gessa, G: Low doses of ethanol inhibit the firing of neurons in the substantia nigra, pars reticulata: A GABAergic effect? Brain Res 360:325, 1985.
60. Miller, L, et al: Chronic benzodiazepine administration: I: Tolerance is associated with benzodiazepine receptor downregulation and decreased gamma-aminobutyric acid$_A$ receptor function. J Pharmacol Exp Ther 246:170, 1988.
61. Mitchell, P and Martin, I: Is GABA release modulated by presynaptic receptors? Nature 274:904, 1978.
62. Morrow, A, et al: Chronic ethanol administration alters gamma-aminobutyric acid, pentobarbital and ethanol-mediated $^{36}Cl^-$ uptake in cerebral cortical synaptoneurosomes. J Pharmacol Exp Ther 246:158, 1988.
63. Murphy, J, et al: Effects of 250 mg% ethanol on monoamine and amino acid release from rat striatal slices. Brain Res Bull 14:439, 1985.
64. Newberry, N and Nicoll, R: Direct hyperpolarizing action of baclofen on hippocampal pyramidal cells. Nature 308:450, 1984.
65. Peinado, J, Collins, D, and Myers, R: Ethanol challenge alters amino acid neurotransmitter release from frontal cortex of the aged rat. Neurobiol Aging 8:241, 1987.
66. Pohorecky, L, Brick, J, and Carpenter, J: Assessment of the development of tolerance to ethanol using multiple measures. Alcoholism: Clinical Experimental Research 10:616, 1986.
67. Rani, V, et al: Acute and short term effects of ethanol on the metabolism of glutamic acid and GABA in rat brain. Neurochem Res 7:297, 1985.
68. Seilicovich, A, et al: Ethanol and hypothalamic GABAergic system. In Racagni, G and Donoso, A (eds): GABA and Endocrine Function. Raven Press, New York, 1986, p 209.
69. Siggins, G, Pittman, Q, and French, E: Effects of ethanol on CA$_1$ and CA$_3$ pyramidal cells in the hippocampal slice preparation: An intracellular study. Brain Res 414:22, 1987.
70. Simler, S, et al: Brain gamma-aminobutyric acid turnover rates after spontaneous chronic ethanol intake and withdrawal in discrete brain areas of C57 mice. J Neurochem 47:1942, 1986.
71. Squires, R, et al: [^{36}S]t-Butylbicyclophosphorothionate binds with high affinity to brain-specific sites coupled to gamma-aminobutyric acid-A and ion recognition sites. Mol Pharmacol 23:326, 1983.
72. Strong, R and Wood, W: Membrane properties and aging: In vivo and in vitro effects of ethanol on synaptosomal gamma-aminobutyric acid (GABA) release. J Pharmacol Exp Ther 229:726, 1984.
73. Supavilai, P and Karobath, M: Ethanol and other CNS depressants decrease GABA synthesis in mouse cerebral cortex and cerebellum in vivo. Life Sci 27:1035, 1980.
74. Suzdak, P, et al: Alcohols stimulate gamma-aminobutyric acid receptor-mediated chloride uptake in brain vesicles: Correlation with intoxication potency. Brain Res 444:340, 1988.
75. Syapin, P and Alkana, R: Chronic ethanol exposure increases peripheral-type benzodiazepine receptors in brain. Eur J Pharmacol 147:101, 1988.
76. Tabakoff, B and Hoffman, P: Biochemical pharmacology of alcohol. In Meltzer, HY (ed): Psychopharmacology: The Third Generation of Progress. Raven Press, New York, 1987, p 1521.
77. Taberner, P and Unwin, J: Behavioural effects of muscimol, amphetamine and chlorpromazine on ethanol tolerant mice. Proceedings of the British Pharmacological Society 74:276, 1981.
78. Takada, R, et al: Ethanol dissociates thiopental and GABA-receptor interaction. Neurochemistry International 10:71, 1987.
79. Tamborska, E and Marangos, P: Brain benzodiazepine binding sites in ethanol dependent and withdrawal states. Life Sci 38:465, 1986.
80. Tarika, J and Winger, G: The effects of ethanol phenobarbital, and baclofen on ethanol withdrawal in the rhesus monkey. Psychopharmacology 70:201, 1980.
81. Tehrani, M and Barnes, E, Jr: GABA down-regulates the GABA/benzodiazepine receptor complex in developing cerebral neurons. Neurosci Lett 87:288, 1988.
82. Thyagarajan, R and Ticku, M: The effect of in vitro and in vivo ethanol administration on [^{35}S]t-butylbicyclophosphorothionate binding in C57 mice. Brain Res Bull 15:343, 1985.
83. Ticku, M, Burch, T, and Davis, T: The interactions of ethanol with the benzodiazepine-GABA receptor-ionophore complex. Pharmacol Biochem Behav (Suppl 1)18:15, 1983.
84. Ticku, M and Kulkarni, S: Molecular interactions of ethanol with GABAergic system and potential of RO15-4513 as an ethanol antagonist. Pharmacol Biochem Behav 30:501, 1988.
85. Ticku, M, Lowrimore, P, and Lehoullier, P: Ethanol enhances GABA-induced $^{36}Cl^-$ influx in primary spinal cord cultured neurons. Brain Res Bull 17:123, 1986.
86. Wafford, K, Harris, R, and Dunwiddie, T: Chloride currents generated by injection of ethanol into xenopus oocytes. Society Neuroscience Abstracts 14:642, 1988.
87. Waldmeier, P, et al: Potential involvement of a baclofen-sensitive autoreceptor in the modulation of the release of endogenous GABA from rat brain slices in vitro. Naunyn Schmiedebergs Arch Pharmacol 337:289, 1988.
88. Wiesner, J, Henriksen, S, and Bloom, F: Ethanol enhances recurrent inhibition in the dentate gyrus of the hippocampus. Neurosci Lett 79:169, 1987.
89. Wixon, H and Hunt, W: Effect of acute and chronic ethanol treatment of gamma-aminobutyric acid levels and on aminooxyacetic acid-induced GABA accumulation. Substance and Alcohol Actions/Misuse 1:481, 1980.
90. Yang, J and Olsen, R: Gamma-Aminobutyric acid receptor binding in fresh mouse brain membranes at 22°C: Ligand-induced changes in affinity. Mol Pharmacol 32:266, 1987.
91. Frye, G, et al: Unpublished data.

CHAPTER 11

A. Leslie Morrow, Ph.D.
Peter D. Suzdak, Ph.D.
Steven M. Paul, M.D.

Ethanol and the GABA/Benzodiazepine Receptor Complex

The biochemical mechanisms underlying the intoxicating, anxiolytic, and sedative properties of ethanol and underlying the development of tolerance and the withdrawal syndrome are poorly understood. Ethanol shares with barbiturates and benzodiazepines several pharmacologic actions, including anxiolytic and sedative activity,[12,21,23] cross-tolerance, and cross-dependence.[4,22] Benzodiazepines and barbiturates effectively alleviate the withdrawal symptoms that occur after chronic ethanol administration,[57] suggesting that all three drugs may share a common mechanism of action. Considerable evidence supports the hypothesis that gamma-aminobutyric acid (GABA)-mediated neurotransmission is involved, at least in part, in the behavioral actions of ethanol.[17] Although ethanol has been shown to affect multiple neurotransmitter systems, including serotonin, norepinephrine, dopamine, and glutamate,[17] the role of these systems in mediating the behavioral effects of ethanol is unclear. By contrast, numerous behavioral studies suggest that GABA receptor activation mediates ethanol's effects. For example, it has been shown that GABAmimetic drugs ameliorate the symptoms of ethanol withdrawal, whereas GABA antagonists potentiate these symptoms.[13] Furthermore, electrophysiologic,[8,39] radioligand binding,[9,61,66,67] and behavioral studies[13,24,30] suggest similarities between ethanol, barbiturates, and benzodiazepines in augmenting GABAergic neurotransmission.

GABA is the most ubiquitous inhibitory neurotransmitter in the brain that interacts with a receptor containing recognition sites for benzodiazepines and barbiturates. These binding sites are linked allosterically to the GABA recognition site, and each site is involved directly or indirectly in the gating properties of an integral Cl^- channel. GABA-receptor-mediated activation of Cl^- conductance results in membrane hyperpolarization and decreased neuronal excitability.[52] Barbiturates and benzodiazepines have been shown to augment the activity of GABA via these specific recognition sites on the GABA receptor complex.[42] By contrast, ethanol interacts very weakly, if at all, with the recognition sites for benzodiazepines and barbiturates,[9,14] suggesting an indirect or non-receptor-mediated interaction of ethanol with the GABA receptor complex.

The most direct evidence that ethanol interacts with the GABA receptor complex to produce its pharmacologic effects comes from recent studies involving subcellular brain preparations and spinal cord cultured neurons,[2,33,49,54,63] where ethanol and other short-chain alcohols have been shown directly to stimulate[53,54] and potentiate GABA-receptor-mediated $^{36}Cl^-$ uptake.[2,33,53,54,63] Ethanol's direct effects are observed at concentrations well within the range observed in acute intoxication (20-60 mM), while subintoxicating concentrations augment muscimol or pentobarbital stimulation of $^{36}Cl^-$ uptake.[2,33,53,54,63] The action of alcohols in stimulating $^{36}Cl^-$ uptake in vitro appears to be mediated by the GABA-coupled Cl^- channel, because the effects are blocked by the specific GABA receptor antagonist bicuculline and by the Cl^- channel antagonist picrotoxin.[33,54] Moreover, the effects of short-chain alcohols on GABA-mediated Cl^- ion flux have been correlated with intoxication potencies in rats and with membrane/buffer partition coefficients.[53]

This chapter reviews the pharmacologic evidence that ethanol interacts with the GABA receptor Cl^- channel complex and that this interaction is antagonized selectively by the imidazobenzodiazepine, Ro15-4513. Also, data are presented that Ro15-4513 antagonizes certain, but not all, ethanol-induced behaviors at concentrations that do not cause intrinsic inverse agonist effects. Finally, we show that subsensitivity of GABA-receptor-mediated Cl^- flux results from chronic administration of ethanol and may explain ethanol tolerance, altered seizure sensitivity, and development of the withdrawal syndrome.

ETHANOL STIMULATION AND POTENTIATION OF GABA-RECEPTOR-MEDIATED Cl⁻ FLUX IN VITRO

Ethanol dose-dependently stimulates $^{36}Cl^-$ uptake into cerebral cortical synaptoneurosomes[53,54,56] and into cultured spinal cord neurons (Fig. 11-1).[33,63] Significant stimulation of $^{36}Cl^-$ uptake is observed at physiologically relevant concentrations (20-70 mM). These effects are biphasic; higher concentrations (>80 mM) cause diminished $^{36}Cl^-$ uptake. The ability of ethanol to increase Cl^- transport is qualitatively similar to that of the barbiturate pentobarbital, which also produces a biphasic concentration response curve (Fig. 11-1).

The ability of alcohols such as ethanol to induce a behavioral state of intoxication correlates with their membrane/buffer partition coefficients and membrane disordering properties.[32,50] Therefore, we investigated the ability of various short-chain alcohols to stimulate GABA-receptor-mediated Cl^- uptake in vitro at "intoxicating" concentrations and found that their potencies were highly correlated with intoxication potencies and membrane/buffer partition coefficents (Fig. 11-2). The stimulatory action of ethanol on Cl^- transport is almost certainly mediated by the GABA receptor complex since bicuculline and picrotoxin inhibit

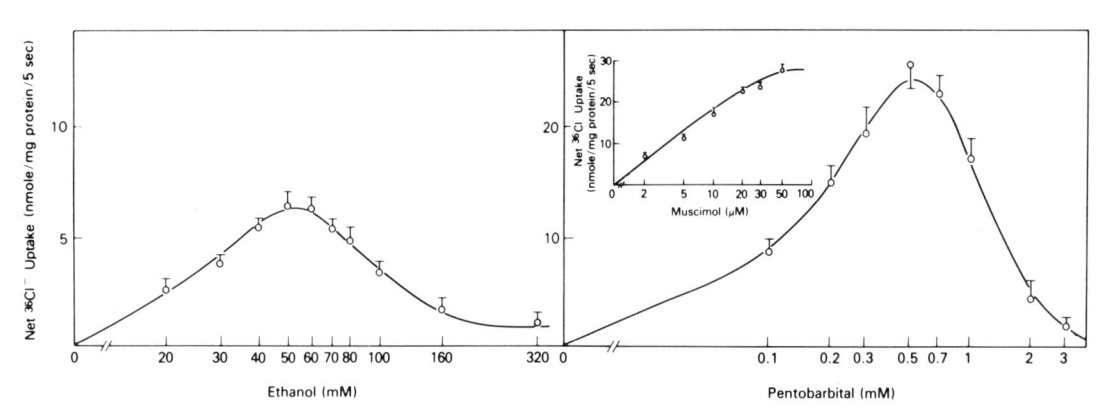

Figure 11-1. Concentration response curves for ethanol- and pentobarbital-stimulated $^{36}Cl^-$ uptake in rat cerebral cortical synaptoneurosomes. Ethanol (20-320 mM) or pentobarbital (0.1-3 mM) was incubated with 0.5 mCi of $^{36}Cl^-$ for 5 sec. Data shown are the mean ± SEM of 3 experiments, each conducted in quadruplicate. (Adapted from Morrow, et al,[36] p. 254.)

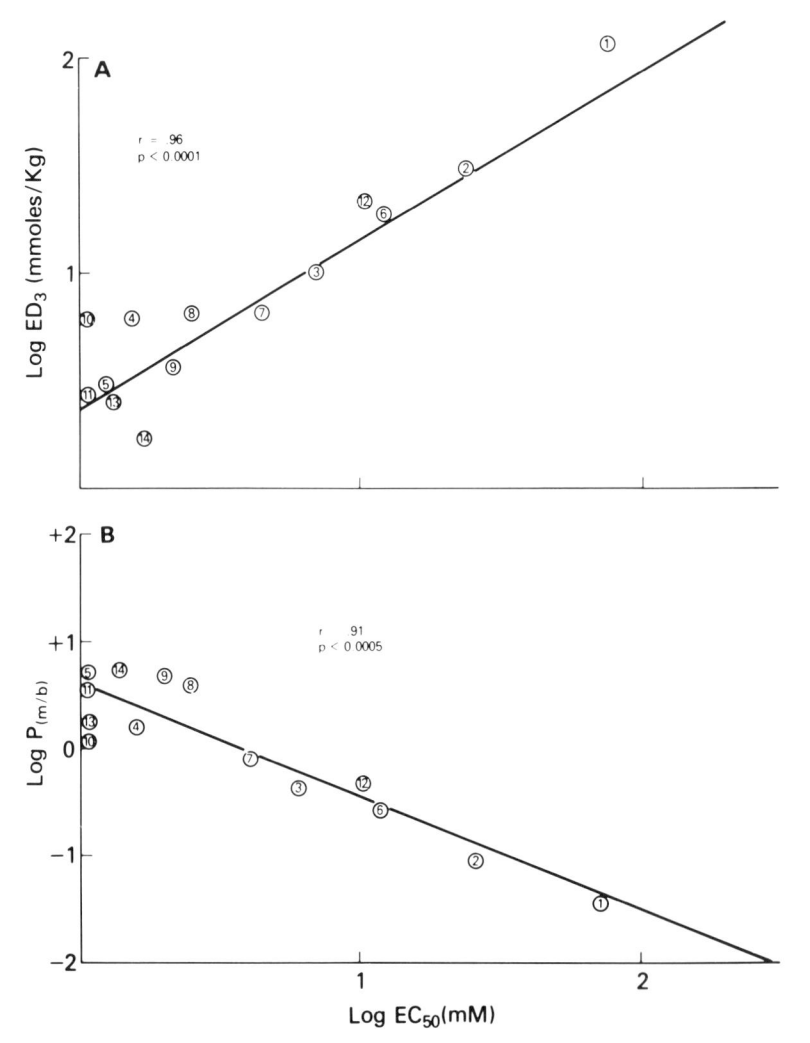

Figure 11-2. The effect of various short-chain alcohols on $^{36}Cl^-$ uptake into rat cerebral cortical synaptoneurosomes: correlation with their intoxication potencies (A) and membrane buffer partition coefficients (B). Individual EC_{50} values for alcohol stimulation of $^{36}Cl^-$ uptake were determined from concentration response curves using a minimum of 6 concentrations for each alcohol. Each point represents the log of mean EC_{50} determined in 3 separate experiments. Alcohols tested were: (1) methanol, (2) ethanol, (3) 1-propanol, (4) 1-butanol, (5) 1-pentanol, (6) 2-propanol, (7) 2-butanol, (8) 2-pentanol, (9) 3-pentanol, (10) isobutanol, (11) iso-amyl alcohol, (12) butanol, (13) t-amyl alcohol, (14) 2-methyl-2 pentanol. (A) Correlation between the log EC_{50} values for stimulation of $^{36}Cl^-$ uptake and their potencies in producing behavioral intoxication (r = 0.96, P < .0001, Pearson's product moment). Behavioral intoxication potencies were taken from McCreery and Hunt.[32] (B) Correlation between the log EC_{50} values for stimulation of $^{36}Cl^-$ uptake and their membrane buffer partition coefficients (r = 0.91, P < .0005, Pearson's product moment). (Adapted from Suzdak, et al,[56] p. 343.)

ethanol's effects.[54] These antagonists had similiar effects on GABA and pentobarbital stimulation of Cl^- flux.[54] Other neurotransmitter receptor antagonists, such as haloperidol, propranolol, verapamil, strychnine, clonidine, and phenoxybenzamine failed to alter ethanol-stimulated Cl^- flux.[54]

The ability of ethanol to directly stimulate Cl^- uptake is relatively weak compared with that of pentobarbital or GABA itself. Like barbiturates, however, ethanol has been shown to potentiate the effects of both GABA and pentobarbital at concentrations between 10-30 mM.[2,53] Ethanol (20 mM) had no effect on basal $^{36}Cl^-$

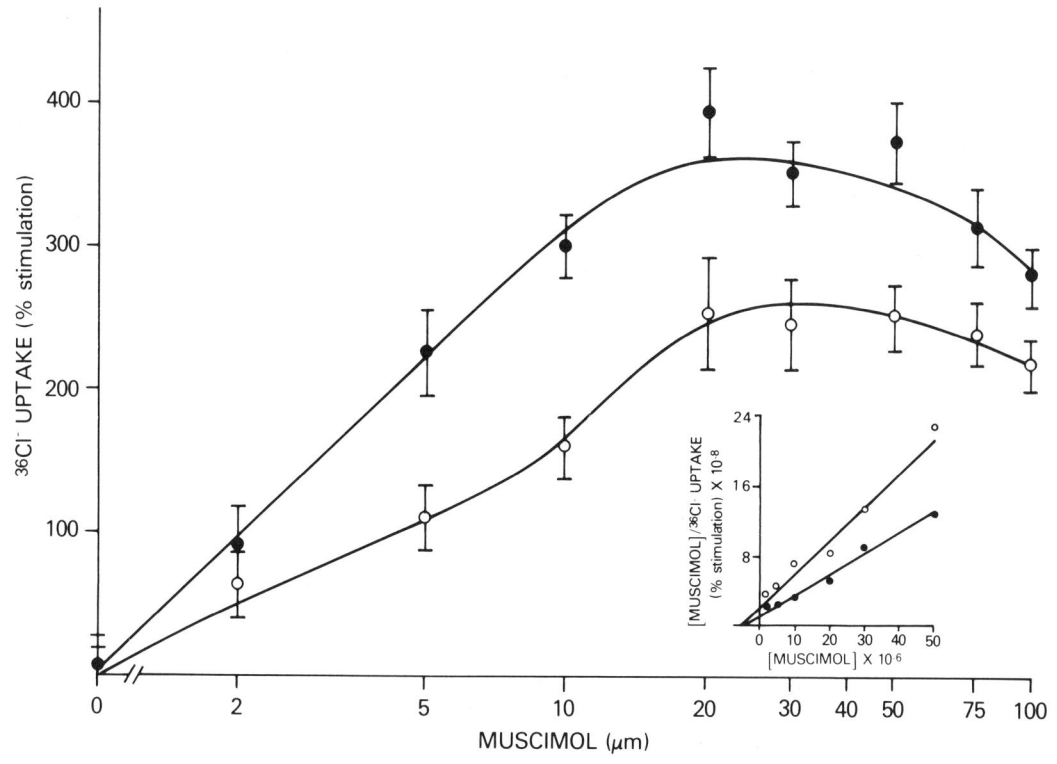

Figure 11–3. Ethanol potentiation of muscimol-stimulated $^{36}Cl^-$ uptake. Increasing concentrations of muscimol (2–100 mM) alone (○) or in combination with ethanol (20 mM) (●) were incubated with synaptoneurosomes and 0.5 mCi $^{36}Cl^-$ for 5 sec. *(Inset)* A Hanes-Woolf plot of the data indicates that ethanol increased the V_{max} for muscimol-stimulated $^{36}Cl^-$ uptake. The apparent K_m for muscimol was not significantly altered in the presence of ethanol. (Adapted from Suzdak, et al,[57] p. 4074.)

uptake, but greatly potentiated muscimol-stimulated $^{36}Cl^-$ uptake (Fig. 11–3). The potentiation of muscimol-stimulated $^{36}Cl^-$ uptake by ethanol appears to result from an increase in the V_{max} of muscimol-stimulated $^{36}Cl^-$ uptake rather than from a change in the apparent K_m.[53] Ethanol at subthreshold concentrations had a similar effect on pentobarbital stimulation of $^{36}Cl^-$ flux, except that ethanol altered both the apparent V_{max} and K_m.[39,49] The findings that relatively low concentrations of alcohol potentiate both GABA-receptor-mediated Cl^- flux,[2,33,53,63] and GABA-mediated electrophysiologic responses[39] and that higher (intoxicating) concentrations directly stimulate the GABA-coupled Cl^- channel, are consistent with previous findings that the actions of ethanol are blocked by bicuculline and picrotoxin.[7,23,24] These data suggest that the anxiolytic and intoxicating properties of ethanol may be mediated, in part, by their interaction with GABA receptors in the central nervous system (CNS).

Ro15-4513 BLOCKS ETHANOL STIMULATION OF GABAergic Cl^- FLUX *IN VITRO*

It has been shown that benzodiazepine agonists dose-dependently, stereospecifically, and reversibly potentiate GABA-mediated Cl^- flux in isolated cerebral cortex vescicles by altering the apparent K_m of muscimol stimulation.[36] Not surprisingly, benzodiazepine inverse agonists have been shown to inhibit muscimol-stimulated $^{36}Cl^-$ uptake by decreasing the apparent K_m for muscimol stimulation of Cl^- flux with no significant effect on the V_{max} (Table 11–1).[36] Therefore, we screened a series of benzodiazepine inverse agonists for their abilities to affect ethanol-stimulated $^{36}Cl^-$ uptake. Of the

Table 11–1. EFFECTS OF BENZODIAZEPINE AGONISTS, INVERSE AGONISTS AND ANTAGONISTS ON MUSCIMOL-STIMULATED $^{36}Cl^-$ UPTAKE *IN VITRO**

Drug	Potentiation or Inhibition of $^{36}Cl^-$ Uptake (nmol/mg Protein)	% Change
B_{10} (+) (1 mM)	7.44 ± 0.91	76
Diazepam (1 mM)	5.81 ± 0.51	59
Flurazepam (10 mM)	4.76 ± 0.37	49
Clonazepam (1 mM)	3.64 ± 0.54	37
Flurazepam (1 mM)	2.43 ± 0.26	25
Ro15-1788 (2 mM)	0.90 ± 0.17	9
Flurazepam (10 mM) + Ro 15-1788	0.50 ± 0.22	5
B_{10} (−) (1 mM)	0.14 ± 0.32	1
Flurazepam (10 mM) + CGS-8216 (2 mM)	0.10 ± 0.30	1
Ro 5-4864 (1 mM)	−1.46 ± 0.45	−15
β-CCE (5 mM)	−3.51 ± 0.26	−36
DMCM (5 mM)	−4.92 ± 0.24	−50

*Drugs were added simultaneously with $^{36}Cl^-$ and muscimol, and incubated for 5 sec. The mean stimulation by muscimol was 9.78 ± 0.92 nmol/mg protein. Potentiation or inhibition of muscimol stimulation represents the actual increase or decrease in $^{36}Cl^-$ uptake compared with the effect of muscimol alone. Data shown are mean ± SEM of 3–7 separate determinations. (Adapted from Morrow and Paul,[36] p. 304.)

benzodiazepine receptor ligands tested, the weak inverse agonist Ro15-4513 proved a very potent antagonist of ethanol-stimulated $^{36}Cl^-$ uptake.[56] At a concentration of 100 nM, Ro15-4513 completely antagonized ethanol-stimulated $^{36}Cl^-$ uptake *in vitro* (Fig. 11–4).[56] However, Ro15-4513 was ineffective in antagonizing pentobarbital- or muscimol-stimulated $^{36}Cl^-$ uptake at concentrations as high as 1 μM (Fig. 11–5). The ability of ethanol to potentiate GABA at subthreshold concentrations was also inhibited by Ro15-4513 (100 nM), but pentobarbital enhancement of muscimol-stimulated Cl^- flux was unaffected. These effects were

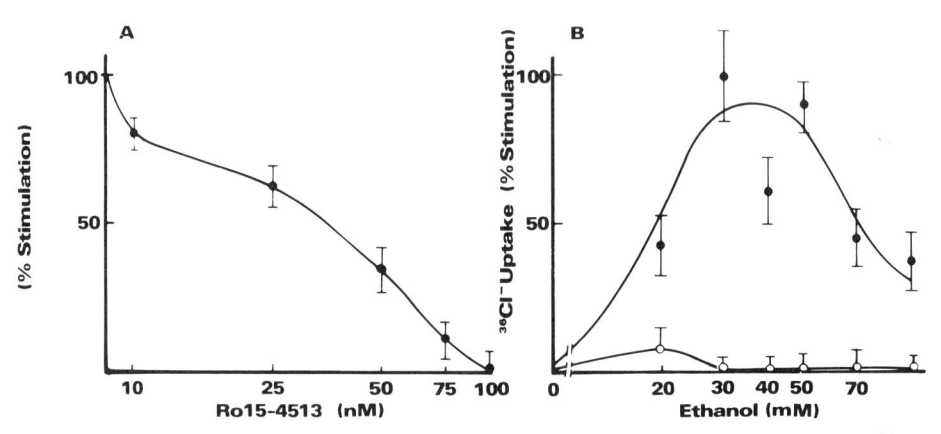

Figure 11–4. The effect of the imidazobenzodiazepine Ro15-4513 on ethanol-stimulated $^{36}Cl^-$ uptake into rat cerebral cortical synaptoneurosomes. (A) Various concentrations of Ro15-4513 (10–100 nM) were added to synaptoneurosomes 5 min before the addition of ethanol (50 mM) and $^{36}Cl^-$. The data shown represent the mean ± SEM of quadruplicate determinations from a typical experiment carried out 3 times with similar results. (B) The effect of various concentrations of ethanol alone (●) or in the presence of Ro15-4513 (100 nM) (○) on $^{36}Cl^-$ uptake into synaptoneurosomes. Ro15-4513 significantly decreased ethanol-stimulated $^{36}Cl^-$ uptake at all concentrations tested ($P < 0.01$, ANOVA followed by Newman-Keuls test). (Adapted from Suzdak, et al.[55])

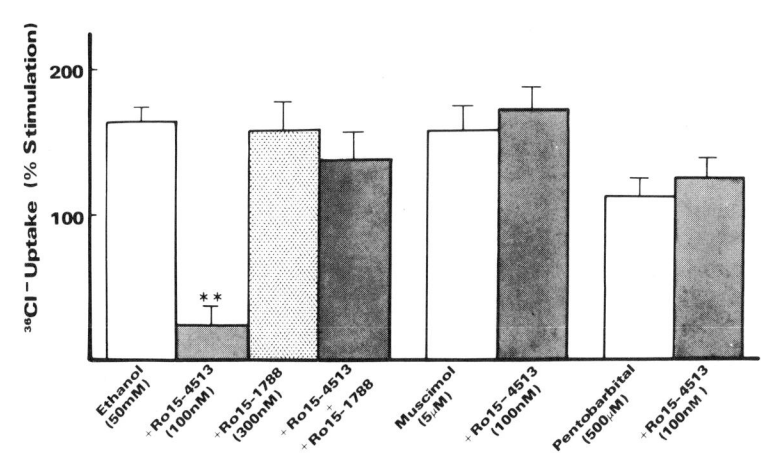

Figure 11-5. The effect of Ro15-4513 on ethanol- (50 mM), muscimol- (5 μM), and pentobarbital- (500 μM) stimulated $^{36}Cl^-$ uptake into rat cerebral cortical synaptoneurosomes. Ro15-4513 (100 nM) was added 5 min prior to the addition of $^{36}Cl^-$ and ethanol, muscimol, or pentobarbital. Ro15-1788 (300 nM) was added simultaneously with $^{36}Cl^-$ and ethanol. Data represent the mean and SEM of quadruplicate determinations from a typical experiment repeated 3 times with similar results. Ro15-4513 significantly blocked ethanol-stimulated $^{36}Cl^-$ uptake ($P < 0.01$, ANOVA followed by Newman-Keuls test). This effect was antagonized by the benzodiazepine receptor antagonist Ro15-1788. In contrast, Ro15-4513 had no effect on either muscimol- or pentobarbital-stimulated $^{36}Cl^-$ uptake. (Adapted from Suzdak, et al,[55] p. 1244.)

not shared by other inverse agonists, including FG-7142, DMCM, and βCCE, at concentrations up to 1 μM (Table 11-2), suggesting that the inhibitory effects of Ro15-4513 on ethanol-mediated Cl⁻ flux may be pharmacologically distinct from its inverse agonist effects. If the effects of Ro15-4513 in antagonizing the action of both high and low concentrations of ethanol were related to its weak inverse agonist properties, then other inverse agonists should also be effective ethanol antagonists. However, none of the other partial or full benzodiazepine receptor inverse agonists tested blocked ethanol-stimulated $^{36}Cl^-$ uptake. The effect of

Table 11-2. THE EFFECT OF BENZODIAZEPINE RECEPTOR ANTAGONISTS AND INVERSE AGONISTS ON ETHANOL-STIMULATED $^{36}Cl^-$ UPTAKE *IN VITRO*

Drug	Concentration	Ethanol Stimulated $^{36}Cl^-$ Uptake (% of ETOH Response)
Ethanol	50 mM	100 ± 12
+ DMCM	1 mM	116 ± 19
+ β-CCE	1 mM	97 ± 16
+ FG-7142	1 mM	103 ± 12
+ CGS-8216	1 mM	109 ± 29
+ Ro15-1788	1 mM	105 ± 26
+ Ro15-4513	0.1 mM	6 ± 12

*Synaptoneurosomes were incubated for 20 min at 30°C and the benzodiazepine antagonists and inverse agonists were added 5 min prior to the ethanol and $^{36}Cl^-$. Uptake was terminated after 5 sec. Each value represents the mean ± SEM of quadruplicate determinations from 3 separate experiments. Only Ro15-4513 significantly decreased ethanol-stimulated $^{36}Cl^-$ uptake ($P < 0.01$, ANOVA followed by Newman-Keuls test.) (Adapted from Suzdak, et al,[36] p. 1246.)

Ro15-4513 appears to be mediated by central benzodiazepine receptors because its ability to inhibit ethanol-stimulated $^{36}Cl^-$ uptake is blocked by the benzodiazepine receptor antagonists Ro15-1788 and CGS-8216.[56] The exact mechanism underlying the specificity of Ro15-4513 in blocking the neurochemical actions of ethanol remains an enigma, but appears to involve a unique interaction with the benzodiazepine recognition site coupled to the GABA receptor complex. Insofar as the ability of alcohols to stimulate Cl^- flux is correlated with their membrane disordering properties, ethanol's effects on Cl^- flux may involve an alteration in the lipid-protein microenvironment of the GABA receptor complex. Thus, ethanol and Ro15-4513 may interact at a common hydrophobic domain of this receptor complex in close proximity to the benzodiazepine recognition site. Further studies will be necessary to elucidate the exact mechanism(s) responsible for the pharmacologic activity of Ro15-4513.

Ro15-4513 ANTAGONIZES ETHANOL-INDUCED BEHAVIORS IN THE RAT

Ethanol is known to produce various behavioral effects. To determine whether Ro15-4513 can modify some of the behavioral actions of ethanol, we first examined its effects using the Vogel anticonflict paradigm and its effects on intoxication produced by ethanol. At relatively low doses, ethanol produces an anticonflict action in several species.[12,21] In the modified Vogel paradigm,[64] ethanol (1 mg/kg) resulted in significant increases in punished responding.[56] Pretreating rats with Ro15-4513 (3 mg/kg) completely blocked the anticonflict actions of ethanol in this paradigm. In contrast, the increased punished responding produced by pentobarbital (4 mg/kg) was not affected by pretreatment with Ro15-4513.[55,56] Ro15-4513 alone did not significantly affect punished or nonpunished responding in these experiments. In contrast, Britton, Ehlers, and Koob, and Koob, Braestrup, and Britton[6,20] found that Ro15-4513 effectively reversed the anticonflict action of ethanol, but only at doses that produced intrinsic effects, that is, doses that caused suppression of both punished and nonpunished responding. This discrepancy may be due to the different sensitivities of the behavioral paradigms employed to study the behavioral effects of ethanol. Specifically, the anticonflict paradigm employed by Suzdak and associates[56] was modified to detect a strong anticonflict effect of ethanol, whereas the paradigm employed by Britton, Ehlers, and Koob[6] was more sensitive to proconflict than anticonflict effects of ethanol.

Using the behavioral rating scale of Majchrowicz,[29] ethanol (1.5–2.5 mg/kg) has produced a level of intoxication in rats characterized by general sedation, staggered gait, and impaired righting reflexes.[26,29,56,58] Ro15-4513 dose-dependently (0.5–10 mg/kg) blocked ethanol intoxication,[26,56,58] and when administered after ethanol, reversed the intoxication produced by ethanol.[56] These effects were antagonized by Ro15-1788 and CGS-8216. The ability of Ro15-4513 to block ethanol-induced intoxication was not shared by other benzodiazepine inverse agonists, including β-CCE and FG-7142.[26,56] Moreover, cotreatment with Ro15-4513 and either FG-7142 or β-CCE[57] blocked the ability of Ro15-4513 to inhibit ethanol-induced intoxication. These data suggest that while Ro15-4513 must bind to the central benzodiazepine recognition site to produce its effect, the ability of Ro15-4513 to block ethanol's effects may not be mediated through this receptor. The fact that other benzodiazepine agonists and inverse agonists and antagonists do not produce the same effect on ethanol-induced behavior suggests that these effects of Ro15-4513 are mediated at a distinct site on the GABA receptor complex.

Higher doses of ethanol (7.5–15 g/kg) are lethal in rodents. Initially, it was reported that Ro15-4513 protected rats against the fatal effects of ethanol.[11] However, a subsequent study failed to confirm these findings.[40] The ability of Ro15-4513 to antagonize various other ethanol-induced behaviors has recently been investigated using concentrations of Ro15-

4513 that do not produce intrinsic inverse agonist effects. For example, Ro15-4513 has been shown to attenuate the discriminative stimulus effects of ethanol but not of pentobarbital in rats;[46] to block oral reinforcement in rats;[48] and to reduce ethanol intake in alcohol-preferring rats.[31] Ro15-4513 reversed the motor incoordination produced by ethanol in the rotorod[5,16] and horizontal wire[43] tests. These latter effects were also blocked by Ro15-1788.

In certain circumstances, Ro15-4513 has been ineffective in blocking ethanol's effects. Low doses of ethanol (1 g/kg) have been shown to increase generalized locomotor activity and wheel-running behavior in rats.[3,19] These behaviors are not antagonized by Ro15-4513. Other actions of Ro15-4513 have been attributed to its inverse agonist properties. For example, Ro15-4513 decreased the number of exploratory head-dippings in a holeboard test as well as the number of head-dips produced by ethanol.[25] However, both these effects are shared by other benzodiazepine inverse agonists.[25] In addition, it has been reported that Ro15-4513 induces seizures in animals that have been withdrawn from ethanol, although it fails to elicit withdrawal itself.[27] In squirrel monkeys, low doses of Ro15-4513 blocked the decrease in locomotor activity produced by ethanol. However, higher doses of Ro15-4513 (>1 mg/kg) caused severe tremors in these monkeys.[34] Thus, the inverse agonist properties of Ro15-4513 probably limit its clinical usefulness.[62]

Ro15-4513 reverses the anticonvulsant effects of ethanol against both bicuculline- and picrotoxin-induced seizures[28] at doses that are not proconvulsant.[41] However, at the same dose, Ro15-4513 failed to reverse the anticonvulsant effect of pentobarbital against picrotoxin-induced seizures.[28] These data also suggest that the ability of Ro15-4513 to antagonize ethanol's effects is specific and not dependent on its inverse agonist activity.

Ro15-4513 has intrinsic pharmacologic actions consistent with its classification as a partial inverse agonist at the central benzodiazepine receptor. These actions include anxiogenic and proconvulsant effects. However, Ro15-4513 is able to reverse many of the behavioral effects of ethanol at concentrations that do not cause intrinsic pharmacologic effects. This ability to reverse selectively certain effects of ethanol (intoxication, anxiolytic and reinforcing effects) suggests that the effects are mediated by the GABA/benzodiazepine receptor complex. Thus, the selectivity of Ro15-4513 seems to depend on both the dose employed and the nature of the behavioral paradigm. Clearly, Ro15-4513 is very useful to delineate the role of the GABA receptor complex in the behavioral effects of ethanol.

CHRONIC ETHANOL ADMINISTRATION DECREASES GABA-RECEPTOR-MEDIATED Cl⁻ FLUX *IN VITRO*

Tolerance to ethanol has been postulated to result from a compensatory decrease in GABA-mediated inhibition in the brain. Subsensitivity of the GABAergic system may also underlie some of the signs and symptoms of the ethanol withdrawal syndrome. Indeed, it has been shown that GABAmimetic drugs ameliorate ethanol withdrawal, whereas GABA antagonists potentiate these symptoms.[13] Alterations in endogenous GABA concentrations and turnover rates following chronic ethanol administration are inconsistent,[17] and probably cannot account for the manifestations of ethanol withdrawal. Radioligand binding studies with [^{3}H]muscimol,[65,66] [^{3}H]flunitrazepam,[9,45,67] and [^{35}S]TBPS[45,60] suggest that the density of GABA receptors in the CNS is not altered by chronic ethanol administration. However, there are suggestions that the sensitivity of both the GABA and benzodiazepine recognition sites to GABA itself may be decreased following chronic ethanol exposure.[10,61]

Tolerance to ethanol has been associated with cross-tolerance to barbiturates.[4,22] Because these drugs interact with the same receptor-coupled Cl⁻ channel,[42,52] any mechanism proposed to account for tolerance to ethanol might also be expected to cause a simultaneous change in sensitivity to barbiturates or GABA. It is interesting that both chronic

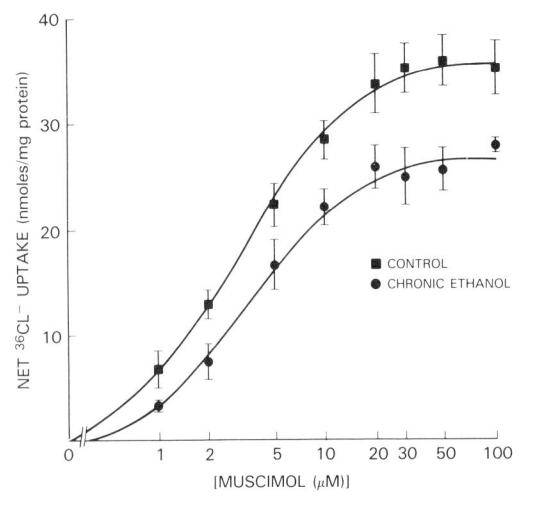

Figure 11-6. Chronic ethanol inhalation decreases the apparent V_{max} of muscimol-stimulated $^{36}Cl^-$ uptake in rat cerebral cortical synaptoneurosomes. Rats were administered ethanol by inhalation (25 mg/l ethanol vapor) for 14 days producing blood ethanol concentrations > 150 mg/%. Chronic ethanol administration produced a 26% decrease (P < 0.01) in the V_{max} of muscimol-stimulated $^{36}Cl^-$ uptake with no significant change in the EC_{50}. Data represent the mean ± SEM of five independent experiments, each conducted in quadruplicate. (Adapted from Morrow, et al,[38] p. 160.)

pentobarbital and ethanol exposure produce the same subsensitive response for GABA and pentobarbital-induced $^{36}Cl^-$ uptake in synaptoneurosomes prepared from cerebral cortices of rats.[35,38] This finding suggests that the synaptoneurosome preparation adequately reflects the overall adaptive responses of the CNS.

Chronic inhalation of ethanol produces physical dependence and tolerance. These effects were associated with a decrease in the sensitivity of the GABA/barbiturate receptor-coupled Cl^- channel when blood ethanol levels produced by the ethanol exposure were greater than 150 mg/dl.[35] This subsensitivity was characterized by a 26 percent decrease in the apparent V_{max} of muscimol-stimulated $^{36}Cl^-$ uptake following chronic ethanol inhalation (Fig. 11-6).[35] In a similar manner, pentobarbital-stimulated $^{36}Cl^-$ uptake was decreased by 25 percent after chronic ethanol treatment (Fig. 11-7). Direct stimulation of $^{36}Cl^-$ uptake by ethanol was not altered by this treatment, as demonstrated in the same tissue preparations where the decreases in muscimol- and pentobarbital-stimulated $^{36}Cl^-$ flux were observed.[35] However, the ability of ethanol (20 mM) to potentiate muscimol-stimulated $^{36}Cl^-$ uptake was completely lost in cerebral cortical synaptoneurosomes[35] and in cerebellar microsacs[1] following chronic ethanol treatment (Fig. 11-8). Thus, it appears that chronic ethanol exposure produces a cellular "desensitization" of the GABA-receptor-coupled Cl^- channel similar to the desensitization of GABA-mediated Cl^- flux that has been demonstrated *in vitro*.[49] The kinetics of the decrease in both muscimol- and pentobarbital-stimulated $^{36}Cl^-$ uptake together with the lack of effects of chronic ethanol ex-

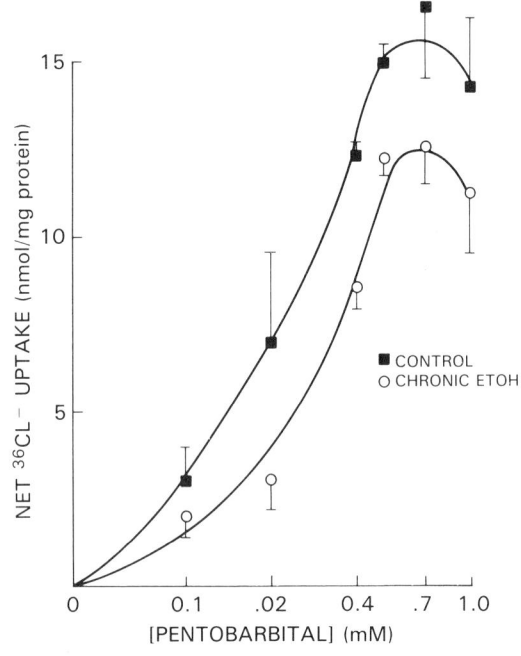

Figure 11-7. Pentobarbital stimulation of $^{36}Cl^-$ uptake is decreased following chronic ethanol administration. Ethanol was administered as in Figure 11-6, and $^{36}Cl^-$ uptake was measured in the same tissue preparations as those used for muscimol-stimulated $^{36}Cl^-$ uptake. The apparent V_{max} of pentobarbital-stimulated $^{36}Cl^-$ uptake was reduced by 25% (P < 0.05) and the EC_{50} was increased 39% (P < 0.05) after chronic ethanol exposure. Data represents the mean ± SEM of 4 independent experiments conducted in quadruplicate. (Adapted from Morrow, et al,[38] p. 160.)

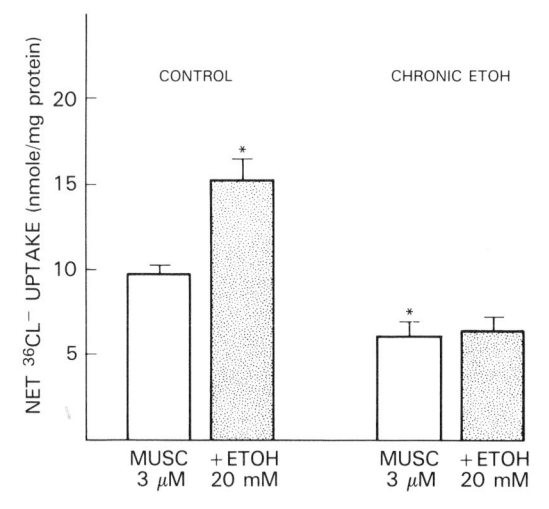

Figure 11-8. Ethanol potentiation of muscimol-stimulated $^{36}Cl^-$ uptake is abolished after chronic ethanol inhalation. Muscimol and ethanol (where indicated) were added simultaneously with $^{36}Cl^-$ and uptake was terminated after 5 sec. There was a small direct effect of ethanol (20 mM) in these experiments. This direct effect was subtracted from total uptake to obtain the net uptake which represents ethanol potentiation. There was a significant potentiation of muscimol stimulation in control synaptoneurosomes (55%, P < 0.001), whereas ethanol did not potentiate muscimol stimulation of $^{36}Cl^-$ synaptoneurosomes prepared from cerebral cortex of ethanol-treated rats. Muscimol (μM) stimulation of $^{36}Cl^-$ uptake was significantly decreased (40%, P < 0.01, n = 6) following chronic ethanol inhalation. (Adapted from Morrow, et al,[38] p. 161.)

posure on receptor density suggest that chronic ethanol administration alters the coupling of the agonist recognition sites to the open state of the Cl^- channel. Loss of the potentiating effect of ethanol on muscimol-stimulated $^{36}Cl^-$ uptake suggests that there may be an alteration in the membrane mechanism(s) by which ethanol interacts with the GABA receptor complex. Chronic ethanol administration has previously been reported to produce tolerance to the membrane disordering effects of ethanol.[18,47,59] However, the observation that there is no change in ethanol's direct effect on $^{36}Cl^-$ uptake suggests that the Cl^- channel itself is not altered in the cerebral cortex following chronic ethanol administration. Thus it appears that the mechanism(s) involved in ethanol's direct effects on $^{36}Cl^-$ flux may be distinct from the mechanisms responsible for its potentiation of GABA- or muscimol-stimulated $^{36}Cl^-$ uptake.

Several days after withdrawal from ethanol, the subsensitivity in both muscimol- and pentobarbital-stimulated $^{36}Cl^-$ uptake is completely reversed.[35] At this time, the signs of ethanol withdrawal have also remitted. This finding is consistent with our suggestion that subsensitivity of the GABA/barbiturate-receptor-coupled Cl^- channel may be involved in the ethanol withdrawal syndrome. Such a hypothesis may also account for the effectiveness of benzodiazepines in the clinical management of ethanol withdrawal reactions.[57] In ethanol withdrawal, benzodiazepines probably compensate for the reduced effectiveness of GABA on Cl^- flux by enhancing GABA's potency, as we have previously demonstrated in vitro.[36]

It has been postulated that tolerance to the behavioral effects of ethanol is related to reduced central GABAergic activity. The effects of chronic ethanol administration on GABA-mediated $^{36}Cl^-$ uptake are consistent with this hypothesis and may also provide a neurochemical explanation for these effects. The development of behavioral tolerance after chronic ethanol administration is characterized by a reduction in ethanol's effect in vivo.[15] This loss in sensitivity may be related in part to the loss of ethanol's ability to potentiate Cl^- flux in vitro. The fact that the direct stimulatory effects of ethanol are unaltered in ethanol-treated rats may account for the fact that the behavioral effects of ethanol are attenuated but not completely lost following chronic ethanol exposure in vivo. It is also highly unlikely that all the behavioral effects of ethanol are attributable to interactions with the GABA receptor complex. However, the fact that ethanol enhancement of muscimol-stimulated $^{36}Cl^-$ uptake is abolished in the same preparations where direct stimulation by ethanol is unaltered after chronic ethanol administration, is consistent with the behavioral characteristics of tolerance to those effects of ethanol that are mediated by this receptor complex. For example, the intoxicating and anxiolytic properties of ethanol appear to be specifically related to GABA receptor function, and these effects are not completely abolished when tolerance to ethanol has developed. We suggest, therefore, that a decrease in GABA-receptor-coupled Cl⁻ conductance may contribute to ethanol tolerance as well as the ethanol withdrawal syndrome.

SUMMARY

Historically, ethanol is one of the psychoactive drugs humans have used most frequently. The exact mechanisms of its anticonflict, anxiolytic, intoxicating, and sedative effects are still under avid and intense investigation. Although it is generally accepted that most of the pharmacologic actions of ethanol result from relatively nonspecific interactions with biologic membranes, there is increasing evidence for some specificity in at least some of the ethanol's actions. For example, the "nonspecific" membrane effects of ethanol appear to result in highly specific effects on the GABA receptor coupled Cl⁻ channel. These effects are blocked specifically and selectively by the novel alcohol antagonist, Ro15-4513. Indeed, the nonspecific membrane effects of alcohols may produce other specific alterations in the conformation of receptors coupled to adenylate cyclase and other ion channels[56] including excitatory amino acid (EAA)-receptor-coupled cation channels.[44] Studies on the physiologic significance of these effects and their relationship to ethanol-induced behavior will be highly valuable.

The development of a biochemical assay for studying the functional interactions of ethanol with the GABA/benzodiazepine Cl⁻ channel complex has been an important tool for elucidating ethanol's mechanism of action in the CNS. Determination of the molecular mechanisms by which ethanol interacts with this receptor complex and produces subsensitive responses to ethanol, pentobarbital, and GABA will be met with substantial interest. The identification of a selective antagonist of ethanol-mediated stimulation and potentiation of GABA-receptor-coupled Cl⁻ flux *in vitro*, as well as intoxication *in vivo*, raises hopes for the future development of a clinically effective ethanol antagonist.

References

1. Allan, AM and Harris, RA: Acute and chronic ethanol treatments alter GABA receptor operated chloride channels. Pharmacol Biochem Behav 27:665, 1987.
2. Allan, AM and Harris, RA: Gamma-aminobutyric acid and alcohol actions: Neurochemical studies of long sleep and short sleep mice. Life Sci 39:2005, 1986.
3. Bixler, MA and Lewis, MJ: The partial inverse benzodiazepine agonist Ro15-4513 potentiates ethanol induced suppression of wheel running in the rat. Neuroscience Abstracts 13:967, 1987.
4. Boisse, NN and Okamoto, M: Ethanol as a sedative-hypnotic: Comparison with barbiturate and non-barbiturate sedative-hypnotics. In Rigter, H and Crabbe, JC (eds): Alcohol Tolerance and Dependence. Elsevier, Amsterdam, 1980, p 265.
5. Bonetti, EP, Burkard, WP, and Gabl, M: A partial inverse benzodiazepine agonist Ro15-1788 antagonizes acute ethanol effects in mice and rats. Br J Pharmacol 86:463P, 1985.
6. Britton, KT, Ehlers, CL, and Koob, GF: Is ethanol antagonist Ro15-4513 selective for ethanol? Science 239:648, 1988.
7. Cott, J, et al: Suppression of ethanol-induced locomotor stimulation by GABA-like drugs. Arch Pharmacol 297:203, 1976.
8. Davidoff, RA: Presynaptic inhibition in an isolated spinal cord preparation. Arch Neurol 28:60, 1973.
9. Davis, WC and Ticku, MK: Ethanol enhances [³H]diazepam binding at the benzodiazepine-GABA receptor ionophore complex. Mol Pharmacol 20:287, 1981.
10. deVries, DJ, et al: Effects of chronic ethanol on the enhancement of benzodiazepine binding to mouse brain membranes by GABA. Neurochem Int 10:231, 1987.
11. Fadda, F, et al: Protection against ethanol mortality in rats by imidazobenzodiazepine Ro15-4513. Eur J Pharmacol 136:265, 1987.
12. Glowa, JR and Barrett, JE: Effects of alcohol on punished and unpunished responding. Pharmacol Biochem Behav 4:169, 1976.
13. Goldstein, DB: Alcohol withdrawal reactions in mice: Effects of drugs that modify neurotransmission. J Pharmacol Exp Ther 186:1, 1978.
14. Greenberg, DA, et al: Ethanol and the GABA-benzodiazepine receptor complex. J Neurochem 42:1062, 1984.
15. Harris, RA, et al: Physical properties and lipid composition of brain membranes from ethanol tolerant mice. Mol Pharmacol 25:401, 1984.
16. Hoffmann, PL, et al: Effect of an imadazobenzodiazepine, Ro15-4513, on the incoordination and hypothermia produced by ethanol and pentobarbital. Life Sci 41:611, 1987.

17. Hunt, WA: The effect of ethanol on GABAergic transmission. Neurosci Biobehav Rev 7:87, 1983.
18. Johnson, DA, et al: Adaptation to ethanol induced fluidization in brain lipid bilayers: Cross tolerance and reversibility. Mol Pharmacol 17:52, 1979.
19. Johnson, HT, June, HL, and Lewis, MJ: The effects of Ro15-4513 on generalized motor activity. Nueroscience Abstracts 13:967, 1987.
20. Koob, GF, Braestrup, C, and Britton, KT: The effects of FG-7142 and Ro15-1788 on the release of punished responding produced by chlordiazepoxide and ethanol in the rat. Psychopharmacology 90:173, 1980.
21. Koob, GF, Strecker, RE, and Bloom, F: Effects of naloxone on the anticonflict properties of alcohol and chlordiazepoxide. Alcohol Actions Misuse 1:447, 1980.
22. Le, AD, et al: Tolerance to and cross tolerance among ethanol, pentobarbital and chlordiazepoxide. Pharmacol Biochem Behav 24:93, 1986.
23. Liljequist, S and Engel, JA: The effects of GABA and benzodiazepine receptor antagonists on the anti-conflict action of diazepam or ethanol. Pharmacol Biochem Behav 21:521, 1984.
24. Liljequist, S and Engel, JA: Effects of GABAergic agonists and antagonists on various ethanol-induced behavioral changes. Psychopharmacology 78:71, 1982.
25. Lister, RG: The benzodiazepine receptor inverse agonists FG-7142 and Ro15-4513 both reverse some of the behavioral effects of ethanol in a holeboard test. Life Sci 41:1481, 1987.
26. Lister, RG, Durcan, MJ, and Linnoilla, M: Antagonism of the ataxic effects of ethanol by drugs acting at benzodiazepine receptors, the picrotoxin site and by alpha-2 receptor antagonists. Neuroscience Abstracts 14:522, 1988.
27. Lister, RG and Karanian, JW: Ro15-4513 induces seizures in DBA/2 mice undergoing ethanol withdrawal. Alcohol 4:409, 1987.
28. Lister, RG and Nutt, DJ: Interactions of the imidazodiazepine Ro15-4513 with convulsants. Br J Pharmacol 93:210, 1988.
29. Majchrowicz, E: Induction of physical dependence upon ethanol and the associated behavioral changes. Psychopharmacologia 43:245, 1975.
30. Martz, A, Deitrich, RA, and Harris, RA: Behavioral evidence for the involvement of gamma-aminobutyric acid in the action of ethanol. Eur J Pharmacol 89:53, 1983.
31. McBride, JW, et al: Effects of Ro15-4513, fluoxetine, and desipramine on intake of ethanol, water, and food on alcohol preferring and non-preferring lines of rats. Pharmacol Biochem Behav 30:1045, 1988.
32. McCreery, MJ and Hunt, WA: Physico-chemical correlates of alcohol intoxication. Neuropharmacology 17:451, 1978.
33. Mehta, G and Ticku, MK: Ethanol potentiation of GABAergic transmission in cultured spinal cord neurons involves γ-aminobutyric acid-gated chloride channels. J Pharmacol Exp Ther 246:558, 1988.
34. Miscek, KA and Weerts, EM: Seizures in drug treated animals. Science 235:1127, 1987.
35. Morrow, AL, et al: Chronic ethanol administration alters γ-aminobutyric acid, pentobarbital and ethanol-mediated $^{36}Cl^-$ uptake in cerebral cortical synaptoneurosomes. J Pharmacol Exp Ther 24:158, 1988.
36. Morrow, AL and Paul, SM: Benzodiazepine enhancement of γ-aminobutyric acid mediated chloride ion flux in rat brain synaptoneurosomes. J Neurochem 50:302, 1987.
37. Morrow, AL, Suzdak, PD, and Paul, SM: Benzodiazepine, barbiturate, ethanol and steroid hormone metabolite modulation of GABA-mediated chloride ion transport in rat brain synaptoneurosomes. In Biggio, G and Costa, E (eds): Chloride Channels and Their Modulation by Neurotransmitters and Drugs: Advances in Biochemical Psychopharmacology, Vol 45. Raven Press, New York, 1988, p 247.
38. Morrow, AL, Suzdak, PD, and Paul, SM: Chronic pentobarbital alters GABA/barbiturate receptor mediated ^{36}chloride uptake in cerebral cortical synaptoneurosomes. Neuroscience Abstracts 12:658, 1986.
39. Nestores, JN: Ethanol specifically potentiates GABA-mediated neurotransmission in the feline cerebral cortex. Science 209:708, 1980.
40. Nutt, DJ, et al: Ro15-4513 does not protect against the lethal effects of ethanol. Eur J Pharmacol 151:127, 1988.
41. Nutt, DJ and Lister, RG: The effect of the imidazobenzodiazepine Ro15-4513 on the anticonvulsant effects of diazepam, sodium pentobarbital and ethanol. Brain Res 413:193, 1987.
42. Olsen, RW: Drug interactions at the GABA receptor ionophore complex. Pharmacol Toxicol 22:245, 1982.
43. Polc, P: Interactions of partial inverse benzodiazepine agonists Ro15-4513 and FG-7142 with ethanol in rats and cats. Br J Pharmacol 86:465P, 1985.
44. Rabe, CS and Tabakoff, B: High sensitivity of NMDA-stimulated calcium uptake to inhibition by ethanol in primary cultures of cerebellar neurons. Neuroscience Abstracts 14:479, 1988.
45. Rastogi, SK, et al: Effect of chronic treatment of ethanol on benzodiazepine and picrotoxin sites on the GABA receptor complex in regions in the brain of the rat. Neuropharmacology 25:1179, 1986.
46. Rees, DC and Balster, RL: Attenuation of the discriminative stimulus properties of ethanol and oxazepam, but not pentobarbital, by Ro15-4513 in mice. J Pharmacol Exp Ther 244:592, 1988.
47. Rottenberg, H, Waring, A, and Rubin, E: Tolerance and cross tolerance in chronic alcoholics: Reduced membrane binding of ethanol and other drugs. Science 213:583, 1981.
48. Samson, HH, et al: Oral ethanol reinforcement in the rat: Effect of the partial inverse benzodiazepine agonist Ro15-4513. Pharmacol Biochem Behav 27:517, 1987.
49. Schwartz, RD, Suzdak, PD, and Paul, SM: GABA and barbiturate receptor mediated $^{36}Cl^-$ uptake in rat brain synaptoneurosomes: Evi-

dence for rapid desensitization of the GABA receptor coupled chloride ion channel. Mol Pharmacol 30:419, 1986.
50. Seeman, P: The membrane actions of anesthetics and tranquilizers. Pharmacol Rev 11:583, 1972.
51. Sellers, EM and Kalant, H: Alcohol intoxication and withdrawal. N Engl J Med 294:757, 1976.
52. Skolnick, P and Paul, SM: Molecular pharmacology of the benzodiazepines. Int Rev Neurobiol 23:103, 1982.
53. Suzdak, PD, et al: Alcohols stimulate GABA receptor mediated chloride uptake in brain vesicles: Correlation with intoxication potency. Brain Res 444:340, 1987.
54. Suzdak, PD, et al: Ethanol stimulates γ-aminobutyric acid receptor mediated chloride transport in rat brain synaptoneurosomes. Proc Natl Acad Sci USA 83:4071, 1986.
55. Suzdak, PD, et al: Response to K.T. Britton, et al. Science 239:649, 1988.
56. Suzdak, PD, et al: A selective imidazobenzodiazepine antagonist of ethanol in the rat. Science 234:1243, 1986.
57. Suzdak, PD, Paul, SM, and Crawley, JN: Effects of Ro15-4513 and other benzodiazepine receptor inverse agonists on alcohol induced intoxication in the rat. J Pharmacol Exp Ther 245:880, 1988.
58. Syapin, PJ, et al: Ethanol intoxication and benzodiazepine antagonists: Dose response of Ro15-4513 and FG-7142. Neuroscience Abstracts 14:521, 1988.
59. Taraschi, TF, et al: Membrane tolerance to ethanol is rapidly lost after withdrawal: A model for studies of membrane adaptation. Proc Natl Acad Sci USA 83:3669, 1986.
60. Thyagarajan, R and Ticku, MK: The effect of in vitro and in vivo ethanol administration of [^{35}S]-t-butylbicyclophosphorothionate binding in C57 mice. Brain Res Bull 15:343, 1985.
61. Ticku, MK and Burch, T: Alterations in γ-aminobutyric acid receptor sensitivity following acute and chronic ethanol treatments. J Neurochem 34:417, 1980.
62. Ticku, MK and Kulkami, SK: Molecular interactions of ethanol with GABAergic system and potential of Ro15-4513 as an ethanol antagonist. Pharmacol Biochem Behav 30:501, 1988.
63. Ticku, MK, Lowrimore, P, and Lehoullier, P: Ethanol enhances GABA induced ^{36}Cl$^-$ flux in primary spinal cord cultured neurons. Brain Res Bull 17:123, 1986.
64. Vogel, JR, Beer, B, and Clody, DE: A simple and reliable conflict procedure for testing anti-anxiety agents. Psychopharmacologia 21:1, 1971.
65. Volicer, L: GABA levels and receptor binding after acute and chronic ethanol administration. Brain Res Bull 5:809, 1980.
66. Volicer, L and Biagioni, TM: Effect of ethanol administration and withdrawal on benzodiazepine receptor binding in the rat brain. Neuropharmacology 21:283, 1982.
67. Volicer, L and Biagioni, TM: Effect of ethanol administration and withdrawal on GABA receptor binding in rat cerebral cortex. Alcohol Actions Misuse 3:31, 1982.

John P. J. Pinel, Ph.D.
Michael J. Mana, Ph.D.
C. Kwon Kim, Ph.D.

CHAPTER 12

Development of Tolerance to Ethanol's Anticonvulsant Effect on Kindled Seizures

Ethanol tolerance and ethanol withdrawal effects are widely presumed to be different manifestations of the same physiologic adaptations. The physiologic adaptations that underlie the development of tolerance to ethanol's effects are presumed to result in withdrawal symptoms, opposite to these effects, once the ethanol is eliminated from the body.[6,10] Proponents of this view make two important predictions about the etiology of ethanol withdrawal seizures: first, that ethanol is a potent anticonvulsant agent, and second, that tolerance develops to ethanol's anticonvulsant effect.

Although there have been numerous demonstrations of ethanol's anticonvulsant actions, until recently there have been few documented attempts to study the development of tolerance to them, despite the fact that such studies may be the key to understanding the etiology of ethanol withdrawal seizures—and hence to treating and preventing them.

Our recent success in the study of tolerance to ethanol's anticonvulsant effect is largely attributable to the adaptation of the kindling model to study the phenomenon. Accordingly, we first review early attempts to study tolerance to ethanol's anticonvulsant effect. Then we describe the kindling model and discuss its advantages and disadvantages. Finally, we review our recent studies of tolerance to ethanol's anticonvulsant effect and discuss the effect-dependency theory of tolerance, which our studies support.

EARLY STUDIES

The first report of the development of tolerance to the anticonvulsant effects of ethanol[8] was the following abstract published in 1949 by Allan and Swinyard:[2]

> After determination of the normal electroshock convulsive seizure threshold, ethyl alcohol was given daily for 20 weeks via stomach tube to a group of white rats. Dosage ranged from 1,000 to 4,000 mg per kilogram of body weight. Similar measurements were made in untreated controls.
>
> The first dose [intubation] of alcohol raised the electroshock seizure threshold from 20% in animals receiving 1,000 mg per kilogram to virtually 100% increase in animals receiving 4,000 mg per kilogram. Following this initial increase a progressive daily decrease occurred until at the end of the third week electroshock seizure threshold was within a normal range. The dose was doubled at the third week and again at the sixth week (maximum dose

8,000 mg per kilogram); this time, however, the maximal elevation of seizure threshold was 20% and 10% respectively. The electroshock seizure threshold of the controls decreased approximately 25% during the first 8 weeks and thereafter remained approximately constant.... (p 419).

Although it was published only in abstract form, the Allan and Swinyard study has been widely cited. Less widely cited have been three studies published in the 1960s and 1970s that failed to confirm their conclusion that tolerance develops to ethanol's anticonvulsant effect. Zarrow, Pawlowski, and Denenberg[39] failed to observe any tolerance to the anticonvulsant effects of ethanol added to the drinking water of their subjects (5 percent or 10 percent solutions) on electroshock seizure thresholds—even after 157 days. McQuarrie and Fingl[24] found no evidence of tolerance to ethanol's anticonvulsant effects on electroshock seizures in mice given alcohol (2 g/kg) by gavage every 8 hours for 14 days. Finally, Chen[4] failed to observe tolerance to ethanol's anticonvulsant effects on audiogenic seizures after 8 days of exposure to ethanol (1.5 g/kg, intraperitoneal [IP]) administered twice per day. Accordingly, by the early 1980s, there was good theoretical reason to believe that tolerance developed to the anticonvulsant effect of ethanol, but the empirical evidence for this hypothesis was hardly overwhelming: one positive report and three negative.

THE KINDLING MODEL AND ETHANOL'S ANTICONVULSANT EFFECT

In 1983, Pinel and colleagues[27] argued that the paucity and inconsistency of earlier studies of tolerance to ethanol's anticonvulsant effect were largely a consequence of the lack of an effective method for studying the subject. They devised a new approach that focused on assessing ethanol's anticonvulsant effect on kindled seizures.

In the broad sense of the term, *kindling* refers to a progressive increase in the motor seizures elicited by a series of periodic convulsive treatments. But in the narrow sense, *kindling* refers to Goddard, McIntyre, and Leech's[9] observation that periodic (e.g., once every 24 hours) low-intensity electrical brain stimulation that initially elicits no convulsive response may gradually come to elicit mild convulsive responses (e.g., head twitches) that progressively increase in intensity with each stimulation until each stimulation elicits a generalized clonic motor convulsion. Although many sites in the brain can be kindled, the amygdala kindles particularly rapidly and reliably and has thus been the preferred stimulation site. Although kindling has been reported in many species, rats have been the most common subjects (see McNamara[23] or Racine[33]).

When assessing anticonvulsant drug effects, kindled seizures have three important advantages over experimental seizures induced by traditional methods. The three most common traditional methods—electroconvulsive shock, pentylenetetrazol (PTZ), and audiogenic stimulation—all elicit convulsions that are extremely variable in form and duration, are difficult to measure, and are often associated with subject injury and fatality. This last problem is particularly serious in studies of tolerance in which anticonvulsant effects are repeatedly assessed in the same subjects,[2] because any systematic change in the apparent anticonvulsant actions of a drug is always confounded by the progressive debilitation and attrition of those subjects experiencing the most severe seizures. In contrast, kindled rats remain healthy and easy to handle for the duration of an experiment and fatalities are extremely rare. Moreover, in well-kindled rats, it is possible to elicit motor seizures that vary little from subject to subject in either form or duration, and baselines can be established in individual animals that display almost no fluctuation from stimulation to stimulation.[27] The importance of such long-term stability in the study of the development of tolerance to ethanol's anticonvulsive effect is obvious, and the stereotyped nature of kindled motor seizures makes the measurement of their intensity a relatively simple matter.

Phases of the Kindling Model

The kindled-seizure model that we use to study the development of tolerance to ethanol's anticonvulsant effect typically involves four phases.

PHASE I: KINDLING

Each rat is first kindled by a series of brief, low-intensity stimulations (1 second, 400 microamps, 60 Hz) through a bipolar stimulation electrode implanted in the amygdala. A regimen of 45 stimulations, administered 3/day, 5 days/week, with at least 2 hours between consecutive stimulations, has been both effective and convenient. Initially there is no behavioral response to each stimulation, but by the end of the kindling phase virtually all rats with accurately implanted electrodes respond to each stimulation with a generalized clonic motor seizure.

PHASE II: BASELINE

Once the rats are kindled, their responses to a series of stimulations delivered according to the schedule that will be used during the treatment phase of the experiment are determined. Most of our studies have employed a bidaily (once every 48 hours) stimulation schedule. Because the amount of time since the last stimulation is an important determinant of the severity of kindled motor seizures, it is important that the interstimulus intervals be regular for the baselines to stabilize.[9,25] We typically administer at least five baseline stimulations. A saline injection is administered 1 hour prior to the last one (the saline baseline test) to establish the baseline with which the effects of the drug injections can be compared.

It is possible to measure the intensity of a kindled motor seizure in a variety of ways. One method is to rate the seizure on an ordinal scale according to its topography (Table 12–1).[28,34] By the end of the baseline phase, most subjects respond to each stimulation with a class 5 or a class 6 motor seizure. Those that do not are dropped from the experiment at this point—they nearly always prove to have faulty or misplaced electrodes. Once the rats have been kindled to the class 6 stage, their responses to each stimulation become very stable, and it is at this point that they can be used most effectively to study the effects of anticonvulsants. But this is not the endpoint of kindling: after several hundred stimulations, there is a further increase in the severity of the elicited motor seizures and the rats begin to display spontaneous motor seizures.[28]

Although motor seizure class is perhaps the most common measure of kindled-seizure intensity, it has the disadvantage of being only an ordinal scale. We have found that the duration of the forelimb clonus component of each motor seizure correlates well with seizure class and various other measures of seizure severity, and it has the advantage of being a continuous ratio scale. Moreover, its consistency is impressive: in study after study

Table 12–1. ORDINAL SCALE FOR RANKING THE SEVERITY OF KINDLED SEIZURES IN RATS

Seizure Class Required	Convulsive Response	Approximate Number of Amygdaloid Stimulations
1	Facial clonus	3
2	Facial clonus with rhythmic head nodding	6
3	Facial clonus; head nodding; forelimb clonus	9
4	Facial clonus; head nodding; forelimb clonus; rearing	12
5	Facial clonus; head nodding; forelimb clonus; rearing; and one falling episode	15
6	Facial clonus; head nodding; forelimb clonus; multiple sequences of rearing and falling	25
7	All of the above with a running fit	300
8	Any of the above with tonus	340
Spontaneously recurring motor convulsions		350

we have found the mean duration of forelimb clonus on the saline baseline test to be within a second or two of 40 seconds, and the baseline duration of seizures in individual rats is almost always within 7 seconds of this value.

Phase III: Treatment

During the treatment phase, the stimulation regimen established during the baseline phase is maintained. Ethanol is administered to each experimental subject, most often by IP injections.

Phase IV: Tolerance Test

Following the treatment phase all subjects receive a test injection of the drug, and their tolerance to its anticonvulsant effects is assessed. The test dose of ethanol is usually 1.5 g/kg IP in a 25 percent solution administered 1 hour before the test stimulation.

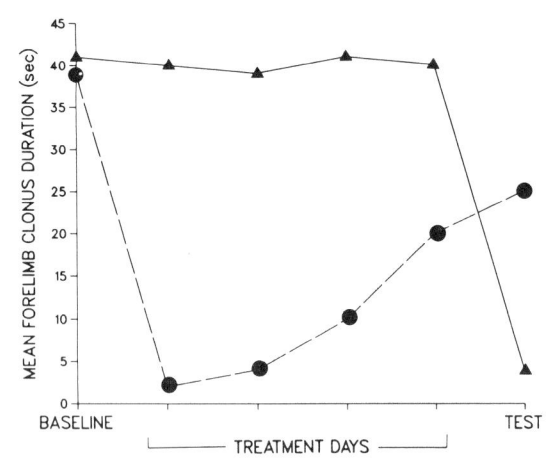

Figure 12–1. The development of tolerance to ethanol's anticonvulsant effect. Kindled rats receiving ethanol (●) demonstrated significant tolerance on the test day, whereas rats receiving saline (▲) did not.

Shortcomings

The kindling model is not without its shortcomings for studying tolerance to the effects of anticonvulsants. Three shortcomings exist. One is the amount of time and effort required to prepare each subject for the treatment phase of an experiment. The surgery, kindling, and baseline phases require about 5 weeks in total. The second is that the necessity of maintaining a regular schedule of stimulations makes it difficult to adapt the model to certain kinds of experimental designs. The third is that there can be a modest amount of subject loss due to inaccurate electrode placement or infection resulting in rejected electrode assemblies. However, these shortcomings are far outweighed by the kindling model's reliability, sensitivity, safety, and control.

TOLERANCE TO THE ANTICONVULSANT EFFECT OF ETHANOL ON KINDLED SEIZURES

The first demonstration of tolerance to ethanol's anticonvulsant effect since Allan and Swinyard's 1949 abstract was published in 1983 by Pinel and associates.[27] Subjects in two treatment groups were stimulated at 24-hour intervals during the baseline and treatment phases of the experiment. During the first 4 treatment days the subjects in the ethanol group received injections of ethanol (1.5 g/kg, IP) twice each day, once 12.5 hours before each stimulation and once 0.5 hours before. The subjects in the saline group received equal volumes of isotonic saline. On the test day, all subjects received injections of alcohol 12.5 and 0.5 hours before the tolerance test stimulation. Figure 12–1 shows that the treatment dose of ethanol initially blocked the seizures normally elicited in the subjects by amygdaloid stimulation and that significant tolerance to this effect developed in the ethanol subjects over the 5 days of alcohol exposure.

DRUG-EXPOSURE AND DRUG-EFFECT THEORIES OF FUNCTIONAL DRUG TOLERANCE

There are two different perspectives on functional drug tolerance: the drug-exposure view and the drug-effect view. Although the drug-exposure view is rarely explicitly stated, it is implicit in most discussions and studies of drug tolerance. It is simply that exposure of the nervous system to a drug is the critical factor in developing tolerance to the drug's effects. From this perspective, the question of whether a drug's effects will manifest themselves is inexorably linked to the question of drug exposure—the possibility that the two may be considered as separate factors is excluded. This oversight represents the basis for what we have called the effect-dependent theory of drug tolerance. From this perspective, drug tolerance is not a consequence of drug exposure *per se;* instead it is an adaptation to the expression of the drug's effects on the ongoing activity of an organism's nervous system—if these effects are not manifested, tolerance cannot develop.

The distinction between the drug-exposure and drug-effect perspectives on functional tolerance can be illustrated with reference to another, better understood form of functional adaptation: the adaptation that occurs to the disruptive effects of visual displacement on visuomotor coordination.[32] When a subject first wears displacing prisms that shift his or her visual world a few degrees to one side, visuomotor coordination is severely disturbed, but after some experience with the prisms, the subject adapts (*i.e.*, becomes tolerant) to the visual displacement and visuomotor coordination returns to normal. What is the factor that leads to this adaptation? Is it exposure to displaced vision (a theory analogous to the drug-exposure theory of tolerance) or is it the experience of the disruption of visuomotor coordination (a theory analogous to the drug-effect theory of tolerance)? The evidence overwhelmingly supports the latter view. Little adaptation develops to the effects of displacing prisms in subjects that do not perform visuomotor tasks while wearing them: it is the experience of the disruptive effects of the prisms on the performance of visuomotor tasks that is critical to the development of tolerance to this effect.[11,35]

CONTINGENT TOLERANCE TO THE ANTICONVULSANT EFFECT OF ETHANOL

Support for the drug-effect theory of drug tolerance comes from reports of contingent drug tolerance. The term *contingent tolerance* was first used in 1971 by Carlton and Wolgin[3] in reference to their observation that tolerance to the anorectic effects of amphetamine did not develop in rats that were not allowed to eat during periods of amphetamine exposure. They adopted this term to emphasize that the development of tolerance was contingent on the repeated experience of the criterion drug effect—in their study the anorectic effect of amphetamine.

This response contingency is an important factor in the development of tolerance to a variety of other drug effects. Rats have been reported not to develop tolerance—or at least not to develop it as rapidly[18]—to: 1) the disruptive effects of ethanol on maze or treadmill running, unless they are allowed to run while intoxicated;[4,18,38] 2) the anorectic effects of quipazine, unless they are allowed to eat while under its influence;[36] 3) the effect of delta-9-tetrahydrocannabinol on lever pressing, unless they are allowed to lever press in the drugged state;[22] 4) the analgesic effects of morphine[15] or ethanol,[12–14] unless the analgesic effects of these drugs are repeatedly experienced; and 5) the hypothermic effect of ethanol, unless they are repeatedly allowed to experience this effect.[1] Similarly, tolerance does not develop to the ethanol-produced acceleration in the decay of postsynaptic potentiation in the abdominal ganglion of Aplysia unless the presynaptic terminal is stimulated in the presence of ethanol.[37] Most recently, Pinel, Pfaus, and Christenson[30] have shown that the development of tolerance to the disruptive effects of alcohol on male sexual behavior is greater when male rats have an opportunity to copulate during periods of ethanol exposure.

The first evidence that tolerance to ethanol's anticonvulsant effect is contingent on the repeated expression of the anticonvulsant effect came from a follow-up to the 1983 study of Pinel and colleagues.[27] In a second experiment reported in the same paper, it was shown that kindled rats that were not stimulated during the treatment phase did not develop tolerance to ethanol's anticonvulsant effect. In this experiment, kindled rats were stimulated once every five days to estab-

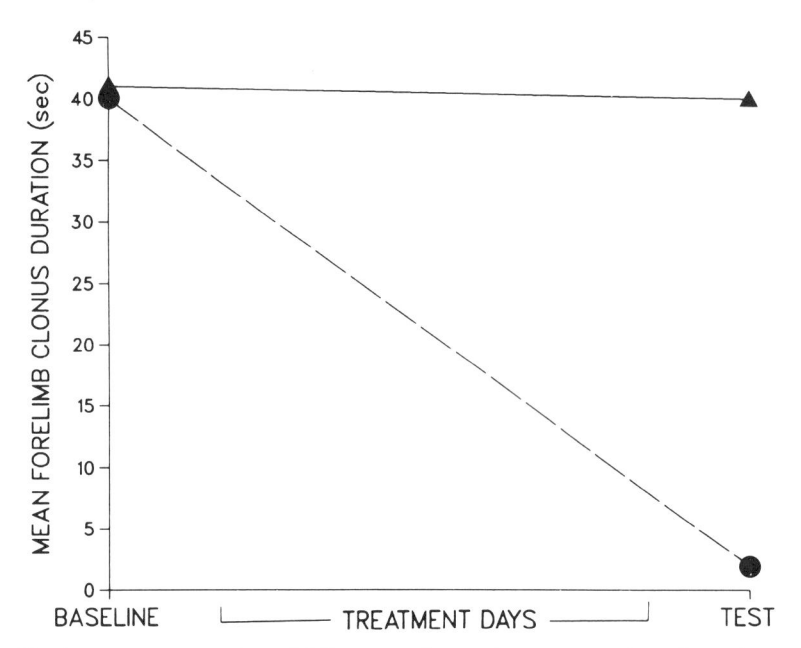

Figure 12–2. Simple exposure to ethanol fails to produce tolerance to ethanol's anticonvulsant effects. Kindled rats that received daily ethanol injections during a five-day stimulation-free period (●) displayed no tolerance; this cannot be due to a baseline shift as there was no change in the forelimb clonus duration in the rats from the saline controls (▲).

lish a five-day-interval pretreatment baseline. Immediately after the last baseline stimulation, the subjects in the alcohol group received the same five-day regimen of ethanol injections used in the first experiment. The last injection occurred 0.5 hour before the next scheduled stimulation, which permitted a test for tolerance to ethanol's anticonvulsant effect. The results of this second experiment are readily apparent in Figure 12-2. Although exactly the same schedule of ethanol injections was administered as in their first experiment, Pinel and colleagues[27] found no evidence of tolerance; the test injection of ethanol almost completely suppressed forelimb clonus (compare Figs. 12-1 and 12-2) in both the ethanol group and in a control group that had received saline injections during the treatment phase. The only difference between the two experiments was that in the first experiment, subjects were stimulated during the periods of ethanol exposure in the treatment phase.

The strongest support for the view that the development of tolerance to a particular drug effect depends on the repeated manifestation of that effect comes from studies using the before-and-after design.[17] Before-and-after experiments involve two groups of subjects. During the treatment phase, subjects in one group receive the drug *before* each test (e.g., before each convulsive stimulation) so that the effect of the drug (e.g., the anticonvulsant effect) can be repeatedly manifested. Subjects in the other group receive the drug *after* each test so that the drug effect cannot be manifested. On the tolerance test, both groups of subjects receive the drug before the test (e.g., the stimulation) so that the effects of the drug on test performance in the two groups can be compared. In such experiments, evidence of greater tolerance in the "before" subjects must be attributable to the drug-effect contingency during the treatment phase because the two groups do not differ in their exposure to either the drug or the test.

Pinel and colleagues[27] conducted a before-and-after experiment to confirm the inference drawn from a comparison of their first two experiments. After establishing a bidaily (once every 48 hour), stimulation baseline, kindled rats were assigned to either an ethanol-before-stimulation group or an ethanol-after-stimulation group. The subjects in both of these groups were then stimulated six more times on the bidaily schedule. The alcohol-before-stimulation subjects were intubated with ethanol (4.5 g/kg in a 30 percent solution) 1.5 hours before each stimulation and a comparable volume of isotonic saline 1.5 hours afterwards. The alcohol-after-stimulation subjects received the same intubations but in the reverse order, that is, the saline before each stimulation and the alcohol after. On the test trial, the rats in both groups were challenged with an IP injection of ethanol (1.5 g/kg in a 25 percent solution, as in the first two experiments) 1.5 hours before the post-treatment test stimulation.

The initial anticonvulsant effect of ethanol, the lack of tolerance development in the ethanol-after-stimulation group, and the substantial tolerance in the ethanol-before-stimulation group are all readily apparent in Figure 12–3. Clearly, the contingency between convulsive stimulation and ethanol exposure plays a major role in the development of tolerance to ethanol's anticonvulsant effects.

Next to the sizable effect of the drug-effect contingency, perhaps the most notable result of Pinel and colleagues'[27] before-and-after experiment was that there was no evidence of tolerance in the ethanol-after-stimulation group: ethanol exposure alone produced no detectable tolerance. The major purpose of two follow-up experiments by these investigators[29] was to demonstrate tolerance to the anticonvulsant effect of ethanol on kindled seizures in the ethanol-after-stimulation condition. They hypothesized that tolerance might develop in the ethanol-after-stimulation condition if they exposed the subjects to higher doses of ethanol (first experiment) or to more administrations of ethanol (second experiment) than those used in the earlier experiment. In the first experiment, rats in three "before" and three "after" conditions received an intubation of 2 g/kg of ethanol, 5 g/kg of ethanol, or saline either 1 hour before or 1 hour after convulsive stimulation on

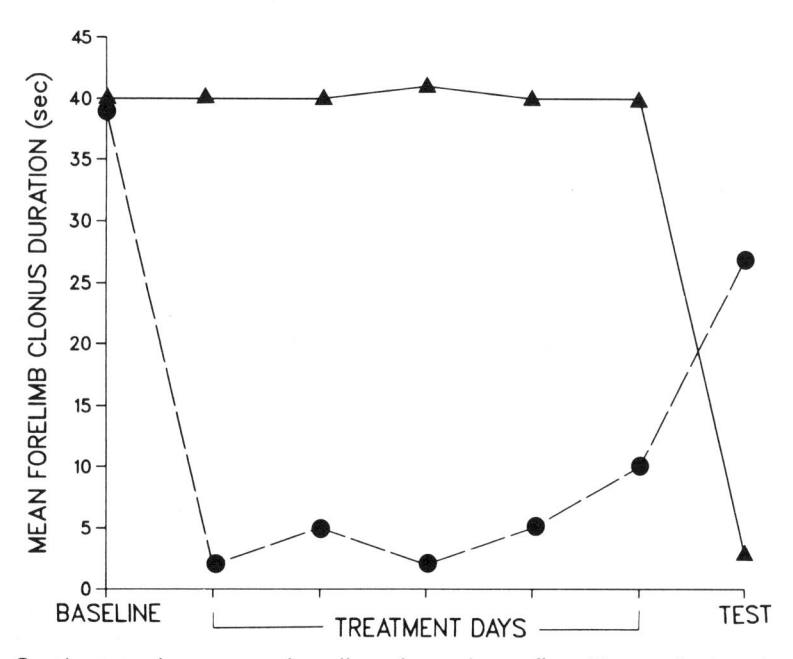

Figure 12–3. Contingent tolerance to ethanol's anticonvulsant effect. The rats in the ethanol-after-stimulation group (▲) demonstrated no tolerance on the test day. In contrast, the rats in the ethanol-before-stimulation group (●) demonstrated significant tolerance, even though they had received the same number and dose of ethanol injections during the treatment phase.

each of five bidaily (once every 48 hours) tolerance-development trials. In the second experiment, rats in three "before" conditions and three "after" conditions received 5, 10, or 20 intubations of ethanol (2 g/kg) on the same bidaily schedule. The results of both these experiments provided strong support for the drug-effect theory of tolerance; all five ethanol-before-stimulation groups developed substantially more tolerance than did their ethanol-after-stimulation controls. Although there was a hint of tolerance in the ethanol-after-stimulation groups, in no case did it achieve statistical significance.[29] Mana, Pinel and Lê[21] subsequently showed that if many (i.e., 20) high-dose (i.e., 5 g/kg) intubations are administered daily (rather than bidaily), tolerance to ethanol's anticonvulsant effect on kindled seizures developed in the absence of a drug-effect contingency; however, it is clear that the response contingency is an important factor in developing tolerance to ethanol's anticonvulsant effect.

GENERALITY OF CONTINGENT TOLERANCE TO ANTICONVULSANT DRUG EFFECTS

During the last 2 years, the kindling model has been used to study the development of tolerance to the anticonvulsant effects of four other anti-epileptic drugs: pentobarbital, diazepam, sodium valproate, and carbamazepine. Each drug was tested in a before-and-after experiment similar to those used to demonstrate contingent tolerance to ethanol's anticonvulsant effect, and in each case the tolerance was shown to be contingent on the occurrence of the drug effect. In each case, tolerance development was almost complete in the drug-before-stimulation condition, and there was little or no evidence of tolerance in the drug-after-stimulation condition.[19,26] Kim, Pinel, and Roese[16] recently showed that cross-tolerance is also contingent on the repeated expression of the drug effect. Only rats exposed to pentobarbital on a drug-before-stimulation regimen subsequently displayed cross-tolerance to the anticonvulsant effect of ethanol; pentobarbital-after-stimulation subjects displayed no cross-tolerance. The same proved true of a transfer of tolerance in the other direction: only rats from an ethanol-before-stimulation group displayed cross-tolerance to pentobarbital's anticonvulsant effect.

CONTINGENT DISSIPATION OF TOLERANCE TO ETHANOL'S ANTICONVULSANT EFFECT

What factors influence the dissipation of tolerance to ethanol's anticonvulsant effect? According to traditional views, the cessation of ethanol exposure should lead to a monotonic decline in tolerance to the effects of alcohol. However, our discovery of the major role played by the drug-effect contingency in the development of tolerance to ethanol's anticonvulsant effect suggested that it might also play a major role in its decline.

To test this hypothesis, kindled rats were rendered tolerant to ethanol's anticonvulsant effect in the usual way, that is, by bidaily ethanol injections (1.5 g/kg, IP), each followed 1 hour later by a convulsive amygdaloid stimulation. They were then assigned to one of six different treatment conditions. The six groups differed in terms of their treatment during a 14-day retention interval. The rats in two groups received an ethanol injection either 1 hour before or 1 hour after each of six bidaily stimulations. Two other groups were treated similarly except that saline rather than alcohol was injected. The rats in a fifth group received the bidaily ethanol injections but no brain stimulations, whereas those in the remaining group received neither stimulation nor ethanol during the retention interval. A single tolerance test was administered to all subjects at the end of the 14-day retention interval. This test was identical to the trials used to induce the development of tolerance; all subjects were stimulated 1 hour after receiving the standard 1.5 g/kg ethanol test injection.

It is clear from Figure 12–4 that the dissipation of tolerance to ethanol's anticonvulsant effect over the 14-day retention

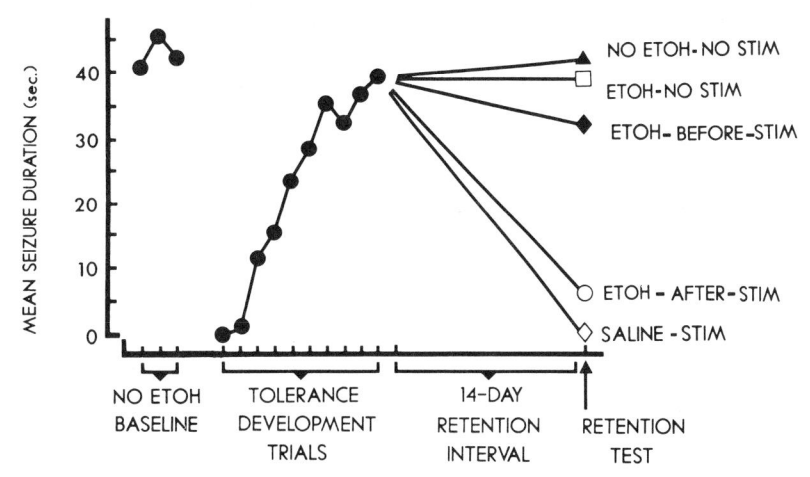

Figure 12-4. Dissipation of contingent tolerance to ethanol's anticonvulsant effect on kindled seizures. After the 14-day retention interval, the no ethanol-no stimulation (▲), the ethanol-before-stimulation, (♦) and the ethanol-no stimulation (□) groups displayed no loss of tolerance. In contrast, tolerance dissipated almost completely in the saline-before-stimulation and saline-after-stimulation groups (combined into a single saline group, ◇) and in the ethanol-after-stimulation group (○).

interval was greatly influenced by the treatment subjects received during this period. In three of the groups—the saline-before-stimulation and saline-after-stimulation groups (results in Figure 12-4), and the ethanol-after-stimulation group—tolerance dissipated almost completely over the retention interval. In contrast, tolerance in the other three groups—the no-ethanol-no-stimulation group, the ethanol-before-stimulation group, and the ethanol-no-stimulation group—did not decline. These results demonstrate quite clearly the inadequacy of the view that the dissipation of ethanol tolerance is a result of the discontinuation of ethanol exposure. The cessation of ethanol injections did not inevitably lead to a decline in tolerance; for example, the subjects that received neither ethanol nor stimulation during the retention interval displayed no loss of tolerance whatsoever. Conversely, continuation of ethanol exposure on the same bidaily schedule associated with the development of tolerance did not ensure that tolerance would be maintained; for example, subjects receiving ethanol *after* each bidaily stimulation displayed no tolerance at all at the end of the 14-day retention period.

What then was the factor that determined whether tolerance to ethanol's anticonvulsant effect dissipated or not? The key factor appears to have been the administration of convulsive stimulation in the absence of ethanol. Tolerance did not decline at all in the two groups receiving no brain stimulation or in the group receiving brain stimulation following an ethanol injection, but it dissipated completely in groups stimulated in the absence of ethanol, even when ethanol was still administered *after* each bidaily stimulation. Just as subjects that have adapted to the effects of vision-displacing prisms must experience the effects of their removal for their adaptation to dissipate, so too subjects tolerant to the anticonvulsant effects of ethanol must experience seizures in the absence of ethanol for the tolerance to dissipate.

SUMMARY

Despite the clinical and theoretical significance of the phenomenon, until recently evidence of tolerance to ethanol's anticonvulsant effect was both scant and equivocal. However, with the application of the kindling model to its study, substantial progress has been made in the last few years. The following conclusions seem firmly established: 1) ethanol is a potent anticonvulsant; 2) tolerance develops to ethanol's anticonvulsant effect; 3) tolerance develops to ethanol's anticonvulsant effect much more readily in subjects repeatedly experiencing its anticonvulsant effects; 4) this effect-contingency plays a major role in the development of tolerance to the anticonvulsant effects of other drugs (i.e., pentobarbital, diazepam, sodium valproate, and carbemazepine); 5) cross-tolerance is effect-contingent; and 6) the dissipation of tolerance to ethanol's anticonvulsant effect is also influenced by the contingency between ethanol exposure and convulsive stimulation.

ACKNOWLEDGMENT

Supported by a Canadian Medical Research Council grant awarded to John P. J. Pinel, and by a Canadian Medical Research Council postgraduate scholarship awarded to Michael J. Mana.

References

1. Alkana, RL, Finn, DA, and Malcolm, RD: The importance of experience in the development of tolerance to ethanol hypothermia. Life Sci 32:2685, 1983.
2. Allan, FD and Swinyard, CA: Evaluation of tissue tolerance to ethyl alcohol by alteration in electroshock seizure threshold. Anat Rec 103:419, 1949.
3. Carlton, PL and Wolgin, DL: Contingent tolerance to the anorexigenic effects of amphetamine. Physiol Behav 7:221, 1971.
4. Chen, CS: A further note on studies of acquired behavioral tolerance to alcohol. Psychopharmacology 27:265, 1972.
5. Chen, CS: A study of the alcohol tolerance effect and an introduction of a new behavioral technique. Psychopharmacology 12:433, 1968.
6. Cicero, TJ: Alcohol self-administration, tolerance and withdrawal in humans and animals: Theoretical and methodological issues. In Rigter, H and Crabbe, JC (eds): Alcohol Tolerance and Dependence. Elsevier/North Holland Biomedical Press, Amsterdam, 1980, p 1.
7. Demelweek, C and Goudie, AJ: An analysis of behavioral mechanisms involved in the acquisition of amphetamine anorectic tolerance. Psychopharmacology 79:58, 1983.
8. Frey, HH: Experimental evidence for the development of tolerance to anticonvulsant drug effects. In Frey, HH, et al (eds): Tolerance to Beneficial and Adverse Effects of Antiepileptic Drugs. Raven Press, New York, 1986, p 7.
9. Goddard, GV, McIntyre, DC, and Leech, CK: A permanent change in brain function resulting from daily electrical stimulation. Exp Neurol 25:295, 1969.
10. Goldstein, DB: Physical dependence on ethanol: Its relation to tolerance. Drug Alcohol Depend 4:33, 1979.
11. Held, R: Plasticity in sensory-motor systems. In Perception: Mechanisms and Models. Readings from Scientific American. WH Freeman, San Francisco, 1972.
12. Jorgenson, HA, Berge, O, and Hole, K: Learned tolerance to ethanol in a spinal reflex separated from supraspinal control. Pharmacol Biochem Behav 22:293, 1985.
13. Jorgenson, HA, Fasmer, OB, and Hole, K: Learned and pharmacologically-induced tolerance to ethanol and cross-tolerance to morphine and clonidine. Pharmacol Biochem Behav 24:1083, 1986.
14. Jorgenson, HA and Hole, K: Learned tolerance to ethanol in the spinal cord. Pharmacol Biochem Behav 20:789, 1984.
15. Kayan, S, Woods, LA, and Mitchell, CL: Experience as a factor in the development of tolerance to the analgesic effects of morphine. Eur J Pharmacol 6:333, 1969.
16. Kim, CK, Pinel, JPJ, and Roese, N: Contingent cross-tolerance between the anticonvulsant effects of pentobarbital and ethanol is bidirectional (submitted for publication).
17. Kumar, R and Stolerman, JP: Experimental and clinical aspects of drug dependence. In Iversen, LL, and Iversen, SD (eds): Principles of Behavioral Pharmacology, Vol 7. Plenum Press, New York, 1977, p 321.
18. LeBlanc, AE, Gibbins, RJ, and Kalant, H: Behavioral augmentation of tolerance to ethanol in the rat. Psychopharmacology 30:117, 1973.
19. Mana, MJ, et al: Contingent tolerance to the anticonvulsant effects of diazepam, carbamazepine, and sodium valproate on kindled seizures in the rat (submitted for publication).
20. Mana, MJ and Pinel, JPJ: Response contingency and the dissipation of ethanol tolerance. Alcohol and Alcoholism Res (Suppl 1):413, 1987.
21. Mana, MJ, Pinel, JPJ, and Lê, AD: Tolerance to the anticonvulsant effect (ACE) of ethanol: Lack of a response contingency. Fourth Congress of the International Society for Biomedical Research on Alcoholism—Abstracts. Alcohol and Alcoholism Res (Suppl):45, 1988.
22. Manning, FJ: Role of experience in acquisition and loss of tolerance to ethanol in the rat. Pharmacol Biochem Behav 5:269, 1974.
23. McNamara, JO: Kindling: An animal model of complex partial epilepsy. Ann Neurol 16:572, 1984.
24. McQuarrie, DG and Fingl, E: Effects of single doses and chronic administration of ethanol on experimental seizures in mice. J Pharmacol Exp Ther 180:203, 1972.
25. Mucha, RF and Pinel, JPJ: Post-seizure inhibition in kindled rats. Exp Neurol 54:266, 1977.
26. Pinel, JPJ, et al: Contingent tolerance and cross-tolerance to anticonvulsant drug effect: Pento-

barbital and ethanol. Psychobiology for publication 1990.
27. Pinel, JPJ, et al: Learned tolerance to the anticonvulsant effect of ethanol. Pharmacol Biochem Behav 18:507, 1983.
28. Pinel, JPJ: Spontaneous kindled motor seizures in rats. In Wada, JA (ed): Kindling 2. Raven Press, New York, 1981, p 179.
29. Pinel, JPJ, Mana, MJ, and Renfrey, G: Contingent tolerance to the anticonvulsant effect of alcohol. Alcohol 2:495, 1985.
30. Pinel, JPJ, Pfaus, JG, and Christensen, B: Contingent tolerance to the disruptive effects of alcohol on the sexual behavior of male rats. Fourth Congress of the International Society for Biomedical Research on Alcoholism—Abstracts (Suppl):47, 1988.
31. Pinel, JPJ, Phillips, AG, and MacNeil, B: Blockage of highly-stable "kindled" seizures in rats by antecedent footshock. Epilepsia 14:29, 1974.
32. Poulos, CX and Hinson, RE: A homeostatic model of Pavlovian conditioning: Tolerance to scopolamine-induced adipsia. J Exp Psychol [Anim Behav] 10:75, 1984.
33. Racine, RJ: Kindling: The first decade. Neurosurgery 3:234, 1979.
34. Racine, RJ: Modification of seizure activity by electrical stimulation. II. Motor seizure. Electroencephalogr Clin Neurophysiol 32:281, 1972.
35. Rock, I and Harris, CS: Vision and touch. In Perception: Mechanisms and Models. Readings from Scientific American. WH Freeman, San Francisco, 1972.
36. Rowland, N and Carlton, J: Different behavioral mechanisms underlie tolerance to the anorectic effects of fenfluramine and quipazine. Psychopharmacology 81:155, 1983.
37. Traynor, A, Schlapfer, W, and Barondes, S: Stimulation is necessary for the development of tolerance to a neuronal effect of ethanol. J Neurobiol 11:633, 1980.
38. Wenger, JR, et al: Ethanol tolerance in the rat is learned. Science 213:575, 1981.
39. Zarrow, MX, Pawlowski, AA, and Denenberg, VH: Electroshock convulsion threshold and organ weights in rats after alcohol consumption. Am J Physiol 203:197, 1962.

CHAPTER 13

John Crabbe, Ph.D.
Ann Kosobud, Ph.D.

Alcohol Withdrawal Seizures: Genetic Animal Models

For most people, alcohol consumption is a benign practice, but for a subset of individuals, excessive alcohol use has serious consequences. Alcohol abuse and alcoholism are frequently accompanied by the development of physical dependence, and a life-threatening withdrawal syndrome may ensue upon abrupt, untreated cessation of drinking. It has been shown that genetic factors play an important role in determining susceptibility to alcoholism. The availability of genetic animal models for the study of alcohol withdrawal is a relatively recent but important development. This chapter reviews the literature on alcohol withdrawal seizures (AWS) in genetic animal models. Suggestions are made regarding how genetic animal models can be used to identify markers of genetic risk for AWS susceptibility. The use of genetic animal models to determine the physiologic basis for AWS is also discussed.

AWS IN ANIMAL STUDIES

Alcohol withdrawal is a state characterized in part by general hyperexcitability of the central nervous system (CNS). The neurobiologic basis for this hyperexcitability is not well understood. Studies of AWS using animal models have revealed some symptoms similar to those humans experience as well as some unique to animals. Friedman[27] summarized the reported characteristics of alcohol withdrawal in humans, monkeys, chimpanzees, dogs, cats, mice, and rats. Tonic-clonic convulsions with recovery and fatal convulsions were among the few signs seen in all species. However, spontaneous seizures occur relatively rarely, and only during severe withdrawal. Hypersensitivity to audiogenic, drug-induced, and electrically induced seizures has been demonstrated in animals withdrawing from alcohol.

Handling-induced convulsions (HICs) were first reported by Goldstein and Pal[35] as a sign of AWS in mice. HICs are elicited by picking up a mouse by its tail. In a mouse withdrawing from a moderate regimen of chronic alcohol treatment, this handling is sufficient to elicit a tonic-clonic or tonic convulsion. If no convulsive sign is elicited by picking up the mouse, it is then twirled gently through a 180° arc. This action frequently elicits convulsive signs. The scale used to score the severity of HICs in mice is presented in Table 13–1, and is adapted from that originally developed by Goldstein.[32] HICs are apparent even after very mild alcohol treatments, for example, several hours after a single injection of alcohol in

Table 13-1. HANDLING-INDUCED CONVULSION RATING SCALE

Symptom	Score
Severe, tonic-clonic convulsion, with quick onset and long duration: spontaneous, or elicited by mild environmental stimulus such as lifting cage top	7
Severe, tonic-clonic convulsion when lifted by the tail, with quick onset and long duration, often continuing for several sec after the mouse is released	6
Tonic-clonic convulsion when lifted by the tail, often with onset delayed by as much as 1–2 sec	5
Tonic convulsion when lifted by the tail	4
Tonic-clonic convulsion after gentle 180° spin	3
No convulsion when lifted by the tail, but tonic convulsion elicited by gentle 180° spin	2
Only facial grimace after gentle 180° spin	1
No convulsion	0

mice.[41] HICs increase in severity with increasing dose or duration of treatment.[32] Graded estimates of withdrawal severity can thus be made over essentially the entire range of withdrawal severity. HICs can be measured repeatedly in the same mice very quickly and simply, with high interrater reliability. Thus, for several reasons, most studies with mice employ HICs to index alcohol withdrawal severity.

Several caveats should be noted. The neurophysiologic and neurochemical bases of HICs are not understood, although the latter have been studied to some degree.[26,30] No electrophysiologic studies of the presumptive seizureform neuronal activity during HICs have been attempted. HICs represent only one aspect of alcohol withdrawal. Thus, if the severity of HICs were found to be elevated in a given experiment, with peak severity occurring after 12 hours, another aspect of withdrawal may have already reached peak severity 6 hours after withdrawal. The HIC scale is ordinal. Although we are confident on the basis of our experience that HIC scale values are ordered correctly (and, furthermore, that the variable "behaves" parametrically), there is no assurance that the different convulsion signs on the HIC scale are measuring the same substrate. For example, the forelimb tonic convulsion elicited by twirling and given a score of 2 may be physiologically independent from the severe tonic-clonic convulsion scored as 6 or 7. Finally, HICs have not been reported in rat experiments. Because most genetic experiments on alcohol and drug withdrawal employ mice, this limitation is not serious for genetic animal model research.

GENETIC DIFFERENCES IN ALCOHOL WITHDRAWAL SEIZURES

Goldstein[31] rendered mice physically dependent on ethanol vapor using the procedure described later in this chapter, in the section "The Model." Mice were scored for HIC severity and then mated. Animals with severe withdrawal HICs were mated, as were those with low withdrawal HIC. When offspring of these matings were subsequently made dependent and withdrawn, the offspring of high-scoring parents had significantly more severe alcohol withdrawal HICs than the offspring of low-scoring parents. This finding strongly suggested that there was significant genetic variability in AWS severity.

A straightforward method for assessing the potential role of genetic factors in determining individual differences in alcohol withdrawal severity is to compare responses of several inbred strains of mice. Because all members of an inbred strain are genetically identical, the differences between strains tested in a controlled environment provide an estimate of the degree of genetic determination of the trait. Early studies reported that DBA/2 strain mice expressed more severe AWS than those of the C57BL/6 strain.[33,36,37,39] Using inbred mouse strains, we tested whether alcohol withdrawal severity, as assessed by HIC scores, differed among many strains chosen for their divergent pedigrees.[22] Twenty inbred strains were tested for alcohol sensitivity, tolerance development, and withdrawal severity. The strains showed significant differences in response to alcohol on each measure, confirming that a high degree of genetic determination of responses to alcohol exists. AWS severity differed 15-fold among strains. When withdrawal seizure scores were corrected by linear regression for blood alcohol levels achieved during chronic exposure, strains still varied eight-fold in HIC severity. Withdrawal seizure severity was negatively correlated with development of tolerance to the hypothermic effect of alcohol, and to a lesser extent with initial hypothermic sensitivity, but with no other tested variables. Thus, withdrawal seizure severity appears to be modulated principally by genes different from those affecting many other responses to alcohol.[22]

Among the inbred strains, C57BL/6 and closely related strains differed significantly in seizure severity from DBA/2 and related strains. We then tested recombinant inbred (RI) strains derived from crosses of C57BL/6 and DBA/2 mice.[15] All but one of the 17 RI strains tested closely resembled one or the other of the two parent strains. This strain distribution pattern suggested the influence of a major gene in determining ethanol withdrawal severity. The gene did not closely resemble any mapped gene, so it was not possible to test this hypothesis more rigorously.[15]

A genetic analysis of several measures of alcohol withdrawal severity in mice included seizures as a variable.[2] Seizure severity was scored similarly to HIC severity, and seizures probably represent the same underlying phenomena. Using a diallel cross of five inbred strains, these investigators found relatively little genetic influence on AWS scores. However, all the genetic variability in seizure scores was additive, indicating that a tendency to be resistant or susceptible to such seizures could be inherited (heritability was 0.14 in males and 0.06 in females).[2]

Thus, several experiments suggested that there was genetic variability in AWS severity as measured by HIC severity. The fact that genetic variability was additive suggested that it would be possible to breed lines of mice genetically selected for differences in AWS severity. Finally, genetic susceptibility to severe withdrawal did not seem to be predictable from equally large genetically determined differences in sensitivity to several other effects of alcohol.

UTILITY OF SELECTED LINES AS GENETIC ANIMAL MODELS

The technique of artificial genetic selection has been used to produce lines of animals that are genetically invariant with regard to the genes determining a particular trait but freely variant at all other segregating gene loci. The first step in establishing selected lines is to test a genetically heterogeneous base population for the trait of interest. Breeding pairs are then chosen on the basis of test scores for maximum expression of the trait of interest, to establish a maximum expression line. The same strategy is used to create a minimum expression line. In succeeding generations, offspring within the maximum line are selected for maximum expression of the trait to continue the line, and offspring within the minimum line are selected to continue that line. There are two primary reasons for developing selected lines. First, after several generations of selection, the divergent lines differ significantly in expressing the selected trait. Selected lines are thus a good tool for testing hypotheses about the neurobiologic mechanisms underlying the selected trait. The second value of selected lines derives from the fact that in a properly executed selection, only those genes underlying the selected trait are affected. Thus, other traits that differentiate the maximum- and minimum-expression lines are presumably controlled by the same genes. Such genetically correlated responses can provide important clues about the paths from gene to trait in the selected lines.

A highly desirable control in a genetic selection is that the entire selection should be replicated: that is, a second subset of mice should be tested, and a second minimum and maximum line established.

This replication constitutes a control for the accidental fixing of genes unrelated to selection, a problem that can occur in the initial choice of breeding pairs or due to inbreeding later in the selection. Replication allows distinction of true genetic correlations between the selected trait and a correlated trait, because a true genetic correlation should appear in both replications. It is very unlikely that random or spurious correlations would appear in both replications. Similarly, inbreeding leads to chance fixation of some alleles irrelevant to the selected trait, resulting in the appearance of a trait in one replicate that appears to be (but is not) a correlated response to selection. It is unlikely, however, that the same alleles would also be fixed by chance in the other replicate. Thus, a difference between both replicates of the maximum and minimum lines in a trait in addition to the selected trait is strong evidence that a genetic correlation exists between the traits.[23] Falconer has published a detailed discussion of the many assumptions and qualifications underlying this logic.[24]

WITHDRAWAL-SEIZURE-PRONE AND WITHDRAWAL-SEIZURE-RESISTANT SELECTED LINES

The Model

The Withdrawal-Seizure-Prone (WSP) and Withdrawal-Seizure-Resistant (WSR) mouse lines were developed by artificial selection as a model of differing genetic susceptibility to the development of alcohol withdrawal. Beginning from independent groups of outbred mice from the HS/Ibg population, two sets of WSP and WSR lines were selected on the basis of HIC severity after withdrawal from chronic ethanol treatment. Mice were made dependent by 72 hours of ethanol inhalation with daily injections of pyrazole, an alcohol dehydrogenase inhibitor, and scored for HIC severity for 24 hours after removal from the inhalation chambers. By selecting for alcohol withdrawal severity over many generations, we have evolved lines of mice that differ principally in allelic frequence of genes relevant to alcohol withdrawal severity as measured by HIC severity, but show no systematic differences for other gene loci. Other characteristics that differentiate WSP from WSR mice can probably be attributed to the expression of genes that determine alcohol withdrawal severity, and, by implication, severity of physical dependence on alcohol.

Response to selection has been robust. After five generations of selection, there was a five-fold difference in HIC severity between the WSP and WSR lines after identical ethanol exposure.[21] After 11 selected generations, a ten-fold difference had developed,[9] and the difference has remained approximately this great. Figure 13-1 shows the typical waxing and waning HIC withdrawal curve for groups of

Figure 13-1. Handling-induced convulsion scores in Withdrawal Seizure Prone (WSP) and Withdrawal Seizure Resistant (WSR) genetically selected mouse lines. All mice were exposed to ethanol vapor for 72 hr. Mean ± SE for 15 WSP and 15 WSR mice from generation 11 of selection are shown. Replicate WSP and WSR lines are pooled.

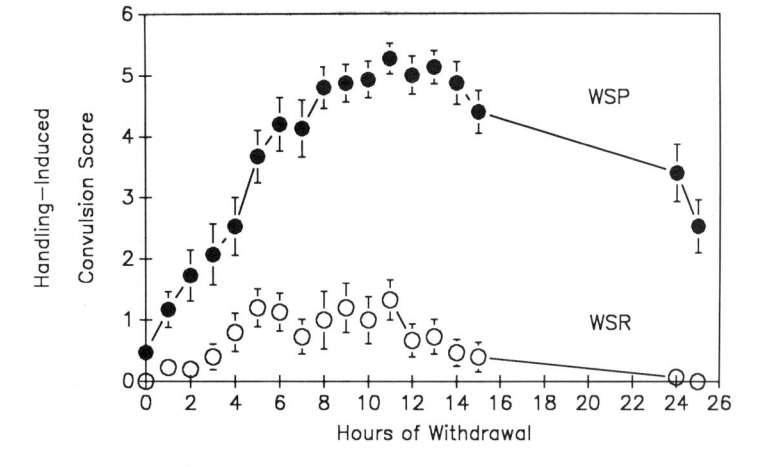

WSP and WSR mice subjected to identical exposure to ethanol vapor for 72 hours. The differences in withdrawal seizure severity were significant in both replicate pairs of WSP and WSR lines. This result confirms that there is a strong genetic influence on alcohol withdrawal severity as measured by HIC severity.

Correlations with Sensitivity and Tolerance

These mice are a useful population for studying variables genetically linked to AWS severity. Interestingly, we found that WSP and WSR mice did not differ in their acute sensitivity to alcohol-induced hypothermia.[20] When alcohol was repeatedly administered, both lines of mice developed tolerance, and there was no significant line difference in magnitude of tolerance development.[20] In addition, they were not differentially susceptible to the hypnotic effects of a higher dose of alcohol. The failure to detect differences was not due to high doses of alcohol, for they also did not differ in sensitivity to alcohol-induced locomotor activation, a response elicited by low alcohol doses.[18] Several other studies of correlated responses in WSP and WSR mice have been reviewed,[11] and in general have reinforced the pattern revealed in the inbred strain studies: genetic control of AWS severity is largely distinct from genetic control of many other responses to alcohol. However, some instructive differences between WSP and WSR mice have been found.

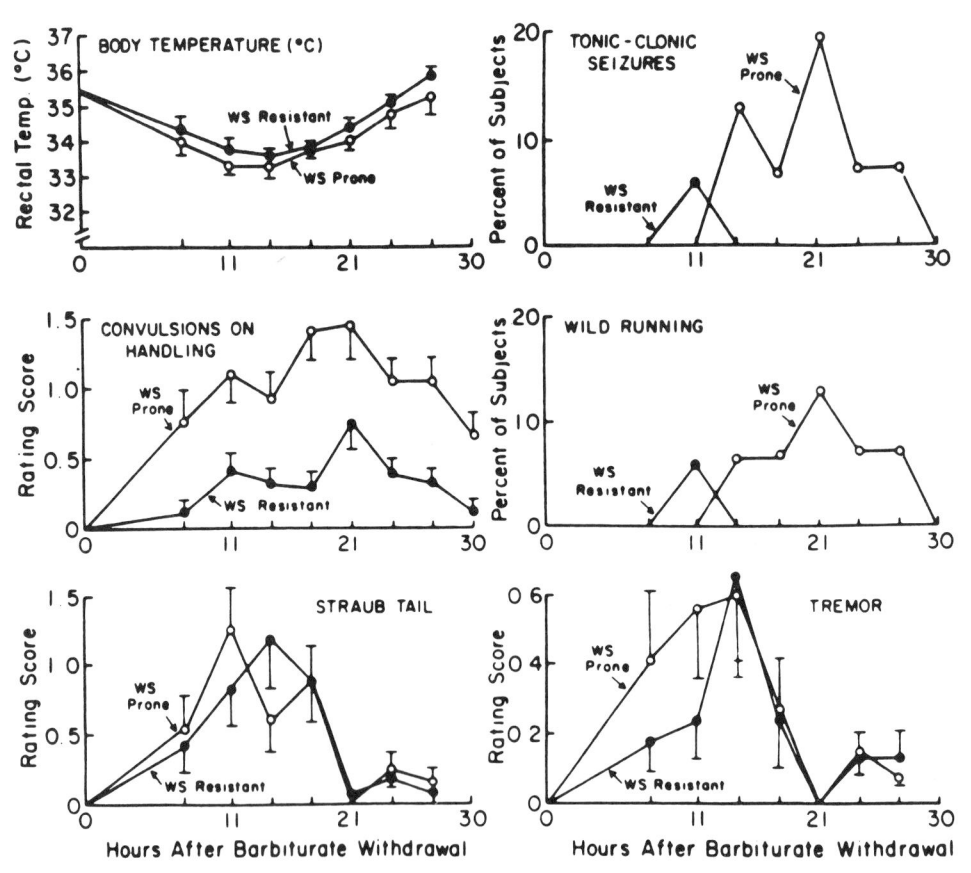

Figure 13–2. Time course for six withdrawal signs monitored following withdrawal from 6.7 days of chronic phenobarbital feeding in an adulterated diet. WSP and WSR mice (15–17 per line) differed significantly on all measures except Straub tail and tremor. Mean ± SE are shown. Replicate WSP and WSR lines are pooled. (From Belknap, et al,[4] p. 169, with permission.)

Genetic Codetermination of Withdrawal from Alcohol and Other Drugs

WSP and WSR mice have been tested for the severity of HIC during withdrawal following chronic treatment with diazepam,[6] nitrous oxide,[5] and phenobarbital.[4] WSP mice had more severe withdrawal HIC than WSR mice following treatment with all three of these drugs. Figure 13-2 shows that spontaneous tonic-clonic and wild-running seizures after barbiturate withdrawal were also more frequent in WSP than in WSR mice. The differences in withdrawal seizures between WSP and WSR mice were present in both replicate pairs of selected lines in each case. This finding suggests that dependence may be induced by similar mechanisms for all these drugs, since phenobarbital, alcohol, and nitrous oxide are thought to produce their anesthetic and sedative actions by similar mechanisms.

Acute Alcohol Withdrawal

Severity of withdrawal is related to dose and duration of treatment in humans[3] and laboratory animals.[32] Even after a single administration of alcohol, a period of increased sensitivity to elicited convulsions can be demonstrated. This effect occurs whether convulsions are elicited using electrical kindling,[49] pentylenetetrazol (PTZ), electroconvulsive shock (ECS),[47] or flurothyl.[50] We had noted that the lowest levels of the HIC sign could be elicited in normal naive mice. When we tested 20 inbred strains, we found that strains differed significantly in the basal levels of HIC severity expressed.[13] When mice were tested hourly for HICs, a slight reduction in HIC severity developed.[16] Therefore, we attempted to use the HIC measure as an assay for acute AWS severity in the WSP and WSR mice. Mice were scored for HIC severity and then injected with a single intraperitoneal (IP) 4 g/kg

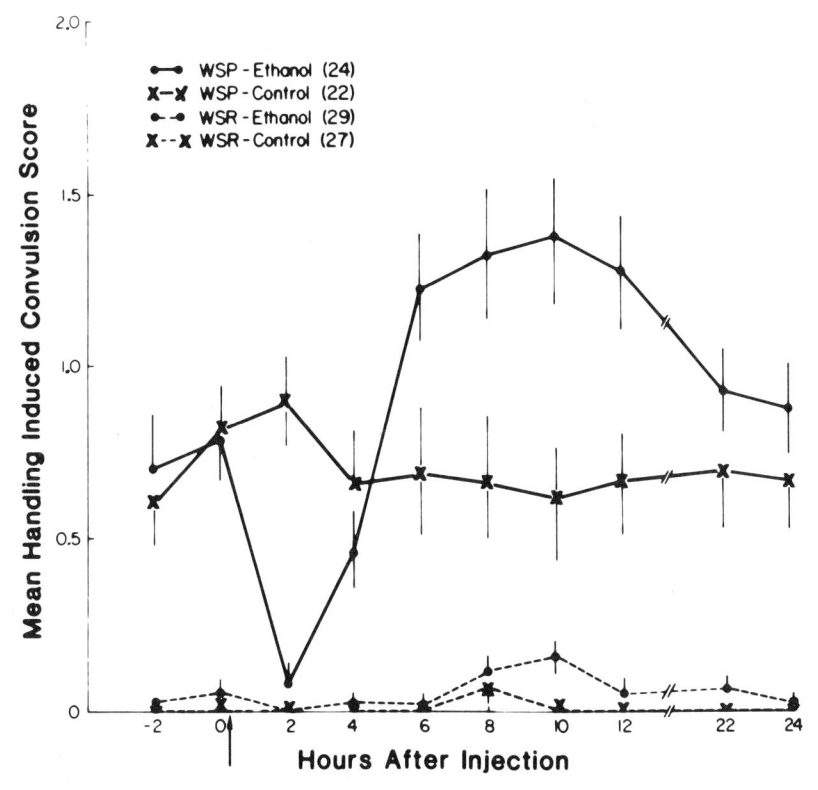

Figure 13-3. Effect of a single IP injection of ethanol (4 g/kg) or saline on handling-induced convulsion scores in WSP and WSR mice. Mean ± SE for HIC scores at intervals before and after injection are shown. Replicate WSP and WSR lines are pooled. (From Kosobud and Crabbe,[41] p. 176, with permission.)

dose of alcohol or saline. Hourly scoring thereafter revealed a clear rebound exacerbation of HIC severity in WSP mice 10 hours after injection; although present, acute withdrawal in WSR mice was minimal (Fig. 13-3). Thus, WSP mice are genetically so predisposed to develop AWS that such seizures occur after a single acute alcohol dose.[41]

Seizure Susceptibility

It is possible that the difference between WSP and WSR mice reflects a general difference in propensity to convulsions. Alcohol dependence could have been the medium for inducing a state of enhanced nervous system excitability, but the specific neurobiologic differences between WSP and WSR mice could have little specifically to do with alcohol dependence *per se*. If the genetic alteration in WSP and WSR mice involves global changes of this sort, then WSP mice could be more sensitive to any convulsant treatment than WSR mice. This difference might be revealed as a difference in threshold sensitivity to a given convulsant. Alternatively, it could lie in differential propagation or termination of the seizure once initiated, and would thus be revealed as a difference in severity or duration of seizure.

Initially, we assessed the first of these possibilities by determining effective median doses (ED$_{50}$) for maximal seizures elicited by ECS, bicuculline, flurothyl, strychnine, PTZ, and picrotoxin in alcohol-naive WSP and WSR mice from the eighth to tenth selected generations. Naive WSP and WSR mice did not differ in sensitivity to these convulsant treatments. However, studies with later selected generations suggested that WSP mice were more sensitive to flurothyl than WSR mice, when latencies to convulse were measured.[25] This finding suggested that a method that involved assessing minimal seizure thresholds might be more sensitive to differences between WSP and WSR mice.

Using naive WSP and WSR mice from both replicates of the 26th and 27th selected generations, we administered several convulsant drugs by tail-vein infusion.[43,44] Drugs presumed to produce convulsions by actions at the GABA/benzodiazepine receptor complex (picrotoxin, TBPS, PTZ, bicuculline, DMCM) and drugs presumed to induce convulsions by other mechanisms (strychnine, CHEB, 4-aminopyridine, kainic acid) were tested. Endpoints studied included myoclonic, clonic, and tonic hindlimb extensor seizures; a particular constellation of endpoints characterized each drug. The purpose for these experiments was two-fold. First, if WSP mice were found generally to be more susceptible to seizures than WSR mice, the specific relationship to alcohol withdrawal of other differences between the lines could be questioned. Second, if WSP and WSR mice were found to differ in sensitivity to a particular agent or class of agents, this finding could provide clues to the neurochemical substrate of AWS.

Consistent differences between WSP and WSR mice were found for picrotoxin, CHEB, and 4-aminopyridine.[43] Figure 13-4 shows the latency to develop a clonic seizure in the four lines of mice tested with picrotoxin. Both WSP lines were more sensitive than the corresponding WSR lines. A similar pattern was seen for CHEB and 4-aminopyridine. These data suggest that sensitivity to some convulsant drugs may be positively correlated

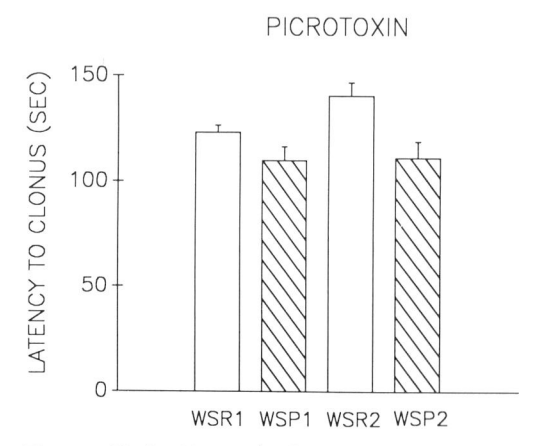

Figure 13–4. Mean ± SE latency to develop clonic convulsions in WSP and WSR mice after tail-vein infusion of picrotoxin. WSP and WSR mice from both replicates of the selection are shown.

with sensitivity to AWS, but the physiologic basis for this difference remains obscure.[43] Picrotoxin blocks neuronal chloride flux, preventing GABA-mediated inhibition.[28] However, the responses of WSP and WSR mice to TBPS and PTZ, which act at least in part at the same binding site as picrotoxin,[52,53] were not the same as their response to picrotoxin. CHEB and 4-aminopyridine are thought to initiate seizures through very different mechanisms of action on neurons. CHEB blocks a calcium-dependent cation flux and directly excites cells,[51] while 4-aminopyridine blocks potassium flux, preventing repolarization of the cell membrane and prolonging the action potential.[54] Rather than a common pharmacologic mechanism of action, the basis for the similar effects of CHEB, 4-aminopyridine, and picrotoxin on WSP and WSR mice may be a particular anatomic site that is involved in propagation or expression of the seizure.

For all other drugs tested, WSP mice of the first replicate were more sensitive than the corresponding WSR mice, but the second replicate pair of lines did not differ. Figure 13–5 shows latency to develop a clonic seizure in the four lines of mice tested with the drug strychnine. A similar pattern was seen for kainic acid, TBPS, DMCM, PTZ, and bicuculline.[43,44]

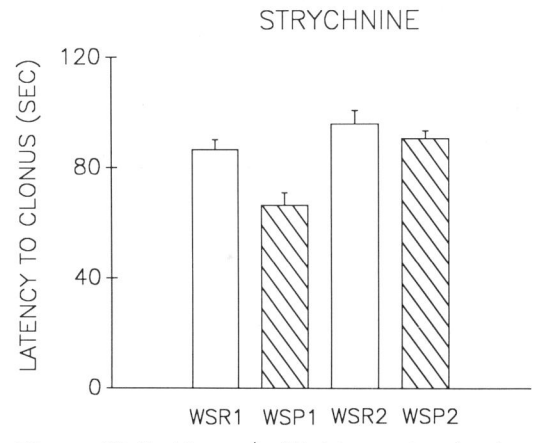

Figure 13–5. Mean ± SE latency to develop clonic convulsions in WSP and WSR mice after tail-vein infusion of strychnine. WSP and WSR mice from both replicates of the selection are shown.

Because differential responsiveness to all tested agents was present in one replicate pair of selected lines only, it may reflect inadvertent selection for seizure sensitivity unrelated to alcohol withdrawal. That is, WSP1 mice may have been fixed for some genes leading to a generalized seizure susceptibility (or WSR1 mice for seizure resistance genes). For the WSP2 and WSR2 lines, however, this is not the case. In all these experiments, the differences between WSP and WSR mice in seizure thresholds were generally rather small relative to differences seen among inbred mouse strains.[42] Thus, genetic selection for alcohol withdrawal severity has neither systematically nor substantially altered the frequencies of genes that determine sensitivity to all convulsant drugs.

Using identical methods, we also tested seizure susceptibility to the above agents in mice from eight to eleven (depending on the agent) different inbred strains. Strains differed significantly in response to each drug.[42] The mean strain sensitivities were then correlated with strain means for ethanol withdrawal HIC values we had previously determined.[22] No significant genetic correlation between sensitivity to any drug and AWS severity was found. Thus, results from WSP and WSR lines were not confirmed in another genetic model. Because genetically selected lines are a more sensitive tool for detecting genetic correlations, the absence of significant correlations in inbred strains does not necessarily invalidate the results with the selected lines, but suggests that the genetic correlations are not strong.

Proconvulsant Sensitivity

We have also examined the sensitivity of WSP and WSR mice to proconvulsant effects of various agents, using HIC severity as an index. Figure 13–6 shows the HIC scores before and after different doses of 3-mercaptopropionic acid in WSP and WSR mice. This GABA synthesis inhibitor produced a dose-dependent, significant increase in HIC scores in both lines, but the WSP line was significantly more sensitive. In similar experiments, we have found relatively greater WSP sen-

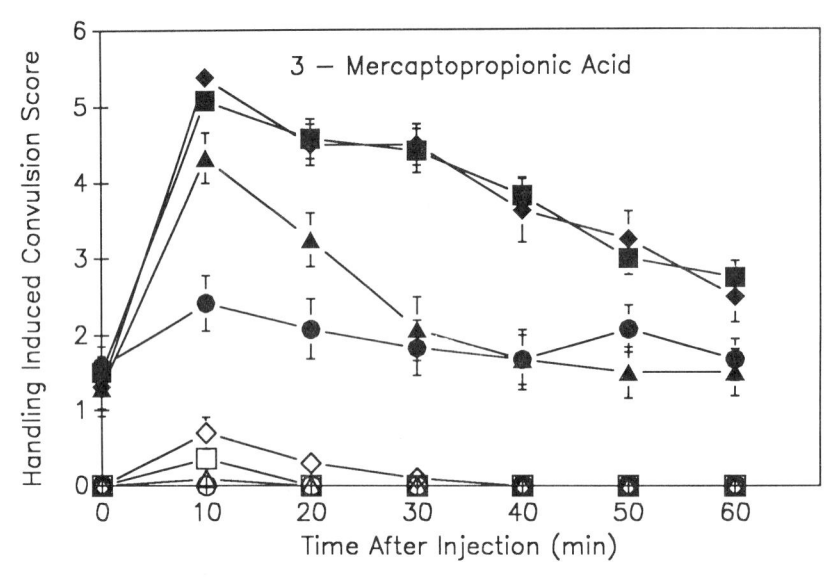

Figure 13–6. Effect of saline or three doses of 3-mercaptopropionic acid on handling-induced convulsion severity before and after injection in WSP and WSR mice. Circles = Placebo; Triangles = 20 mg/kg; Squares = 30 mg/kg; Diamonds = 40 mg/kg. Mean ± SE are shown. Open symbols = WSR mice; Closed symbols = WSP mice. Replicate WSP and WSR lines are pooled.

sitivity to the proconvulsant effects of picrotoxin, bicuculline, and PTZ,[26] as well as the benzodiazepine inverse agonists Ro-15-4513 and FG-7142.[17] Genetic differences in sensitivity to these compounds could not be attributed clearly to the GABA system, for neither the binding of flunitrazepam nor its enhancement by GABA were different in whole brain preparations from the selected lines. Density and affinity of TBPS binding sites in several brain areas also did not differ between WSP and WSR mice.[26]

Sensitivity to Anticonvulsant Treatments

Although WSP and WSR mice do not differ in threshold for seizures elicited by ECS, WSR mice are more sensitive to ethanol-induced elevation of ECS seizure thresholds.[48] Therefore, we assessed the generality of this genetic difference in anticonvulsant sensitivity.[10] We found that relative to WSP mice, WSR mice were approximately twice as sensitive to the anticonvulsant effects of the first five straight-chain alcohols. WSR mice were approximately three times as sensitive to the anti-ECS effects of the depressants ethchlorvynol and methyprylon, and two- to four-fold more sensitive when tested after the administration of barbital, phenobarbital, pentobarbital, and diazepam. Similar differential protection was seen after administration of phenytoin and valproic acid.[10] Figure 13–7 shows the results after administration of 15 mg/kg carbamazepine. The physiologic substrate for the difference in anticonvulsant response is not known. Tests of the selected lines for differences in sensitivity to ethanol-induced elevations of maximum seizure ED_{50}s for several convulsant drugs did not reveal such a substantial sensitivity difference. WSR mice tended to be more protected by ethanol against seizures elicited by flurothyl and strychnine, but not against those elicited by the GABA-related drugs picrotoxin, PTZ, and bicuculline.[48] All the WSP/WSR differences cited were significant in both replicates of the selection. Thus, the difference in sensitivity to all anticonvulsants tested suggests that some common mechanisms of gene action facilitate anticonvulsant sensitivity and reduce AWS severity.

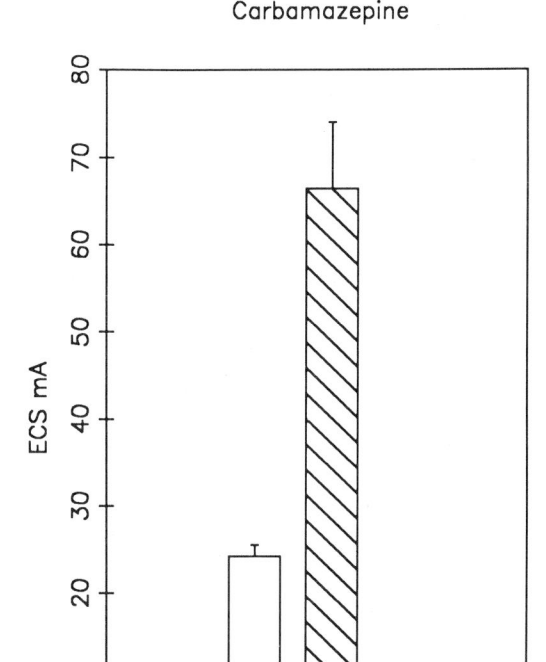

Figure 13–7. Mean and 95 percent confidence interval for the electroconvulsive shock amperage effective in inducing tonic hindlimb extensor seizures in 50 percent of the tested mice in each group. Mice were tested 60 minutes after administration of 15 mg/kg carbamazepine; WSP and WSR mice were previously shown not to differ in sensitivity to ECS after placebo administration.[10,48] Groups of 16 to 18 WSP and WSR mice are shown. Replicate WSP and WSR lines are pooled.

Conclusions from Studies with WSP and WSR mice

We conclude that the selection program has generally not produced significant differences in seizure susceptibility between WSP and WSR mice. Thus, these lines remain a viable genetic animal model for examining potential correlates of AWS mechanisms. On the other hand, studies of sensitivity to particular convulsants in these lines have not been fruitful in identifying the critical neurobiologic differences between WSP and WSR mice that lead to substantial differences in AWS susceptibility and characteristics. The differences between the lines in seizure susceptibility appear small compared with seizure susceptibility differences among a number of inbred strains. Given the large, generalized differences in anticonvulsant sensitivity between the lines, it seems more likely that exploration of these differences will be useful.

WITHDRAWAL SEIZURES IN OTHER GENETIC ANIMAL MODELS

Studies with Severe-Ethanol-Withdrawal and Mild-Ethanol-Withdrawal Mice

Following the principles outlined previously in this chapter, Severe-Ethanol-Withdrawal (SEW) and Mild-Ethanol-Withdrawal (MEW) lines have been developed by selective breeding. In this program, mice are made dependent by 9 days of exposure to an alcohol-adulterated liquid diet as their only food source. They are selected using a multivariate index of withdrawal severity. Hutchins and associates[38] assessed multiple behavioral and physiologic measures of withdrawal. On the basis of a principal component analysis, seven measures were selected.[45] These measures included three measures of activity, two indices of seizure severity (HICs and spontaneous seizures), body temperature, and alcohol consumption. The experiment is replicated.

After five generations, SEW and MEW lines showed approximately 1.5-fold divergence in one replicate, but little divergence in the other.[1] After ten generations, divergence was present in both lines, although it remained small.[55] Like the WSP and WSR lines, SEW and MEW mice did not differ in acute hypnotic or hypothermic response to alcohol.[55] SEW and MEW lines were also tested for withdrawal severity following chronic treatment with phenobarbital. In contrast to WSP and WSR mice, SEW and MEW mice did not differ on this measure, although a difference could appear as selection continues to influence relevant genes and the lines diverge further.[7] Recently, the group developing the SEW and MEW lines has reported that alcohol consumption has been eliminated from the selection index and that response to selection appears to be increasing.[8] They have also reported a genetic analysis of the selection index confirming a negative genetic correlation between voluntary alcohol consumption and alcohol withdrawal severity. This finding is consistent with our finding that WSR mice voluntarily consume more alcohol than WSP mice when given the choice between water and alcohol-water solutions.[40]

Studies with Other Selected Lines

Lines of mice have also been genetically selected for differences in initial sensitivity to alcohol. Long-sleep (LS) and Short-sleep (SS) mice differ significantly in the duration of loss of the righting reflex following a single IP administration of alcohol.[46] These lines were made dependent by 3 days of exposure to alcohol vapor with pyrazole treatment, and were then withdrawn and scored for HIC severity.[34] LS mice showed milder withdrawal than SS mice, suggesting a possible negative genetic correlation between sensitivity to alcohol-induced loss of righting reflex and alcohol withdrawal severity. However, this result differs from results with inbred strains,[22] where no correlation was indicated. Furthermore, WSP and WSR mice do not differ in loss of righting reflex sensitivity to alcohol.[20]

Lines of mice sensitive (DS) and resistant (DR) to the effect of diazepam to induce ataxia on a rotarod have also been developed.[29] After seven generations of selection, there is no overlap in the two populations of animals, with DS mice averaging over 200 minutes of impairment and DR mice averaging less than 30 minutes after a standard dose of 20 mg/kg diazepam. There is a clear shift in dose-effect curves, with the DS mice 8–15-fold more sensitive than the DR mice across a range of doses.[29] We have rendered DS and DR mice physically dependent on alcohol using the inhalation procedure described. Upon withdrawal, DR mice had significantly more severe HICs than DS mice, although they had been exposed to identical chronic levels of alcohol. This suggests that diazepam-induced ataxia, a response blocked by Ro15-1788 and therefore presumably receptor mediated, is controlled by some of the same genes controlling resistance to alcohol withdrawal severity.[19]

We have also selected lines of mice sensitive (COLD) and resistant (HOT) to the acute hypothermic effects of ethanol.[12] When replicate COLD and HOT mice were tested for severity of AWS, HOT mice of one replicate had more severe withdrawal seizures than their paired COLD line, but this difference was not seen in the other pair of lines.[18] Nonetheless, this finding is consistent with the negative genetic correlation between hypothermic sensitivity and withdrawal severity we had earlier reported in inbred strains.[22] Finally, we have developed lines of mice that are responsive (FAST) and unresponsive (SLOW) to the locomotor-activating properties of an acute ethanol injection.[14] These lines did not differ in withdrawal seizure severity.[18] This finding is consistent with the genetic independence of locomotor activation and withdrawal observed in the inbred strain study.[22]

FUTURE UTILITY OF GENETIC ANIMAL MODELS: FINDING OUT WHAT IS INHERITED

Although the literature on genetic determinants of AWS in animal models is not extensive, it provides a relatively consistent picture. Significant genetic control of AWS severity has been demonstrated in a variety of ways: with inbred strains, recombinant inbred strains, and selectively bred lines. The use of genetic animal models allows identification of genetically correlated traits. Thus, patterns of common genetic influence may be determined using one method and verified with the others. The availability of genetically selected lines makes it possible to explore possible neurochemical and neurophysiologic determinants of withdrawal seizures in populations genetically tooled to express very large differences in these traits. Because the existing genetic animal models of AWS were developed rather carefully in the genetic sense, they are excellent material for systematically exploring the relative contributions of genetic predisposition and environmental modulation. Clearly, not all animals (or humans) genetically predisposed to severe alcohol withdrawal develop symptoms of withdrawal. Studies of gene-environment interactions are critically important and are virtually nonexistent in most areas of behavior genetic research, including this one. The practical problem is identifying individual levels of risk, rather than statistical estimates of risk characterizing populations. Such individualized risk markers almost certainly depend upon the identification of individual genes, themselves predictive of AWS severity. Genetic animal models allow us to study such predictors in a laboratory setting where the roles of genes and environment may be controlled.

SUMMARY

Genetic animal models offer several advantages for studying mechanisms underlying AWS susceptibility. Early experiments demonstrated that there was significant genetic control of withdrawal severity in mice made physically dependent on alcohol. Inbred strains differ greatly in withdrawal severity. Studies with recombinant inbred mice suggest that a single gene may play a significant role in alcohol withdrawal. Because genetically selected lines are bred to differ maximally in a trait of interest, other effects of genes determining the selected response are also highly accentuated. Thus, mechanisms underlying observable responses are revealed. WSP and WSR mice were bred to display, respectively, maximal and minimal HICs after withdrawal from chronic alcohol treatment. WSP mice show more severe withdrawal HICs than WSR mice after chronic phenobarbital, diazepam, and nitrous oxide treatment. This finding suggests that there is a general genetic predisposition to dependence on CNS-depressant drugs. WSP mice show more pronounced withdrawal HICs than WSR mice after a single injection of alcohol. WSP and WSR mice do not differ significantly in their initial sensitivity to alcohol, or in the development of tolerance to alcohol. This finding suggests that genetic control of AWS severity is largely distinct from genetic control of other responses to alcohol.

WSP and WSR mice do not differ in maximal seizure thresholds when subjected to a variety of convulsant treatments. However, when tested for threshold responses to convulsants, WSP mice are more sensitive than WSR mice to picrotoxin, CHEB, and 4-aminopyridine, but not to a number of other drugs acting at a variety of sites (bicuculline, DMCM, kainic acid, PTZ, TBPS, strychnine). Proconvulsant sensitivity can be revealed by administering low doses of drugs and scoring HIC severity. In this test, WSP mice are more sensitive than WSR mice to the proconvulsant effects of 3-mercaptopropionic acid, picrotoxin, bicuculline, PTZ, Ro15-1788, and FG 7142. WSR mice are much more sensitive than WSP mice to the anticonvulsant effects of depressants as assessed by the elevation of MES levels. Several alcohols, barbiturates, diazepam, ethchlorvynol, methyprylon, carbamazepine, phenytoin, and valproic acid all were more effective in WSR mice. Thus, some common mechanism of gene action may facilitate anticonvulsant sensitivity and reduce AWS sensitivity. Other genetic animal models for alcohol-related traits have been developed, and the limited data available on their relative seizure susceptibilities are generally consistent with the differences between WSP and WSR mice. In summary, research using genetic animal models suggests a specific relationship between sensitivity to anticonvulsants and reduced ethanol withdrawal seizure severity; such models may prove useful in determining the neurobiologic mechanisms underlying these phenomena.

References

1. Allen, DL, et al: Selective breeding for a multivariate index of ethanol dependence in mice: Results from the first five generations. Alcoholism: Clin Exp Res 7:443, 1983.
2. Allen, DL, et al: Genetic effects on various measures of ethanol dependence in mice: A diallel analysis. Drug Alcohol Depend 13:125, 1984.
3. Ballenger, JC and Post, RM: Kindling as a model for alcohol withdrawal syndromes. Br J Psychiatry 133:1, 1978.
4. Belknap, JK, et al: Ethanol and barbiturate withdrawal convulsions are extensively codetermined in mice. Alcohol 5:167, 1988.
5. Belknap, JK, Laursen, SE, and Crabbe, JC: Ethanol and nitrous oxide produce withdrawal-induced convulsions by similar mechanisms in mice. Life Sci 41:2033, 1987.
6. Belknap, JK, Crabbe, JC, and Laursen, SE: Ethanol and diazepam withdrawal convulsions are extensively codetermined in WSP and WSR mice. Life Sci 44:2075, 1989.
7. Cole-Harding, S, Wilson, JR, and Schlesinger, K: Phenobarbital withdrawal in mice selectively bred for differences in ethanol withdrawal severity (abstr). Alcoholism: Clin Exp Res 10:108, 1986.
8. Corley, R and Allen, D: Multivariate diallel analysis of ethanol withdrawal symptoms in mice. Alcoholism: Clin Exp Res 12:99, 1988.
9. Crabbe, JC, et al: Bidirectional selection for sensitivity to ethanol withdrawal seizures in Mus musculus. Behav Genet 15:521, 1985.
10. Crabbe, JC, et al: Genetic differences in anticonvulsant sensitivity in mouse lines selectively bred for ethanol withdrawal severity. J Pharmacol Exp Ther 239:154, 1986.
11. Crabbe, JC: Genetic models of alcohol dependence. Alcohol and Alcoholism (Suppl) 1:103, 1987.
12. Crabbe, JC, et al: Genetic selection of mouse lines sensitive (COLD) and resistant (HOT) to acute ethanol hypothermia. Alcohol Drug Res 7:163, 1987.
13. Crabbe, JC, et al: Handling induced convulsions in twenty inbred strains of mice. Substance and Alcohol Actions/Misuse 1:149, 1980.
14. Crabbe, JC, et al: Mice genetically selected for differences in open-field activity after ethanol. Pharmacol Biochem Behav 27:577, 1987.
15. Crabbe, JC, et al: Polygenic and single-gene determination of response to ethanol in BXD/Ty recombinant inbred mouse strains. Neurobehav Toxicol Teratol 5:181, 1983.
16. Crabbe, JC, et al: Pyrazole exacerbates handling-induced convulsions in mice. Neuropharmacology 20:605, 1981.
17. Crabbe, JC: Unpublished material, 1988.
18. Crabbe, JC, et al: Use of selectively bred mouse lines to study genetically correlated traits. In Kuriyama, K, Takada, A, and Ishii, H (eds): Biomedical and Social Aspects of Alcohol and Alcoholism. Excerpta Medica, Amsterdam, 1988.
19. Crabbe, JC and Gallaher, ES: Unpublished material, 1987.
20. Crabbe, JC and Kosobud, A: Sensitivity and tolerance to ethanol in mice bred to be genetically prone (WSP) or resistant (WSR) to ethanol withdrawal seizures. J Pharmacol Exp Ther 239:327, 1986.
21. Crabbe, JC, Kosobud, A, and Young, ER: Genetic selection for ethanol withdrawal severity: Differences in replicate mouse lines. Life Sci 33:955, 1983.
22. Crabbe, JC, Young, ER, and Kosobud, A: Genetic correlations with ethanol withdrawal severity. Pharmacol Biochem Behav 18:544, 1983.
23. Deitrich RA and Spuhler K: Genetics of alcoholism and alcohol actions. In Smart, RG, et al (eds): Research Advances in Alcohol and Drug Problems, Vol 8. Plenum Press, New York, 1984, p 47.
24. Falconer, DS: Introduction to Quantitative Genetics, ed 2. Longman, New York, 1983.
25. Feller, DJ and Crabbe, JC: Unpublished material, 1987.
26. Feller, DJ, Harris, RA, and Crabbe, JC: Differences in GABA activity between ethanol withdrawal seizure prone and resistant mice. Eur J Pharmacol 157:147, 1988.
27. Friedman, HJ: Assessment of physical dependence on and withdrawal from ethanol in animals. In Rigter, H and Crabbe, JC (eds): Alcohol Tolerance and Dependence. Elsevier/North Holland Biomedical Press, Amsterdam, 1980, p 93.
28. Galindo, A: GABA-picrotoxin interaction in the mammalian central nervous system. Brain Res 14:763, 1969.
29. Gallaher, EJ, et al: Mouse lines selected for genetic differences in diazepam sensitivity. Psychopharmacology 93:25, 1987.
30. Goldstein, DB: Alcohol withdrawal reactions in mice: Effects of drugs that modify neurotransmission. J Pharmacol Exp Ther 186:1, 1973.
31. Goldstein, DB: Inherited differences in intensity of alcohol withdrawal reactions in mice. Nature 245:154, 1973.
32. Goldstein, DB: Relationship of alcohol dose to intensity of withdrawal signs in mice. J Pharmacol Exp Ther 180:203, 1972.
33. Goldstein, DB and Kakihana, R: Alcohol withdrawal reactions and reserpine effects in inbred strains of mice. Life Sci 15:415, 1974.
34. Goldstein, DB and Kakihana, R: Alcohol withdrawal reactions in mouse strains selectively bred for long or short sleep times. Life Sci 17:981, 1975.
35. Goldstein, DB and Pal, N: Alcohol dependence produced in mice by inhalation of ethanol: Grading the withdrawal reaction. Science 172:288, 1971.
36. Grieve, SJ, Griffiths, PJ, and Littleton, JM: Genetic influence on the rate of development of ethanol tolerance and the ethanol physical withdrawal syndrome in mice. Drug Alcohol Depend 4:77, 1979.
37. Griffiths, PJ and Littleton, JM: Concentrations of free amino acids in brains of mice of different strains during the physical syndrome of withdrawal from alcohol. Br J Exp Pathol 58:391, 1977.

38. Hutchins, JR, et al: Behavioral and physiological measures for studying ethanol dependence in mice. Pharmacol Biochem Behav 15:55, 1981.
39. Kakihana, R: Alcohol intoxication and withdrawal in inbred strains of mice: Behavioral and endocrine studies. Behav Neural Biol 26:97, 1979.
40. Kosobud, A, Bodor, AS, and Crabbe, JC: Voluntary consumption of ethanol in WSP, WSC and WSR selectively bred mouse lines. Pharmacol Biochem Behav 29:601, 1988.
41. Kosobud, A and Crabbe, JC: Ethanol withdrawal in mice bred to be genetically prone or resistant to ethanol withdrawal seizures. J Pharmacol Exp Ther 238:170, 1986.
42. Kosobud, A and Crabbe, JC: Genetic correlations among inbred strain sensitivities to convulsions induced by nine convulsant drugs. Brain Res, in press.
43. Kosobud, A and Crabbe, JC: Sensitivity to convulsant drugs in WSP and WSR selectively bred mice (submitted for publication).
44. Kosobud, A, Cross, S, and Crabbe, JC: Neurosensitivity to pentylenetetrazol convulsions in inbred and genetically selected mice. (submitted for publication).
45. McClearn, GE, et al: Selective breeding in mice for severity of the ethanol withdrawal syndrome. Substance and Alcohol Actions/Misuse 3:135, 1982.
46. McClearn, GE and Kakihana, R: Selective breeding for ethanol sensitivity: Short-sleep and long-sleep mice. In McClearn, GE, Deitrich, RA, Erwin, VG (eds): Development of Animal Models as Pharmacogenetic Tools. US Department of Health and Human Services–NIAAA, Washington, DC, 1981, p 147.
47. McQuarrie, DG and Fingl, E: Effects of single doses and chronic administration of ethanol on experimental seizures in mice. J Pharmacol Exp Ther 124:264, 1958.
48. McSwigan, JD, Crabbe, JC, and Young, ER: Specific ethanol withdrawal seizures in genetically selected mice. Life Sci 35:2119, 1984.
49. Mucha, RF and Pinel, JPJ: Increased susceptibility to kindled seizures in rats following a single injection of alcohol. J Stud Alcohol 40:258, 1979.
50. Sanders, B: Withdrawal-like signs induced by a single administration of ethanol in mice that differ in ethanol sensitivity. Psychopharmacology 68:109, 1980.
51. Skerrit, JH and MacDonald, RL: Multiple actions of convulsant barbiturates on mouse neurons in cell culture. J Pharmacol Exp Ther 230:82, 1984.
52. Squires, RF, et al: Convulsant potencies of tetrazoles are highly correlated with many actions on GABA/benzodiazepine/picrotoxin receptor complexes in brain. Life Sci 35:1439, 1984.
53. Squires, RF, et al: [^{35}S]t-butyl bicyclophosphorothionate binds with affinity to brain specific sites coupled to γ-aminobutyric acid-A and ion recognition sites. Mol Pharmacol 23:326, 1982.
54. Thesleff, S: Aminopyridines and synaptic transmission. Neuroscience 5:1413, 1980.
55. Wilson, JR, et al: Ethanol dependence in mice: Direct and correlated responses to ten generations of selective breeding. Behav Genet 14:235, 1984.

PART III

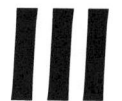

Classification and Diagnosis of Syndromes

CHAPTER 14

Richard H. Mattson, M.D.

Alcohol-Related Seizures

The relationship between alcohol use and seizures dates to earliest recorded literature.[20] The Romans used the term *morbus convivialis* to describe in part alcohol-related seizures.[14] Though we are aware of the relationship, we do not yet possess a full understanding of the clinical syndromes. The various reasons for seizure occurrence in persons using alcohol in varying amounts and in persons with alcoholism have been described in several reviews[2,7,15] and are detailed in subsequent chapters in this section.

A major effort was made in 1939 to review critically the current understanding of the effects of alcohol on humans. A Research Council on Problems of Alcohol was organized in affiliation with the American Academy for the Advancement of Science to review the world literature, including 100,000 books, pamphlets, and papers about the effects of alcohol. Substantive medical works ultimately reviewed included 5,500 publications pertinent to understanding how alcohol affects humans. Bowman and Jellinek[1] cited 33 papers dating to 1874 that reported cases related to "alcoholic epilepsy." Based on eight studies, epilepsy was reported to occur in 25% of alcoholic patients. Five other studies reported that 15% of epileptic patients were "abnormal drinkers," although Lennox's[14] careful study found a lower percent. Regardless of the reported frequency of alcoholism and seizures or seizures occurring with heavy alcohol use, the association far exceeded what might be expected by chance alone. A variety of causes were proposed, including the following: alcohol was a precipitant but not a cause of latent epilepsy, that is, a genetic predisposition was brought out by alcoholism; alcoholism produced cerebral damage (brain lesions) causing epilepsy; and alcohol precipitated episodes simulating epilepsy but not truly epileptic in charater.[1] Alcohol withdrawal was not mentioned.

In the past half century these concepts have become better defined. This chapter categorizes the various clinical syndromes. Categorization helps facilitate diagnosis and management. Two major groups can be identified: persons with alcoholism who have seizures, and persons with epilepsy who use alcohol. Table 14-1 outlines the groups.

ALCOHOLISM AND SEIZURES

Alcohol Withdrawal

For many years, alcohol was considered a toxic substance that precipitated seizures.[14,20] Such a conclusion logically evolved from observing seizures occurring in persons using alcohol in excess. Although a withdrawal effect had long been supported by European studies, at the time of Bowman and Jellinek's[1] review little credence was given in the United

Table 14-1 ALCOHOL-RELATED SEIZURES

I. ALCOHOLISM
   A. Acute cerebral or medical disorders
      1. Metabolic (hypoglycemia, hyponatremia, hypomagnesemia, uremia, hepatic encephalopathy)
      2. Toxic (cocaine, narcotic, and so forth)
      3. Infection (meningitis, encephalitis)
      4. Trauma (subdural, subarachnoid hemorrhage)
      5. Coincidental disorders (stroke, neoplasm, AVM)
   B. Withdrawal syndrome
   C. Epilepsy (seizures during prolonged abstinence)
      1. Symptomatic of long-term effects of disorders noted in IA
      2. Coincidental symptomatic epilepsy*
      3. Latent epilepsy unmasked by alcoholism
      4. Epilepsy due to neuronal damage caused by alcohol?
      5. Epilepsy due to kindled effect of repeated withdrawal seizures?
II. EPILEPSY
   A. Alcoholism developing in patients with epilepsy
   B. Seizures precipitated by alcohol use in nonalcoholic patients with epilepsy (rebound withdrawal)
   C. Latent epilepsy unmasked by alcohol use
   D. Seizures induced by direct effect of alcohol?

*Generalized idiopathic epilepsy appears at a much younger age than alcoholism.

States to the theory that withdrawal played a significant role in "alcoholic epilepsy" or delirium tremens. Despite this thinking, in 1942 Kalinowsky[13] emphasized that many neurologic complications of alcoholism occurred during a phase of withdrawal. This concept was consistent with the fact that similar effects are elicited by discontinuing other substances, such as barbiturates.[13] In the prior year, Lennox[14] studied a large population of patients with epilepsy, including a small number who drank heavily. He noted that "rum fits occur most often, not during the period of maximal concentration of alcohol in the body, but during the sobering up process."

A decade later, Victor and Adams[21] reviewed their experience at the Massachusetts General Hospital and carefully defined an alcohol withdrawal syndrome (AWS), emphasizing that seizures were part of an early manifestation of this syndrome. The unique studies of Isbell and associates[11] supported this finding. A group of persons hospitalized for substance abuse at the United States Public Health Service Hospital in Lexington, Kentucky agreed to consume heavy amounts of alcohol for up to 12 weeks, followed by abrupt discontinuation. Clinical changes and in some cases electroencephalographic (EEG) changes were observed. Two subjects developed seizures during the withdrawal period. Paroxysmal EEG discharges were observed in some patients in the group.[23]

These important studies were followed by Victor and Brausch's[22] landmark publication reporting data from a large series of alcoholic patients who experienced seizures during phases of withdrawal. The clinical characteristics of AWS were carefully defined, and the definitions have stood the test of time. Victor and Brausch[22] reported that after periods of prolonged heavy alcohol intake, and in the absence of other systemic causes or cerebral disease, seizures occurred during the period when alcohol levels were decreasing or in the next few days. AWS usually occurred after years of steady and prolonged alcohol intake. Withdrawal seizures usually were generalized in type, few in number, self limited, and often did not recur even without anti-epileptic drug therapy. In addition, the EEG revealed abnormal photic sensitivity (photomyogenic or photoconvulsive response) in about half the patients during withdrawal.[22] In the Lexington study, Wikler and associates[23] also noted some paroxysmal changes. This finding has not been consistently reproduced. Vossler and Browne (see Chapter 17) and Hauser, Nicolosi, and Anderson[8] have found this response much less frequently. The variation may be explained partly by technical factors such as light intensity, darkness of the room, distance from the flash, and timing of the test. Use of therapeutic agents such as benzodiazepines or paraldehyde before the EEG greatly attenuates this abnormal response and may account in part for more recent negative reports.

Hillbom's experience in Helsinki (see Chapter 19) has demonstrated similar but not identical AWS patterns. Heavy drinking only on weekends was followed by the occurrence of seizures during the first one or two days of the week. Hillbom concluded that long-term, continuous drinking was not necessary to cause seizures.

The recent epidemiologic study by Ng and associates[16] suggests that the occurrence of seizures specifically during alcohol withdrawal cannot be defined, although they found a statistically significant direct relationship between quantity of alcohol used and frequency of occurrence of seizures. These data differ from that generated by other investigations, as reviewed by Victor in Chapter 32.

Specific Cerebral and Systemic Causes

The major studies of Victor and Adams[21] and Victor and Brausch[22] on the important role of alcohol withdrawal in causing alcohol-related seizures may have led some physicians to be insufficiently aware of other reasons seizures may occur in patients who use alcohol.[4,7,9,15,18] Patients with alcoholism are susceptible to the many causes of seizures in the general population (Table 14–1). In fact, the lifestyle of heavy alcohol users puts them at special risk. Head injury, central nervous system (CNS) infections, neoplasms, and strokes, all of which cause seizures, are more frequent in patients with alcoholism. Heavy alcohol intake also may induce seizures by causing acute metabolic derangements, including hypoglycemia, hyponatremia, and hypomagnesemia. Hypoglycemia often is a consequence of the depletion of enzymes necessary for gluconeogenesis in alcoholic patients who have been relying on ethanol for caloric intake and have consumed relatively little else. The intake of toxic substances or drugs of abuse such as cocaine also may precipitate seizures.

Diagnosis of these disorders is beyond the scope of this review and is covered in more detail in subsequent chapters. However, in addition to history and physical examination, analysis of blood chemistries and cells, cerebrospinal fluid, EEG studies, computed tomography (CT) or magnetic resonance imaging (MRI), or even invasive angiographic studies might be considered, depending on the clinical presentation. Failure of the patient promptly to recover consciousness and orientation, abnormal findings on any of the diagnostic studies, or focal abnormalities on neurologic examination or in the EEG provide important signals of potentially serious and correctable medical and neurologic disorders.

Symptomatic Epilepsy in Alcoholics

A variety of cerebral insults in the patient with alcoholism may produce symptomatic epilepsy with partial or secondarily generalized seizures. These persons then run as great a risk for seizures as persons with symptomatic epilepsy from other causes. They are also more likely than other epilepsy patients to have seizures precipitated by alcohol withdrawal independent of the epileptic lesion. Finally, alcoholic patients with symptomatic epilepsy may have seizures exacerbated from the epileptic focus as a rebound from moderate to heavy alcohol intake, as reported for nonalcoholic patients with epilepsy (see Chapter 22).

Alcohol-Induced Epilepsy

It has not been established whether chronic alcoholism and the specific effects of alcohol can cause neuronal changes or permanent damage leading to epilepsy during periods of prolonged abstinence. Dam and associates[3] reported that no etiology other than a history of heavy alcohol use was apparent in 23 percent of all cases of new-onset epilepsy. Changes such as a cerebral and cerebellar atrophy with development of organic brain syndrome or ataxia are probably directly due to ethanol toxicity, at least in part. It has been proposed that after prolonged heavy alcohol use, changes may occur in susceptible tissue such as hippocampus, leading to epilepsy development.[7] Such changes have yet to be clearly demonstrated either in human or animal experimental models.

EPILEPSY AND ALCOHOL USE

Alcoholism in People with Epilepsy

A certain number of patients with epilepsy may use excessive amounts of alcohol or become alcoholic for the same reasons that lead to alcoholism in the general population. In addition, the psychosocial stresses many patients with epilepsy experience theoretically place this population at greater risk. However, little evidence indicates that alcoholism is any more frequent in patients with epilepsy than in the general population. Indeed, Lennox[14] found the prevalence of alcoholism to be lower in this group. Nevertheless, heavy alcohol intake in patients with epilepsy is quite likely to exacerbate the seizure problem and make them especially susceptible to seizures during the withdrawal phase. The reasons are the same as those described for the alcoholic patient who later develops epilepsy.

Nonalcoholic Epilepsy Patients

The close relationship between alcoholism and seizures has led to the theory that any intake of alcohol in patients susceptible to seizures poses a significant risk. Abstinence has often been advised for these patients.[10] Despite this general belief, several studies have found that light intake of alcohol has little or no effect on seizure occurrence[6,10,14] (see Chapters 21 and 22). On the other hand, moderate or heavy alcohol intake, even if practiced only infrequently, was found to be followed by exacerbation of seizures in 85 percent of patients with epilepsy (see Chapter 22). Little evidence from either human or experimental animal studies indicates that alcohol directly increases or precipitates seizures[5,10,19] (see Chapter 22). Indeed, both animal and human studies suggest that alcohol has transient anticonvulsant properties.[7,17]

Unmasking of Latent Epilepsy

In early reports, the occurrence of seizures in patients who drank heavily was often thought to be due to a genetic predisposition to epilepsy. Subsequent studies have demonstrated that multiple causes can be found for seizures in patients with heavy alcohol use and alcoholism does not simply unmask epilepsy. Some nonalcoholic patients experience occasional seizures, usually of the generalized tonic-clonic type. These persons often have a history of moderate to heavy intake and sleep deprivation associated with some festive occasion the night before the seizure. Replication of the circumstances in a laboratory may disclose generalized spike and wave activity or other epileptiform pattern[18] (see Chapter 22). Giove and Gastaut[6] have described this event as "activation par la fête," which may be freely translated as "activation by celebration." It is likely that such persons have very mild or latent epilepsy elicited only by these seizure-inducing factors.

SUMMARY

Multiple reasons exist for the occurrence of seizures in association with alcohol use. Careful diagnostic evaluation is important to delineate the cause in order to select the optimal treatment. Since Bowman and Jellinek[1] reviewed the world literature 50 years ago, basic and clinical scientists have advanced our understanding of alcohol-related seizures. Jellinek[12] noted: "In the course of our readings we have come across some investigations devised with such careful foresight as only the most competent scientists can accomplish and carried out with accuracy reflecting only the finest workmanship. But the conclusions drawn from these excellently devised and performed experiments have sometimes been in direct though surely unconscious contradiction to the experimental data." In clinical studies, Jellinek[12] found, "some accepted conclusions have come from poorly devised experiments or from numerically inadequate material and in some instances have been based on a misapplication of statistical methods to laboratory data." Jellinek emphasizes that abundant shortcomings can be found in existing clinical studies and that much more clarification is needed. Clinical issues to resolve include the following: Is there a frequency or quantity of drinking that by itself causes epilepsy? Does alcohol produce cerebral changes that cause or increase the potential for seizures to occur, independent of all other intercurrent causes? Are there groups of people for whom acute alcohol use elicits a paradoxical epileptic response? Are there subgroups of epileptic patients for whom even modest intake of alcohol poses significant risks? This brief list suggests that much is yet to be learned about the association between alcohol use and seizures.

ACKNOWLEDGMENT

Research supported by the Veterans Administration Medical Research Service and NINDS Grant 5PONSO6208-22.

References

1. Bowman, K and Jellinek, E: Alcohol addiction and its treatment. In Jellinek, E (ed): Alcohol Addiction and Chronic Alcoholism. Yale University Press, New Haven, 1942, p 3.
2. Chan, WK: Alcoholism and epilepsy. Epilepsia 26:323, 1985.
3. Dam, AM, et al: Late onset epilepsy: Etiologies, types of seizure, and value of clinical investigation, EEG and computerized tomography scan. Epilepsia 26:227, 1985.
4. Earnest, MP and Yarnell, P: Seizure admissions to a city hospital: The role of alcohol. Epilepsia 17:387, 1976.
5. Essig, CF and Lam, RC: Convulsions and hallucinatory behavior following alcohol withdrawal in the dog. Arch Neurol 18:626, 1968.
6. Giove, G and Gastaut, H: Epilepsie alcoolique et d'enclenchement alcoolique des crises chez les epileptiques. Rev Neurol (Paris) 113:347, 1965.
7. Hauser, WA, Ng, SK, and Brust, JC: Alcohol, seizures, and epilepsy. Epilepsia 29:S66, 1988.
8. Hauser, WA, Nicolosi, RS, Anderson, VE: Electroencephalographic findings in patients with ethanol withdrawal seizures. Clin Neurophysiol 52:64, 1982.
9. Hillbom, ME: Occurrence of cerebral seizures provoked by alcohol abuse. Epilepsia 21:459, 1980.
10. Hoppener, RJ, Kuyer, A, and van der Lugt, PM: Epilepsy and alcohol: The influence of social alcohol intake on seizures and treatment in epilepsy. Epilepsia 24:459, 1983.
11. Isbell, H, et al: An experimental study of the etiology of "rum fits" and delerium tremens. Quarterly Journal of the Study of Alcohol 16:1, 1955.
12. Jellinek, EM: Scope and method of the study. In Jellinek, E (ed): Alcohol Addiction and Chronic Alcoholism. Yale University Press, New Haven, 1942, p xv.
13. Kalinowsky, LB: Convulsions in nonepileptic patients on withdrawal of barbiturates, alcohol and other drugs. Archives of Neurology and Psychiatry 48:946, 1942.
14. Lennox, WG: Alcohol and epilepsy. Quarterly Journal of Studies on Alcohol 2:1, 1941.
15. Mattson, RH: Seizures associated with alcohol use and alcohol withdrawal. In Browne, TR and Feldman, RG (eds): Epilepsy: Diagnosis and Management. Little, Brown & Co. Boston 1983, p 325.
16. Mattson, RH, Pratt, KL, Calverley, JR: Electroencephalograms of epileptics following sleep deprivation. Arch Neurol 13:310, 1965.
17. McQuarrie, DG and Fingl, E: Effects of single doses and chronic administration of ethanol on experimental seizures in mice. J Pharmacol 124:264, 1958.
18. Ng, KC, et al: Alcohol consumption and withdrawal in new-onset seizures. N Engl J Med 319:666, 1988.
19. Rodin, EA: Effects of acute alcohol intoxication on epileptic patients. Arch Neurol 4:103, 1961.
20. Tempkin, O: The Falling Sickness, ed 2. Johns Hopkins Press, Baltimore, 1971.
21. Victor, M and Adams, RD: The effect of alcohol on the nervous system. Research Publication of the Association for Research on Nervous and Mental Diseases 32:526, 1953.
22. Victor, M and Brausch, J: The role of abstinence in the genesis of alcoholic epilepsy. Epilepsia 8:1, 1967.
23. Wikler, A, et al: Electroencephalographic changes associated with chronic alcoholic intoxication and the alcohol abstinence syndrome. Am J Psychiatry 113:106, 1956.

CHAPTER 15

Maurice Victor, M.D.

Alcohol Withdrawal Seizures: An Overview

Any discussion of alcohol withdrawal seizures (AWS) is predicated on the assumption that such a disorder exists, that is, that there is a seizure state causally related not simply to the abuse of alcohol, but specifically to the cessation of drinking (withdrawal) following a period of chronic intoxication. My purpose is not to challenge the validity of the withdrawal theory; indeed, all our observations support it. But it is noteworthy how readily this concept is accepted now, and how the very term *alcohol withdrawal syndrome* has become a standard part of medical language. This was not always the case; validation and universal acceptance of the withdrawal theory are relatively recent developments.

THE CONCEPT OF AWS

The notion that certain seizures in the alcoholic patient are related to the withdrawal of alcohol was probably first expressed by Huss,[20,23] who recognized that convulsions were frequent among alcoholics. More importantly, he drew a distinction between convulsions in epileptics who drank and convulsions that were brought about by the cessation of drinking. The relationship of seizures to the cessation of drinking was also commented upon by others in the last century.[6,12] In 1901, Bonhoeffer[2] stated that the sudden withdrawal of alcohol was an important factor in the genesis of delirium tremens, a view that was subsequently affirmed by other physicians, including Hare,[17] Osler,[31] and Kalinowsky.[24]

However, this view failed to prevail. Perhaps it was because the alcohol withdrawal theory rested only on isolated observations and statements, unsupported by careful clinical or animal experimental studies. Statements that denied the causative role of alcohol withdrawal in the genesis of delirium tremens came to carry as much weight as those affirming it, and gradually the former view gained wider acceptance. Some investigators[3,4] rejected the withdrawal theory on the grounds that only a small proportion of their alcoholic patients developed delirium tremens after being jailed or admitted to the hospital. (This is hardly surprising, considering that only 5 percent of patients hospitalized for serious alcoholic illnesses develop delirium tremens.[38])

An article that was quoted frequently to discredit the withdrawal theory is that of Piker,[32] who stated after questioning 275 patients with *delirium tremens* that 74.5 percent had the onset of their symptoms while still drinking. It should be noted that Piker's data were derived from patients' statements, following their recovery, with no corroboration from independent sources. Furthermore, Piker apparently did not distinguish between cases of fully developed delirium tremens and cases with milder symptoms, such as tremulousness and hallucinosis; nor did he consider the possible effects of relative abstinence or a falling blood alcohol level in the genesis of the latter symptoms.

Another notion that gained considerable popularity in the 1930s was that "abstinence is in itself an expression of the beginning of delirium." Originally stated by Bumke and Kant,[7] this view was elaborated by Noyes[30] and by Bowman, Wortis, and Keiser.[5] The latter authors regarded "disgust for alcohol" as well as nausea and vomiting consequent to gastritis and hepatitis, as the initial symptoms of delirium tremens, rather than possible precipitating factors. The protagonists of this idea neglected the fact that delirium tremens need not develop in a setting of nausea, vomiting, and "disgust for alcohol," and that it often occurs in the absence of these symptoms, following the abrupt imposition of abstinence by injury, infection, admission to the hospital for elective surgery, and so forth.

Implicit in the view of Bumke and Kant was the idea that delirium tremens and related disorders simply represent the most severe form of alcohol intoxication—an untenable notion. The symptoms of intoxication, consisting of slurred speech, uninhibited behavior, staggering gait, stupor, and coma, are quite distinctive and different from the symptom complex of tremor, hallucinations, fits, and delirium. The former group of symptoms is associated with a high blood alcohol level, whereas the latter symptoms become evident only with a reduction of blood alcohol from a previously higher level. Symptoms of intoxication increase in severity as more alcohol is consumed, so that drowsiness, for example, may progress to a state of coma and respiratory depression. On the other hand, symptoms such as tremor and hallucinations, or even full-blown delirium tremens, may be nullified by the administration of alcohol.

Despite the illogicality of equating the tremulous-hallucinatory-convulsive state with intoxication and the dearth of evidence upon which this notion was based, Bowman and Jellinek[4] wrote in 1941 that the withdrawal theory had been virtually discarded in the United States. In Europe, this theory was also relegated to obsolescence.[1,7] This was certainly the prevailing point of view at the Boston City Hospital in 1949, at which time we undertook our studies of alcoholism. That such an attitude would prevail at this institution is all the more remarkable when one considers the vast numbers of alcoholics that were available for study there. In a survey that we conducted in 1951, more than half the adult men and 15 percent of the women showed the medical or neurologic effects of severe alcoholism.

Our observations clearly indicated that the most constant and the one indispensable factor in the genesis of tremulous-hallucinatory-convulsive-delirious symptoms was the withdrawal of alcohol following a period of chronic intoxication. The clinical evidence to support this concept was first presented in 1952 and published the following year.[38] These data are summarized briefly below.

The shaded area in Figure 15–1 represents the period of drinking and is, for purposes of illustration, greatly foreshortened; the periodic notches in the baseline portray the initial and mildest manifestations of abstinence—the morning tremulousness, uneasiness, nausea, and retching that occur after the period of abstinence represented by a night's sleep. The patient can suppress these symptoms by taking a drink or two, after which he or she is able to drink in the usual manner for the rest of the day, only to have the symptoms reassert themselves the following morning. After a variable period of time and for a variety of reasons, this pattern of drinking ends and the patient can no longer maintain or reestablish the previous blood alcohol level. The symptoms of intoxication subside, usually over a period of 6 or 7 hours, and a new group of symptoms, those of abstinence or withdrawal, then becomes manifest. In addition to the recurring morning tremulousness, three major groups of abstinence symptoms can be recognized: 1) a state characterized mainly by tremor and hallucinations, which peaks in intensity 24 hours after the cessation of drinking; 2) convulsive

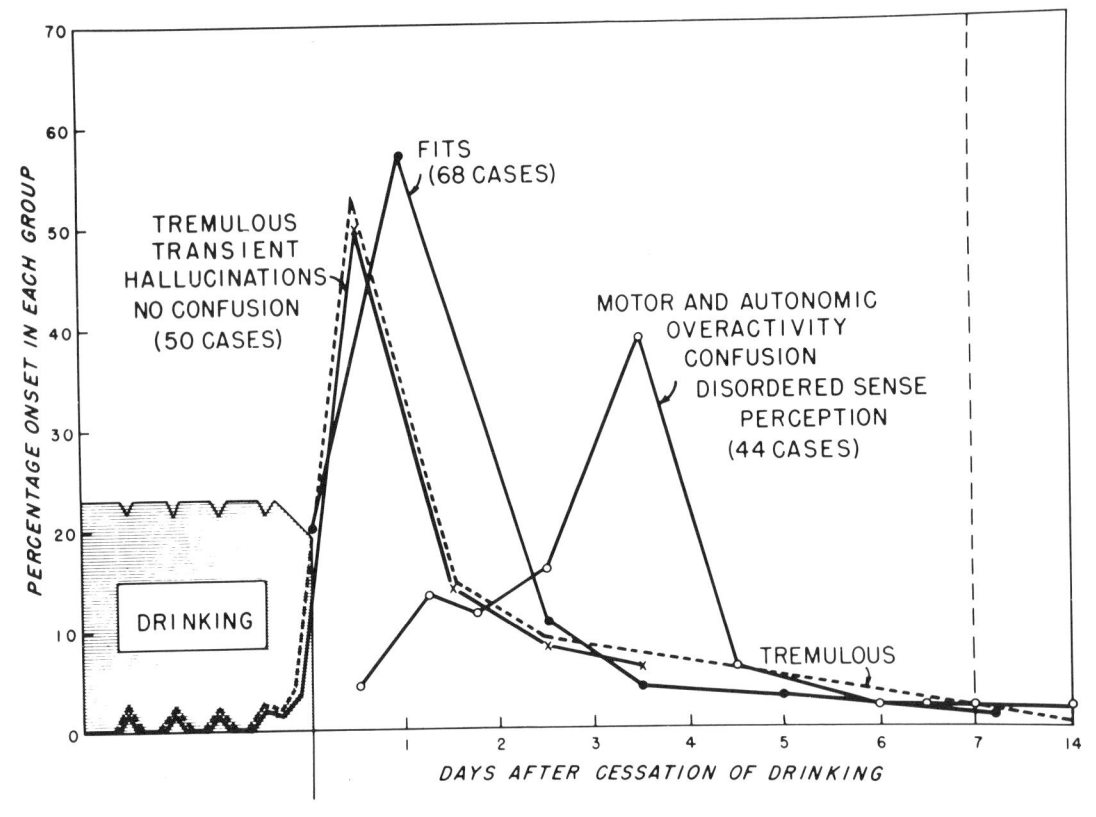

Figure 15–1. The relationship between cessation of drinking and the onset of tremulousness, hallucinations, seizures, and delirium tremens. (Adapted from Victor and Adams.[38])

seizures, usually grand mal in type, that occur singly or in short bursts, and in the majority of cases, between 7 and 48 hours after withdrawal, with a peak incidence at 24 hours; and 3) a state characterized by gross tremor and agitation, disorders of sense perception, and increased psychomotor and autonomic nervous system activity. The latter syndrome, for which we believe the term *delirium tremens* should be reserved, has its onset between the 72 and 96 hours after the cessation of drinking.

Each syndrome may occur more or less by itself, but more often they occur in combination, in which case they appear in a predictable sequence. Characteristically, delirium tremens is preceded by tremulousness and transient hallucinations, and the latter symptoms may even subside considerably before the delirium becomes manifest. Similarly, when seizures and delirium tremens occur in the same patient, the seizures invariably precede the delirium. Also, it is evident that the severity of the clinical symptoms is related to the degree and duration of drinking. The mildest degree of the syndrome, taking the form of tremulousness, anorexia, nausea, and general irritability, may occur after a few days of drinking and after a relatively short period of abstinence (*e.g.*, after a night's sleep); the most severe form of the syndrome, that is, delirium tremens, occurs after many weeks or months of drinking, becoming apparent only after several days of abstinence.

These observations, derived from the study of alcoholic patients on the wards of a large city hospital, were virtually duplicated by Isbell and coworkers[21] in a carefully controlled study of chronic intoxication and withdrawal in a group of ten volunteer subjects. Alcohol was administered orally, at 1- to 2-hour intervals, in a dose of 266 to 489 ml/day for 7 to 87 days. Convulsions and delirium did not appear during the period in which the patients consumed alcohol in sufficient amounts to maintain high blood alcohol levels. Following alcohol withdrawal, patients who drank for only a few weeks showed tremulousness, nausea, perspiration, and insomnia of brief duration. Six patients who drank for 48 to 87 days showed similar symptoms, only more severe; two of them also had transient hallucinations, two had seizures, and three developed delirium tremens—the former manifestations preceding the latter. Clearly demonstrated here was the typical sequence of the withdrawal symptoms as well as the relationship of the intensity of the withdrawal symptoms to the amount of alcohol consumed and the duration of the period of intoxication. It was also interesting that the manifestations of alcohol withdrawal in these subjects were very much the same as those induced by chronic intoxication and withdrawal from barbiturates.[21]

In the decade or two that followed these clinical observations, the concept of an alcohol withdrawal syndrome was amply confirmed by a series of animal studies. The most noteworthy are those of McQuarrie and Fingl,[26] Essig and Lam,[11] Freund,[13] Goldstein,[14,15] and Ellis and Pick.[9,10] These studies are particularly significant with respect to AWS insofar as seizure activity—both clinical and electroencephalographic—is the most readily recognized feature and measurable index of withdrawal in animals. The first animal experiments to support the withdrawal concept were those of McQuarrie and Fingl.[26] Using mice, they demonstrated that single doses of alcohol temporarily raised the seizure threshold, followed by a brief but definite lowering of the threshold below normal. Administration of high doses of alcohol for an extended period produced a more marked and prolonged drop in the seizure threshold after alcohol withdrawal. Essig and Lam[11] described convulsions following the abrupt withdrawal of ethanol after a two-month administration through surgically implanted gastric cannulae. A withdrawal syndrome was also reported in weight-controlled mice following a five-day period of intoxication produced by consuming an ethanol-containing liquid diet.[13]

Subsequently, Ellis and Pick[9,10] induced a state of physical dependence upon alcohol in rhesus monkeys. The progression of withdrawal signs in the monkeys was very similar to that observed in humans.[21,38] These studies in monkeys were particularly important because they demonstrated that signs of abstinence depended upon a decline in the blood alcohol level from a previously higher level in the brain and not necessarily upon the complete disappearance of alcohol from the blood. Thus, the onset of tremulousness occurred at levels as high as 200 mg/100 ml, behavioral changes at 50 to 150 mg/100 ml, and convulsions at 85 mg/100 ml. In humans also, early signs of abstinence have been observed with blood alcohol concentrations as high as 100 mg/100 ml.[21,28]

These clinical and experimental studies adequately answer most of the arguments that have been made against the withdrawal theory. One can readily comprehend that a reduction in alcohol intake and a fall in the blood alcohol level will result in the emergence of withdrawal signs despite the fact that the patient is still drinking. In fact, in these circumstances, the patient drinks mainly to suppress withdrawal symptoms; because such a patient may have the odor of alcohol on his or her breath, these symptoms have been attributed erroneously to the effects of intoxication. It is also apparent that delirium tremens occurs in only a small proportion of hospitalized or incarcerated alcoholics, because this complication requires a background of heavy drinking sustained for many weeks or months; casual, short-term, or weekend drinking, even though it may result in arrest for drunkenness, will not result in serious withdrawal symptoms. Finally, it should be noted that some patients suffer practically no clinical signs of withdrawal, although the amount and duration of their drinking appears to be more or less comparable to that of patients with abstinence symptoms. One would surmise that alcohol withdrawal following a period of chronic intoxication, although a necessary factor in the genesis of delirium tremens and related disorders, is not in itself a sufficient factor in all cases. The additional factor(s) that may or may not be involved in withdrawal symptoms are considered later in this chapter.

CONVULSIVE SEIZURES IN THE ALCOHOLIC: ANALYSIS OF THE CLINICAL FEATURES OBSERVED IN HOSPITALIZED PATIENTS

That a close relationship exists between the abuse of alcohol and the occurrence of convulsive seizures is generally acknowledged. Over the years a wide variety of opinions have been expressed about this relationship, most of them with no meaningful supporting data.[36] As part of our original study of the effects of alcohol on the nervous system, we analyzed 266 consecutive adult patients who were hospitalized with obvious alcoholic neurologic illnesses.[38] In 32 (12 percent), a convulsive seizure or several seizures had complicated the alcoholic illness. Moreover, in the majority of alcoholics with seizures, there appeared to be a close relationship to the withdrawal of alcohol, as depicted in Figure 15–1.

These early observations prompted a more systematic and detailed investigation of the question of "alcoholic epilepsy." The clinical data were derived from the study of 241 alcoholic patients who presented with convulsive seizures or, in some cases, with other types of alcoholic illness that in turn were complicated by seizures. In each case, the history of the patient's drinking habits and the occurrence of seizures were substantiated by a person(s) other than the patient and who was deemed reliable. Independent corroboration of this type was an unwavering condition for inclusion of a patient in this study. We quickly realized that the patient alone was an untrustworthy witness, particularly for events in the hours and days preceding his or her admission. Parenthetically, it may be mentioned that strict adherence to these criteria accounted for the fact that it took us 15 years to complete this study; we estimated that for every patient included there were approximately nine others for whom the clinical data were insufficiently secure to permit inclusion. The details of this study are presented elsewhere.[36,40] Here, only the general features are discussed.

Clinical observations of 241 alcoholic patients who presented with convulsive seizures permitted the delineation of three distinct epileptic syndromes. By far the most common syndrome, in the briefest terms, took the following form: The patient was a serious drinker for many years, whose seizures began in adult life. The seizures occurred in relation to an episode of sustained drinking, not during the period of chronic intoxication, but only after the cessation of drinking, or alcohol withdrawal. The convulsive attack consisted of a single seizure or of several seizures occurring over several hours. The seizures themselves were grand mal in type and the electroencephalogram (EEG), except in immediate relationship to the convulsive seizures, was normal. (In the relatively small number of patients with focal seizures, there were usually focal EEG changes and other evidence of focal cerebral lesions; see below.) In almost one third of the patients, the seizures were followed by delirium tremens; invariably, the seizures had terminated before the onset of the delirium. About half the patients showed an abnormal sensitivity to photic stimulation in the form of photomyoclonus or photoconvulsions. The period of vulnerability to photic stimulation bore roughly the same temporal relationship to alcohol withdrawal as did the spontaneous seizures.

A second and surprisingly small group (7 of 241 cases) consisted of patients with idiopathic epilepsy, who only became alcoholic many years after the onset of their seizures. Subsequent observations suggested that these patients are more numerous than our original study had indicated.

The third and least clearly defined group comprised 21 patients in whom cerebral trauma and alcoholism were associated. This group was distinguished by the fact that the seizures were frequently focal and accompanied by focal EEG abnormalities. In the patients with idiopathic and post-traumatic epilepsy, seizures occurred during periods of sobriety as well as in relation to drinking, but they were far more frequent and severe in the latter circumstance. The period of intoxication that precipitated seizures was not necessarily prolonged; in some cases, a weekend or even a single evening of drinking was sufficient.

Thus, our observations indicated that the main factor in the precipitation of seizures was the withdrawal of alcohol following a period of sustained intoxication. This factor was operative not only in the usual form of alcoholic epilepsy, but also in cases of idiopathic and post-traumatic epilepsy, although less uniformly and after shorter periods of intoxication. The data supporting this are illustrated in Figure 15-2.

There were remarkably few cases in which the seizures seemed to be unassociated with abstinence from alcohol. In four patients, seizures occurred within a few hours of the last drink, at a time when they were allegedly still intoxicated. There is no ready explanation for these instances, but they do not negate the findings in 157 other patients in whom a significant period of abstinence (longer than six hours) preceded the onset of seizures. Another exceptional case, of a different type, was that of a patient who had his first seizure 20 days after drinking ceased, long after the other signs of alcohol withdrawal had disappeared.

An impressive feature of our study was the small proportion (16 percent) of patients who showed EEG abnormalities. If the overt instances of post-traumatic and idiopathic epilepsy are excluded, as well as several cases that reverted to normal within 2 weeks, then the proportion is reduced to 9 percent. This incidence compares very closely with that found in a large series of alcoholics who were tested within 2 weeks of admission to the hospital,[8] and also with that in the normal male population. In contrast, we found EEG abnormalities in 50 percent of non-alcoholic patients with idiopathic epilepsy while Greenblatt, Levin, and DeCorli[16] detected abnormalities in 75 percent.

Our study provided no information about the EEG during the course of alcoholic intoxication, but this subject has been studied extensively in both animals and humans.[36] It is generally agreed that

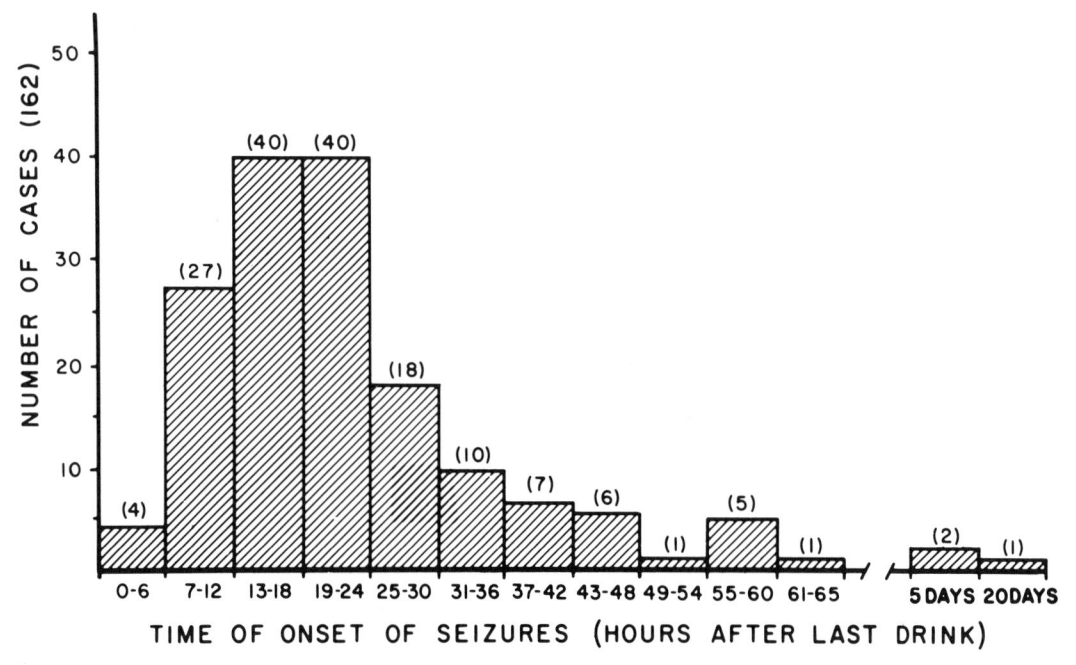

Figure 15-2. The relationship between cessation of drinking and the onset of convulsive seizures. (Adapted from Victor and Brausch.[40])

rising concentrations of alcohol reduce the frequency of brain waves, and that slowing in the EEG usually appears at about the concentration at which the signs of intoxication become obvious. Of greater interest, however, are those studies in which EEGs have been made serially during chronic intoxication and in the period immediately following withdrawal. In one subject who had been maintained at a high blood alcohol level for 5 days, paroxysmal high-voltage slow activity appeared 48 hours after the abrupt withdrawal of alcohol.[29] Wikler and coworkers[42] followed the EEG changes in three patients during chronic intoxication and withdrawal under controlled experimental conditions. Mild degrees of slowing occurred during the period of chronic intoxication. After alcohol withdrawal, sharp waves, spikes, and paroxysmal changes appeared, but these changes were transient and occupied only the 15th to 19th hours of the abstinence period. This period coincides with the peak incidence of spontaneous seizures in our patients (Fig. 15-1), and the transient nature of the EEG abnormalities is in keeping with the brevity of the convulsive attacks. The observations of Wikler and coworkers would also explain the normality of the EEG in a group of chronically intoxicated subjects who were tested 31 to 34 hours after their last drink,[41] as well as in our patients who were tested at variable periods after their seizures.

The EEG evidence does not support the notion that seizures in the alcoholic represent latent epilepsy made manifest by alcohol, or that alcohol simply precipitates convulsive attacks in patients who are subject or constitutionally predisposed to seizures. Insofar as the EEG is a record of physiologic activity of the cerebral cortex, it reflects a characteristic series of changes engendered by alcohol itself—mild slowing during chronic intoxication, a rapid return to normal immediately after cessation of drinking, mild but definite dysrhythmias occupying a discrete period in the withdrawal phase, and again a return to normal. Except for this very transient period following alcohol withdrawal, the incidence of EEG abnormalities in patients with alcoholic epilepsy is not greater than in the normal population—in sharp contrast to patients who are indeed subject to seizures.

How is the very common, highly stereotyped convulsive syndrome designated in the alcoholic? The term "rum fits" or "whiskey fits" is as suitable as any other, and has been used for years by alcoholics themselves. It clearly sets apart seizures that begin in adult life, that occur in particular relationship to sustained inebriety and withdrawal from alcohol, and that are associated with transient EEG abnormalities and photic sensitivity, from those that occur with or without drinking and are associated with persistent EEG abnormalities. In making this distinction, we do not deny that idiopathic, post-traumatic, and other types of seizures are adversely affected by alcohol. They are; it should be noted, however, that with certain qualifications these seizures bear the same relationship to intoxication and withdrawal as do "rum fits."

The Cause of "Rum Fits"

It is evident that the one indispensable factor in the genesis of "rum fits" is the withdrawal of alcohol, following a period of chronic intoxication.[22] Alcohol withdrawal in itself may be an insufficient factor in producing "rum fits" and related disorders, however. Additional mechanisms may be operative. It is our belief that two factors, hypomagnesemia and respiratory alkalosis, are particularly important in this respect. The data describing the role of these factors in the genesis of withdrawal symptoms have been previously reported.[43-45]

Early in our studies of alcoholism it became apparent that patients with severe alcohol withdrawal symptoms, particularly those with seizures, were remarkably sensitive to photic stimulation. This sensitivity took the form of tonic-clonic convulsion with loss of consciousness (photoconvulsion) or, more frequently, of coarse clonic movements of the face and neck, spreading to involve the trunk and limbs, without loss of consciousness (photomyoclonus). The latter response was usually accompanied by a paroxysmal EEG discharge and frequently culminated in a major generalized seizure, particularly if photic stimulation was continued after the onset of myoclonus. A systematic investigation of large numbers of hospitalized alcoholics disclosed that photoconvulsions or photomyoclonus could be induced in about half the patients during the early stages of alcohol withdrawal, and that these responses had the same temporal relationship to cessation of drinking as did spontaneous seizures (Fig. 15-3). In contrast, such responses to photic stimulation were practically never produced in normal persons and only rarely in patients with idiopathic epilepsy.[19,36,40]

In assessing the role of hypomagnesemia[25] and other agents in the genesis of withdrawal seizures, advantage was taken of yet another attribute of the photomyoclonic response. It was found that in photic-sensitive patients, characteristic responses could be induced over many hours or even days, and that photic stimulation could be repeated at frequent intervals over 30 to 60 minutes without altering the seizure threshold (the number of flashes/second and the duration of the stimulus required to produce myoclonus). Thus, it was possible to judge the effects of administration of magnesium (or other agents) upon the photomyoclonus threshold in patients with alcohol withdrawal symptoms.

The frequency of hypomagnesemia in alcohol withdrawal states has been noted by many investigators.[18,28,33,35] Our initial observations of this relationship were made in a group of 18 alcoholic patients who were free of hepatic or renal disease, diabetes mellitus, hypocalcemia, malabsorption, and other diseases that might have had a primary effect on magnesium metabolism.[44] Each patient was subjected to stroboscopic stimulation at the time of his or her admission to the hospital and at 8-hour intervals thereafter, until the alcohol withdrawal symptoms had abated. Ten subjects responded with photomyoclonus while eight did not. Five of the ten patients who responded also had spontaneous seizures. Eight of the ten patients who showed photomyoclonus in the withdrawal period were given magnesium sulfate (MgSO$_4$) intravenously in doses of 206 g (16.7-50 mEq). In three patients, administration of 3 g of MgSO$_4$ abolished the response at all frequencies within minutes. In the other five patients, all of whom had much lower magnesium levels, the photomyoclonus threshold following the MgSO$_4$ administration was significantly elevated.

The foregoing study disclosed another consistent alteration in the withdrawal

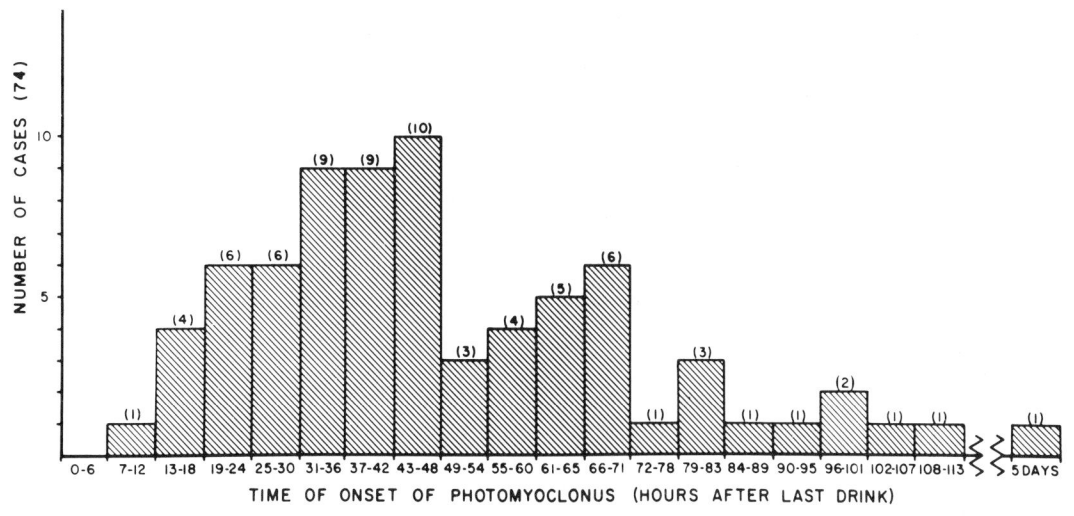

Figure 15-3. The relationship between alcohol withdrawal and the occurrence of photomyoclonus. (Adapted from Victor and Brausch.[40])

period, namely, the rapid evolution of an alkalotic state. This finding was consistent with the observations of Sereny, Rapoport, and Husdan,[34] who noted a transient rise in the arterial pH of eight alcoholic subjects during the initial 48 hours of hospitalization. The alkalemia characterizing the withdrawal state and its relation to hypomagnesemia and photomyoclonus were investigated initially in four volunteer subjects who drank for 60 days, after which they were withdrawn abruptly.[45] The rise in arterial pH values, which could be detected as early as 8 hours after alcohol withdrawal, was often concomitant with a fall in the serum magnesium level and an increased sensitivity to photic stimulation. These features are illustrated in Figures 15-4 and 15-5. Tremor and hyperreflexia, prominent during the period of hypomagnesemia and alkalosis, abated as the serum magnesium and arterial pH values returned to normal. It is noteworthy that the serum calcium values in these four patients were normal (4.5–5.5 mEq/liter) throughout the intoxication and withdrawal periods.

These investigations served as the basis for a more elaborate study designed to explain the nature of the alkalosis that characterizes the alcohol withdrawal state.[43] Nine alcoholics, observed under controlled conditions of drinking and abstinence, were the subjects of the latter study. Following a control period of observation, these patients consumed between one and two pints of 100-proof bourbon daily *ad lib*, in addition to an adequate diet and supplemental vitamins. Four of the patients drank in this way for 60 days, and five for 14 days. The rise in arterial pH that followed the abrupt withdrawal of alcohol was accompanied by a fall in pCO_2 values—the pH abnormality proved to be a pure respiratory alkalosis resulting from tachypnea and increased depth of respiration. The severity of the withdrawal symptoms correlated with the magnitude of change of the arterial pH and pCO_2. Only the patients with relatively large changes in pH and pCO_2 (with one exception these were the patients who drank for 60 days) showed spontaneous seizures, photomyoclonus, and severe

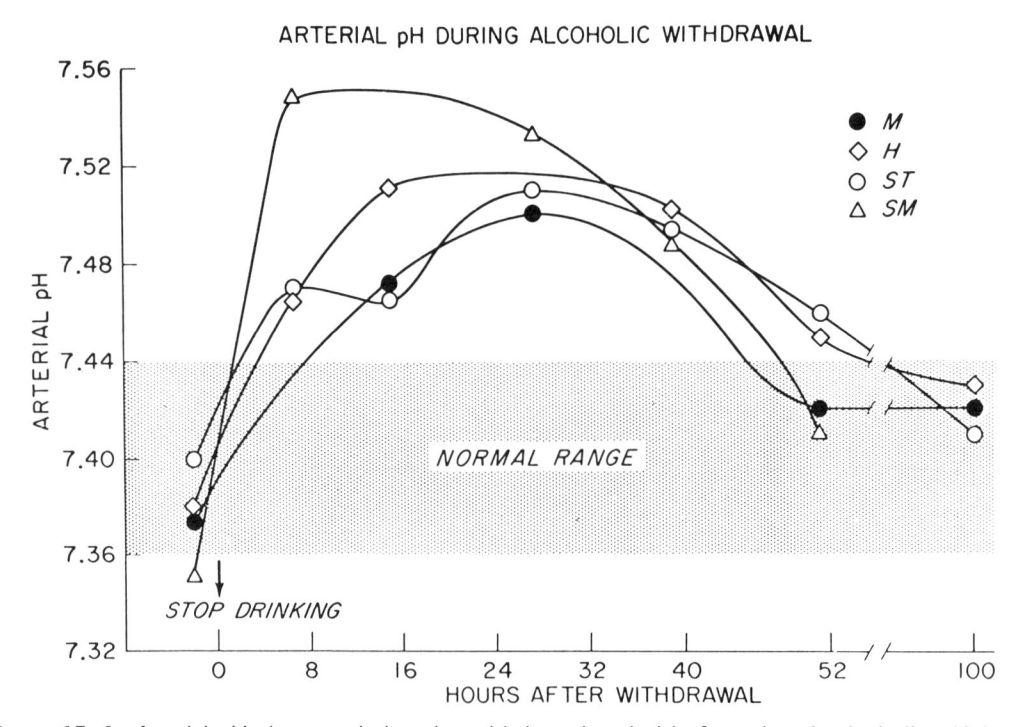

Figure 15–4. Arterial pH changes during the withdrawal period in four chronic alcoholics. (Adapted from Wolfe and Victor.[44])

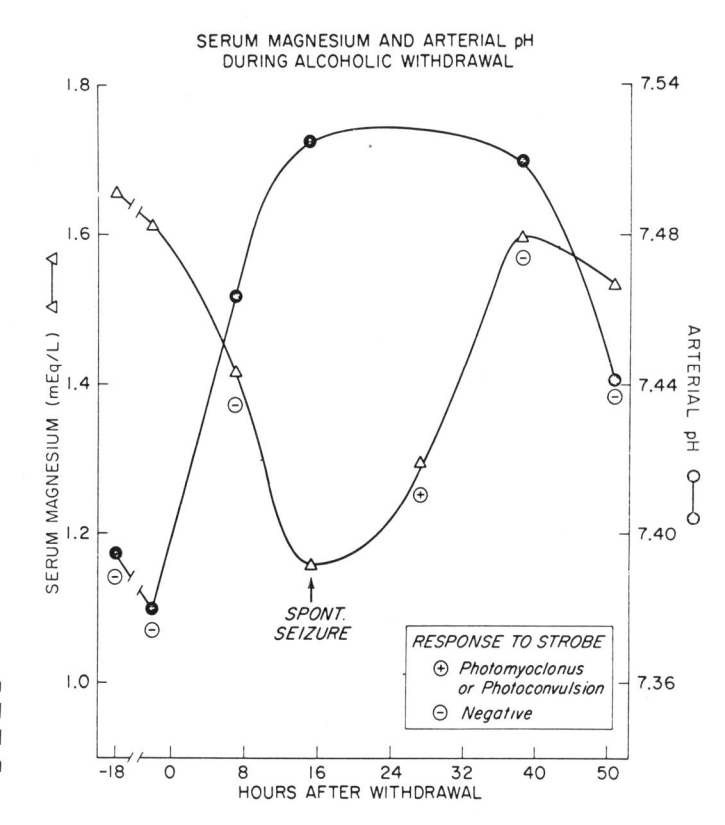

Figure 15–5. Relationship between arterial pH, serum magnesium, and photic sensitivity during the alcohol withdrawal period. (Adapted from Wolfe and Victor.[44])

tremulousness. The fall in serum magnesium levels during the withdrawal period was much greater in the patients who drank for 60 days than in those who drank for 14 days (an average fall of 0.41 mEq/liter in the former, and 0.10 mEq/liter in the latter). Serum calcium levels remained in the normal range in all nine patients throughout the study, and only two patients developed acute hypokalemia during withdrawal.

These observations, which were made of patients in a metabolic ward during control, drinking, and withdrawal periods, were extended in another study of 31 alcoholics who were admitted to the Cleveland Metropolitan General Hospital from the emergency ward.[45] The withdrawal symptoms in the latter group were much more severe than those of the previously studied patients. We made observations in nine cases of delirium tremens as well as in 22 patients with the earlier signs of withdrawal (13 with tremor or hallucinations or both, and nine with seizures).

This latter study provided additional evidence that the early phase of alcohol withdrawal is consistently associated with respiratory alkalosis and that the severity of the clinical manifestations correlated closely with the magnitude of this biochemical derangement (Fig. 15–6 and Fig. 15–7). The respiratory alkalosis was maximal between 12 and 21 hours after withdrawal, and the occurrence of seizures and hallucinations coincided with the maximal degree of respiratory alkalosis. The reduction in pCO_2 and rise in arterial pH were greater in the patients with seizures than in those with tremor and hallucinations. The respiratory alkalosis had largely corrected itself within 50 hours of withdrawal, at which time the symptoms were minimal or absent.

Apart from the changes in serum magnesium, arterial pH, and pCO_2, no consistent biochemical abnormalities were associated with withdrawal symptoms. Measurements of SGOT and SGPT were normal, and values of serum proteins, sodium, chloride, calcium, potassium, and

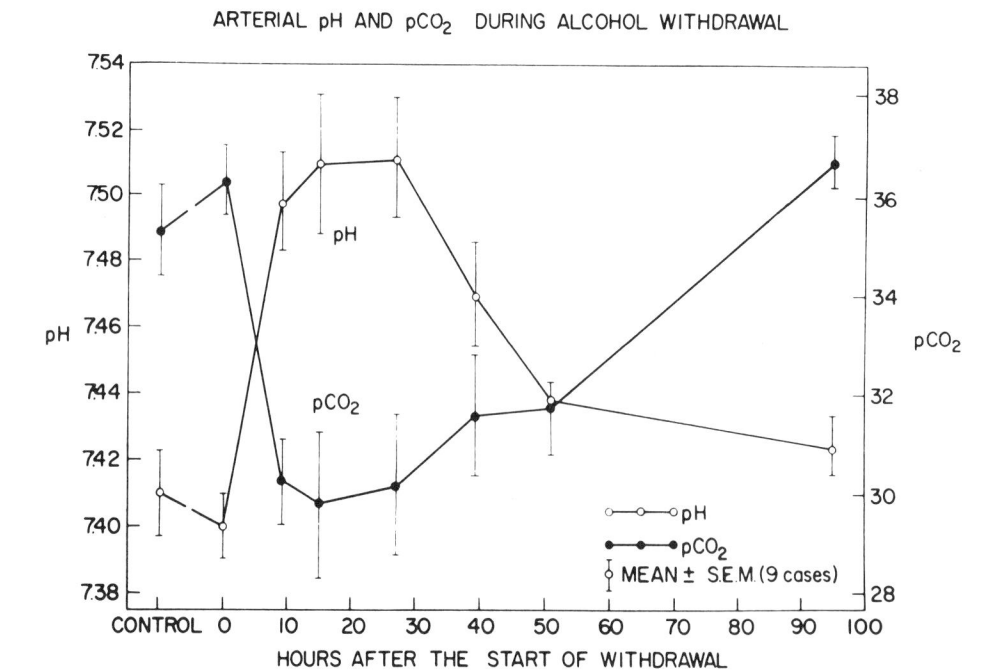

Figure 15–6. Arterial pH and CO$_2$ values during the alcohol withdrawal period in nine subjects. Control values were obtained before drinking began; values at 0 hour were obtained just prior to the last drink (withdrawal of alcohol). (Adapted from Wolfe, et al.[43])

glucose, estimated repeatedly during the intoxication and withdrawal periods, disclosed only a few instances of hyperglycemia and a slight depression of the serum potassium level in eight of the 31 patients.

It may be concluded from these studies that all but the mildest forms of alcohol withdrawal are associated with acute transient hypomagnesemia and with respiratory alkalosis, which is most likely the result of hyperventilation.[37] In the initial phase of the withdrawal period, that is, for approximately 48 hours following cessation of drinking, the severity of the withdrawal symptoms is closely correlated to the magnitude of change of these biochemical abnormalities. Further, we observed that administering magnesium raises the seizure threshold in the withdrawal period and that it may also improve other abstinence symptoms. Additionally, correcting respiratory alkalosis may have a salutary effect on withdrawal symptoms, but more data are required to be certain.

In addition to these relationships, there is considerable indirect evidence that hypomagnesemia and respiratory alkalosis may be important in causing withdrawal symptoms. Manifestations of both central and peripheral nervous system irritability have been described repeatedly in states of magnesium deficiency. It is commonly observed that hyperventilation may precipitate seizures in patients with epilepsy and cause slowing of the EEG even in normal persons. A striking example of the effects of hyperventilation occurs in patients with chronic obstructive lung disease who have high arterial pCO$_2$ and normal or slightly decreased pH values. When these patients are mechanically hyperventilated, the pCO$_2$ decreases and arterial pH increases, and, if such treatment is prolonged or excessive, they may become disoriented and develop hallucinations, tremor, hyperreflexia, generalized muscular irritability, and seizures. Symptoms may be quickly relieved by simply allowing pCO$_2$ to increase.

It is postulated that hypomagnesemia and alkalosis, each of which is known to be associated with hyperexcitability of the

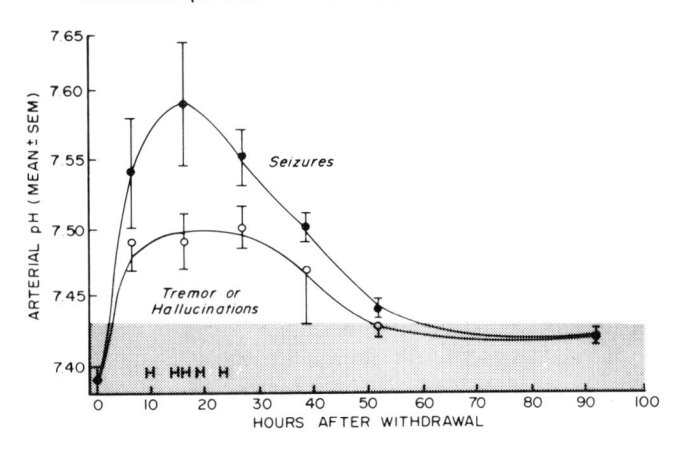

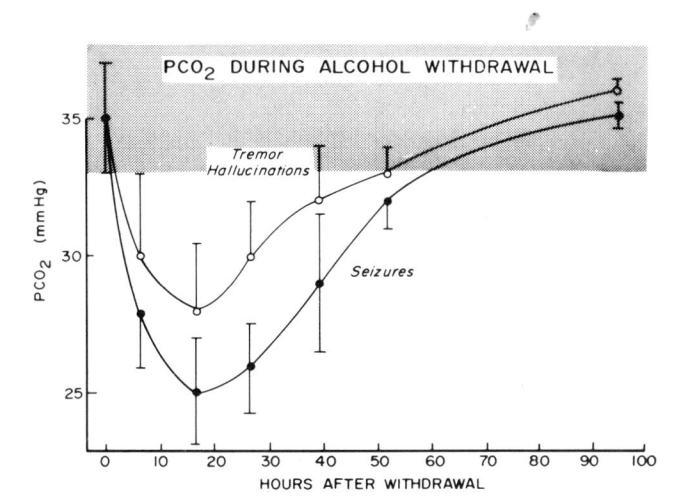

Figure 15–7. Arterial pH values (top) and pCO$_2$ (bottom) during the alcohol withdrawal period in 13 patients with tremor or hallucinations (or both) and 9 patients with seizures (1 patient had several seizures). (Adapted from Wolfe and Victor.[45])

nervous system, are compounded to produce photomyoclonus, spontaneous seizures, and perhaps other symptoms that characterize the early phase of alcohol withdrawal. The precise relationship between hypomagnesemia and alkalosis is not understood. Possibly, the latter may be responsible for the former by causing a shift of magnesium into bone and other intracellular sites, just as alkalemia causes a shift of potassium from extra- to intracellular compartments. The specific mechanism by which alcohol intoxication and withdrawal produce respiratory alkalosis is a matter of speculation. The effect of chronic alcohol intoxication on the respiratory center is to cause a decrease in ventilatory response to carbon dioxide. Possibly, removal of the depressant effect of alcohol is followed by a rebound phenomenon, resulting in an increased sensitivity of the respiratory center to carbon dioxide and hyperventilation.

SUMMARY

This overview has covered mainly our own investigations into the problem of alcohol and epilepsy and, more specifically, into the role of alcohol withdrawal in the genesis of convulsive seizures. It was thought that such a review, based as it is on a series of sequential studies over a period of 35 years, would be more interesting than an attempt to review the many divergent views of this subject. This approach to the subject was not intended to minimize the work of others or ideas that are not concordant with our own. A full expression of these varying views is found in other chapters in this volume.

References

1. Bleuler, E: Textbook of Psychiatry (authorized translation by Brill, AA). Macmillan, New York, 1951, p 327.
2. Bonhoeffer, K: Die akuten Geisteskrankheiten der Gewohnheitstrinker. Eine klinische Studie VIII. Fisher, Jena, 1901, p 226.
3. Bostock, J: Alcoholism and its treatment. Med J Aust 26:136, 1939.
4. Bowman, KM and Jellinek, EM: Alcoholic mental disorders. Quarterly Journal of the Study of Alcohol 2:312, 1941.
5. Bowman, KM, Wortis, H, and Keiser S: The treatment of delirium tremens. JAMA 112:1217, 1939.
6. Bratz, D: Alkohol und Epilepsie. Allgemeine Zeitschrift für Psychiatrie 56:334, 1899.
7. Bumke, O and Kant, F: Trunksucht und Chronisher Alkoholismus. In Bumke, O, Foerster, O (eds): Handbuch der Neurologie. Springer, Berlin, 1936, Vol 13, p 828.
8. Dyken, M, Grant, P, and White, P: Evaluation of electroencephalographic changes associated with chronic alcoholism. Diseases of the Nervous System 22:284, 1961.
9. Ellis, FW and Pick, JR: Ethanol-induced withdrawal reactions in rhesus monkeys. Pharmacologist 11:256, 1969.
10. Ellis, FW and Pick, JR: Experimentally induced ethanol dependence in rhesus monkeys. J Pharmac Exp Ther 175:88, 1970.
11. Essig, CF and Lam, RC: Convulsions and hallucinatory behavior following alcohol withdrawal in the dog. Arch Neurol 18:626, 1968.
12. Fere, E: L'Epilepsie. Gauthier-Villars et Fils, Paris, 1896, p 227.
13. Freund, G: Alcohol withdrawal syndrome in mice. Arch Neurol 21:315, 1969.
14. Goldstein, DB: An animal model for testing effects of drugs on alcohol withdrawal reactions. J Pharmacol Exp Ther 183:14, 1972.
15. Goldstein, DB: Relationship of alcohol dose to intensity of withdrawal signs in mice. J Pharmacol Exp Ther 180:203, 1972.
16. Greenblatt, M, Levin, S, and DeCorli, F: The electroencephalogram associated with chronic alcoholism, alcoholic psychosis, and alcoholic convulsions. Arch Neurol Psychiatry 52:290, 1944.
17. Hare, F: Alcohol and delirium tremens. Br Med J 1:446, 1915.
18. Heaton, FW, et al: Hypomagnesaemia in chronic alcoholism. Lancet 2:802, 1962.
19. Hughes, JR, Curtin, MJ, and Brown, VP: Usefulness of photic stimulation in routine clinical electroencephalography. Neurology 10:777, 1960.
20. Huss, M: Chronische Alcohol-Krankheit. Fritze, Stockholm, 1852.
21. Isbell, H, et al: Chronic barbiturate intoxication: experimental study. Arch Neurol Psychiatry 64:1, 1950.
22. Isbell, H, et al: An experimental study of the etiology of "rum fits" and delirium tremens. Quarterly Journal of the Study of Alcohol 16:1, 1955.
23. Jellinek, EM: Classics of the alcohol literature: Magnus Huss' Alcoholismus Chronicus. Quarterly Journal of the Study of Alcohol 4:85, 1943.
24. Kalinowsky, LB: Convulsions in non-epileptic patients on withdrawal of barbiturates, alcohol, and other drugs. Arch Neurol Psychiatry 48:946, 1942.
25. Klingman, WO, et al: Role of alcoholism and magnesium deficiency in convulsions. Transactions of the American Neurological Association 80:162, 1955.
26. McQuarrie, DG and Fingl, E: Effects of single doses and chronic administration of ethanol on experimental seizures in mice. J Pharmacol Exp Ther 124:264, 1958.
27. Mendelson, JH et al: Serum magnesium in delirium tremens and alcoholic hallucinosis. Journal of Nervous and Mental Diseases 128:352, 1959.
28. Mendelson, JH and LaDou, J: Experimentally induced chronic intoxication and withdrawal in alcoholics. II. Psychophysiological findings. Quarterly Journal of the Study of Alcohol (Suppl) 2:14, 1964.
29. Newman, HW: The effect of alcohol on the electroencephalogram. Stanford Medical Bulletin 17:55, 1959.
30. Noyes, AP: Modern Clinical Psychiatry, ed 2. WB Saunders, Philadelphia, 1939, p 218.
31. Osler, W: Principles and Practice of Medicine, ed 8. D Appleton, New York, 1917, p 398.
32. Piker, P: On the relationship of sudden withdrawal of alcohol to delirium tremens. Amer J Psychiatry 92:1387, 1937.
33. Randall, RE, Rossmeisl, EC, and Bleifer, KH: Magnesium depletion in man. Ann Intern Med 50:257, 1959.
34. Sereny, G, Rapoport, A, and Husdan, H: The effect of alcohol withdrawal on electrolyte and acid-base balance. Metabolism 15:896, 1966.
35. Suter, C and Klingman, W: Neurologic manifestations of magnesium depletion states. Neurology 4:691, 1955.
36. Victor, M: The pathophysiology of alcoholic epilepsy. Res Publ Assoc Res Nerv Ment Dis 46:431, 1968.
37. Victor, M: The role of hypomagnesemia and respiratory alkalosis in the genesis of alcohol-withdrawal symptoms. Ann NY Acad Sci 215:235, 1973.

38. Victor, M and Adams, RD: The effect of alcohol upon the nervous system. Res Publ Assoc Res Nerv Ment Dis 32:526, 1953.
39. Victor, M and Adams, RD: On the etiology of the alcoholic neurologic diseases: With special references to the role of nutrition. Am J Clin Nutr 9:379, 1961.
40. Victor, M and Brausch, CC: The role of abstinence in the genesis of alcoholic epilepsy. Epilepsia 8:1, 1967.
41. Weiss, AD, et al: Experimentally induced chronic intoxication and withdrawal in alcoholics. Electroencephalographic findings. Quarterly Journal of the Study of Alcohol (Suppl 2, pt 7):96, 1964.
42. Wikler, A, et al: Electroencephalographic changes associated with chronic alcoholic intoxication and the alcohol abstinence syndrome. Am J Psychiatry 113:106, 1956.
43. Wolfe, SM, et al: Respiratory alkalosis and alcohol withdrawal. Trans Assoc Am Physicians 82:344, 1969.
44. Wolfe, SM and Victor, M: The physiological basis of the alcohol withdrawal syndrome. In Mello, NK, Mendelson, JH (eds): Recent Advances in Studies of Alcoholism. US Government Printing Office, Washington, DC, 1971, p 188.
45. Wolfe, SM and Victor, M: The relationship of hypomagnesemia and alkalosis to alcohol withdrawal symptoms. Ann NY Acad Sci 162:973, 1969.

Stephen K. C. Ng, M.D., Dr.P.H.

CHAPTER 16

Alcohol-Related Seizures: A Diversity of Mechanisms?

There is no universally accepted definition of alcohol-related seizures, although seizures among heavy alcohol users are well recognized clinical phenomena. Some investigators consider most seizures in current alcohol users to be alcohol-related[33,69] Thus, seizures that are secondary to cerebral tumors, vascular malformation, aneurysms, and so forth, are nonetheless labeled alcohol related if the subject has used alcohol shortly before the seizure.[33] Because multiple factors besides alcohol can lead to seizures, a more reasonable approach is to consider seizures alcohol related only if alcohol is likely to have led to their genesis or precipitation.

Seizure genesis refers to a protracted lowering of seizure threshold (usually in terms of months or years). Such a lowering may be permanent. The clinical manifestations are recurrent seizures long after the responsible factor or event has occurred. Seizure precipitation, on the other hand, refers to an acute and reversible lowering of seizure threshold. Seizures recur only in the presence of precipitating factors or events. It is theoretically important to distinguish between the role of alcohol in the genesis as opposed to the precipitation of a seizure, because different mechanisms and prognosis may be involved. In practice, such a distinction is not always possible. Additionally, alcohol may lead to seizure genesis in some cases and seizure precipitation in others.

When a seizure disorder predates any alcohol use, the role of alcohol is most likely that of seizure precipitation. It is often believed that alcohol exacerbates seizures in patients with epilepsy, and some epileptics report that their seizures have often followed alcohol use, especially during the "sobering up" period.[39,44,69] Mechanisms for seizure exacerbation include, among others, the stimulant effect of alcohol, alcohol withdrawal, and enchancement of anticonvulsant metabolism due to hepatic enzyme induction by alcohol. Experimental studies, however, have failed to demonstrate that social drinking has any substantial effect on clinical seizure activity, although some studies connect social drinking with neurophysiologic changes on electroencephalograms (EEG).[35,44,54]

With regard to seizure genesis, alcohol use might play either a sufficient or insufficient role. Whether alcohol use alone is sufficient for seizure genesis has not been adequately studied. Chronic alcoholism is associated with cerebral atrophy and cerebellar degeneration and it is possible that these changes themselves cause seizures. The insufficient role, on the other hand, is illustrated by joint action of alcohol with trauma, stroke, or infection. Alcohol intoxication often leads to head trauma, which can in turn cause seizures. Heavy alcohol use is also linked to stroke and increased susceptibility to infections, both of which also can cause seizures. Head trauma has been thought to be the cause of many so-called alcohol-related seizures. However, its role in these seizures remains speculative, because most patients with alcohol-related seizures do not have localized abnormalities on physical examination, EEG, or computed tomography (CT) scan.

It is commonly believed that alcohol use only precipitates seizures in the great majority of cases. These seizures are generally considered to be temporary aberrations of the central nervous system (CNS) and not to reflect any underlying prolonged increase of seizure susceptibility. They therefore require no treatment other than giving up alcohol. Although there are reports that acute alcohol intoxication can precipitate seizures,[13,64,66,73] the conventional wisdom is that the majority of alcohol-precipitated seizures are the result of alcohol withdrawal.[69] The withdrawal hypothesis suggests that after prolonged heavy drinking, cessation of alcohol intake results in a decline of blood alcohol level (BAL), which initiates a chain of physiologic changes leading to seizures. These changes include electrolyte imbalances,[69] calcium channel activity,[9,31,40] disturbances of cell membranes,[1] and alterations in gamma-aminobutyric acid (GABA) and other neurotransmitters.[14,21,36]

Clinically, alcohol withdrawal seizures (AWS) are mostly major motor tonic-clonic (grand mal), occurring within 7 to 48 hours of stopping alcohol intake, and are usually associated with other signs and symptoms of alcohol withdrawal.[69] Typically the EEGs of these patients are normal or show only nonspecific changes.

Several lines of evidence support the withdrawal hypothesis. The most often cited are Victor's observational studies (see Chapter 15), which document that 88 percent of seizures in a series of alcohol abusers occurred within 7 to 48 hours of stopping alcohol intake. The human experiment by Isbell and associates[37] is also believed by many to be crucial to the hypothesis. Lastly, many animal experiments appear to confirm what Isbell found in humans[17–20,28,42,46,51–53,74]

CRITIQUE OF PAST STUDIES

Observational Studies

The observation of Victor and Brausch[69] that 88 percent of seizures among alcohol abusers occur within 7 to 48 hours of a last drink does not necessarily imply that seizures are related to alcohol withdrawal. Two major problems affect the interpretation of their data—the probability of chance events and selection bias. Because drinking is cyclical and repetitive, the interval between seizure and last drink is interpretable only if one knows the frequency and quantity of a person's alcohol use. For example, if a person drinks regularly once every 24 hours, no event in his or her life can occur more than 24 hours after a last drink. It is not surprising, therefore, that in a group of heavy drinkers, many of whom drank on a daily basis, few seizures occurred more than 48 hours after a last drink. The possibility of such an artefact is suggested by the fact that among drinkers, seizures due to cerebral tumor, vascular accident, or aneurysm also tend to occur during the withdrawal period.

There may also be important selection bias in the sample of patients Victor and Brausch[69] studied. Their 241 patients were recruited over a period of 15 years from three different hospitals in two cities. A strict recruitment requirement was the independent corroboration of a subject's drinking history. Many alcoholics who had no family or friends to provide independent corroboration were therefore excluded from the study. The 241 patients included represent a 10 percent nonsystematic sample of over 2000 potential candidates seen by the study team.[68] Unknown selection factors may lead to serious confounding and internal validity problems. Generalization of the results is also greatly limited by such a selection process.

Human Experiments

Isbell and associates' human experiment, in which two out of ten former morphine addicts developed seizures after alcohol withdrawal, has not been successfully replicated by others.[47] Their experimental setting was highly artificial and the drinking pattern studied was unlike that of free-living alcoholics. One of the two persons who developed seizures had a history suggestive of previous seizures. On the other hand, other human experiments demonstrate that temporal lobe spikes, psychomotor seizures, and convulsions can be induced within minutes of alcohol administration with no interval for withdrawal.[43,64,66] Indeed, more human experiments support seizure development on acute alcohol administration than on withdrawal. Neither of these experimental results, however, explain clinical alcohol-related seizures, because it is generally believed that years of alcohol use must pass before alcohol-related seizures develop.

Animal Experiments

Animal studies seem to support the notion that seizures are integral components of the alcohol withdrawal phenomenon. The evidence is less conclusive than it first appears, however. For example, one of the many hazards of cross-species extrapolation from animal experiments is that most seizure manifestations in animals are not the same as those in humans. In many of the studies under review, species were selected for genetic susceptibility to seizures provoked by either sound or handling. Several other areas are not strictly coherent with the human experience. Thus the proportion of animals that developed seizures on withdrawal (close to 100 percent)[17,20] is much higher than that observed in humans. Brief exposures to alcohol (including a single injection) have been reported to induce seizures,[42] in contrast to the years of alcohol abuse required in humans. Investigators report very high mortality in animals during both alcohol intoxication and withdrawal,[18,20] a phenomenon not found in humans. While in humans seizures can occur up to 2 weeks after alcohol withdrawal, in animals seizures are either not observed or not reported after a short period following withdrawal. Seizures during the intoxication phase and before withdrawal may sometimes be missed; in most experiments reviewed, observation was not continuous but focused on withdrawal (animals were often found dead in tonic postures in their cages in the morning,[10,26] even though some of them, e.g., mice, were nocturnal feeding animals and had been drinking alcohol water during the night[10]).

Additional Considerations

Other observations also suggest that seizures related to alcohol may not all be simple withdrawal seizures. First, withdrawal seizures are thought to be triggered by a falling BAL after alcohol intake is stopped. Because BAL is close to zero 24 hours after a last drink, a falling BAL is unlikely to be the cause of seizures that occur more than 24 hours after a last drink. Human studies showed poor correlation between BAL and withdrawal symptoms.[37,47] Moreover, in an experiment in mice, "withdrawal" symptoms were related to the total dose of alcohol received and not to the BAL achieved.[27] Thus, as long as the total amount was similar, low doses of alcohol administered over a long period of time produced the same intensity of "withdrawal" symptoms as high doses administered over a short time, even though these two methods of alcohol administration produce very different BALs. Thus, these symptoms are more compatible with a direct dose-related effect of alcohol than with alcohol withdrawal.

Second, subjects who have had a previous alcohol-related seizure are at increased risk of further alcohol- and non-alcohol-related seizures.[34,48,56] The risk of recurrence following a first alcohol-related seizure is 30 percent in 3 years, a risk similar to the risk of other unprovoked seizures.[32] This fact suggests either that alcohol seizures lower a person's seizure threshold permanently, or that persons with alcohol seizures have an underlying seizure predisposition similar to that postulated for other unprovoked seizures.

Third, alcoholics with no other known seizure risk factor continue to have seizures long after they have stopped drinking. This fact is compatible with the earlier definition of seizure genesis. Various investigators have attributed between 23 to 37 percent of epileptic cases in adults to chronic alcohol abuse.[12,13,25]

Fourth, the long period of alcohol abuse necessary for seizure development (on average 10 years or more[13]) provides the strongest evidence that alcohol-related seizures may be a chronic disease. Because most people develop tolerance to alcohol within days and physical dependence within weeks of continued drinking,[47] it is difficult to understand why seizures thought to be related to these phenomena do not occur more frequently and after a much shorter duration of alcohol use, considering that alcohol withdrawal of 8 to 10 hours duration occurs almost daily even among the heaviest drinkers (*e.g.*, when they go to sleep).

Finally, studies of alcoholics in detoxification programs treated prophylactically with anticonvulsants provided intriguing results. In some randomized studies anticonvulsants such as phenytoin administered for 5 to 10 days were successful in reducing the number of patients having seizures after alcohol cessation.[48,56] They did not, however, prevent all seizures. Whereas seizures among untreated subjects occurred within the first week of alcohol cessation, subjects treated with anticonvulsants developed seizures in the second week of alcohol cessation after anticonvulsant therapy had been discontinued.[56] Because other alcohol withdrawal symptoms had long subsided, it is questionable whether these late seizures are related to alcohol withdrawal.

There are thus enough unresolved questions to warrant careful examination of alcohol-related seizures. Little is known about the relative risk alcohol use poses for seizure development. The relationship of neither duration, magnitude, nor type of alcohol use to the risk of incurring seizures has been studied. The interval between cessation of drinking and onset of seizure has been carefully documented in only one previous study.[69] No formal test of the withdrawal hypothesis using a large data set has ever been conducted, and data correlating the frequency and amount of alcohol use with the interval between last drink and seizure have never been published. We therefore carried out a study at Harlem Hospital to address these issues.

THE HARLEM STUDY

A case-control study involving adults with new onset seizures (cases) and adults admitted for the first bout of a surgical emergency (controls) was carried out at Harlem Hospital in New York City between December 1981 and February 1984.

Methods

CASES

Cases were drawn from Harlem Hospital in New York City, the sole municipal hospital for about 120,000 poor blacks living in the central Harlem section of the city. Persons aged over 15 years admitted with first seizures were eligible (n = 341). Hospital policy, sustained by constant communication between project and medical staff, was to admit all such patients for a complete neurologic work-up. Ninety-five percent of eligible subjects were found by searching the computerized daily admissions log for all patients with first seizures and other suspicious diagnoses (*e.g.*, syncope, hypoglycemia, and coma) and by reviewing their charts; 5 percent appeared among referrals to the neurology service after admission (these referrals were also screened).

A *first seizure* was defined as the first single seizure (or cluster of seizures within a 24-hour period) ever experienced by a person. The definition was relaxed on two counts: childhood febrile seizures did not invalidate the diagnosis of first seizure (n = 4), and patients with a recurrence of seizures that had begun within the previous year but for which the patient had not sought medical care were also accepted (n = 59). In 90 percent, eyewitnesses described the seizures; in the remaining 10 percent, the diagnosis met three of four criteria (loss of consciousness; urinary or fecal incontinence; tongue or cheek laceration; postictal confusion or Todd's paralysis). Among 341 eligible cases, 308 (90.3 percent) were interviewed; 16 (4.7 percent) died; 9 (2.6 percent) were discharged, and 6 (1.8 percent) signed out against medical advice before interview; and two (0.6 percent) were not mentally competent to give informed consent.

Controls

Subjects in the control group gave no history of afebrile seizures. They were patients over age 15 admitted to Harlem Hospital for the first time for an acute surgical condition with symptom onset within 1 year of admission (Table 16–1). Patients with diagnoses connected to alcohol abuse (e.g., acute pancreatitis, traffic accident injuries) were excluded. Of 345 eligible control subjects identified from admission logs, 294 (85.2 percent) were interviewed; 33 (9.6 percent) were discharged and 1 (0.3 percent) died before interview; 14 (4 percent) refused participation; 1 (0.3 percent) discharged himself against medical advice; and 2 (0.6 percent) were mentally incompetent. Controls were not matched to cases.

Interviews and Data Quality

Patients were interviewed after giving informed consent, usually within 72 hours of admission. The questionnaire covered medical and medication history, present illness, use of alcohol, tobacco, and illicit drugs, and family history of seizure disorder. Alcohol use in the 6 months before admission (or, for those who had stopped drinking, in the 6 months before they stopped) was described separately for wine, beer, and liquor in terms of usual frequencies and volumes. Duration of chronic use, frequency of heavy drinking (>5 drinks per occasion), and changes of pattern within two weeks of hospital admission were ascertained. For cases, the time that elapsed between the last drink and the seizure was noted. Information gathered by interview was generally consistent with the histories in medical charts.

Missing data (for any variable less than 4 percent, but slightly more frequent among cases) were handled in three ways, all conservative with respect to the estimate of seizure risk from alcohol use. For categorical exposure variables, missing entries were classified as unexposed. For frequency of alcohol use, missing entries (15 cases and 8 controls) were classed as nil. For volume of alcohol intake, the group mean of subjects who reported the same frequency of use as the person with the missing value (8 cases and 7 controls)

Table 16–1. ADMITTING DIAGNOSIS OF CONTROLS

Diagnosis	Percent	(Number)
Acute appendicitis	24.2	(71)
Acute cholecystitis	13.6	(40)
Intestinal obstruction	11.2	(33)
Perianal abscess	9.9	(29)
Hematuria	7.1	(21)
Rectal bleeding	4.8	(14)
Abdominal pain	4.4	(13)
Tonsillitis	3.4	(10)
Epididymitis or testicular torsion	2.7	(8)
Pneumothorax	2.4	(7)
Diverticulitis	1.7	(5)
Miscellaneous	14.6	(43)
Total	100.0	(294)

was substituted without regard to case/control status. Because consumption was higher for subjects in the case group, the substitution lowered estimated intake for cases and raised estimated intake for controls.

CLASSIFICATION OF SEIZURES

Seizures were classed by type as generalized onset major motor (n = 193), partial (n = 89), or unclassified (n = 26), and by etiology either as provoked (26 percent) or unprovoked (74 percent) on the basis of joint chart reviews (blind to interview data) by the project director and by a neurologist. To be considered provoked, a seizure must have had powerful and immediately antecedent provocations such as: metabolic derangements (e.g., serum glucose >500 mg/dl or <50 mg/dl or uremia) (n = 17); strokes or intracranial bleeding within 7 days of seizure onset (n = 29); central nervous system (CNS) infection (n = 9); brain tumor (n = 14); intravenous epileptogenic drugs within 1 hour of seizure (n = 5); body temperature >40.5°C (n = 2); head trauma involving loss of consciousness, skull radiographs, or hospital admission within 7 days before seizure onset (n = 5). Other than these exceptions, no assumptions were made about the effects of factors under study, including alcohol use and withdrawal; thus "withdrawal seizures" were classified as unprovoked.

STATISTICAL ANALYSIS

Respondents were classed as *non-drinkers* (drank less than once a year), *ex-drinkers* (previously drank at least once a month and had abstained for at least one year), and *current drinkers* (all others). Drinking was quantified in terms of frequency per week, volume per occasion, and duration in years. Group differences were evaluated nonparametrically by the two-tailed Wilcoxon rank sum test and the Kruskal-Wallis test.[11] The product of frequency, volume, and absolute alcohol content for each beverage consumed was calculated to obtain an average daily intake in grams of absolute alcohol (ADAA). Allocations of absolute alcohol by weight were for wine 15 percent, for beer 4.5 percent, and for liquor 45 percent.[38] The volume of a single *drink* of liquor has been variously considered as one or two ounces.[24,29,58,72] Our own nonsystematic inquiry among patients and in bars in Harlem led us to count a *drink* of liquor as two ounces. ADAA is presented primarily as a categorical variable, although it was examined also as a continuous variable. Multiple logistic regression[57] was used to estimate the adjusted odds ratios (OR) and 95 percent confidence limits (CL) of alcohol for seizures while controlling for confounders in this study, namely age, sex, history of hypertension, head injury, stroke, and chronic heroin use (six months or longer). Life-table method was used to analyze the interval between last drink and seizure (abstention time) among current drinkers. The probabilities of remaining seizure free after the last drink were plotted against duration of abstention. The resulting curves were used to compare subgroups among seizure patients (unprovoked *vs.* provoked seizures; unprovoked seizures with prior head injury or stroke *vs.* unprovoked seizures without such histories; among unprovoked seizures with no prior head injury or stroke, those with generalized onset major motor *vs.* partial seizures; and those whose drinking had increased, decreased, stopped, or remained unchanged in the two weeks before admission) using the two-tailed Peto-Peto Wilcoxon test.[57]

Also, expected probabilities of remaining seizure free after a last drink were plotted on the null hypothesis that seizures occur randomly and independent of the time of the last drink. These expected probabilities—functions of the frequency of drinking and amount of alcohol consumed at each drinking episode—were calculated using two assumptions derived from the literature:[37,47,67] 1) people can tolerate an average intake of one ounce of absolute alcohol/hour, and 2) on any given day drinking is continuous, up to a maximum of 18 hours. The first assumption was varied both up and down to test its robustness.

Table 16–2. DEMOGRAPHIC CHARACTERISTICS OF PATIENTS WITH SEIZURES (CASES) AND CONTROLS

Characteristic	Cases (n = 308)	Controls (n = 294)
Mean age ± SD (ye)***	50.2 ± 17.6	41.7 ± 20.6
Male**	64%	49%
Black	94%	95%
Completed high school**	36%	46%
Currently married	17%	18%
Currently employed*	27%	35%
Using Harlem Hospital as primary source of health care	54%	58%

***$p < .001$
**$p < .01$
*$p < .05$

(From Ng, SK, et al: Alcohol consumption and withdrawal in new-onset seizures. N Engl J Med 319:666, 1988, with permission.)

Results

SOCIODEMOGRAPHIC CHARACTERISTICS

Cases and controls differed in age, sex, employment, and education (Table 16–2). Education, however, was not a risk factor for seizures in multivariate analysis. The 59 patients with untreated first seizures in the 12 months before admission were combined with true incident cases because they did not differ in sociodemographic or exposure variables and, on separate analyses, yielded identical results.

PATTERN OF ALCOHOL CONSUMPTION

Distribution of Drinkers. Compared with male controls, a smaller proportion of male cases were non-drinkers (11 percent versus 21 percent) (Table 16–3). Among women, proportions of non-drinkers were larger (42 percent versus 50 percent). The proportions of ex-drinkers were similar among cases and controls of both sexes.

Ex-drinkers. Among ex-drinkers, length of abstinence among male cases and controls averaged 3.8 and 6.3 years, respectively, and among women 7.2 and 6.7 years, respectively. Duration of chronic alcohol use before quitting did not differ between cases and controls of either sex. Especially among controls, ex-drinkers had been heavy drinkers. However, after adjustment for confounders, neither previous daily alcohol intake (OR = 0.9/100 g, CL = 0.7, 1.2) nor length of abstinence (OR = 0.6/10 years, CL = 0.2, 1.8) had significant associations with seizures. In the absence of elevated seizure risk from previous alcohol use, we excluded ex-drinkers from further analysis. Two hundred eighty-three cases and 267 controls remained.

Table 16–3. ALCOHOL USE ACCORDING TO SEX IN PATIENTS WITH SEIZURES AND CONTROLS

	Men		Women	
	Cases, No. (%)	Controls, No. (%)	Cases, No. (%)	Controls, No. (%)
Non-drinker	21 (11)	30 (21)	47 (42)	75 (50)
Current drinker	158 (80)	98 (68)	57 (52)	64 (42)
Ex-drinker	18 (9)	15 (11)	7 (6)	12 (8)
Total	197 (100)	143 (100)	111 (100)	151 (100)

(From Ng, SK, et al: Alcohol consumption and withdrawal in new-onset seizures. N Engl J Med 319:666, 1988, with permission.)

Table 16–4. TYPES OF ALCOHOLIC BEVERAGE USED BY CURRENT DRINKERS AMONG CASES AND CONTROLS OF EACH SEX

Type of Alcoholic Beverage	Men Cases, No. (%)	Men Controls, No. (%)	Women Cases, No. (%)	Women Controls, No. (%)
Wine only	15 (9.5)	7 (7.1)	3 (5.3)	11 (17.2)
Beer only	6 (3.8)	14 (14.3)	12 (21.0)	10 (15.6)
Liquor only	39 (24.7)	14 (14.3)	19 (33.3)	17 (26.6)
Wine and beer only	5 (3.2)	6 (6.1)	1 (1.8)	6 (9.4)
Wine and liquor only	13 (8.2)	10 (10.2)	1 (1.8)	6 (9.4)
Beer and liquor only	31 (19.6)	20 (20.4)	6 (10.5)	9 (14.0)
Wine and beer and liquor	49 (31.0)	27 (27.6)	15 (26.3)	5 (7.8)
Total	158 (100)	98 (100)	57 (100)	64 (100)

(From Ng, SK, et al: Alcohol consumption and withdrawal in new-onset seizures. N Engl J Med 319:666, 1988, with permission.)

Current Drinkers: Duration, Type, Frequency, and Volume. The mean duration of chronic alcohol use, adjusted for age and sex, was similar for case and control current drinkers (18.1 versus 17.5 years). After adjusting for ADAA, duration of drinking carried no significant risk for seizures in multivariate analysis (OR = 1.1/10 years; CL = 0.9, 1.2). Cases favored liquor (alone or combined with other types of alcohol) more than controls (men, 83.5 percent versus 72.5 percent respectively; women, 71.9 percent versus 57.8 percent respectively); consistent with preference, cases drank liquor significantly more often, and in larger volume per occasion. Overall alcohol intake was clearly greater among cases. Fifty-three percent of cases and 18.5 percent of controls drank every day. Frequency of drinking was closely correlated with volume for all types of alcoholic beverage in both cases and controls (correlation coefficients between 0.4 and 0.7). Binge drinking, measured by sporadic heavy drinking (5 drinks or more a day), was rare among ordinarily light drinkers. Only 14 subjects (4 cases, 10 controls) whose regular intake was 4 drinks or less engaged in heavy drinking more often than once a year. Only 1 of the 14 engaged in such binges more often than once a month. Tables 16–4 and 16–5 summarize these data.

Table 16–5. ALCOHOL CONSUMPTION ACCORDING TO AVERAGE FREQUENCY (OCCASIONS PER WEEK) AND VOLUME (OUNCES PER OCCASION) AMONG CURRENT DRINKERS IN PATIENTS WITH SEIZURES AND CONTROLS OF EACH SEX[t]

Beverage	Men Frequency Cases (n = 158)	Men Frequency Controls (n = 98)	Men Volume Cases (n = 158)	Men Volume Controls (n = 98)	Women Frequency Cases (n = 57)	Women Frequency Controls (n = 64)	Women Volume Cases (n = 57)	Women Volume Controls (n = 64)
Wine	2.3	0.9	20.4	8.0	0.7	0.5	3.9	3.3
Beer	2.2	2.2	20.7*	26.2	2.0*	0.8	32.9*	10.2
Liquor	3.6***	1.5	14.4***	7.3	2.3***	0.6	8.3***	2.9

[t]Because multiple comparisons were made, cautious interpretation in these univariate comparisons could assign statistical significance only to p-values of less than .001.
*p < 0.05   ***p < 0.001 Wilcoxon rank sum test (2-tailed)
(From Ng, SK, et al: Alcohol consumption and withdrawal in new-onset seizures. N Engl J Med 319:666, 1988, with permission.)

Dose-Effect of Alcohol Intake

Unprovoked Seizures. With ADAA as a categorical variable, cases and controls did not differ in exposure to alcohol below 50 g/day. Above 50 g/day, increasingly larger proportions of cases were exposed, compared with controls. Thus, the odds of exposure among cases tripled that of controls between 51 and 100 g/day, rose eight-fold between 101 and 200 g/day, almost 20-fold between 201 and 300 g/day, above which there was no further increase in odds. This pattern was similar between the sexes but less stable in women because there were fewer heavy drinkers. When ADAA was treated as a continuous variable (with intakes below 51 g and above 300 g recoded as 0 and 300 g respectively), every additional 100 g of daily alcohol intake almost tripled the odds for a first unprovoked seizure (OR = 2.8/100 g, CL = 2.1, 3.8). Women had higher odds ratios than men (OR = 11.4/100 g, CL = 3.3, 38.9; and OR = 2.4, CL = 1.8, 3.2 respectively). Table 16–6 summarizes these data.

Provoked Seizures. Odds of exposure to alcohol were again higher for cases with this class of seizures than controls, but the odds ratios became significantly different from 1 only with intakes above 200 g/day. These ratios were in general about half as large as those for unprovoked seizures, but again did not rise further at intakes above 300 g/day. With ADAA analyzed as a continuous variable, OR for women was 3.9/100 g (CL = 1.1, 13.8) and for men 1.7/100 g (CL = 1.1, 2.6). For both sexes together, every additional 100 g of daily alcohol intake between 51 g and 300 g doubled the odds for a first provoked seizure (OR = 1.9/100 g, CL = 1.4, 2.8). Table 16–6 summarizes these data.

Last Drink and Seizure Onset. Information on abstention time (Fig. 16–1) was obtained from 184 (85.6 percent) of the 215 current drinkers. Abstention ranged from 1 minute (assigned when the person had a seizure *while* drinking) to 8 months. Within 24 hours of the last drink, 61.4 percent of seizures had occurred: 19 percent (n = 35) in the first hour; 25.6 percent (n = 47) from 2 to 12 hours, and 16.8 percent (n = 31) from 13 to 24 hours. After that, subjects reported abstention times in days only, producing clusters at 48 and 72 hours. Only 38.6 percent of seizures (n = 71) occurred between 7 and 48 hours; 16.3 percent of seizures (n = 30) occurred between 15 days and 8 months.

In analyses of abstention time to elicit

Table 16–6. ADJUSTED ODDS RATIOS FOR RISK OF SEIZURE AND ALCOHOL INTAKE IN MEN, WOMEN, AND BOTH SEXES COMBINED

	Men		Women		Both Sexes
Alcohol Intake (g/day)	Cases/Controls	Odds Ratio (95% Confidence Limits)	Cases/Controls	Odds Ratio (95% Confidence Limits)	Odds Ratio (95% Confidence Limits)
Unprovoked seizures					
None	15/30	1	29/75	1	1
1–50	30/65	1.1 (0.5, 2.4)	21/59	1.5 (0.7, 3.4)	1.3 (0.8, 2.3)
51–100	17/15	2.2 (0.8, 5.7)	4/4	3.4 (0.7, 17.8)	2.8 (1.3, 6.3)
101–200	23/9	4.7 (1.7, 13.3)	9/1	37.1 (4.1, 333)	7.9 (3.3, 18.7)
201–300	22/4	11.2 (3.2, 39.3)	6/0		19.5 (6.1, 62)
>300	38/5	14.3 (4.5, 45.8)	2/0		19.2 (6.6, 56.4)
Provoked seizures					
None	6/30	1	18/75	1	1
1–50	8/65	0.9 (0.2, 3.1)	9/59	0.9 (0.3, 2.5)	1 (0.5, 2.2)
51–100	7/15	2.4 (0.6, 9.9)	0/4	0	2.3 (0.7, 7.2)
101–200	3/9	1.2 (0.2, 6.6)	1/1		1.4 (0.3, 5.8)
201–300	6/4	11.7 (1.9, 70.6)	2/0		10.1 (2.3, 43.8)
>300	4/5	3.5 (0.6, 20)	3/0		7.4 (1.8, 30.5)

(From Ng, SK, et al: Alcohol consumption and withdrawal in new-onset seizures. N Engl J Med 319:666, 1988, with permission.)

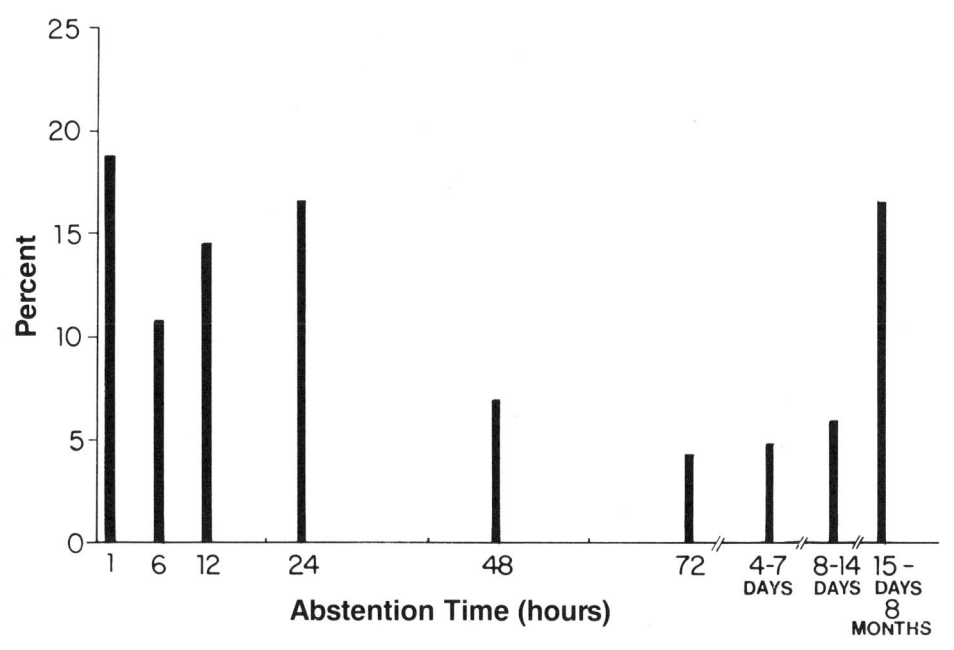

Figure 16-1. Frequency distribution of interval between last drink and first seizure (abstention time) for 184 seizure patients. (From Ng, SK, et al: Alcohol consumption and withdrawal in new-onset seizures. N Engl J Med 319:666, 1988, with permission.)

the withdrawal phenomenon, seizures occurring more than two weeks after the last drink (n = 30) were dropped, because such seizures are not ordinarily attributed to alcohol withdrawal. Abstention time patterns of unprovoked seizures (n = 130) and provoked seizures (n = 24) (Fig. 16-2) did not differ (χ^2 = 1.19, p = 0.27). Among unprovoked seizures, subjects who had histories of head injury or stroke (n = 47) had the same abstention patterns as subjects without such histories (n = 83) (χ^2 = 1.4, p = 0.24). Among unprovoked seizures with no prior head injury or stroke, generalized onset major motor seizures (n = 60) and partial seizures (n = 14) did not differ (χ^2 = 3.16, p = .08). Likewise, the patterns of patients who, in the 2 weeks before admission, had decreased drinking (n = 31) or kept their drinking unchanged (n = 91) did not differ (χ^2 = 1.26, p = 0.26). Compared with patients whose drinking was unchanged, however, those whose drinking increased (n = 17) had seizures sooner after the last drink (χ^2 = 7.36, p < .001) and those who had stopped drinking (n = 15) had them later (χ^2 = 14.39, p < .001). Patients who had the shortest abstention time were the heaviest drinkers, in terms of both average frequency and volume (Table 16-7). ADAA declined as length of abstention increased, and was significantly different among the groups with different abstention times (χ^2 = 10.4, p = .015).

Probability Models. The expected probabilities of remaining seizure free in successive intervals after the last drink under the random occurrence hypothesis were calculated separately for unprovoked and provoked seizures (Fig. 16-2), and for patients grouped according to changes in drinking behavior in the two weeks before admission (Fig. 16-3). Patients who had kept their drinking unchanged had expected probabilities that were remarkably similar to their observed patterns. Patients who had increased their drinking had seizures earlier than expected under the random occurrence hypothesis. Conversely, patients who had decreased or stopped drinking had seizures later. These curves were quite robust to changes in model assumptions, such as the hourly rate of alcohol intake (Fig. 16-4).

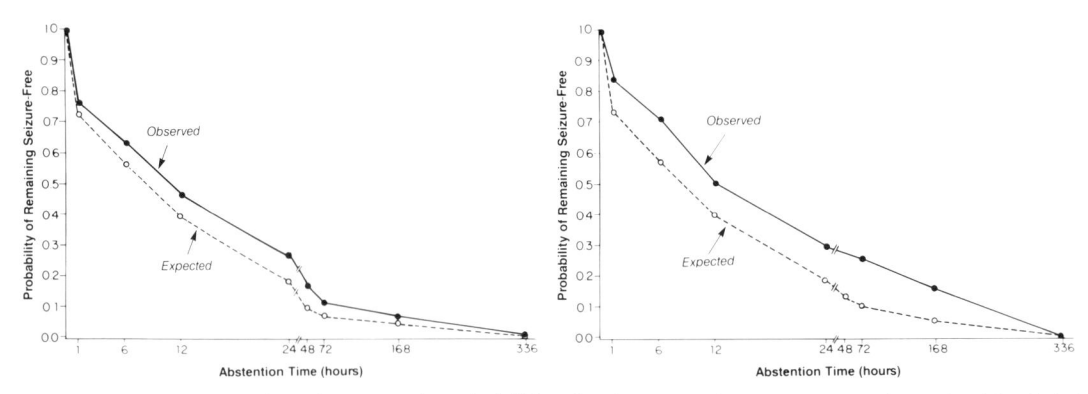

Figure 16–2. Observed and expected probabilities (under a random-occurrence hypothesis) of *(left panel)* remaining free or unprovoked or, *(right panel)* provoked seizures in successive intervals after the last drink (assuming intake of 1 oz per hour). (From Ng, SK, et al: Alcohol consumption and withdrawal in new-onset seizures. N Engl J Med 319:666, 1988, with permission.)

Discussion

The substantial difference in alcohol intake between patients with incident seizures and patients in a comparable control group in this study confirms for the first time, in epidemiologic terms, a longstanding clinical observation. Both the number of drinkers and amount of drinking among cases substantially exceeded that among controls. Cases drank more often, drank larger quantities on each occasion, and favored liquor. On a summary measure of intake (ADAA), unprovoked seizures related to alcohol more strongly (OR = 2.8/100 g) than provoked seizures (OR = 1.9/100 g).

Although alcohol use differed between men and women, similar risk patterns held. Seizure risk appeared only above a threshold value of 50 g of absolute alcohol (about 2 drinks of liquor) per day. Between 50 and 300 g/day, the risk of unprovoked seizures rose almost 20-fold and of provoked seizures about 10-fold. Above 300 g/day, risk rose no further. Every additional 100 g of daily alcohol intake between 51 g and 300 g (measured by ADAA) tripled the risk of unprovoked seizures and doubled the risk of provoked seizures.

Although most cases were long-term alcohol users, controls did not differ in this regard. Lack of risk attached to duration of use could mean: Our data on duration are too imprecise to detect differences;

Table 16–7. ALCOHOL CONSUMPTION PATTERN AMONG CURRENT DRINKERS WITH SEIZURE, ACCORDING TO INTERVAL SINCE LAST DRINK

	Interval Since Last Drink			
	< 1 Hour (n = 35)	1–11 Hour (n = 47)	12–47 Hour (n = 44)	48–336 Hour (n = 28)
Wine (frequency/week)	3.1	2.5	1.7	1.1
Beer (frequency/week)	2.7	2.2	2.7	1.7
Liquor (frequency/week)	3.2	4.1	3.8	2.7
Wine/occasion (oz)	24.7	23.9	14.6	9.3
Beer/occasion (oz)	33.8	17.9	25.6	33.9
Liquor/occasion (oz)	19.6	11.4	12.7	8.2
ADAA* (g)	306.7	226.8	219.1	134.9

*p = .015 Kruskal-Wallis test, (2-tailed)
(From Ng, SK, et al: Alcohol consumption and withdrawal in new-onset seizures. N Engl J Med 319:666, 1988, with permission.)

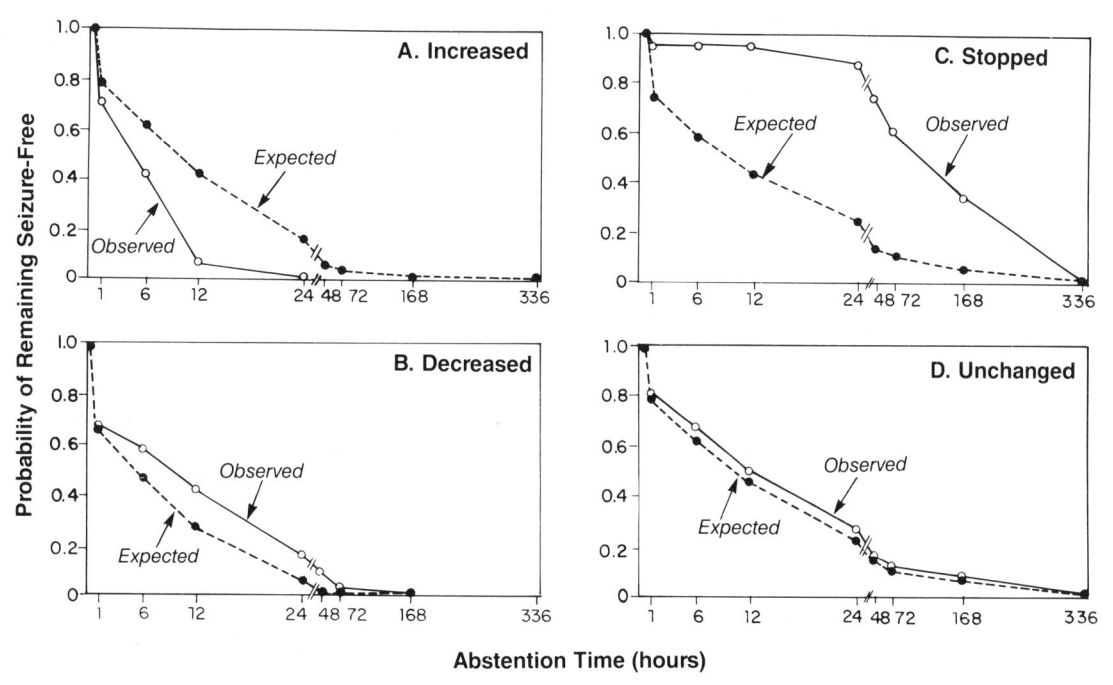

Figure 16–3. Observed and expected probabilities (under a random-occurrence hypothesis) of remaining seizure-free in successive intervals (hours) after the last drink when drinking in the two weeks before admission was (A) increased, (B) decreased, (C) stopped, or (D) unchanged. (From Ng, SK, et al: Alcohol consumption and withdrawal in new-onset seizures. N Engl J Med 319:666, 1988, with permission.)

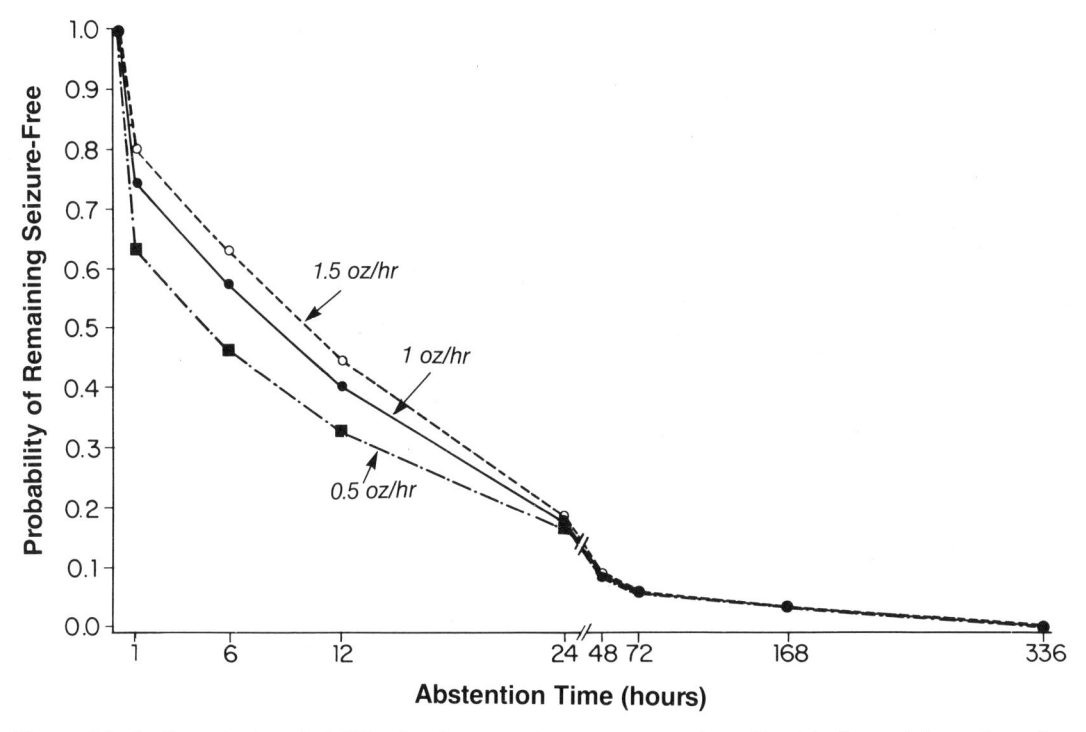

Figure 16–4. Expected probabilities (under a random-occurrence hypothesis) of remaining seizure-free in successive intervals (hours) after the last drink assuming different hourly rates of alcohol intake in patients with unprovoked seizures.

duration of *chronic* use and of *heavy* use do not correspond (detailed data cover only the 6 months before admission or cessation; before that habits might have differed); or when alcohol use is the norm and begins early, heavy and light drinkers differ in the amount but not the duration of alcohol use, and seizure risk is attached *only* to chronic heavy drinking. We favor the last explanation.

We do not think our findings result from improper control selection or difficulties of measuring intake. Hospital patients with first seizures are a select subsample of first seizures in the community. A hospital control series, however, provides suitable comparison at least insofar as the entry to medical care reflects unknown confounding factors. With regard to intake, the 6-month period covered before admission minimizes, especially among controls, the effect of changes in drinking habits as their disease progressed. Although interviews about alcohol use involve suspect self-reports of undesirable social behavior, the consensus is that no measure, including biologic measures, is superior.[2,6,15,23,24,41,50,59-63,70,71]

The amount of alcohol used by our subjects was impressive—several times higher, for example, than that reported in a recent British study.[24] Underreporting was discouraged, first because questions on alcohol use were a small and unobtrusive part of a comprehensive interview, and second because heavy use of alcohol in the hospital population studied carries little evident stigma. The estimate of risk would be biased only if the validity of reported alcohol intake differed systematically between cases and controls.

The true risk from alcohol is likely to be higher than reported here because our analytic strategies have been conservative and hospital controls are known to have a high prevalence of alcoholism.[3,30,45,49] The dose-response pattern, the consistency of the results between men and women, the more pronounced associations with unprovoked rather than provoked seizures, and the decline in risk as the time of exposure recedes with lengthening abstention all point to heavy alcohol use as a cause of seizures.

SEIZURE AND ALCOHOL WITHDRAWAL

This analysis omits controls because most controls had no reference point as well defined as a seizure episode to which they could relate the last drink before admission, and because the prodrome of illnesses among controls could have altered drinking habits before admission.

One hundred eighty four cases reported on the time of the last drink before seizure; 16.3 percent of these seizures (n = 30) occurred 2 weeks after abstention, and hence do not relate to conventional conceptions of alcohol withdrawal. Among the 154 remaining candidates for withdrawal seizures, seizures occurred within 1 hour of the last drink in 35, by which time withdrawal has usually not supervened (in the first hour, blood alcohol would have fallen by no more than 20-35 mg/dl[67] and in some might have been rising[47]). They were nonetheless retained in the analysis because they may represent relative abstinence, as suggested by Victor and associates.[69] In extensive analysis, we could find no support for the withdrawal phenomenon as an explanation for seizures.

Only 30 percent of the 154 patients (n = 46) had stopped or decreased their drinking within 2 weeks of hospitalization. The majority of patients had either maintained or increased their regular intake.

Among the 154 candidates, withdrawal seizures could not be separated by the subjects' abstention patterns. Thus unprovoked seizures (most commonly attributable to withdrawal) were indistinguishable from provoked seizures by abstention time; among unprovoked seizures, subjects with a history of head injury or stroke and those without were also indistinguishable; and among unprovoked seizures not involving prior head injury or stroke, generalized onset major motor seizures were indistinguishable from partial seizures. One possibility is that all seizures in alcohol users are withdrawal seizures. Even if we entertain this possibility, provoked seizures should still be associated with distinct abstention patterns if seizure onset after the last drink is determined by some physiologic mechanism that lowers seizure threshold, since there were additional risk factors working in conjunction with alcohol to lower the threshold. There are two additional possibilities: withdrawal seizures are too few for a pattern to be detected; or the relation of withdrawal seizures and last drink is determined by characteristics shared by all drinkers with seizures.

If the majority of seizures in alcohol users are due to withdrawal, we should find a high concentration of seizures occurring within the withdrawal period (between 7 and 48 hours). A test for the withdrawal hypothesis is therefore to compare the observed distribution of seizures with an expected distribution based on the null hypothesis that seizures occur randomly, taking into consideration individual drinking patterns. Because some withdrawal seizures may occur outside the conventional 7 to 48 hour period, a liberal criterion to reject the null hypothesis is to consider any seizure clustering within 2 weeks after the last drink *not anticipated by the random occurrence model* as evidence for withdrawal seizures. We were not able to demonstrate any meaningful departure from our models of random occurrence. Only 38.6 percent of seizures occurred between 7 and 48 hours, a proportion in accordance with the random occurrence model. There was no unexpected clustering of seizures within the 2-week period after the last drink. When in the 2 weeks before admission drinking remained unchanged, observed and expected probabilities were practically identical. When drinking behavior changed, the models remained plausible; the observed probabilities deviated in the anticipated degree and direction from those based on alcohol use before the change: an increased intake led to earlier seizures because the nondrinking phase was shortened and overall abstention time decreased. The reverse was true for decreased intakes.

The seizure-free probabilities after a drinking episode calculated under the randomness hypothesis are quite robust. Thus, changes in our first assumption about the rate of drinking hardly alter the shape of the hypothetical curves. Changes in our second assumption (for any reported intake drinking is continuous up to a maximum of 18 hours per day) decrease the longest possible continuous abstention time in a given day allowed by the model. Although the expected probabilities will be less accurate for seizures occurring after longer abstentions, in the majority abstention time was very short (24 hours in 61.4 percent), and loss of accuracy should be small.

As abstention time before a first seizure was greater, so was alcohol use less in the previous 6 months. Thus, patients whose seizures followed closely upon drinking were heavier drinkers than those whose seizures occurred after longer periods of abstention. The hypothesis of random occurrence predicts such a result: heavy drinkers have their seizures either while drinking or shortly after a last drink because there are no prolonged nondrinking periods.

Although we offer new interpretations of our own and other investigators' data, the configurations of these can be made congruent. We confirm what other investigators have observed: many alcoholics who develop seizures after recent alcohol use have other risk factors for seizures. Because withdrawal seizures are mainly diagnosed by exclusion, as work-up of these patients becomes more sophisticated, fewer seizures are attributed to alcohol withdrawal. Thus the reported proportion of withdrawal seizures among alcohol users decreased from 88 percent[69] to 59 percent[16] to 31 percent.[33] It is also not a new observation that the timing of seizures after the last drink is not unique to or even typical of withdrawal seizures.[22] With regard to the seizure types associated with alcohol, too, in Victor and Brausch's series,[69] as in ours, several types occurred indiscriminantly: subjects with focal seizures, prior epilepsy, prior head trauma, and prior parietal infarct all have seizures within the "withdrawal" period.

A review of the major differences between our study and that of Victor and Brausch is relevant to the interpretation of these results. While the Harlem study enrolled over 90 percent of eligible cases in less than 3 years in a single hospital, Victor and Brausch's[69] patients were a 10 percent nonsystematic sample recruited over 15 years in three different hospitals. Their strict requirement of independent corroboration of alcohol history excluded 90 percent of potential study subjects. Self-reports of alcohol drinking have been found to be quite reliable and correlate well with biologic markers.[6,15,23,59,60,70,71] Among heavy drinkers there is no evidence that collateral informants provide better alcohol history than study subjects.[41] The stringent requirement of Victor and Brausch was therefore probably unnecessary and led only to unknown selection biases and inability to generalize.

Despite the requirement of independent corroboration, information on the interval between seizure and last drink was obtained in only 61 percent of Victor and Brausch's patients. In contrast, this information was obtained in 85 percent of the current drinkers in the Harlem study.

Victor and Brausch's patients were selected for both seizures and alcoholism. The association between heavy drinking and seizure is therefore predetermined. No information on the effects of light and moderate drinking on seizures was available. In contrast, the Harlem study recruited cases only on the basis of seizures. We thus have a more representative picture of alcohol use among seizure patients, including light and occasional drinking.

While the majority of the Harlem patients had "a first ever" seizure, the proportion of recurrent to first seizures in Victor and Brausch's study is unclear. Factors that affect survival and seizure recurrence will thus be inseparable from factors that initiate seizure onset in their study.

SUMMARY

Alcohol-related seizures are not homogeneous and result from diverse mechanisms. It is likely that alcohol leads to both genesis and precipitation of seizures. Although there is evidence that some of these seizures may be related to alcohol withdrawal, the proportion due to withdrawal is probably much smaller than is commonly believed. The long *incubation period* and the dose-response relation of seizure risk with alcohol suggest that these seizures result from chronic and possibly cumulative effects of alcohol exposure. While we readily accept the harmful structural effects of alcohol on organs such as the liver and the heart, we tend to overlook the possibility of direct or indirect structural brain damage from excessive alcohol use. Chronic alcoholism is often associated with nutritional cerebral disorders, such as the Wernicke-Korsakoff syndrome. There is also radiologic evidence of cerebral atrophy manifested as widening of sulci and dilatation of ventricles.[7,8,9,55,65] Alcoholics show various degrees of impairment on neuropsychologic tests of cerebral function,[5] and cerebellar degeneration is a known complication of alcoholism. It has recently been suggested that the effect of alcohol on calcium channels may be the basis of cardiac myopathy, and alcohol also appears to affect calcium channels in brain cells in a similar manner.[31] Chronic alcoholics also have decreased cerebral blood flow.[4] Any of these mechanisms can explain the long-term effect of alcohol on the brain and may lead eventually to seizures. It is time to look beyond the withdrawal paradigm and resolve some of the unanswered questions about alcohol-related seizures.

References

1. Alling, C: Alcohol effects on cell membrane. Epilepsia 29:492, 1988.
2. Armor, DJ, Polich, JM, and Stambul, HB: Alcoholism and Treatment. Prepared for the US National Institute on Alcohol Abuse and Alcoholism. Rand Corporation, Santa Monica, 1976.
3. Barchha, R, Stewart, MA, and Guze, SB: The prevalence of alcoholism among general hospital ward patients. Am J Psychiatry 125:681, 1968.
4. Berglund, M and Ingvar, D: Cerebral blood flow and its regional distribution in alcoholism and Korsakoff's psychosis. J Stud Alcohol 37:586, 1976.
5. Bergman, H, et al: Computed tomography of the brain and neuropsychological assessment of male alcoholic patients. In: Richter, D. (ed): Addiction and Brain Damage. Croom Helm, London, 1980, p 201.
6. Bernadt, MW, et al: Comparison of questionnaire and laboratory tests in the detection of ex-

cessive drinking and alcoholism. Lancet 1:325, 1982.
7. Cala, LA, and Mastaglia, FL: Computerized tomography in chronic alcoholics. Alcohol 5:283, 1981.
8. Carlen, PL, et al: Reversible cerebral atrophy in recently abstinent chronic alcoholics measured by computerized tomography scans. Science 200:1076, 1978.
9. Carlen, PL, Rogier-Naquet, I, and Reynolds, J: Alterations of neuronal calcium and potassium ionic currents during alcohol administration and withdrawal. Epilepsia 29:493, 1988.
10. Collins, AL: Personal communication, 1988.
11. Conover, WJ: Practical Nonparametric Statistics, ed 2. John Wiley & Sons, New York, 1980.
12. Dam, AM, et al: Late-onset epilepsy: Etiologies, types of seizures, and value of clinical investigation, EEG, and computerized tomography scan. Epilepsia 26:227, 1985.
13. Devetag, F, et al: Alcoholic epilepsy: Review of a series and proposed classification and etiopathogenesis. Ital J Neurol Sci 3:275, 1983.
14. Diamond, I, Mochly-Rosen, D, and Gordon, A: Reduced adenosine receptor activation in alcoholism: Implications for alcohol-withdrawal seizures. Epilepsia, 29:493, 1988.
15. Dunbar, JA, et al: Drivers, binge drinking, and gammaglutamyltranspeptidase. Br Med J 285:1083, 1982.
16. Earnest, MP and Yarnell, PR: Seizure admissions to a city hospital: The role of alcohol. Epilepsia 17:387, 1976.
17. Ellis, FW, and Pick, JR: Experimentally induced ethanol dependence in rhesus monkeys. J Pharm Exp Ther 175:88, 1970.
18. Essig, CF and Lam, RC: Convulsions and hallucinatory behavior following alcohol withdrawal in the dog. Arch Neurol 1968; 18:626, 1968.
19. Falk, JL, Samson, HH, and Winger, B: Behavioral maintenance of high concentration of blood ethanol and physical dependence in the rat. Science 177:811, 1972.
20. Freund, G: Alcohol withdrawal syndrome in mice. Arch Neurol 21:315, 1969.
21. Frye, GD: Gamma-aminobutyric (GABA) changes in alcohol withdrawal. Epilepsia 29:493, 1988.
22. Gerson, IM and Karabell, S: The use of the electroencephalogram in patients admitted for alcohol abuse with seizures. Clin Electroencephalogr 10:40, 1979.
23. Gill, GV, et al: Acute biochemical responses to moderate beer drinking. Br Med J 285:1770, 1982.
24. Gill, JS, et al: Stroke and alcohol consumption. N Engl J Med 315:1041, 1986.
25. Giroire, H, et al: Remarques sur l'etiologie de 200 cas d'epilepsie generalisée à debut tardif (importance de facteur alcoolique). Rev Neurol 94:634, 1956.
26. Goldstein, DB: Personal communication, 1987.
27. Goldstein, DB: Relationship of alcohol dose to intensity of withdrawal signs in mice. J Pharm Exp Ther 180:203, 1972.
28. Goldstein, DB and Pal, N: Alcohol dependence produced in mice by inhalation of ethanol: Grading the withdrawal reaction. Science 172:288, 1971.
29. Gordon, T and Doyle, JT: Drinking and mortality. Am J Epidemiol 125:263, 1987.
30. Green, JR: The incidence of alcoholism in patients admitted to medical wards of a public hospital. Med J Aust 1:465, 1965.
31. Greenberg, DA, et al: Calcium channel changes during alcohol withdrawal. Epilepsia 29:492, 1988.
32. Hauser, WA, et al: Clinical findings, seizure recurrence, and sibling risk in alcohol-withdrawal seizure patients. Epilepsia 23:422, 1982.
33. Hillbom, ME: Occurrence of cerebral seizures provoked by alcohol abuse. Epilepsia 21:459, 1980.
34. Hillbom, ME and Hjelm-Jager, M: Should alcohol withdrawal seizures be treated with anti-epileptic drugs? Acta Neurol Scand 69:39, 1984.
35. Hoppener, RJ, Kuyer, A, and van der Lugt, PJM: Epilepsy and alcohol: The influence of social alcohol intake on seizures and treatment in epilepsy. Epilepsia 24:459, 1983.
36. Hunt, WA: The effect of ethanol on GABAergic transmission. Neurosci Behav Rev 7:87, 1983.
37. Isbell, H, et al: An experimental study of the etiology of "rum fits" and delirium tremens. Quarterly Journal of Studies on Alcohol 16:1, 1955.
38. Khavari, KA and Farber, PD: A profile instrument for the quantification and assessment of alcohol consumption: The Khavari alcohol test. J Stud Alcohol 39:1525, 1978.
39. Lennox, WG: Alcohol and epilepsy. Quarterly Journal of Studies on Alcohol 2:759, 1941.
40. Littleton, JM: Calcium channel activity in alcohol dependency and withdrawal seizures. Epilepsia 29:492, 1988.
41. Maisto, SA, Sobell, LC, and Sobell, MB: Comparison of alcoholics' self-reports of drinking behavior with reports of collateral informants. J Consult Clin Psychol 47:106, 1979.
42. Majchrowicz, E: Induction of physical dependence on alcohol and the associated metabolic and behavioral changes in rats. Psychopharmacologia (Berlin) 43:245, 1975.
43. Marinacci, AA: A special type of temporal lobe (psychomotor) seizures following ingestion of alcohol. Bulletin of the Los Angeles Neurological Society 27:241, 1963.
44. Mattson, RH, et al: Effect of alcohol intake in nonalcoholic epileptics. Neurology 25:361, 1975.
45. McCusker, J, Cherubin, C, and Zimberg, S: Prevalence of alcoholism in general municipal hospital population. NY State J Med 71:751, 1971.
46. McQuarrie, DG and Fingle, E: Effects of single doses and chronic administration of ethanol on experimental seizures in mice. J Pharm Exp Ther 124:264, 1958.
47. Mendelson, JE: Experimentally induced chronic intoxication and withdrawal in alcoholics. Quarterly Journal of Studies on Alcohol 2:1, 1964.
48. Newsom, JA: Withdrawal seizures in an in-patient alcoholism program. In Galanter, M (ed): Currents in Alcoholism, Vol 6, Treatment and

Rehabilitation and Epidemiology. Grune & Stratton, New York, 1979, p 11.
49. Nolan, JP: Alcohol as a factor in the illness of university service patients. Am J Med Sci 249:135, 1965.
50. Orford, J: A comparison of alcoholics whose drinking is totally uncontrolled and those whose drinking is mainly controlled. Behav Res Ther 11:565, 1973.
51. Pieper, WA and Skeen, MJ: Induction of physical dependence on ethanol in rhesus monkeys using oral acceptance technique. Life Sci 11:989, 1972.
52. Pieper, WA, et al: The chimpanzee as an animal model for investigating alcoholism. Science 176:71, 1972.
53. Richter, CD: Production and control of alcoholic cravings in rats. Neuropharmacology 3:39, 1956.
54. Rodin, EA, Frohman, CE, and Gottlieb, JS: Effect of acute alcohol intoxication on epileptic patients. Arch Neurol 4:115, 1961.
55. Ron, MA, Acker, W, and Lishman, WA: Morphologic abnormalities in the brains of chronic alcoholics: A clinical, psychological, and computerized axial tomographic study. Acta Psychiatr Scand 62(Suppl 286):41, 1980.
56. Sampliner, R and Iber, F: Diphenylhydantoin control of alcohol withdrawal seizures: Results of a controlled study. JAMA 230:1430, 1974.
57. SAS Institute, Inc: SUGI Supplemental Library User's Guide, Version 5 ed. Cary, North Carolina, 1986.
58. Schatzkin, A, et al: Alcohol consumption and breast cancer in the epidemiologic follow-up study of the first national health and nutrition examination survey. N Engl J Med 316:1169, 1987.
59. Shaper, AG, et al: Alcohol and ischaemic heart disease in middle aged British men. Br Med J 294:733, 1987.
60. Shaper, AG, et al: Biochemical and haematological response to alcohol intake. Ann Clin Biochem 22:50, 1985.
61. Sobell, LC, et al: Reliability of alcohol abusers' self-reports of drinking behavior. Behav Res Ther 17:157, 1979.
62. Sobell, LC and Sobell, MB: Outpatient alcoholics give valid self-reports. J Nerv Ment Dis 161:32, 1975.
63. Sobell, LC and Sobell, MB: Validity of self-reports in three populations of alcoholics. J Consult Clin Psychol 46:901, 1978.
64. Thompson, GN: The electroencephalogram in acute pathological alcoholic intoxication. Bulletin of the Los Angeles Neurological Society 28:217, 1963.
65. Torvik, A, Lindboe, CF, and Rodge, S: Brain lesions in alcoholics: A neuropathological study with clinical correlations. J Neurol Sci 56:233, 1982.
66. Tukue, I, Okamoto, T, and Kashiwagi, T: A case of chronic alcoholism showing a picture of alcholic epilepsy following intravenous infusion of alcohol. Hiroshimaigaku 21:171, 1968.
67. Ugarte, G, et al: Influence of alcohol intake, length of abstinence and meprobamate on the rate of ethanol metabolism in man. Quarterly Journal of Studies on Alcohol 33:698, 1972.
68. Victor, M: Overview on alcohol withdrawal seizures. Presented at the International Symposium on Alcohol and Seizures, Washington, DC, September 30, 1988.
69. Victor, M and Brausch, C: The role of abstinence in the genesis of alcoholic epilepsy. Epilepsia 8:1, 1967.
70. Whitehead, TP, Clarke, CA, and Whitfield, AGW: Biochemical and haematological markers of alcohol intake. Lancet 1:978, 1978.
71. Whitfield, JB: Alcohol-related biochemical changes in heavy drinkers. Aust NZ J Med 11:132, 1981.
72. Willett, WC, et al: Moderate alcohol consumption and the risk of breast cancer. N Engl J Med 316:1174, 1987.
73. Yamane, H and Katoh, N: Alcoholic epilepsy: A definition and a description of other convulsions related to alcoholism. Eur Neurol 20:17, 1981.
74. Yanai, J and Ginsburg, BE: Audiogenic seizures in mice whose parents drank alcohol. J Stud Alcohol 37:1564, 1976.

CHAPTER 17

David G. Vossler, M.D.
Thomas R. Browne, M.D.

The Electroencephalogram in Patients with Alcohol-Related Seizures

Management of cases involving recent seizures and alcohol use may be difficult when the patient's clinical history is insufficient. Electroencephalography (EEG) is an important tool in the evaluation of such cases. Numerous animal and clinical studies on this subject have been published in the last 50 years. In this chapter, we review the EEG changes observed during the administration of ethanol to animals and humans. We compare reported EEG findings in animals during the acute phase of alcohol withdrawal with reported EEG findings in humans with chronic alcoholism during the early and late stages of abstinence. We also analyze several studies that have described EEG patterns in patients with alcohol-related seizures. If clinicians are aware of these findings, the EEG can help distinguish patients with epilepsy and alcohol abuse (who may require long-term anticonvulsant medications) from patients whose seizures relate solely to alcohol withdrawal.

EFFECTS OF ETHANOL ON EEG ACTIVITY

Acute Administration

ANIMAL STUDIES

In studies of the direct effects of alcohol in five cats, Perrin, Kalant, and Livingston[55] (using visual EEG analysis) observed an initial increase in the frequency and amplitude of activity recorded from cortical surface electrodes but an opposite effect on mesencephalic reticular formation (MRF) activity at the start of a 1 g/kg infusion. As the infusion of ethanol continued, a progressive decline ensued in both frequency and amplitude at all locations except the hippocampus (which showed no change despite marked flattening elsewhere). Using 25 intact cats with cortical and depth electrodes and three animals with *cerveau isolé* preparations, Dolce and Decker[15] (using power density spectral analysis) also found increased beta (>13 Hz) activity in the cortex after small (10–50 mg/kg) doses. At doses of 50–500 mg/kg, more theta (4–7 Hz) and less beta power in the cortex but more beta power in the hippocampus and MRF were observed. Over 2 g/kg there was a substantial loss of power in all frequency bands.

A study of ethanol-naive rhesus monkeys showed that a single 1.25 g/kg dose of alcohol produced EEG activation and acceleration but 3 to 8 g/kg daily for up to 2 months caused a consistent slowing of at least one component of the EEG.[1] Earlier experiments on cats[26,27,60] and monkeys[29] also support the generalization that higher frequency activity occurs with acute small doses of alcohol, but slower activity occurs with larger amounts. Because the effects were similar in intact cats and *cerveau isolé* preparations, it was suggested that these changes result from a direct influence of alcohol on the forebrain.[15,60]

Human Studies

Several groups of investigators have examined the effects of short-term administration of measured quantities of ethanol on the EEG of humans. Zilm and associates[72] gave eight male volunteers a 1 g/kg dose of ethanol daily for 10 days. Daily EEGs were performed 3 days before, 3 days after, and throughout the alcohol administration phase. Power density spectral analysis of the EEG showed no statistically significant changes during either of the baseline periods or during the alcohol period, but this finding may have been related to the relatively low dose of alcohol used.

Other investigators report substantial effects. Nagy and associates[49] examined the EEGs of 30 persons with maximal blood alcohol levels (BALs) of 99-228 mg/dl, and noted prominent slowing of frequencies and increased amplitudes. Naitoh[50] administered ethanol to alcoholics and noted that "low" doses of alcohol were accompanied by an increased abundance, and somewhat diminished amplitude, of alpha (8-13 Hz) activity (although it slowed by approximately one Hz). Kotani[40] studied nine "complex" (with delirium or hallucinations) and seven "simple" chronic alcoholics without a history of seizures, recording EEGs before and after administering 100 g of intravenous (IV) ethanol. He observed an initial slowing of alpha frequencies, followed by a decrease in amplitude. Changes occurred earlier and were greater in the "complex" group.

These findings are consistent with the results of earlier work as well. Lolli, Nencini, and Misiti[44] reported the effects of dry red wine and dry martinis (0.4 g ethanol/kg body weight) on 20 normal men. They calculated the index (number of waves and their amplitudes in a given frequency range) of the subjects' EEGs and found that most changes were nonsignificant at low BALs, but dry wine produced more *alpha* (8-14 Hz), theta (4-7/Hz), and *delta* (2-3 Hz) activity than martinis. Little beta activity resulted from consuming either beverage, but larger amplitudes and slower activity developed as the patients became intoxicated. In seven normal volunteers who received acute administration of ethanol, Newman[51] found a rough correlation between slowing of alpha activity and BAL; with higher BALs bursts of 4- to 8-Hz waves appeared. Holmberg and Mårtens[30] gave ten normal control subjects and ten alcoholics a 1.25 g/kg dose of ethanol. A decrease in mean alpha frequency of 1.4 and 1.5 Hz occurred in the alcoholic and normal groups, respectively. In a later reanalysis by Begleiter and Platz,[4] no statistically significant differences between the groups were detected, but there were large variations between individuals in both groups. Interestingly, neither the maximum BAL nor the degree of ataxia correlated with the extent of EEG slowing.

Engel and Rosenbaum[17] reported on seven normal subjects and four patients with alcohol-related seizures given 1 to 2 g/kg ethanol after an overnight fast. The degree of intoxication and impairment of consciousness corresponded to the change in mean alpha frequency (gross changes were associated with a decrease of 2-3 Hz) compared with baseline, but did not correspond with the absolute frequency reached. Subjects with fast-normal or abnormally fast EEG activity before drinking showed more "normal" patterns during intoxication. The latter result may simply reflect the relaxation effect of alcohol. In addition, all patients felt sober before their EEG returned to the pre-alcohol pattern.

Finally, Davis and associates[11] gave six normal persons 2 ml/kg of 100 percent ethanol over 1 hour and noted a parallel slowing of frequencies and rising BAL. Less "fast alpha" (10-13 Hz) and more 6- to 7-Hz activity occurred at "low BAL," and more 4- to 8-Hz spectral energy developed at higher BALs. The maximal slowing occurred after the level began to fall, and it decreased more slowly than the BAL curve. The peak alpha frequency (about 10 Hz) did not change, but there was a shift to slower alpha frequencies.

These experiments indicate that low-dose ethanol administration produces both an increased abundance of alpha activity and a slowing of the mean alpha frequency (by 1-3 Hz) in humans regardless of a history of seizures or alcoholism. As higher BALs are reached, progressive EEG slowing (increased theta and delta activity) occurs.

The presence of interictal epileptiform patterns (spikes and sharp waves and their variants as defined by Chatrian and associates[7]) during human alcoholic intoxication has been examined. Mattson and associates[46] studied 14 nonalcoholic patients with epilepsy and various seizure types, using EEGs during the oral intake of light to moderate amounts of ethanol (0.5-1 ml/kg). In six cases with interictal discharges on the baseline EEG, a transient "anticonvulsant effect" manifested by marked suppression of spikes occurred during rising or peak BALs. No prominent discharges were observed during the test, but "rebound" was noted in two cases 12 hours later. Rodin, Frohman, and Gottlieb[57] examined 25 patients with epilepsy. EEGs were recorded half an hour, 3 hours, 1 day, and 3 days after subjects consumed 6 oz of 50 percent ethanol; BALs of 30 to 284 mg/dl were reached. Diffuse theta activity occurred in 15 patients (especially 3 hours after the dose), a slight increase of beta activity occurred in two patients, and "electrical seizures" occurred in four patients, particularly the day after the administration of ethanol (two had increased temporal sharp waves and two had "paroxysmal activity"). Bach-y-Rita, Lion, and Ervin[3] gave 150 to 300 ml of 25 percent ethanol IV to ten men with a history of violent behavior during intoxication and to two persons with epilepsy (the latter had depth electrodes implanted in the amygdaloid regions). No discharges were seen in the former group (with so-called "pathologic intoxication"), but increased sharp activity appeared in both amygdaloid areas (but not in the cortex) in the seizure patients. To our knowledge, the latter finding has not been replicated, but it suggests that subcortical structures may also play a role in the generation of epileptiform activity during alcohol intoxication in humans.

These studies suggest that epileptiform discharges are rare in scalp EEGs during ethanol intake and contrast with earlier findings by Marinacci,[45] who gave varying amounts of beer or liquor to 402 patients with "pathologic intoxication." During intoxication, 14 percent of these patients were said to have anterior temporal lobe spikes, and 4 percent had "psychomotor episodes." This report is difficult to analyze because it is not clear what proportion of these "spikes" were present on the shorter baseline EEGs, and because some "spikes" may have been activity now regarded as "patterns of uncertain significance"[7] (e.g., small sharp spikes, 6-Hz spike-and-slow-waves, 14- and 6-Hz positive burst).

Chronic Administration

Animal Studies

After 5 weeks of ethanol administration (1.5 g/kg one, two, or three times/day), Perrin, Kalant, and Livingston[55] observed the appearance of high-amplitude spike-like activity in the hippocampi and cortex of normal cats. This observation may have actually been made during early alcohol withdrawal since the two cats without spike-like discharges were the only ones receiving ethanol three times per day (see below). Earlier work by Guerro-Figueroa and associates[26] using cats with epileptogenic foci showed increased numbers of discharges in subcortical structures during the first 2 to 5 days of alcohol administration, but a gradual decrease in cortical and subcortical discharges later (days 10-30). A similar time course was noted for clinical seizures in the latter animals (no seizures occurred in ten normal cats).[26] Thus, the timing of interictal epileptiform patterns and clinical seizures during ethanol intoxication in cats appears to depend on the presence of an epileptogenic lesion.

Human Studies

Ten inmates without histories of epilepsy were given ethanol daily for 24 days by Weiss and colleagues.[69] Significant slowing of the alpha rhythm (from 10 to 8

Hz) occurred between days 14 and 24, but 2 days after withdrawal it rose to 10.5 Hz. Hyperventilation had no clear effect and no "seizure patterns" were seen at any time. In addition, the normal driving response to photic stimulation was significantly suppressed between days 14 and 24, but returned to normal by the second day of withdrawal. Wikler and associates[71] gave 458 to 489 ml of 95 percent ethanol to three former narcotic addicts daily for 48 to 55 days. None had previously experienced seizures, and all EEGs were normal before the study. Initially, changes consisted of diffuse slowing with an increased proportion of 4- to 6-Hz activity, an increased abundance of occipital alpha activity, and a slowing of the mean alpha frequency. Over days the EEG showed a partial return to normal, suggesting the development of a type of tolerance. A small (5 percent) increase in alcohol dose reinstituted the early changes. In addition, the subject's degree of behavioral intoxication did not display a consistent relationship to EEG slowing.

Höppener, Kuyer, and van der Lugt[31] examined EEG changes in 29 epileptic subjects who consumed "social" quantities of ethanol for 16 weeks (about 20 g twice weekly). EEGs were recorded the morning after an evening dose. No changes occurred in either background activity or responses to hyperventilation and photic stimulation during the alcohol period compared with baseline. Moreover, the "total epileptic activity" was not greater than in a nondrinking control group (n = 23) with epilepsy.

Thus, chronic high-dose ethanol consumption produces EEG slowing, but a degree of EEG "tolerance" may develop. By contrast, long-term consumption of "social" quantities by patients with epilepsy appears to have no lasting effect on EEGs recorded the day after drinking.

EEG FINDINGS DURING WITHDRAWAL

Most patients with alcohol-related seizures are sent to the EEG laboratory when they are sober. Therefore, although one must be aware of the effects discussed above, knowledge of the EEG changes occurring during withdrawal is more important in managing these cases.

Early Period of Abstinence

ANIMAL STUDIES

In a report by Poldrugo and Snead,[56] 20 rats were intoxicated for two successive 18-day periods and subsequently withdrawn for EEG monitoring. In the first withdrawal period, spikes were most abundant 4 hours after the last dose of ethanol and were most frequent in the hippocampus. They were less frequent in the cortex and thalamus, and least numerous in the amygdala. During the second alcohol withdrawal period, spikes were significantly ($p < 0.05$) more abundant. They appeared in the same relative distribution and reached a maximum in 2 to 3 hours, yet were absent about 5 hours after withdrawal (Fig. 17-1). BALs fluctuated widely during the second alcohol addiction phase, and it was hypothesized that the increased frequency of spikes during the second withdrawal phase was due to a kindling effect of repeated minor withdrawals.[56]

The importance of subcortical, cerebellar, and brainstem structures in the development of epileptiform activity had been postulated earlier by Hunter and associates.[32,33] Chronically intoxicated rats were withdrawn from ethanol while EEG recordings were made from the frontal cortex, amygdala/hippocampus, diencephalon, and MRF.[32] Low-amplitude spikes progressing to paroxysms of spindle-like spikes appeared before clinical seizures in limbic, mesencephalic, and nonspecific diencephalic structures significantly more frequently than in the cortex or specific diencephalic areas. During audiogenic convulsions, discharges began in the amygdala or MRF and spread, with some delay and lower amplitude, to other areas. With multiple seizures, ictal discharges nearly always began in the MRF and showed much less spread to the cortex.[32] In subsequent experiments, these investigators found a time-dependent increase in spikes in caudate and red nuclei, substantia nigra, and pontine reticular formation

SPIKE FREQUENCY ANALYSIS

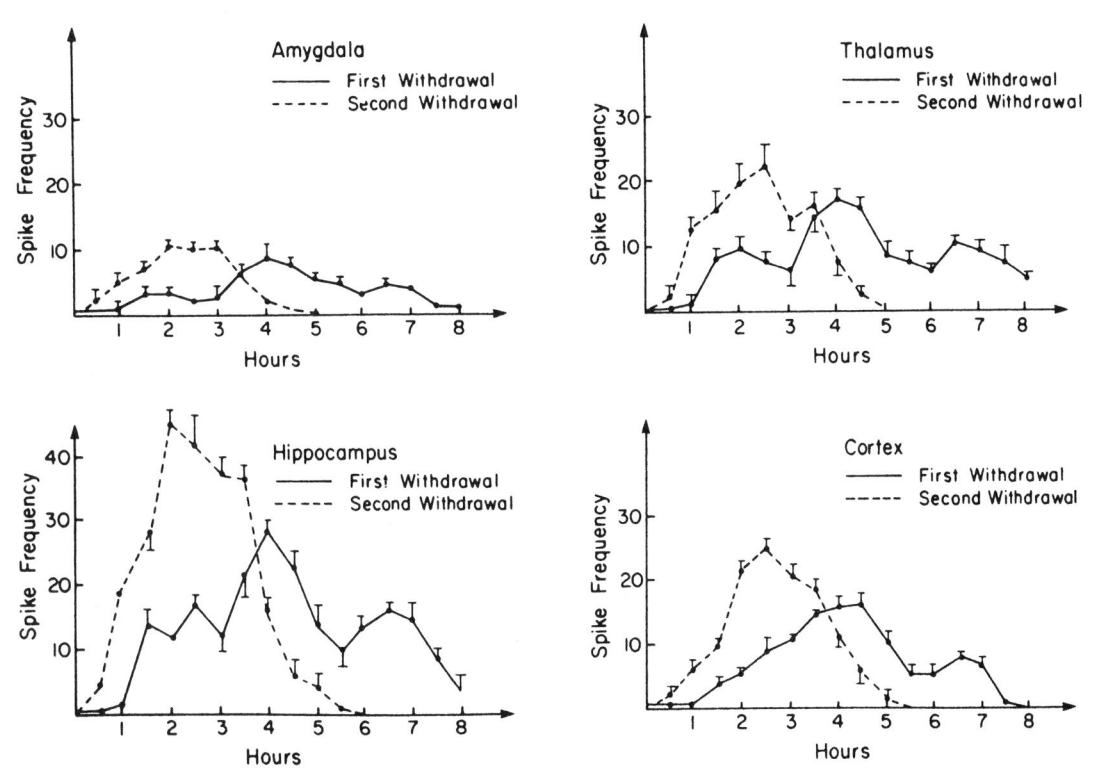

Figure 17–1. Epileptiform discharges in rats during early withdrawal. Average spike frequency at 4 sites in rats during 8 hours of a first (*solid line*) and second (*dashed line*) ethanol withdrawal period. All spike frequencies were significantly ($p < 0.05$) greater during the second withdrawal. (From Poldrugo and Snead,[56] p. 143, with permission.)

in rats withdrawing from chronic intoxication.[33] They believed that the development of epileptiform discharges during alcohol withdrawal might involve interactions between the thalamus and the striatum, substantia nigra, red nucleus, and cerebellum.

Further evidence of subcortical discharges during alcohol withdrawal is found in studies on other species. Maxson and Sze[48] were unable to record spikes from the cortex of mice during audiogenic convulsions after alcohol withdrawal, but Walker and Zornetzer[68] recorded single spike events leading to sustained seizure discharges in the cortex, thalami, hippocampi, and septal nuclei of mice during alcohol withdrawal. They also observed that subclinical and clinical ictal discharges were more severe during a second withdrawal period.[68] In experiments with five healthy cats, Perrin, Kalant, and Livingston[55] observed spike-like hippocampal activity, and in three of five animals, bursts of spike-like activity in cortical areas during withdrawal. A 1 g/kg "challenge dose" of IV alcohol reduced discharges in both these areas. An earlier study with cats withdrawing from chronic, large doses of ethanol also described the appearance of prominent cortical, MRF, amygdala, and hippocampal spikes and ictal discharges in "normal" animals and animals rendered epileptic.[26] These discharges were enhanced with photic stimulation and non-REM sleep. All cortical and subcortical epileptiform activity in "normal" cats and all secondary discharges in cats with epileptogenic foci were abolished by treatment with diazepam.[26]

In summary, epileptiform patterns appear in cortical and subcortical sites during alcohol withdrawal in animals. They are more prominent during repeated alcohol withdrawal periods and photic stimulation, and can be diminished or abolished by alcohol or diazepam.

HUMAN STUDIES

Abnormalities

Our experience and other published findings suggest that the EEG is normal in most persons during alcohol withdrawal. Hauser and associates[28] reviewed the EEGs of 117 patients with withdrawal seizures and found normal or nonspecifically abnormal records in 97 percent of these cases (but found them in only 58 percent of patients with idiopathic or remote seizures). Wessely[70] found normal EEGs in 64 percent of 258 chronic alcoholics with a history of seizures, and Victor and Brausch[66] noted that 84 percent of 130 patients presenting to the hospital with alcohol-related seizures had normal EEGs. Arentsen and Sindrup[2] noted that 69 percent of EEGs in 317 chronic alcoholics (abstinent for more than 1 week; two thirds were receiving disulfiram) were normal; 87 percent of a subgroup with only excessive social drinking and no central nervous system (CNS) complications had normal recordings. Although disulfiram may produce EEG slowing, the dose was low and the percentage of abnormal EEGs was similar in patients receiving and patients not receiving disulfiram. Funkhouser, Nagler, and Walke[21] compared recordings from 81 patients with uncomplicated alcoholism (no seizures, psychosis, or delirium tremens) with recordings from 74 persons with unselected alcohol-related seizures, and found 79 percent and 59 percent normal EEGs, respectively. The EEGs of 34 patients with uncomplicated alcoholism abstinent for 1 or 2 days were compared with those of 55 "normal controls" by Little and McAvoy;[42] 80 percent of the former and 84 percent of the latter were normal. Finally, Greenblatt, Levin, and DiCori[25] tested 157 hospitalized chronic alcoholics and found that 95 percent of those without psychosis under age 30 and 83 percent of the 24 subjects with alcohol withdrawal seizures (AWS) (as the only seizure type) had normal EEGs (compared with 25 percent of 115 patients with a history of idiopathic epilepsy).

Beta Activity

A common EEG finding in early alcohol withdrawal is diffuse, low-amplitude beta activity. Although a "low voltage EEG"[7] is not abnormal *per se*, it occurs in only a small proportion of recordings from normal persons. Frank, Heber, and Fritsch[19] performed visual and quantitative (power density spectral) EEG analysis in two groups of alcoholics with differing durations of abstinence (1–10 days and 11–21 days) and in a control group. They noted that both alcoholic groups showed significantly ($p < 0.01$) more beta frequency power in central and occipital areas than the control group, but no substantial differences were detected between the alcoholic groups. Kaplan and associates[35] used spectral analysis to compare the EEGs of 56 alcoholics abstinent for 2 to 48 days with those of nonalcoholics and found significantly ($p < 0.05$) more fast beta (18–31 Hz) activity over the left frontotemporal and right occipital areas within 7 days after the last drink. Patients receiving chlordiazepoxide had both excessive slow beta (13–17 Hz) and fast beta activity; a finding consistent with the well-known effect of benzodiazepines on the EEG. Similar results were noted by Spehr and Stemmler,[62] who used power spectral analysis and Hjorth's time domain descriptors to quantitatively examine the EEGs of alcoholics 1.8 days after admission to an alcohol detoxification unit. EEGs during the acute withdrawal stages of impending or early delirium tremens showed extremely low-amplitude activity over the middle and posterior scalp regions in 14 of 15 cases.[61] In another investigation, low-voltage beta activity was noted on spectral analysis of the EEG over the anterior areas in 15 alcoholics 3 or 4 days after the start of abstinence, but these investigators reported no details about medications administered.[10] Romerio and associates[58] examined the EEGs of 150 chronic (>5 years) alcoholics within one week of admission. These patients had never experienced seizures and had no history of head injury or cerebrovascular events. Prominent beta (and diminished alpha) activity was noted in 41 percent. Other early reports using visual EEG analysis support these findings.[21,37,41] Unfortunately, statistical comparisons with control groups, blinded EEG interpretation, and control for the effects of medications and drug abuse were not performed in many of these clinical studies.

Alpha Activity

Lower amplitude, less abundant alpha activity is also a common finding in the early phase of alcohol withdrawal. Although spectral analysis showed insignificantly less occipital alpha power in abstinent alcoholics than in controls in one recent study,[19] other studies using this technique have noted significantly ($p < 0.05$) less relative alpha power compared with alcoholics in treatment for 4 to 6 weeks[10] or nonalcoholic controls.[35] The timing of the recordings may have been a factor in the former study;[19] Spehr and Stemmler[62] found that both relative and absolute alpha power and the dominant alpha frequency significantly ($p = 0.001$) increased in EEGs recorded 18 days after an EEG recorded in early abstinence. Numerous other investigations have also shown both less abundant and lower-amplitude alpha activity (with or without a slowing of the mean frequency) in the early stages of alcohol withdrawal in patients with and without seizures.[11,20,21,37,41,42,58,61,64,71] Although these studies were based on visual EEG analysis, a few used manual quantification methods such as calculation of the "alpha index."[11,37,42] Some but not all of these investigators made comparisons with appropriate control groups. To what degree this increased beta and decreased alpha activity reflect a nonspecific hyperalert state in early alcohol withdrawal is unclear.

Theta and Delta Activity

Diffuse slow activity occurs in a small proportion of alcoholics during the early stages of abstinence. Kaplan and associates[35] found that hospitalized alcoholics (n = 56) showed significantly ($p < 0.001$) increased 1- to 4-Hz frequency interhemispheric coherence and spectral power, compared with nonalcoholics. The degree of coherence correlated negatively with the patient's brain age quotient score measured by neuropsychologic testing. Spehr and Stemmler[62] studied 48 chronic alcoholics (15 of whom had AWS) and noted a significantly ($p < 0.004$) slower mean delta (< 4 Hz) frequency and greater percentage of delta activity within 2 days of admission than 18 days later. Devetag and associates[14] observed focal and generalized slowing in 6 percent and 30%, respectively, of patients with AWS, compared with 2 percent and 9 percent of patients with "alcoholic epilepsy" (alcoholics with seizures not related to withdrawal or massive intake of alcohol and no risk factors for or previous history of epilepsy). Romerio and associates[58] studied chronic alcoholics without known CNS lesions, using both EEG and hepatic blood tests performed within a week of admission; subjects showed a 22 percent incidence of diffuse slow activity. Although some patients with severe liver dysfunction had normal EEGs, slowing of EEG activity was observed in only 16 percent with normal liver function and 29 percent with severe dysfunction. In one report, 10 percent of 258 chronic alcoholics with a history of seizures showed theta activity over the anterior head regions.[70] In an earlier report by Victor and Brausch,[66] the EEGs of 12 of 130 AWS patients contained diffuse slowing (four later reverted to normal) and two showed bilateral frontotemporal slow activity. Diffuse theta activity mixed with background rhythms was seen in 20 percent of another group of chronic alcoholics more than a week after hospitalization.[2] The authors argue that the latter finding was related not to disulfiram administration, head trauma, or age, but rather to a history of delirium tremens or seizures.[2] Lafon and associates[41] found a correspondence between diffuse EEG abnormalities and generalized atrophy as shown by pneumoencephalography. Similarly, in a study of 11 chronic alcoholics, Newman[52] detected a relationship between cerebral atrophy (by computed tomography [CT] scan) and generalized slowing, but only in patients over age 60. Wikler and associates[71] observed that 15 to 20 hours after sudden withdrawal from an experimental period of chronic intoxication, three subjects demonstrated moderate- to high-voltage rhythmic theta activity coincident with a drop in the percentage of alpha activity and a BAL of 0 mg/dl, and clinical agitation. One of these subjects had a seizure 41 hours after withdrawal, and another experienced delirium tremens after 4 days of abstinence. From these varied reports, no single etiology for the generalized slowing during early abstinence emerges. The contributions of drowsiness and illness and the effects of medications are unclear.

Focal Slowing

Focal slow waves are observed less often than generalized slow activity.[14] In a group of 14 patients with a history of AWS and head injury, the eight with focal episodes all had focal EEG abnormalities and the six with generalized spells had no focal abnormalities.[66] A second group (n = 4) with focal AWS but no history of head trauma had EEGs showing focal abnormalities.[66]

Epileptiform Patterns

An important feature of the EEG in patients with alcohol-related seizures is interictal epileptiform patterns. Chan[6] surveyed the literature and found that most investigators have reported a low (usually <10 percent) incidence of epileptiform activity in alcoholics who had seizures only during withdrawal, but a high (35 to 90 percent) incidence in nonalcoholic patients with epilepsy. Schear[61] found no discharges in the EEGs of 15 patients with impending delirium tremens. Similarly, in the series of Romerio and associates[58] "paroxysmal abnormalities" were seen in only one of 150 alcohol abusers without seizures. That patient had severe hepatic dysfunction. Wessely[70] noted a 7 percent incidence of "definite paroxysms" and a 19 percent frequency of "dysrhythmias with outbursts of sharp waves and spikes" in 258 alcoholics with histories of seizures. Of 130 alcoholics presenting with seizures, EEGs showed focal slowing or spikes in five patients (two had previous head injuries) and diffuse slow activity and spikes in two patients with idiopathic epilepsy.[66] Giove and Gastaut[24] found no epileptiform patterns in 31 patients with only alcohol-related seizures and no history of head injury. Pentylenetetrazol (PTZ) produced generalized and focal discharges in one and six patients, respectively; three of these patients had generalized tonic-clonic seizures.[24] Wikler and associates[71] observed that all of three subjects undergoing chronic experimental intoxication displayed "random spikes" and paroxysmal slow wave bursts after 15 to 48 hours of alcohol withdrawal. BALs were maintained around 200 mg/dl during intoxication, but fell to 0 after 15 to 19 hours of abstinence. One of the three had a generalized seizure after 41 hours of alcohol withdrawal. Funkhouser, Nagler, and Walke[21] noted "paroxysmal dysrhythmias" (epileptiform patterns and bursts of slow activity) in 0 percent of 81 patients with uncomplicated alcoholism and in 7 percent of 74 patients with convulsions during alcohol withdrawal. The latter group was not divided into persons with both epilepsy and alcoholism and those with only AWS.

Effects of Sleep and Sleep Deprivation

Van Sweden[63] has stated that EEGs recorded during sleep have only limited informative value and add little to the data offered by the waking recording in alcoholics presenting with seizures. He found no activation of epileptiform discharges in recordings made following sleep deprivation in six patients 1 day after or in four patients about 10 days after waking EEGs were recorded. The statistical significance of this data was not tested and the number of patients believed to suffer from epilepsy was not stated.

In contrast, Deisenhammer, Klinger, and Trägner[13] published a detailed EEG study in which 590 patients were divided into six groups based on the presence of alcohol abuse, seizures of any etiology (except group I), and risk factors for epilepsy (acquired brain damage, epilepsy prior to the onset of alcohol abuse, or a family history of epilepsy) (Table 17–1). They excluded patterns of uncertain significance (small sharp spikes, 14- and 6-Hz positive burst) as well as photoparox-

Table 17-1. FOCAL AND GENERALIZED EPILEPTIFORM DISCHARGES BEFORE AND AFTER SLEEP DEPRIVATION

History*	n	Focal Before Sleep Deprivation	Focal After Sleep Deprivation	Generalized Before Sleep Deprivation	Generalized After Sleep Deprivation
I. Alcohol, withdrawal seizures	52	3.8%	3.8%	1.9%	7.7%
II. Alcohol, seizures, risk factors	128	18.7%	23.4%	17.2%	28.1%
III. Alcohol	24	0%	0%	0%	4.2%
IV. Alcohol, risk factors	32	15.6%	9.3%	3.1%	6.2%
V. Seizures	117	14.5%	16.2%	16.2%	27.4%
VI. Seizures, risk factors	237	26.6%	32.9%	12.2%	20.3%

*Groups of patients divided according to history of alcoholism, seizures of any etiology (except group I, which included patients with seizures during withdrawal only), and risk factors for epilepsy. (From Deisenhammer, Klinger, and Trägner,[13] p. 528, with permission.)

ysmal and photomyogenic responses. Focal and generalized discharges appeared on a waking EEG in 4 percent and 2 percent, respectively, of 52 patients with pure AWS (group I), and in only 4 percent and 8 percent, respectively, on EEGs recorded after sleep deprivation a few (mean = 6) days later. The differences between waking and sleep EEGs were not significant. In contrast, a group (II) of 128 patients with alcoholism, seizures, and risk factors for epilepsy had focal and generalized discharges in 19 percent and 17 percent, respectively, of waking EEGs, and 24 percent and 28 percent of recordings after sleep deprivation. The increase in generalized discharges after sleep deprivation in this group was statistically significant. The incidence of discharges in group II was comparable to that observed in the group with epilepsy but no history of alcoholism (group VI). Group II showed significantly ($p < 0.005$) more focal and generalized discharges (both before and after sleep deprivation) than group I, and significantly ($p < 0.005$) more generalized discharges than group IV (with alcoholism and risk factors, but no seizures). Thus, EEGs recorded during wakefulness can help distinguish sober patients with seizures due to alcohol withdrawal alone from patients with seizures related to an underlying epileptic disorder. Furthermore, sleep deprivation is more likely to activate epileptiform patterns in patients with epilepsy when they are sober than it is in persons with AWS.

Periodic Lateralized Epileptiform Discharges

Periodic lateralized epileptiform discharges (PLEDs) consist of continuous sharp waves or spikes recurring at fairly regular intervals and confined to one area or, more commonly, lateralized over one hemisphere. In the initial description of this pattern, Chatrian, Shaw, and Leffman[8] examined multiple EEGs of 33 patients with PLEDs. All patients exhibited symptoms and signs of impaired neurologic function and 29 patients experienced seizures during the course of their illness. It was suggested that alcohol withdrawal played a role in generating both PLEDs and partial seizures in some of the 12 patients with chronic alcoholism in this series. More recently, Chu[9] described this pattern in four patients with partial motor seizures during alcohol withdrawal. In all cases, PLEDs appeared over a pathologically or radiologically verified lesion, but CT scans demonstrated, in each of the cases, respectively: a persistent right temporal lobe abnormality; no abnormalities except transient focal enhancement during a Todd's paralysis; generalized atrophy; and normal findings. The first patient displayed right sided PLEDs two days after alcohol withdrawal (Fig. 17-2A). Five months later, persistent

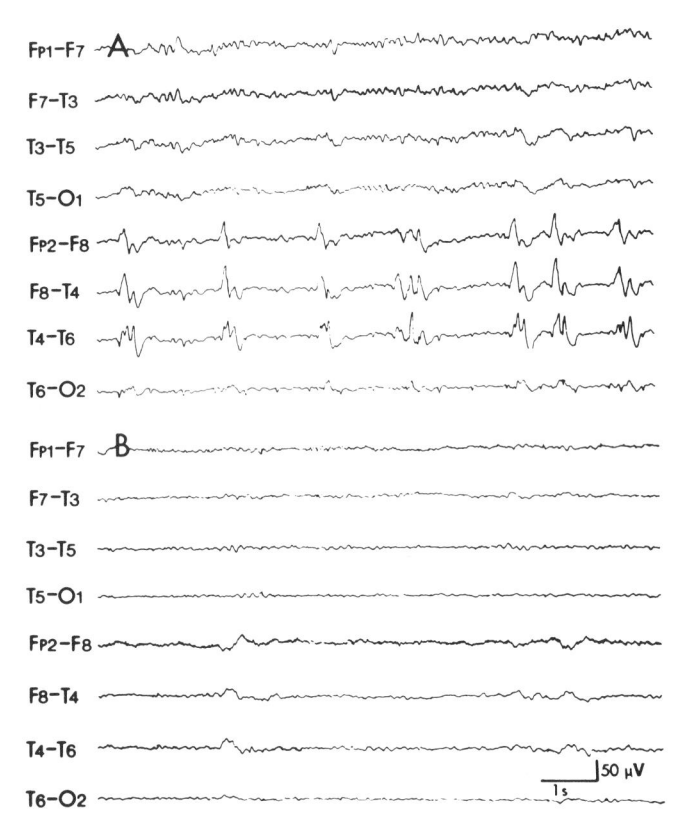

Figure 17–2. Periodic lateralized epileptiform discharges in early withdrawal. A 53-year-old woman experienced left sided partial motor seizures 2 days after discontinuing 2 months of daily vodka intake. A CT scan revealed a well-demarcated area of lucency in the right temporal lobe. (A) EEG showing periodic lateralized epileptiform discharges best developed in the right frontotemporal area. (B) Slow wave focus in the same region 5 months later. A repeat CT scan was unchanged. (From Chu,[9] p. 552, copyright 1980, American Medical Association, with permission.)

focal slow activity was apparent in the EEG (Fig. 17–2B). The second patient had a history of head trauma, and in the latter two cases, autopsy revealed "old" infarctions. Niedermeyer and associates[53] also described this pattern in ten chronic alcohol abusers with motor seizures and neurologic deficits, but in whom CT, magnetic resonance imaging (MRI), and arteriography findings were "mostly normal." Finally, Dauben and Adams[12] reported PLEDs 1 and 7 days after a stroke associated with a partial seizure in one patient. This EEG later returned to normal, but one month later (after eight days of heavy alcohol use) the patient became mute and PLEDs were again noted. These findings suggest that alcohol withdrawal can trigger PLEDs, neurologic deficits, and repetitive partial seizures in persons with pre-existing focal hemispheric lesions. Lesions may or may not be detected with neuroimaging techniques.

Response to Photic Stimulation

Exaggerated responses to photic (stroboscopic) stimulation during alcohol withdrawal were first reported by Lafon and associates.[41] One chronic alcoholic admitted for detoxification demonstrated diffuse multiple spike patterns with 15-Hz and a "grand mal" convulsion with 10-Hz light flashes. These findings are examples of the photoparoxysmal response (PPR), which is defined by the occurrence of bilaterally synchronous, symmetrical, and generalized spike-and-slow-wave and multiple spike-and-slow-wave complexes and may include associated impairment of consciousness and brisk jerks involving the musculature of the whole body (but predominantly of the head and arms).[7] The term PPR is preferred to the photoconvulsive response (PCR) because clinical convulsions frequently do not accompany this pattern. Lloyd-Smith and Gloor,[43] Karpati and associates,[36] and Giove and Gastaut[24] noted that PPR (with or without focal and generalized seizures) could be induced in alcohol abusers only during alcohol withdrawal. This response was noted several hours after the experimental administration of alcohol as well.[49] Although abnormal, PPR is nonspecific because it can be seen upon withdrawal from sedatives (most notably, barbiturates) as well.

Gastaut, Trevisan, and Naquet[22] described a "fronto-polar recruiting response of muscular origin" in 26 percent of chronic alcoholics, but reported that it did not occur with greater abundance or prominence in persons with alcohol-related seizures. This pattern is similar to what was once called the photomyoclonic response and is currently termed the *photomyogenic response (PMR)*. PMR is characterized by the appearance of brief repetitive muscle spikes over the anterior regions of the head that cease when the stroboscopic stimulus is withdrawn. It may encompass the simultaneous occurrence of eyelid myoclonus, vertical ocular oscillation, and discrete jerking largely involving the head and facial musculature.[7] It is a quantitatively, but not qualitatively, abnormal response.

Victor and Brausch[66] studied 84 patients using EEGs and photic stimulation during acute alcohol withdrawal. Of those, 19 of the 44 subjects with AWS and 16 of the 40 without seizures, but with signs of alcohol withdrawal prior to testing, showed excessive photic sensitivity (eyelid myoclonus was excluded). The latter included "photomyoclonus, photoconvulsions, and/or other paroxysmal EEG activity." The maximum sensitivity occurred 43 to 48 hours after the last drink. This 42 percent incidence of PPR and PMR is substantially higher than that reported in normal persons (4 percent).[39] In a later report, Victor[65] found PMR in 56 percent of 18 alcohol withdrawal patients (six of whom had "spontaneous seizures") tested with EEGs on admission to the hospital and every 8 hours thereafter. Patients with PMR were significantly ($p < 0.01$) more hypomagnesemic than patients without PMR. Treatment of eight of these patients with $MgSO_4$ abolished the response in 38 percent and elevated the threshold in another 62 percent. A PMR persisted in one patient tested 1.5 hours after receiving both 50 mg chlordiazepoxide and 3 g $MgSO_4$, but was absent 1 hour after a second IV dose of $MgSO_4$. A relationship between transient hypomagnesemia, respiratory alkalosis, seizures, and abnormal photic responses was noted in four patients withdrawing from 60 days of chronic intoxication.[65]

Hauser and associates[28] compared the EEGs of 117 patients with recent seizures related to the reduction or cessation of alcohol consumption with those of adults with idiopathic first seizures. Recordings were made within 48 hours of the seizure; only one alcohol withdrawal patient had a PPR. In the series of Devetag and associates,[14] the group with AWS showed no abnormal response to photic stimulation, but 3.6 percent of those with "alcoholic epilepsy" showed PPRs. These and other studies[23,69] contrast with those mentioned above, but the time between the start of alcohol withdrawal and the recording of the EEG and the medications (if any) patients received before the EEG were rarely specified. More recently, Fisch and associates[18] studied 37 untreated patients with mild to moderately severe withdrawal symptoms (but not seizures) within 72 hours of their last drink, using diffuse and patterned stroboscopic stimulation. Two patients displayed PMR, but no PPRs. This finding contrasts with Victor and Brausch's[66] findings about the group without seizures. Possible explanations for these discrepancies include: differences in severity of alcohol withdrawal symptoms, duration of alcohol abuse, nutritional status and race; a greater incidence of polysubstance abuse; and adherence to more recent definitions of PMR and PPR.[7]

We reviewed the EEGs of 40 consecutive patients meeting the following criteria: 1) EEG preceded by seizure(s) and within 96 hours of last drink; 2) treatment with benzodiazepines (BZPs) alone or combined with phenytoin (PHT); 3) no $MgSO_4$, paraldehyde, or other anti-epileptic drugs; 4) no alcohol-unrelated seizures; and 5) alcohol as the only substance of abuse. In 18 patients, 19 EEGs were obtained after treatment with a single (n = 14) or two (n = 5) BZPs. The time (mean ± standard deviation) since last drink was 52 ± 22 hours and since last seizure was 33 ± 22 hours. EEGs were recorded in 22 patients after treatment with a single (n = 15), or two (n = 7) BZPs, plus PHT. Time from last drink was 62 ± 22 hours and from last seizure was 45 ± 22 hours. None of the patients in either group had

Table 17–2. PHOTIC SENSITIVITY IN PATIENTS WITH SIGNS OF ALCOHOL WITHDRAWAL

Study	n	Time of EEG Recording	Number of Patients (%) with PMR or PPR
Victor and Brausch[66]			
AWS(s)	44	Soon after admission	19 (43)
No seizure(s)	40		16 (40)
Victor[65]			
AWS(s)	6	On admission and	5 (83)
No seizure(s)	12	every 8 hr	5 (42)
Vossler and Browne[67]			
Group I*	18	52 hr‡	0 (0)
Group II†	22	61 hr‡	0 (0)

*Patients with seizures related only to alcohol withdrawal receiving benzodiazepines (BZPs) prior to the EEG.
†Patients with AWS receiving both BZPs and PHT prior to the EEG.
‡Mean time between patient's last drink and EEG.

PPR or PMR (see Table 17–2). Although this study does not address the current incidence of these responses in untreated persons, it suggests that they are rare among AWS patients who receive BZP(s) either alone or combined with PHT prior to the EEG.[67]

Recently, we studied a 61-year-old woman with a history of chronic alcohol abuse but no history of seizures or risk factors for epilepsy. Approximately 12 hours after her last drink, she experienced a single seizure that began with upward deviation of the head and eyes, followed by generalized tonic-clonic activity. The BAL was 0 mg/dl and her neurologic examination and CT scan findings on admission were normal. Nine hours after the seizure, an EEG revealed a PPR at multiple frequencies of light flashes (Fig. 17–3A). Five hours later the EEG still showed a PPR; with 14-, 16-, and 18-Hz flashes she exhibited a few brief generalized jerks of the upper and lower extremities during the stimulation. With 18-Hz stimulation she also experienced the visual hallucination that her daughter and other familiar persons were standing around her bed in the EEG laboratory. Minutes later, when tested again with 14-Hz flashes, she experienced a 55-second generalized tonic-clonic seizure that began with upward and leftward head and eye deviation (Fig. 17–3B). She received no BZPs, other sedatives, anti-epileptic drugs, $MgSO_4$, or paraldehyde before either recording. Ten minutes after the photically induced seizure she was given 1 mg lorazepam IV. Thirty minutes after the seizure, stimulation at 14-, 16-, and 18-Hz produced only photic driving responses (Fig. 17–3C). Although it can be suggested that the seizure blunted the PPR when the patient was retested, she was alert and fully oriented, and her background EEG activity had returned to baseline at that time. This case provides direct evidence that BZPs can abolish abnormal responses to photic stimulation.

Mattson[47] reported similar results with the acute administration of alcohol. He found that ethanol could abort both PMR and PPR; the latter returned 24 hours later. He also noted that paraldehyde reversed photic sensitivity as promptly as alcohol intake.[47] Similarly, Klinger and Wessely[38] gave 60 ml of brandy to subjects displaying PMRs and PPRs and noted that PPRs were "extinguished."

Later Period of Abstinence

Saletu and associates[59] examined quantitative EEGs of 42 chronic alcoholics undergoing alcohol withdrawal before, during, and after a 3-week treatment period with short- and long-acting BZPs. Im-

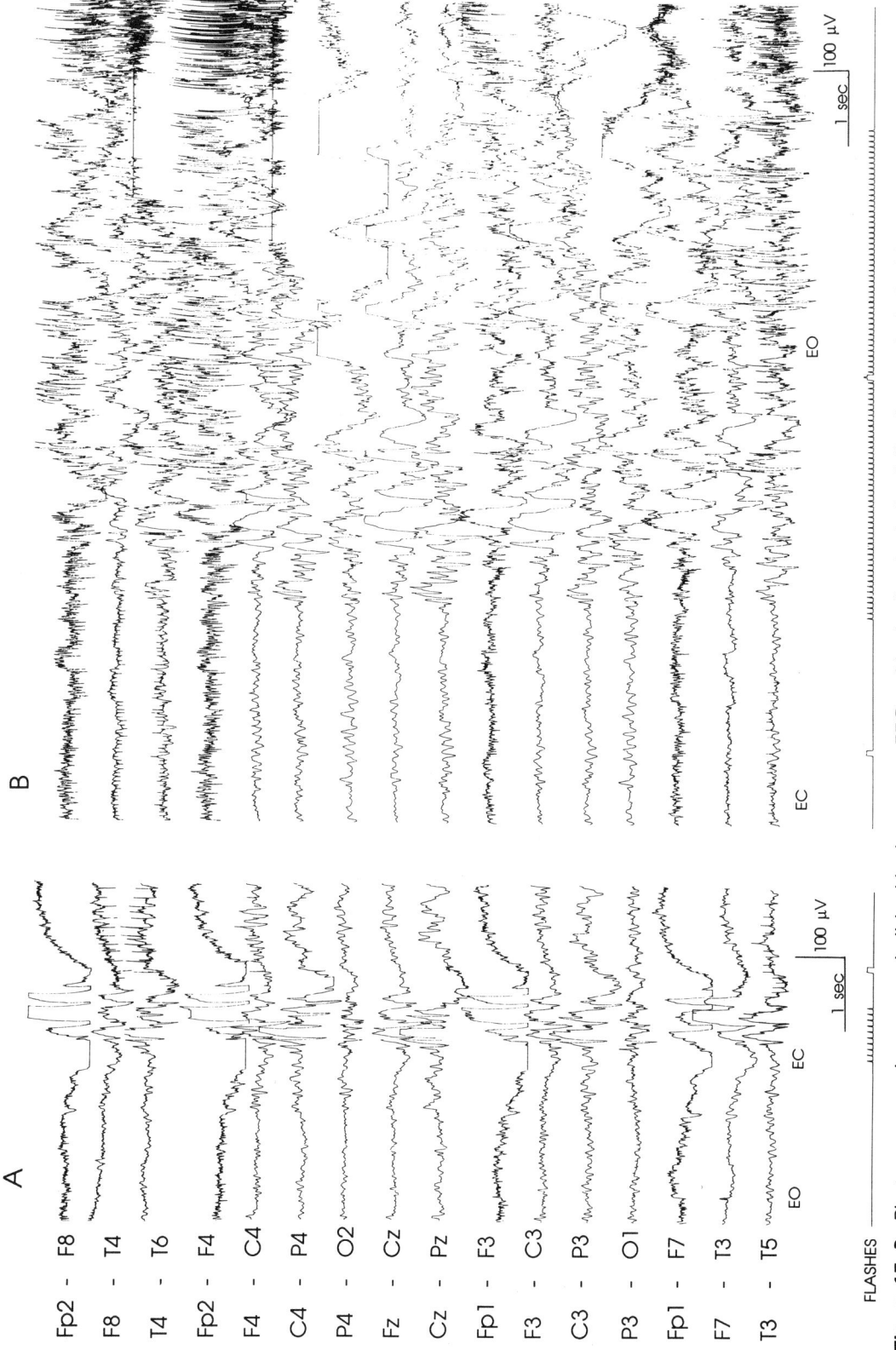

Figure 17–3. Photoparoxysmal response abolished by lorazepam. EEGs with photic stimulation following an alcohol withdrawal seizure. A 61-year-old woman with a history of cardiac disease and chronic alcohol abuse experienced one generalized tonic-clonic seizure about 12 hours after the cessation of drinking. Medications included isosorbide dinitrate and diltiazem. (*A*) 9 hours after the seizure, a photoparoxysmal response (PPR) is elicited by 13-Hz photic stimulation. (*B*) 5 hours later the PPR persists with 14-Hz light flashes and evolves into a generalized seizure (see text for details).

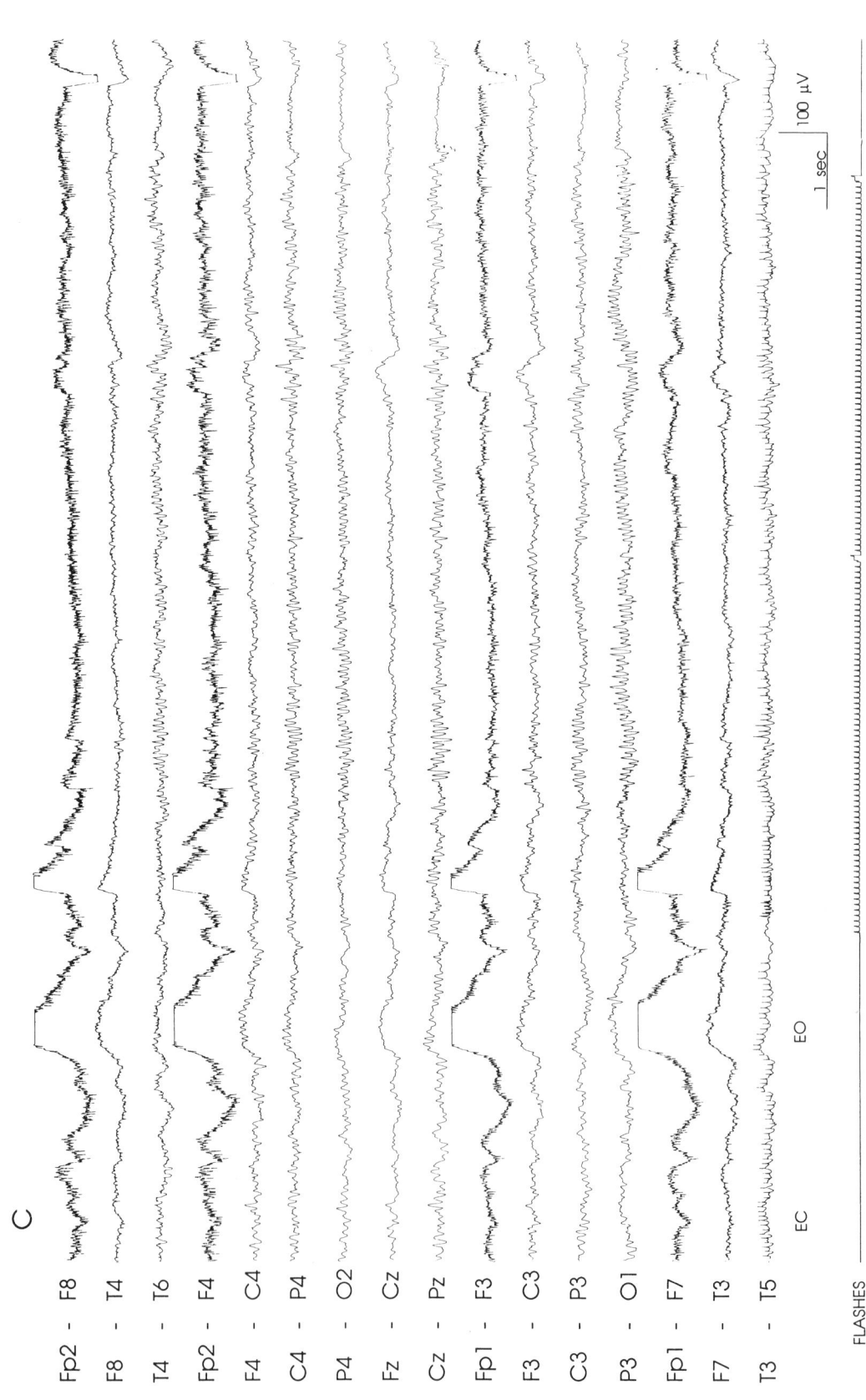

Figure 17–3. *(continued)* (C) 20 minutes after 1 mg i.v. lorazepam (30 min after the seizure) the PPR is extinguished and, instead, a well-developed normal photic driving appears with 14-Hz strobe.

proved alpha and diminished beta activity were seen with the short-acting drug (lopirazepam) after three weeks, but an "anxiolytic profile" (increased beta power) was observed both with the longer-acting agent (prazepam) and immediately after a dose of lopirazepam. Additional reports on EEGs examined visually or with spectral analysis reveal that the quantity and frequency of alpha activity more than one week after withdrawal is higher than alpha abundance and frequencies measured during early abstinence or are no different from alpha quantity and frequencies measured in controls.[10,16,37,61,64,72] These studies indicate that although alpha activity may be reduced in amount and frequency during the early period of alcohol withdrawal, it improves with continued abstinence.

Frank, Heber, and Fritsch[19] found no difference in relative beta power in alcoholics during days 11 to 21 compared with days 1 to 10 of abstinence, but noted increased beta power in both groups versus that measured in controls. However, other reports indicate that although the spectral power of beta activity more than four weeks after withdrawal is greater in patients with neuropsychologic impairment, it diminishes substantially in persons whose cognitive scores improve.[10,70]

A recent study by Olivennes[54] noted spikes in 25 percent of 11 patients with a history of alcoholism and seizures, but the relationship between the latter is difficult to evaluate, and their observation of spikes in 40 percent of the EEGs of a group of patients with heroin addiction with no apparent history of epilepsy seems higher than expected. In contrast, Brumback, Kelly, and Staton[5] gave 20 male alcoholics abstinent for 1 month 100 mg of methohexital by rapid IV injection. Spike activation occurred in only one alcoholic (with a history of epilepsy following a stroke) and three epileptic control patients. This low incidence of epileptiform discharges corroborates a report by Johannesson, Berglund, and Ingvar,[34] who found none among the EEGs of 50 alcoholics tested 16 ± 11 days of abstinence. One limiting factor in the latter report is that the patients were given some type of medication for a week prior to the EEG and 50 percent of EEGs showed nonspecific slowing. A study by Gerson and Karabell[23] found four patients with multifocal spikes or diffuse spike-and-slow-wave discharges among 148 patients who were untreated prior to the EEG and had alcohol-related seizures (some occurred before the withdrawal period). One of the patients with diffuse discharges had a history of idiopathic epilepsy. Therefore, epileptiform activity seems to be infrequent not only immediately after an alcohol-related seizure, but also during longer periods of abstinence.

USEFULNESS OF EEGs IN ALCOHOL-RELATED SEIZURES

From the studies presented, several observations can be made about the EEG findings in persons with alcohol-related seizures. The EEG is normal or reveals nonspecific changes (increased beta and decreased alpha activity; diffuse slowing) in the majority of patients who have had seizures due solely to alcohol withdrawal. Epileptiform discharges are uncommon (<10 percent) in these patients, but are present in 35–90 percent of (sober) patients with epilepsy. In persons with epilepsy who have discharges when sober, epileptiform activity may decrease as BALs rise and increase as they fall. Sleep deprivation is more likely to activate generalized epileptiform discharges in sober patients with epilepsy than in persons with only AWS. Alcohol withdrawal can trigger a PLEDs pattern and repetitive partial seizures in patients with pre-existing focal hemispheric lesions (some of which may not be seen on imaging studies). Focal slow or sharp wave activity suggests the presence of a structural lesion (e.g., traumatic scar, subdural hematoma). Photic sensitivity (PPR and PMR) may occur in more than one third of untreated persons who have recently had an alcohol-related seizure. BZPs (alone or combined with PHT), ethanol, paraldehyde, and $MgSO_4$ can abolish this photic sensitivity. The presence of PPR or PMR in a patient after a first unexplained tonic-clonic seizure suggests the possibility of surreptitious alcohol abuse as the etiology.

The EEG can provide important diagnostic information for clinicians who are aware of these findings and are managing patients presenting with alcohol-related seizures. Evaluation should include recording a waking EEG with photic stimulation soon after the seizure, and recording an EEG following sleep deprivation after the hyperalert state of alcohol withdrawal has subsided.

SUMMARY

The EEG of animals shows greater fast-frequency activity with small doses of ethanol. Large amounts produce slowing and loss of amplitude. Humans display an increased abundance of alpha activity with small doses, but prominent theta and delta slow activity with large amounts. During chronic administration of large doses, a partial return to the baseline EEG has been reported.

Spike-like activity was seen in cats with epileptogenic foci during the first few days of chronic intoxication, but in normal cats only after weeks of ethanol intake. The latter occurrence may have been due to brief alcohol withdrawal. In two reports, patients with epilepsy had fewer spikes and sharp waves while acutely intoxicated than during recovery.

During alcohol withdrawal, EEGs are normal in most patients with seizures from no other cause, but patients with both epilepsy and alcoholism often have abnormalities. In early alcohol withdrawal patients with and without seizures commonly show low-voltage recordings with increased beta activity and less abundant, lower amplitude alpha waves. After long periods of abstinence, diminished beta activity and increased alpha abundance and mean frequency have been reported.

Generalized EEG slowing is infrequent in patients during early alcohol withdrawal; multiple factors may be responsible. Focal slow activity is even less common and has been associated with partial seizures, which suggest the presence of a structural brain lesion.

Several animal species display prominent epileptiform patterns and ictal discharges in cortical and especially subcortical and brainstem structures during alcohol withdrawal. They are enhanced by photic stimulation and repeated withdrawal periods, and are suppressed by alcohol or diazepam. Focal and generalized epileptiform patterns are uncommon in alcoholics both with and without AWS, but are significantly more frequent during early abstinence in patients who have seizures not related to alcohol withdrawal and who have risk factors for epilepsy. Sleep deprivation is more likely to elicit epileptiform patterns in (sober) persons with epilepsy than in patients with only AWS. Periodic lateralized epileptiform discharges and repetitive partial seizures may be triggered by alcohol withdrawal in patients with pre-existing focal hemispheric lesions.

PPRs and PMRs may occur in patients with alcohol-related seizures. We never observed these responses among AWS patients treated with BZPs before the EEG was recorded. An untreated patient no longer had a PPR after we administered lorazepam. Alcohol, $MgSO_4$, and paraldehyde may also abolish these responses.

We conclude that the EEG is a useful test in the clinical evaluation of patients with alcohol-related seizures.

ACKNOWLEDGMENT

This work was supported in part by the Veterans Administration.

References

1. Altshuler, HL, et al: Changes in the rhesus monkey's EEG responses to ethanol during chronic exposure. Pharmacol Biochem Behav 13:233, 1980.
2. Arentsen, K and Sindrup, E: Electroencephalographic investigation of alcoholics. Acta Psychiatr Scand 38:371, 1963.
3. Bach-y-Rita, G, Lion, JR, and Ervin, FR: Pathological intoxication: Clinical and electroencephalographic studies. Am J Psychiatry 127:698, 1970.
4. Begleiter, H and Platz, A: The effects of alcohol on the central nervous system in humans. In Kissin, B and Begleiter, H (eds): The Biology of Alcoholism, Vol 2. Plenum Press, New York, 1972, p 293.

5. Brumback, RA, Kelly, MJ, and Staton, RD: Abnormal electroencephalograms in male alcoholics after methohexital (brevital) injection: A pilot study. Currents in Alcoholism 8:57, 1981.
6. Chan, AWK: Alcoholism and epilepsy. Epilepsia 26:323, 1985.
7. Chatrian, GE, et al: A glossary of terms most commonly used by clinical electroencephalographers. Electroencephalogr Clin Neurophysiol 37:538, 1974.
8. Chatrian, GE, Shaw, C-M, and Leffman, H: The significance of periodic lateralized epileptiform discharges in EEG: An electrographic, clinical and pathological study. Electroencephalogr Clin Neurophysiol 17:177, 1964.
9. Chu, N-S: Periodic lateralized epileptiform discharges with preexisting focal brain lesions: Role of alcohol withdrawal and anoxic encephalopathy. Arch Neurol 37:551, 1980.
10. Coger, RW, et al: EEG difference between male alcoholics in withdrawal and those stabilized in treatment. Currents in Alcoholism 8:85, 1981.
11. Davis, PA, et al: The effects of alcohol upon the electroencephalogram (brain waves). Quarterly Journal of Studies on Alcohol 1:626, 1941.
12. Dauben, RD and Adams, AH: Periodic lateralized epileptiform discharges in EEG: A review with special attention to etiology and recurrence. Clin Electroencephalogr 8:116, 1977.
13. Deisenhammer, E, Klinger, D, and Trägner, H: Epileptic seizures in alcoholism and diagnostic value of EEG after sleep deprivation. Epilepsia 25:526, 1984.
14. Devetag, F, et al: Alcoholic epilepsy: Review of a series and proposed classification and etiopathogenesis. Ital J Neurol Sci 3:275, 1983.
15. Dolce, G and Decker, H: The effects of ethanol on cortical and subcortical electrical activity in cats. Res Commun Chem Pathol Pharmacol 3:523, 1972.
16. Emmerson, RY, et al: EEG, visually evoked and event related potentials in young abstinent alcoholics. Alcohol 4:241, 1987.
17. Engel, GL and Rosenbaum, M: Delirium: Electroencephalographic changes associated with acute alcoholic intoxication. Arch Neurol Psychiatry 53:44, 1945.
18. Fisch, BJ, et al: The EEG response to diffuse and patterned light stimulation during acute alcohol withdrawal. Electroencephalogr Clin Neurophysiol 64:76P, 1986.
19. Frank, H, Heber, G, and Fritsch, M: Analyse des EEGs alkoholkranker in der ersten phase der abstinenz. Nervenarzt 56:730, 1986.
20. Funderburk, WH: Electroencephalographic studies in chronic alcoholism. Electroencephalogr Clin Neurophysiol 1:369, 1949.
21. Funkhouser, JB, Nagler, B, and Walke, ND: The electro-encephalogram of chronic alcoholism. South Med J 46:423, 1953.
22. Gastaut, H, Trevisan, C, and Naquet, R: Diagnostic value of electroencephalographic abnormalities provoked by intermittent photic stimulation. Electroencephalogr Clin Neurophysiol 10:194, 1958.
23. Gerson, IM and Karabell, S: The use of the electroencephalogram in patients admitted for alcohol abuse with seizures. Clin Electroencephalogr 10:40, 1979.
24. Giove, G and Gastaut, H: Épilepsie alcoolique et déclenchment alcoolique des crises chez les épileptiques, Rev Neurol 113:347, 1965.
25. Greenblatt, M, Levin, S, and DiCori, F: The electroencephalogram associated with chronic alcoholism, alcoholic psychosis and alcoholic convulsions. Arch Neurol Psychiatry 52:290, 1944.
26. Guerro-Figueroa, R, et al: Electrographic and behavioral effects of diazepam during alcohol withdrawal stage in cats. Neuropharmacology 9:143, 1970.
27. Hadji-Dimo, AA, Ekberg, R, and Ingvar, DH: Effects of ethanol on EEG and cortical blood flow in the cat. Quarterly Journal of Studies on Alcohol 29A:828, 1968.
28. Hauser, WA, et al: Electroencephalographic findings in patients with ethanol withdrawal seizures. Electroencephalogr Clin Neurophysiol 54:64P, 1982.
29. Hogans, AF, Moreno, OM, and Brodie, DA: Effects of ethyl alcohol on EEG and avoidance behavior of chronic electrode monkeys. Am J Physiol 201:434, 1961.
30. Holmberg, G and Mårtens, S: Electroencephalographic changes in man correlated with blood alcohol concentration and some other conditions following standardized ingestion of alcohol. Quarterly Journal of Studies on Alcohol 16:411, 1955.
31. Höppener, RJ, Kuyer, A, and van der Lugt, PJM: Epilepsy and alcohol: The influence of social alcohol intake on seizures and treatment in epilepsy. Epilepsia 24:459, 1983.
32. Hunter, BE, et al: Ethanol dependence in the rat: Role of non-specific and limbic regions in the withdrawal reaction. Electroencephalogr Clin Neurophysiol 45:483, 1978.
33. Hunter, BE and Walker, DW: Ethanol dependence in the rat: Role of extrapyramidal motor systems in the withdrawal reaction. Exp Neurol 62:374, 1978.
34. Jóhannesson, G, Berglund, M, and Ingvar, DH: EEG abnormalities in chronic alcoholism related to age. Acta Psychiatr Scand 65:148, 1982.
35. Kaplan, RF, et al: Power and coherence analysis of the EEG in hospitalized alcoholics and nonalcoholic controls. J Stud Alcohol 46:122, 1985.
36. Karpati, G, et al: Graded photic hyperexcitability and cerebral seizures in alcohol withdrawal syndromes. Electroencephalogr Clin Neurophysiol 15:1051, 1963.
37. Kennard, MA, Bueding, E, and Wortis, SB: Some biochemical and electroencephalographic changes in delirium tremens. Quarterly Journal of Studies on Alcohol 6:4, 1945.
38. Klinger, D and Wessely, P: Influence of alcohol on photomyoclonic and photoconvulsive responses. Electroencephalogr Clin Neurophysiol 43:272P, 1977.
39. Kooi, KA, Thomas, MH, and Mortensen, FN: Photoconvulsive and photomyoclonic responses in adults. Neurology 10:1051, 1960.
40. Kotani, K: EEG studies on endogenous psychoses and alcohol intoxication. Bull Osaka Med Sch Suppl 12:303, 1967.

41. Lafon, R, et al: L'épilepsie tardive de l'alcoolisme chronique. Rev Neurol 94:624, 1956.
42. Little, SC and McAvoy, M: Electroencephalographic studies in chronic alcoholism. Quarterly Journal of Studies on Alcohol 13:9, 1952.
43. Lloyd-Smith, D and Gloor, P: Abnormal photic sensitivity in alcohol withdrawal syndrome. Electroencephalogr Clin Neurophysiol 13:496, 1961.
44. Lolli, G, Nencini, B, and Misiti, R: Effects of two alcoholic beverages on the electroencephalographic and electromyographic tracings of healthy men. Quarterly Journal of Studies on Alcohol 25:451, 1964.
45. Marinacci, AA: A special type of temporal lobe (psychomotor) seizures following ingestion of alcohol. Bulletin of the Los Angeles Neurological Society 28:241, 1963.
46. Mattson, RH, et al: Effect of alcohol intake in nonalcoholic epileptics. Neurology 25:361, 1975.
47. Mattson, RH: Seizures associated with alcohol use and alcohol withdrawal. In Browne, TR and Feldman, RG (eds): Epilepsy: Diagnosis and Management. Little, Brown & Co, Boston, 1983, p 325.
48. Maxson, SC and Sze, PY: Electroencephalographic correlates of audiogenic seizures during ethanol withdrawal in mice. Psychopharmacology 47:17, 1976.
49. Nagy, L, et al: Cerebral electrical phenomena elicited by alcohol. Z Rechtsmed 73:185, 1973.
50. Naitoh, P: The value of electroencephalography in alcoholism. Ann NY Acad Sci 215:303, 1973.
51. Newman, HW: The effect of alcohol on the electroencephalogram. Stanford Medical Bulletin 17:55, 1959.
52. Newman, SE: The EEG manifestations of chronic ethanol abuse: Relation to cerebral cortical atrophy. Ann Neurol 3:299, 1978.
53. Niedermeyer, E, et al: Subacute encephalopathy with seizures in alcoholics (SESA). Epilepsia 28:605, 1987.
54. Olivennes, A: Éléments de comparaison du tracé électro-encéphalographique de veille des éthyliques et des héroïnomanes: Étude de 2 groupes de 70 et 51 patients. Ann Med Psychol 145:546, 1987.
55. Perrin, RG, Kalant, H, and Livingston, KE: Electroencephalographic signs of ethanol tolerance and physical dependence in the cat. Electroencephalogr Clin Neurophysiol 39:157, 1975.
56. Poldrugo, F and Snead, OC: Electroencephalographic and behavioral correlates in rats during repeated ethanol withdrawal syndromes. Psychopharmacology 83:140, 1984.
57. Rodin, EA, Frohman, CE, and Gottlieb, JS: Effect of acute alcohol intoxication on epileptic patients. Arch Neurol 4:115, 1961.
58. Romerio, C, et al: Studio elettroencefalografico su 150 casi di alcoolisti ospedalizzati. Minerva Med 71:1081, 1980.
59. Saletu, M, et al: Clinical symptomatology and computer analyzed EEG before, during and after anxiolytic therapy of alcohol withdrawal patients. Neuropsychobiology 9:119, 1983.
60. Sauerland, EK and Harper, RM: Effects of ethanol on EEG spectra of intact and isolated forebrain. Exp Neurol 27:490, 1970.
61. Schear, HE: The EEG pattern in delirium tremens. Clin Electroencephalogr 16:30, 1985.
62. Spehr, W and Stemmler, G: Postalcoholic diseases: Diagnostic relevance of computerized EEG. Electroencephalogr Clin Neurophysiol 60:106, 1985.
63. Van Sweden, B: The EEG in alcohol addicts presenting with seizures. Clin Neurol Neurosurg 85:12, 1983.
64. Varga, B and Nagy, T: Analysis of alpha-rhythm in the EEG of alcoholics. Electroencephalogr Clin Neurophysiol 12:933, 1960.
65. Victor, M: The role of hypomagnesemia and respiratory alkalosis in the genesis of alcohol-withdrawal symptoms. Ann NY Acad Sci 215:235, 1973.
66. Victor, M and Brausch, C: The role of abstinence in the genesis of alcoholic epilepsy. Epilepsia 8:1, 1967.
67. Vossler, DG and Browne, TR: Absence of EEG photoparoxysmal responses in alcohol withdrawal seizure patients treated with benzodiazepines. Neurology 38(Suppl 1):404, 1988.
68. Walerk, DW and Zornetzer, SF: Alcohol withdrawal in mice: Electroencephalographic and behavioral correlates. Electroencephalogr Clin Neurophysiol 36:233, 1974.
69. Weiss, AD, et al: Experimentally induced chronic intoxication and withdrawal in alcoholics: Electroencephalographic findings. Quarterly Journal of Studies on Alcohol (Suppl) 2:96, 1964.
70. Wessely, VP: Das EEG bei alkoholikern mit epileptischen manifestationen. Wein Klin Wochenschr 86:618, 1974.
71. Wikler, A, et al: Electroencephalographic changes associated with chronic alcoholic intoxication and the alcohol abstinence syndrome. Am J Psychiatry 113:106, 1956.
72. Zilm, DH, et al: EEG correlates of the alcohol-induced organic brain syndrome in man. Clinical Toxicology 16:345, 1980.
73. Zilm, DH, Kaplan, HL, and Capell, H: Electroencephalographic tolerance and abstinence phenomena during repeated alcohol ingestion by nonalcoholics. Science 212:1175, 1981.

Michael P. Earnest, M.D.

CHAPTER 18

Etiologies of Acute Alcohol-Related Seizures

Seizures occurring as a complication of alcoholism pose a diagnostic problem.[18,19] Such convulsions often are caused by uncomplicated withdrawal from chronic alcohol abuse.[1] In that situation no tests are required and no anticonvulsant treatment is given because the seizures resolve spontaneously.[10]

However, some alcoholic patients with acute seizures have an important medical process or brain lesion causing the seizures.[6–9] Electrolyte imbalance, hypoglycemia, meningitis, subdural hematomas, cerebral contusions, and traumatic subarachnoid hemorrhage are common medical complications of alcoholism. Alcoholics also may ingest other toxins, for example, methanol, and some may abuse other drugs (such as cocaine or amphetamines) that can cause seizures. The alcoholic patient also may have an occult neurologic process such as pre-existing epilepsy, a traumatic brain lesion, cerebral vascular malformation, stroke, or may have a tumor that lowers the seizure threshold so that alcohol withdrawal concomitantly precipitates the seizures.[7,9,11,12] Many of the non-alcohol-withdrawal causes of seizures require treatment to abort potentially serious medical or neurologic complications and to prevent further seizures.

PRIOR STUDIES OF SEIZURES ASSOCIATED WITH ALCOHOL ABUSE

Victor and Brausch's[24] seminal 1967 paper was the first large series in which alcohol-related seizures were analyzed in detail (although Victor and Adams[23] had previously reported some cases). Victor and Brausch reported "241 alcoholic patients who either presented with convulsive seizures or with other symptoms of alcoholism . . . complicated by seizures."[24] Their cases seemed to fall into three categories. The large majority represented a syndrome currently known as alcohol withdrawal seizures (AWS), in which an adult who had been drinking for many years significantly reduced his or her intake after an episode of heavy consumption. A few to 48 hours thereafter, one or several generalized convulsions occurred within a span of a few hours. The second category of patients, and a small minority (seven), had pre-existing epilepsy complicated by alcoholism. The third group consisted of 21 patients with seizures, alcoholism, and prior head trauma. Unfortunately, the authors reported no clinical laboratory or radiologic data except electroencephalograms (EEGs) to elucidate the prevalence of significant but occult metabolic, toxic, or intracranial processes.

Hillbom[9] reviewed 277 cases in which patients presented to an emergency room with seizures and recent alcohol intoxication. His study excluded cases involving diabetes with hypoglycemia or acute head trauma and children under age 16. Extensive laboratory and radiologic tests and EEGs were performed. Etiologies defined by clinical and laboratory criteria included head trauma (36 percent), alcohol abuse (31 percent), presumably meaning uncomplicated AWS, cerebrovascular disease (6 percent), and central nervous system (CNS) neoplasms and infections (4 percent). The author did not describe the criteria by which he defined head trauma as the cause of the seizures, but he commented on the frequency of seizures complicated by "acute brain injuries" and noted "that the presence of the abstinence syndrome [confusion, tremor, agitation] sometimes masked ... such diseases as chronic subdural hematoma, brain contusion and even acute brain infarction."[9] Forty-four of his cases (15.8 percent) had "new diseases" disclosed by the diagnostic work-up.

Feussner and associates[8] evaluated the diagnostic yield of computed tomographic (CT) brain scanning in 151 cases of probable AWS. Their retrospective review summarized both neurologic examination and CT scan findings. The CT scans showed focal cerebral lesions in 15.2 percent, hydrocephalus in 2.0 percent, and diffuse atrophy in 34.4 percent. However, if cases were separated into those with focal neurologic deficits on examination and those without, the former group had a 30 percent prevalence of focal structural brain lesions and the latter only 6 percent. If only potentially reversible lesions were considered, the ratio between the two patient groups was 18 percent to 1 percent. They concluded that " ... in the absence of either focal deficits on neurologic examination or signs of acute head trauma, CT brain scanning does not improve the evaluation of patients with alcohol withdrawal seizures."[8]

Other series have attempted to relate seizures to duration and severity of alcohol abuse.[3,28] Ng and associates have challenged the connection between seizures and withdrawal from alcohol.[28] Other investigators have tried to distinguish types of "alcoholic epilepsy" or define an underlying metabolic, physiologic, or brain defect.[2,5,13–17,19–22,25–27] However, no studies other than Hillbom's and ours have studied a large unselected series of patients with alcoholism and acute seizures to define the prevalence of metabolic, toxic, and CNS processes.

ALCOHOL-RELATED SEIZURES IN PATIENTS ADMITTED TO A MUNICIPAL HOSPITAL

A retrospective chart review was done to define etiologies of seizures in patients admitted to a municipal hospital for evaluation and treatment of convulsions.[7] Patients who had been admitted to the neurology department because of seizures were selected from the admissions log. The charts were reviewed and data collected about age, sex, racial or ethnic group, history of alcohol abuse, type of seizure, prior seizures, final etiologic diagnosis, and the results of all appropriate laboratory, EEG, and radiologic evaluations. CT scans were not available for the period of the study.

Results

A total of 472 admissions for seizures were reviewed, of which alcohol-related seizures comprised 195 cases (41.3 percent). The alcohol-related cases predominantly involved men (80.5 percent) and these patients were older than the nonalcoholic patients, with a median age range of 45 to 55 years for alcoholic patients, compared with 25 to 35 years for nonalcoholic patients. In the alcohol-related group 126 (65 percent) had generalized seizures; 47 (24 percent) had focal seizures, defined as a focal onset of motor activity; and 21 (11 percent) had unknown type. There were no cases of psychomotor (complex partial) seizures.

Etiologies were defined by the discharge diagnosis in the chart (Table 18-1). A toxic-metabolic cause was found in 115

Table 18-1. ETIOLOGIES OF SEIZURES IN 195 PATIENTS ADMITTED FOR ALCOHOL-RELATED SEIZURES*

Etiology	Cases†	Percent†
Toxic-metabolic	115	59
Unknown	47	24
Trauma	38	20
Cerebrovascular disease	9	5
Tumor	3	2
Idiopathic epilepsy	3	2
Other	5	3

*Adapted from Earnest and Yarnell,[7] p 388.
†The total numbers and percent are greater than 195 and 100% because in some cases seizures were ascribed to multiple etiologies.

(59 percent) of the 195 alcohol-related cases. That category included AWS, drug overdose, and all endogenous metabolic disorders that might cause a seizure (e.g., hypoglycemia, hyponatremia, hepatic failure). In that group 105 cases (91 percent) were ascribed to alcohol withdrawal. An unknown-cause group comprised 47 (24 percent) of the cases, trauma caused 38 (20 percent), and cerebrovascular disease 9 (4.6 percent). The unknown-cause category included many patients who may have had AWS but whose history or laboratory evaluation findings were not fully consistent with uncomplicated alcohol withdrawal. The trauma category included patients with significant old or recent head injuries. Six patients had subdural hematomas and one a probable contusion shown by angiography, but few patients had angiograms done. Overall 13 (6.7 percent) had clinically important intracranial processes, including stroke, tumor, traumatic lesions, and intracranial infection, shown by clinical and radiologic evaluations.

Clinical Correlations

Focal seizures occurred in 47 of the alcohol-related seizures, including 16 cases with a toxic-metabolic etiology. Presumably those patients had an occult focal cerebral lesion (possibly a cortical scar or acute contusion from trauma) that caused a focal-onset seizure during withdrawal from alcohol. Eight other cases (17 percent) with focal seizures had intracranial structural lesions; six were cerebrovascular lesions, one a traumatic hematoma, and one a tumor. Five of the patients with cerebrovascular disease were over age 55, and the patient with a tumor was over 50.

Conclusions

In this series of patients admitted to the neurology department of a municipal hospital, alcohol-related seizures were predominantly (54 percent) AWS, and many others were suspected to be. Other toxic-metabolic conditions were rare. However, trauma (20 percent) and cerebrovascular disease (4.6 percent) were important other causes. Overall, 6.7 percent had clinically significant intracranial processes. Focal seizures occurred in 24 percent of all cases and were a marker for intracranial lesions, but at a low level of probability (17 percent). Patients over age 50 had a higher prevalence of intracranial lesions.

INTRACRANIAL LESIONS IN PATIENTS WITH AN APPARENT FIRST AWS

The value of a CT scan as part of the laboratory evaluation of AWS has been questioned.[8] We conducted a study to evaluate the diagnostic yield of a CT scan in patients having a first AWS and to determine the correlation of clinical signs on examination with CT findings.[6]

Methods

All patients seen in the emergency department of the Denver General Hospital with an apparent first AWS were included. Neurology residents evaluating the cases enrolled in the study patients who had generalized convulsions precipitated by sudden abstinence or reduction of consumption following chronic ingestion of large quantities of alcohol. Patients were excluded from the study who had *status epilepticus*, prominent focal signs, coma, a major acute head injury, a severe toxic or metabolic disorder, systemic infection, or any apparent cause of seizures other than alcohol withdrawal. Patients with prior recurrent alcohol-related seizures or known epilepsy also were excluded. The goal was to include only patients with an apparent first AWS who had no clinical features or signs on examination indicating an intracranial process.

The evaluating physician completed a data sheet for each case including demographic information, alcohol consumption history, neurologic and general medical history, medical and neurologic examination findings, and laboratory results. A CT scan was then obtained. The subsequent clinical course, final clinical diagnosis, and treatment selected were also recorded.

A retrospective study was also conducted by identifying cases of AWS from the neurology department admissions log. Inclusion and exclusion criteria were identical to those used for the prospective study. Charts were reviewed and a data sheet identical to the prospective study form was completed for each case.

CT scan results were tabulated as normal; generalized enlargement of cerebrospinal fluid (CSF) spaces; anterior lobe cerebellar atrophy; focal brain abnormality due to an old injury; and possible active structural intracranial lesion. Each case involving a possibly active intracranial lesion was then evaluated in detail. The CT scan itself was examined and the chart reviewed to determine the treating physician's diagnostic impression about the CT lesion and what management was adopted. Lesions were considered "clinically significant" if further diagnostic tests were done, treatment for the lesion was recommended, a neurosurgery consultation was ordered or plans were made for follow-up in the outpatient clinic.

Correlations between the presence of a clinically significant CT lesion and the findings on neurologic history and examination were sought. Statistical tests used were chi-square with Yate's correction, stepwise multifactorial discriminant analysis, and loglinear logistic regression analysis.

Results

A total of 259 cases were studied, 137 in the prospective emergency department series and 122 in the retrospective neurology admissions chart review. Because there were no significant differences in demographic or clinical features, the data from the two groups were combined when analyzing the results.

The average age of the patients was 41.7 years and 214 (82.6 percent) were men (Table 18–2). A single seizure occurred in 188 (72.6 percent) parents, and 249 (96.1 percent) had three or fewer seizures. The onset of seizures was between 8 and 71 hours in 156 (72.9 percent) cases, with 12.7 percent earlier and 14.4 percent later in onset. All patients had a CT scan, but only 242 (93.4 percent) had contrast enhancement.

CT findings were abnormal in 151 (58.3 percent) cases (Table 18–3). Generalized enlargement of CSF spaces and cerebellar atrophy were the predominant abnormalities in 112 cases, and focal brain lesions due to old trauma, surgery, or known brain infarction were found in 13 cases. Thirty patients had possibly active brain lesions revealed by the first CT scan.

Further review of the clinical course and management of the 30 cases involving possibly active lesions disclosed that in 11

Table 18–2. DEMOGRAPHIC AND CLINICAL FEATURES OF 259 CASES OF FIRST ALCOHOL-RELATED SEIZURES*

Average age	41.7 years
Male sex	214 (82.6%)†
Number of seizures	
1	188 (72.6%)
3 or less	249 (96.1%)
Onset of seizures	
Under 8 hr	27 (12.7%)
8–71 hr	156 (72.9%)
Over 71 hr	31 (14.4%)
History of head trauma	66 (25.4%)
Clinical signs	
Minor head trauma	52 (20.1%)
Depressed alertness	26 (10.0%)
Minor focal signs	38 (14.7%)

*Adapted from Earnest et al,[6] Table 1.
†Percentages based on cases with data available.

Table 18-3. HEAD CT SCAN FINDINGS IN PATIENTS WITH APPARENT ALCOHOL WITHDRAWAL SEIZURES

Clinical Findings	Earnest et al[6] (n = 259)	Feussner et al[8] (n = 151)
Normal	108 (42%)	73 (48%)
Cerebral atrophy	99 (38%)	52 (34%)
Active intracranial lesion	16 (6%)	11 (7%)†
Old focal brain injury	13 (5%)	12 (8%)*
Cerebellar atrophy	13 (5%)	—
Hydrocephalus	3 (1%)	3 (2%)

*Cerebral infarctions (11 cases) and temporal lobe atrophy (1 case).
†Subdural hematomas (7), hygromas (2), and intracranial hemorrhages (2).

cases the CT abnormality was considered by the treating physicians to be clinically insignificant and no further evaluation was done. The final diagnoses in those cases were focal lesion probably due to old trauma (four cases), possible small cortical lesions (three cases), possible communicating hydrocephalus (three cases) and unusual prominence of a middle cerebral artery (one case). In three other cases, reviews of the original CT scans or repeat CT studies generated findings judged to be normal.

Sixteen patients (6.2 percent) were considered to have clinically significant intracranial lesions. Four had subdural collections consistent with chronic subdural hematomas, three had probable bifrontal subdural hygromas, two had neurocysticercosis, and two had vascular malformations. There were single cases of subacute subdural hematoma, skull fracture with subarachnoid blood, middle cerebral artery aneurysm without subarachnoid hemorrhage, possible frontal lobe glioma, and a low-density occipital lesion without mass effect, probably an infarction.

Clinical management was changed by the CT scan result in ten cases (3.9 percent). The middle cerebral artery aneurysm was surgically ablated; one patient with cysticercosis was given praziquantel; for the patient with a probable tumor, the two with vascular malformations, and five with subdural collections, further radiologic studies and neurosurgical consultations were conducted. The patient with a fracture and subarachnoid blood underwent a lumbar puncture. One patient with a large subdural hematoma declined surgical intervention and three others left the hospital against medical advice before scheduled angiography was performed. The other cases were managed by outpatient clinical follow-up alone.

Correlation of Clinical Features with CT Scan Findings

Among the 16 patients with clinically significant lesions, five had a history of past head trauma, four had signs of recent head trauma, four were disoriented, three had minor focal neurologic signs, two had depressed alertness, and two suffered headache. However, none of those clinical features was significantly associated with intracranial lesions on CT (positive CT findings) when tested statistically. Neither sex, age, number of seizures, nor seizure type (generalized, focal motor, focal motor with secondary generalization, and "other") correlated with a positive CT.

In addition, patients were grouped by multiple factors for analysis. The presence of any one or more of the features of history of head trauma, signs of recent head trauma, focal neurologic signs, depressed alertness, or headache did not correlate with positive CT findings. Likewise, the absence of all those clinical features did not significantly correlate with negative CT finding.

Conclusions

Of 259 patients with a first AWS, CT scan revealed clinically significant intracranial processes in 6.2 percent. The presence of depressed alertness, minor focal signs, or history or signs of minor head trauma or headache did not predict positive CT findings, that is, an intracranial lesion. Conversely, the absence of all those features did not predict negative CT findings. Thus, a CT scan is an important test to identify occult intracranial processes in patients with a probable first AWS even when the clinical history and examination do not indicate an intracranial lesion.

ETIOLOGIES OF ACUTE ALCOHOL-RELATED SEIZURES

The etiologies of acute seizures in alcohol-abusing patients have been most completely defined in three series, by Victor and Brausch,[24] Earnest and Yarnell[7] and Hillbom[9] (Table 18-4). The most common etiology seems to be true AWS. However, through the 13 years spanned by the three studies, the percentage of cases diagnosed as AWS dropped from 88 percent to 31 percent. That decline probably reflects the selection criteria for patients in the three studies, as well as more extensive clinical laboratory and radiologic evaluation of cases in the latter two series, including CT scans in the most recent one. Nonetheless, it is my continuing experience that over half the cases involving alcohol-related seizures eventually are diagnosed true AWS. Although many of these patients have had prior head injuries from falls, assaults, and other traumas, the seizures probably still represent AWS.

The second most common etiology of alcohol-related convulsions seems to be head trauma. The clinical series describing trauma as a frequent etiology in alcohol-related seizures do not clearly distinguish between an old and an acute head injury, nor describe the criteria according to which the trauma was judged etiologic.[7,9] In the Earnest and Yarnell[7] series, trauma cases involved predominantly old trauma that had required medical care, including some necessitating craniotomy. A small minority (seven of 38) trauma cases involved acute intracranial lesions.[7] Hillbom did not clarify how he defined cases as having a traumatic etiology.[9] If the AWS and trauma categories are combined for both series, about 70 percent of all cases are attributable to those causes.

It is difficult to diagnose a seizure occurring during the alcohol withdrawal period as being due to trauma rather than alcohol withdrawal itself. A majority of alcoholic patients probably will admit to old head trauma, if a detailed history is taken. Many of them also have had a recent head injury during a binge of inebriation. To ascribe the seizure to the old or recent trauma rather than to alcohol withdrawal is a nearly arbitrary clinical decision. The seizure may be reasonably as-

Table 18–4. ETIOLOGY OF ACUTE SEIZURES IN ALCOHOL-ABUSING PATIENTS: 3 CLINICAL SERIES

Etiology	Victor and Brausch[24]* (n = 241)	Earnest and Yarnell[7]† (n = 195)	Hillbom[9]‡ (n = 277)
Alcohol withdrawal	88%	54%	31%
Trauma	7%	20%	36%
Other toxic/metabolic	—	5%	3%
Stroke	—	5%	6%
Nontraumatic intracranial lesions	—	2%	4%
Epilepsy	4%	2%	4%
Unknown	—	24%	15%

*No CT scans done, no clinical tests reported other than EEGs.
†No CT scans done.
‡Excluded cases with hypoglycemia and acute head trauma.

cribed to trauma if: the seizures are focal in onset and the focality is appropriate to the location of known brain injury; CT scan shows an acute brain contusion or acute intracranial hematoma; an EEG shows a focal abnormality representative of a known traumatic injury; or the patient had a prior head injury causing an intracranial lesion (e.g., cerebral contusion or subdural hematoma) leading to neurologic deficits or surgery.

Other etiologies are far less common. Only 5 percent or fewer of cases involve nonalcoholic toxic or metabolic causes; about 5 percent involve an old or recent stroke; 2 percent to 4 percent involve other intracranial lesions; and the same proportion involve epilepsy independent of alcohol abuse. Fifteen to 20 percent involve an unknown cause, in many cases probably AWS in which the history or clinical details confuse the diagnosis. I have observed that in the current decade, many alcohol-abusing patients also have a history of abusing other substances, especially cocaine, benzodiazepines, and amphetamines. Their seizures may be caused by acute drug toxicity (e.g., cocaine or amphetamines) or withdrawal from CNS-depressant drugs other than alcohol.

The Value of Clinical Laboratory and Radiologic Tests

Laboratory and radiologic evaluation discloses a non-AWS, nontrauma etiology in 15 percent to 20 percent of cases of alcohol-related seizures.[6-9] A few of the occult processes are disclosed by metabolic and toxicologic screening tests. EEGs show epileptic discharges in a small percent of cases.[4,7,24] Skull x-rays have been marginally useful and have been supplanted by CT scanning.

CT scanning is the most available and effective procedure to demonstrate or rule out an otherwise occult intracranial process.[6,8,9] About half the patients are found to have anatomically normal brains and a third to have diffuse atrophy (Table 18-3).[6,8] However, the CT scan shows an old brain lesion, usually infarction, in another 5 percent to 10 percent of cases, and in an additional 5 percent to 10 percent a more acute lesion is demonstrated, including subdural hematoma or hygroma, traumatic contusion, vascular malformation, or infection.[6,8] Few of the more acute lesions necessitate immediate medical or surgical treatment, but knowledge of their presence guides subsequent management.

Implications for Diagnostic Work-up

Patients with alcohol-related seizures should probably routinely undergo hematologic studies, biochemical and toxicologic screening, and routine as well as toxicologic urinalysis. If there is clinical evidence of significant metabolic imbalance, serum calcium and magnesium measurements are important. Suspicion of infection necessitates lumbar puncture. At least one EEG should be done after a first-ever seizure to rule out epileptic discharges, the presence of which implies a seizure disorder independent of alcohol withdrawal.[4,7,24] The presence or absence of somnolence or headache, minor head trauma, or minor focal signs or focal seizures do not correlate with the presence or absence of intracranial lesions.[6] Thus, a CT scan probably should be performed in every case involving a first alcohol-related seizure, regardless of the history and examination findings.[1] If the patient has acute seizures and has previously had alcohol-related seizures, careful clinical evaluation should guide the decision about obtaining a CT scan.

SUMMARY

The patient with acute alcohol-related convulsions may have uncomplicated AWS or may have a life-threatening intracranial process. A retrospective study of 195 cases of alcohol-related seizures in which patients were admitted to a municipal hospital neurology department disclosed that 116 (59 percent) had a toxic-metabolic etiology, in virtually all cases the alcohol withdrawal state. Another 38 (20 percent) involved a history or current evidence of brain trauma; 9 (5 percent) involved vascular brain lesions; and 3 (2 percent) involved tumors. Forty-seven cases (24 percent) involved focal seizures; 8 (17 percent) of those involved a structural intracranial lesion. A prospective study of CT head scans of 259 patients with a first alcohol-related seizure included only cases involving generalized convulsions, recent abstinence from alcohol abuse, and no obvious etiology for seizures other than alcohol withdrawal. The CT scans disclosed that 16 (6.2 percent) of cases involved intracranial lesions. These lesions included subdural hematomas (five), subdural hygromas (three), vascular malformations (two), neurocysticercosis (two), and single cases of traumatic subarachnoid hemorrhage, unruptured aneurysm, possible glioma, and cerebral infarction. Clinical management was altered by the scan result in ten cases (3.9 percent). History or signs of minor head trauma, headache, level of consciousness, and focal seizures or focal neurologic signs on examination did not correlate significantly with an abnormality detected on CT. The absence of those features likewise did not predict benign CT findings.

ACKNOWLEDGMENTS

The author gratefully acknowledges the contributions of Drs. Phillip Yarnell, John Marx, Howard Feldman, Mark Biletch, and Larry Sullivan for the two clinical studies cited from Denver General Hospital. Special thanks to James Harris, B.S., and Gary Knapp, M.A., for data analysis and to Ms. Susan Padilla for preparing the manuscript.

References

1. Berner, J and Earnest, MP: Alcohol withdrawal syndromes. Topics in Emergency Medicine 6:39, 1984.
2. Chu, NS and Yarnell, PR: Alcoholic cerebellar disease and seizures. Surg Neurol 5:29, 1976.
3. Danesin, A: Epileptic seizures in chronic alcoholics (abstr). Electroencephalogr Clin Neurophysiol 28:214, 1970.
4. Deisenhammer, E, Klingler, D, and Tragner, H: Epileptic seizures in alcoholism and diagnostic value of EEG after sleep deprivation. Epilepsia 25:526, 1984.
5. Devetag, F, et al: Alcoholic epilepsy: Review of a series and proposed classification and etiopathogenesis. Ital J Neurol Sci 3:275, 1983.
6. Earnest, MP, et al: Intracranial lesions shown by CT scans in 259 cases of first alcohol-related seizures. Neurology 38:1561, 1988.
7. Earnest, MP and Yarnell, PR: Seizure admissions to a city hospital: The role of alcohol. Epilepsia 17:387, 1976.
8. Feussner, JR, et al: Computed tomography brain scanning in alcohol withdrawal seizures: Value of the neurologic examination. Ann Intern Med 94:519, 1981.
9. Hillbom, ME: Occurrence of cerebral seizures provoked by alcohol abuse. Epilepsia 21:459, 1980.
10. Hillbom, ME and Hjelm-Jager, M: Should alcohol withdrawal seizures be treated with anti-epileptic drugs? Acta Neurol Scand 69:39, 1984.
11. Hillbom, M and Kaste, M: Alcohol intoxication: A risk factor for primary subarachnoid hemorrhage. Neurology 32:706, 1982.
12. Hillbom, M and Kaste, M: Does ethanol intoxication promote brain infarction in young adults? Lancet 2:1181, 1978.
13. Hunter, BE and Walker, DW: The neural basis of ethanol dependence: Is the withdrawal reaction mediated by localized changes in synaptic excitability? Adv Exp Med Biol 126:251, 1980.
14. Isbell, H, et al: An experimental study of the etiology of "rum fits" and delirium tremens. Quarterly Journal of the Study of Alcohol 16:1, 1955.
15. Johnson, R: Medical review series 5: Alcohol and fits. Br J Addict 80:227, 1985.
16. Kalinowsky, LB: Convulsions in nonepileptic patients on withdrawal of barbiturates, alcohol and other drugs. Archives of Neurology and Psychiatry 48:946, 1942.
17. Klupp, VM: Zerebrale Krampfanfalle bei chronischem Alkoholismus. Fortschr Med 45:1777, 1980.
18. McMicken, D: Seizures in the alcohol-dependent patient: A diagnostic and therapeutic dilemma. J Emerg Med 1:311, 1984.
19. Morris, JC and Victor, M: Alcohol withdrawal seizures. Emerg Med Clin North Am 5:827, 1987.
20. Newsom, JA: Withdrawal seizures in an in-patient alcoholism program. Curr Alcohol 6:11, 1979.
21. Ottonello, GA, Regesta, G, and Tanganelli, P: Withdrawal seizures in alcoholics: A transverse and longitudinal investigation. Ital J Neurol Sci 2:191, 1983.
22. Tartara, A, Manni, R, and Mazzella, G: Epileptic seizures and alcoholism: Clinical and pathogenetic aspects. Acta Neurol Belg 83:88, 1983.
23. Victor, M and Adams, RD: The effect of alcohol on the nervous system. Res Publ Assoc Res Nerv Ment Dis 32:526, 1953.
24. Victor, M and Brausch, C: The role of abstinence in the genesis of alcoholic epilepsy. Epilepsia 8:1, 1967.
25. Wolfe, SM, et al: Respiratory alkalosis and alcohol withdrawal. Trans Assoc Am Physicians 82:344, 1969.

26. Wolfe, SM and Victor, M: The relationship of hypomagnesemia and alkalosis to alcohol withdrawal symptoms. Ann NY Acad Sci 162:973, 1969.
27. Yamane, H and Katoh, N: Alcoholic epilepsy: A definition and a description of other convulsions related to alcoholism. Eur Neurol 20:17, 1981.
28. Ng, SKC, et al: Alcohol consumption and withdrawal in new-onset seizures. N Engl J Med 319:666, 1988.

CHAPTER 19

Matti E. Hillbom, M.D., Ph.D.

Alcohol Withdrawal Seizures and Binge Versus Chronic Drinking

Before it was clear that there was a direct causal relationship between alcohol consumption and seizures,[50] both the epidemiology and pathogenesis of alcohol withdrawal seizures (AWS) had been investigated. One of the earliest observations was the frequent occurrence of seizures soon after cessation of prolonged heavy drinking.[24] However, investigators have long known that even short periods of intoxication can exacerbate seizures after alcohol withdrawal, at least among persons with pre-existing or acquired seizure disorders.[27]

The frequency of acute seizures seems to increase during the course of an alcoholic career. This finding suggests that the duration of alcohol consumption may play an important role in the genesis of AWS. However, the intensity of intoxication may be even more important than its duration, and little is known about the effect of repeated alcohol withdrawals. This chapter reviews AWS in relation to drinking habits.

OBTAINING INFORMATION ON ALCOHOL AND DRUG INTAKE

Because the vast majority of alcoholic patients, especially young ones, have normal findings on physical examination and because most of the available laboratory markers of alcohol consumption lack specificity and sensitivity, data on alcohol consumption must be obtained by carefully interviewing the patient and supplemented, if necessary, by interviewing people who know the patient. However, laboratory tests and clinical signs are more objective in diagnosing alcoholism than self-reports. I recommend the reader review a recent report evaluating 108 potential indicators of alcohol abuse including clinical signs and medical history items in relation to diagnostic accuracy.[41]

Drinking History

The aim of taking the drinking history is to quantify the amount of alcohol consumed by the subject within a given period of time. A day-to-day inquiry about the week preceding the acute seizure(s) should be conducted, and intake of various types of alcoholic beverages (including light beer) should be determined separately. It is important to know the duration of the last drinking bout and whether the daily alcohol intake was consistent. If the patient is a periodic drinker, one might ask how many days he or she has been sober during the past year, and how many drinking bouts have occurred?

Because the most common cause of bias in self-reported alcohol consumption is forgetting, it is very important to interview relatives and friends of the patient. Another cause of bias is selective reporting, which is particularly common among general hospital patients who are afraid of the stigma associated with excessive alcohol use. In my experience, however, it has been relatively simple to obtain a reliable drinking history from patients being treated at a detoxification unit. Patients admitted to the emergency ward or internal medicine department of a general hospital, however, often give an unreliable drinking history. Therefore, laboratory markers of heavy drinking should also be studied.

Laboratory Markers

At present, the most useful laboratory marker of recent heavy drinking is serum gamma-glutamyltransferase (GGT) level. The increased activity of this enzyme is a sensitive sign of alcohol abuse, but the literature includes variable data on its selectivity. Elevated values have been observed after a binge of only 2 or 3 days and after repeated alcohol challenges.[14] According to a recent report, the sensitivity of GGT was not less than 81 percent among 107 inpatients at a detoxification center.[47] Unfortunately, GGT is not a specific marker, and elevated values are also usually seen in patients with diabetes or nonalcoholic liver disease and in subjects taking anti-epileptic drugs.

Another widely used laboratory marker of alcoholism is macrocytosis (elevated erythrocyte mean corpuscular volume [MCV]). However, this parameter cannot be used as a marker of binge drinking, because it is insensitive and is frequently elevated in chronic alcoholics with liver disease or nutritional deficiencies. In addition, MCV lacks specificity.

An ideal laboratory marker of excessive drinking would be both sensitive and specific. A candidate for such a marker is the desialylated transferrin that can easily be measured in serum by chromatofocusing and radioimmunoassay for transferrin.[44] Preliminary results have shown that this assay detects 90 percent of persons who have consumed more than 100 g of alcohol daily for at least 2 months. Moreover, this test did not yield false positives in subjects with diabetes or nonalcoholic liver disease.[43] Desialylated transferrin was originally tested as a laboratory marker of alcoholism in Sweden, and it was found that using anti-epileptic drugs does not give false positives.[42] This finding is important because many patients who are not known to be alcoholics are prescribed anti-epileptic drugs and referred to outpatient departments for treatment of epilepsy.

Finally, it has been suggested that antibodies formed against acetaldehyde adducts may help identify alcohol consumption.[25]

Binge Versus Chronic Drinking

Drinking habits are strongly influenced by cultural factors. For example, in Scandinavia, drinking is mainly a leisure activity, and drinking for intoxication is an accepted way of having fun that is not prohibited by religious or moral attitudes. Accordingly, drinking occasions tend to cluster on weekends and holidays. Most alcoholics, especially younger ones, are periodic drinkers. By contrast, in wine-drinking countries consumption of alcoholic beverages is more evenly distributed during the week, and continuous drinking is more prevalent. In addition, drinking to the point of intoxication is not popular and most alcoholics drink every day.

Because the length of a binge, the total dose of alcohol consumed, and the state of intoxication achieved can all be considered to influence the occurrence of AWS, it is probable that there are differences between countries in the epidemiology of AWS. However, this theory has not yet been substantiated.

The temporal pattern of alcohol consumption has been studied in both Finland[40] and the United States,[2] and drinking habits in each appear to be similar. Accordingly, the available epidemiologic data on AWS from these two countries will be considered.

Earnest and Yarnell[12] were the first to

emphasize the high percentage of AWS among seizure patients in a primary emergency hospital (Denver General Hospital). At least 41 percent of their patients had a history of alcohol abuse, and among those admitted for seizures 24 percent had seizures that were considered a direct consequence of alcohol withdrawal. These findings contrasted with many previous reports of much smaller percentages.[8] The study did not address the temporal distribution of AWS or the effect of drinking behavior, but it stimulated other researchers to study these problems.

Although AWS was first found to be most frequent among the socioeconomically disadvantaged urban population of Denver, similar observations were later made about patients admitted to the University Central Hospital of Helsinki. This is the primary emergency hospital of Helsinki, and patients admitted come from all social classes. Striking similarities were found between seizure admissions to the Denver and Helsinki hospitals. For example, sex distribution of the patients suggests that men suffer AWS more frequently than women (Table 19-1). During the 1970s men drank four fifths of all the alcohol consumed in Finland.[39] Data are lacking, but probably in Colorado men also drank more than women at that time. A recent study[2] has shown that drinking occasions cluster on weekends and evenings in the United States, as in Finland.[39]

In countries where weekend and holiday drinking is more prevalent than daily drinking, the effect of binge drinking on AWS can be seen. In a study from Helsinki, the weekly rhythms of AWS unrelated to alcohol consumption, and seizures occurring after alcohol withdrawal in known epileptics were compared and considered in light of alcohol consumption statistics for the general population. Analyses revealed that AWS are more frequent on Mondays than any other day, while seizures unrelated to alcohol consumption are evenly distributed throughout the week.[20] Interestingly, the frequency of alcohol-related seizures among epileptics peaked on both Sundays and Mondays. Seizures were found to be provoked after even short periods of drinking (1-6 days), and in many cases neither signs and symptoms of the alcohol withdrawal syndrome nor any other apparent cause of epilepsy were seen.

Further analysis showed that while AWS occur most frequently on Mondays, seizures of unknown etiology but provoked by either alcohol ingestion or withdrawal occur most frequently on Sundays (Fig. 19-1). Even seizures precipitated after a very short drinking bout (24 hours) peak on Sundays. These data suggest that the weekly rhythm of drinking is definitely correlated with seizure occurrence. Probably, the occurrence of "rum fits" on Mondays coincides with the start of a new work week. When people try to stop drinking in order to go to work, the associated rapid withdrawal provokes seizures. On the other hand, seizures accumulating on Sundays are mainly induced by a short drinking binge, that is, from Friday evening to Saturday night, and many of the people affected are known epileptics who imbibe alcohol during their leisure time. The cause of other fits provoked by withdrawal from a short binge of drinking remains unknown in the absence of clear alcohol withdrawal signs and symptoms. The fact that the majority of seizures occurred during withdrawal from drinking and only a few occurred

Table 19-1. EFFECT OF ALCOHOL CONSUMPTION ON THE GENDER DISTRIBUTION OF SEIZURE

| | Sex Ratio (Males:Females) | | |
Series	Alcohol-Related	Alcohol-Unrelated	Total
Earnest and Yarnell[12]	4.1:1.0	1.0:1.0	1.7:1.0
Hillbom[20]	4.8:1.0	1.1:1.0	2.0:1.0

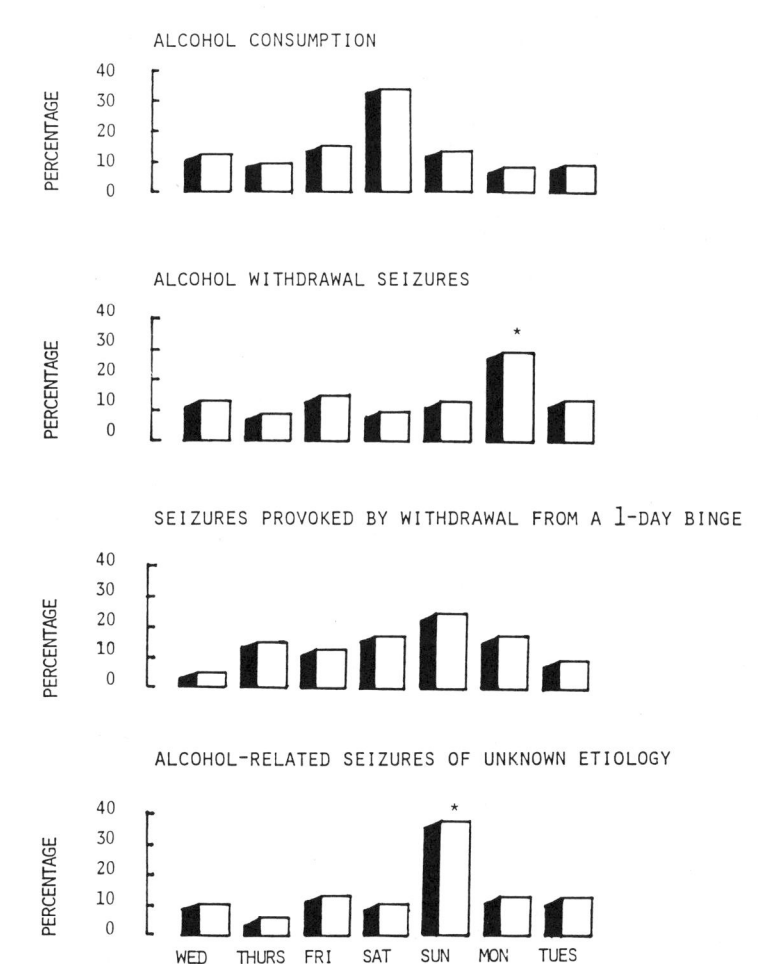

Figure 19–1. Temporal relationships between the peak occurrences of alcohol consumption (n=2988), alcohol withdrawal seizures (n=97), seizures provoked by withdrawal from a one day binge (n=82) and alcohol-related seizures of unknown etiology (n=40). Altogether 664 consecutive seizure admissions to the primary emegency hospital in Helsinki were retrospectively analyzed. *p < 0.05 for differences between the observed and expected (even) distributions along the week (chi-square test with Yates correction).

during intoxication suggests that these seizures were not so-called true "alcoholic epilepsy."[51]

Erratic Drug Taking and Drug Abuse

Many sedatives and hypnotics effective in treating alcohol withdrawal, particularly the benzodiazepines, are misused by alcoholics, and rapid withdrawal from these drugs can precipitate seizures. Unfortunately, in many countries such drugs are prescribed for alcoholics who are attempting to abstain from alcohol. This policy has led to a new problem, combined drug and alcohol abuse. Persons suffering this problem seem to be at increased risk for developing seizures, compared with traditional alcoholics. Indeed, their seizures develop several days after alcohol withdrawal—later than those of alcoholics who do not abuse drugs.[33]

Another factor that seems to increase the occurrence of seizures among alcoholics is erratic use of nonsedative anticonvulsants, such as phenytoin and carbamazepine.[21] It is well-known that drug treatment of outpatient alcoholics is strongly hampered by their poor compliance. Alcoholics are prone to take drugs irregularly, take them in overdose, or fail completely to take prescribed drugs when they are drinking. They use anti-epileptics in a manner that may lead to gradual development of a lowered seizure threshold. Further studies are needed to prove how erratic drug taking increases alcoholics' seizure susceptibility.

According to Aminoff and Simon,[1] the single most common cause of status epilepticus is noncompliance with anticonvulsant drug regimens. On the other hand, status epilepticus among subjects admitted to a primay emergency hospital in Helsinki was found to be preceded by alcohol abuse in one third of the cases.[35] Use of nonsedative anticonvulsants may provoke even fatal complications.[22] The half-life of phenytoin is shortened by alcohol abuse,[26] and alcoholics are frequently treated with disulfiram, an inhibitor of phenytoin metabolism.[48] These data all suggest that nonsedative anticonvulsants should not be prescribed for alcoholics.[19]

OBTAINING INFORMATION ON SEIZURES AND ALCOHOL WITHDRAWAL

In evaluating the role of drinking behavior as a factor that influences the occurrence of AWS, it is important accurately to diagnose both seizures and alcohol withdrawal as well as other possible causes of seizures.

Diagnosis of Cerebral Seizures

The diagnosis of cerebral seizures is not necessarily simple, because seizures usually occur outside the hospital. AWS is not unique in this respect. In the absence of a reliable case history, laboratory tests may help. Serum levels of aspartate aminotransferase and particularly creatine kinase are frequently slightly elevated in patients who have had a grand mal seizure or burst of seizures the previous day. Fresh sores on the tongue and lips as well as signs of incontinence also suggest cerebral seizures.

Signs and Symptoms of Alcohol Withdrawal

Withdrawal from prolonged drinking provokes a whole series of gastrointestinal, cardiovascular, neurologic, and psychologic symptoms.[18] The most useful clinical signs and symptoms are elevated pulse rate and blood pressure, slight to moderate fever in the absence of infection, tremor, sweating, dilated pupils, and diarrhea. Of course, these symptoms are not specific to acute alcohol withdrawal, but if some occur with a history of recent heavy drinking or laboratory data that suggest alcoholism, the diagnosis is very likely.

These signs and symptoms usually disappear within a couple of days of hospital admission. Sometimes profound agitation, anxiety, hallucinations (auditory, visual, or tactile), disorientation or clouding of consciousness develops, suggesting delirium tremens.[28]

Respiratory alkalosis is a common finding in alcohol withdrawal, and some data have suggested that the rapid development of hypokalemia may precede delirium.[46] A quickly disappearing metabolic acidosis (within 1–2 hours) may be caused by grand mal seizures that have occurred just prior to blood sampling.[34]

Diagnosis of Underlying Disease

The cause of seizures should not be ascribed to alcohol withdrawal until other etiologies have been excluded. Unfortunately, many physicians neglect this task because they believe the alcohol withdrawal diagnosis certain if the patient appears to be a heavy drinker. However, heavy drinkers are at risk of developing acute brain injuries, cerebral infections, and intracranial hematomas. These problems can occur in the absence of focal deficits on neurologic examination. Even hidden brain tumors can be silent in this respect.

All acute seizure problems necessitate a careful clinical neurologic examination supplemented with measurements of sodium, calcium, and glucose in the serum. Other diagnostic aids include specialist consultation, cerebrospinal fluid (CSF) examination, computed tomography (CT) brain scanning, and electroencephalography (EEG). According to one study, CT brain scans in the absence of focal deficits on neurologic examination or signs of acute head trauma do not improve the evaluation of AWS.[13] However, when focal neurologic deficits are absent, 6 percent of CT scans show focal structural lesions. In another study in which seizures provoked by alcohol or its withdrawal were not excluded, CT scans revealed tumors in 3 percent of subjects having their first seizure problem.[23] It was not noted whether any of these patients was a heavy drinker, but in another study, two of 277 subjects exhibiting alcohol-related seizures (mainly AWS) had intracranial neoplasms.[20]

A normal EEG is common in alcoholics who have AWS, provided that it is not performed during a seizure. However, abnormalities suggest that there may be undiagnosed disease, and such a finding usually warrants brain CT scans. Accordingly, EEG and CT scans, although not necessary in all cases of AWS, frequently reveal new diseases even in alcoholics.

DRINKING HABITS AND ALCOHOL WITHDRAWAL SEIZURES

There is no convincing clinical evidence that binge drinking differs from continuous heavy drinking with respect to AWS occurrence. Both drinking patterns are known to precipitate seizures during withdrawal. It has often been mentioned in the literature that seizures are associated with lengthy alcohol abuse. However, the exact reason for this fact is unknown. Alcoholics are at greater risk of suffering traumatic brain injuries and cerebrovascular accidents than nonalcoholics. Many alcoholics have focal seizures that may or may not correlate with structural brain lesions.[12] Accordingly, causes of epilepsy other than heavy drinking may account for at least part of the increased seizure frequency among alcoholics with a long history of alcohol abuse.

The Kindling Hypothesis of Withdrawal Seizures

Ballenger and Post[4] have hypothesized that the duration and intermittency of alcohol abuse are related to the development of increasingly severe alcohol withdrawal symptoms, including seizures. In other words, convulsive symptoms occurring in alcoholics may gradually develop and intensify after repeated alcohol withdrawals. As a matter of fact, ethanol concentration in brain tissue, where some adaptive changes are thought to occur, greatly fluctuates during even one drinking bout. For example, falling asleep every 24 hours leads to short periods of withdrawal. Theoretically, these periods can be considered to kindle withdrawal symptoms. On the other hand, longer periods of withdrawal may also potentiate withdrawal symptoms.

Clinical Observations

Alcoholics with a long and intense drinking history,[15] alcoholics with brain atrophy,[3] and elderly alcoholics[11] seem to be particularly prone to AWS. However, thus far there is no experimental data to prove that seizures are kindled by repeated withdrawals in humans. Data are scarce because it is not considered ethical to give large amounts of alcohol to volunteers. Reliable follow-up studies with alcoholics are also difficult, and we do not know whether seizures are becoming more frequent and long lasting solely because of repeated withdrawals.

Some evidence to support this concept comes from a recent study[5] comparing the number of previous detoxifications among alcoholics with (n = 25) and without (n = 25) a history of seizures (Fig. 19-2). It appeared that the seizure group was significantly younger than the nonseizure group. However, the alcoholic careers were equally intense and of similar duration, although drinking habits were unknown. The data suggest that some alcoholics are more prone to develop seizures than others, but cannot address whether the seizure group was more frequently detoxified, simply because seizures were already present in their history. Such patients are detoxified as inpatients in many centers.

The fact that even short periods of intoxication lead to seizures during alcohol

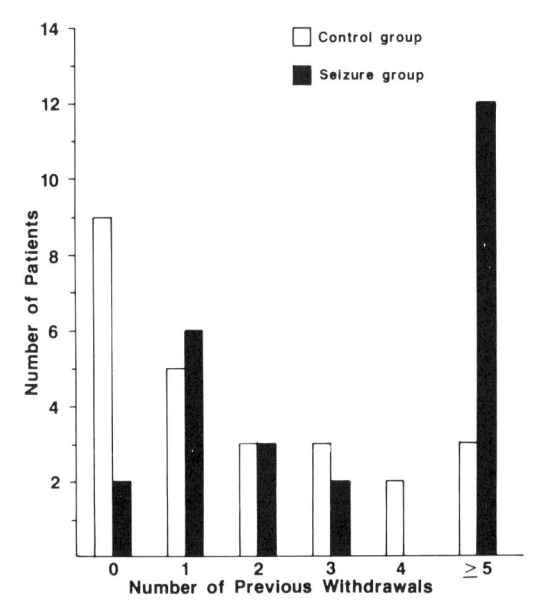

Figure 19–2. Number of previous withdrawals (detoxifications) in the seizure and control groups. (From Brown, et al,[5] p. 507, with permission.)

withdrawal, particularly in subjects with scars, tumors, or other irritative factors in brain tissue, indirectly correlates kindling with AWS. However, further studies are needed to prove whether repeated withdrawals can increase the number of seizure occasions.

Experimental Evidence

Many of the questions that have arisen and remain unanswered by clinical studies can be explored in animal experiments. Among the earliest findings was that the longer the duration and the greater the intoxication achieved, the greater the intensity of the subsequent alcohol withdrawal symptoms.[16] Later studies demonstrated that seizures are precipitated following withdrawal from a short period (4 days) of intense intoxication.[6,29] Observations from animal experiments agree with many clinical observations.[20,31,49]

Majchrowicz and Hunt[30] speculated that one reason it might take alcoholic humans longer than alcoholic rats to reach a state of physical dependence (withdrawal state) is their inability to sustain severe degrees of intoxication for prolonged periods without becoming unconscious. Experimental animals can easily be kept unconscious for prolonged periods by forced ethanol administration. These investigators also considered the possibility that a short interruption (24 hours) of continuous intoxication might prolong the time needed to develop physical dependence. This idea was supported by the findings of Goldstein.[16,17]

Pinel, Van Oot, and Mucha[37] were the first to demonstrate that repeated electrical stimulation of the brain potentiates the effect of subsequent alcohol withdrawal. Both amygdaloid kindling and electroconvulsive shocks produced the same effect.[36] A single dose of ethanol rendered mice and rats more susceptible to seizures elicited by pharmacologic and electrical stimulations.[32,38] Increases in the duration of kindled motor seizures and after-discharges were detected following the metabolism of a single intoxicating injection of ethanol.

Whether prior exposure to alcohol decreases the number of stimulations required to induce a kindled seizure has also been studied. The results demonstrate that the effect on kindling of alcohol is dose dependent, and that low doses do not affect kindling.[7]

Finally, multiple short periods of repeated alcohol intoxication (two days) and subsequent withdrawal (five days) were shown to lower the seizure threshold of rats.[9] These findings support the kindling hypothesis of withdrawal seizures.

CONCLUSIONS

Clinical studies have failed to demonstrate a significant difference in seizure occurrence between binge drinkers and chronic drinkers. However, they clearly suggest that some alcoholics are more prone to develop AWS than others. Even nonalcoholics seem to be stricken by seizures after short binges of drinking, which suggests that a lowered seizure threshold and a severe state of intoxication can be contributory factors. We lack evidence that repeated short episodes of intoxication and withdrawal result in increased seizure susceptibility in humans. The evidence that does support this effect is indirectly obtained and is far from convincing.

By contrast, more exact data have been derived from animal experiments. In accordance with clinical studies, these studies have shown that the duration and intensity of intoxication are important factors contributing to the occurrence of AWS. Furthermore, animal studies have demonstrated that several types of stimulation of brain tissue can potentiate the effects of alcohol withdrawal, and that prior exposure to alcohol can facilitate the development of kindled seizures. These findings agree with clinical observations that epileptics easily develop seizures after very short but intensive drinking bouts.

Animal experiments have suggested that very short interruption of intoxication attenuates rather than enhances the development of seizure susceptibility. On the other hand, a drinking pattern mimicking the human weekend of drinking was found to increase seizure susceptibility.

Unanswered Questions

No comparisons have been made of AWS among countries where drinking habits differ. We do not know whether withdrawal seizures are less prevalent in wine-drinking countries, that is, in countries where continuous drinking is the most common drinking pattern, than in countries where binge drinking is typical, like Scandinavian countries. Reliable drinking histories may be difficult to obtain in wine-drinking countries and laboratory markers of alcoholism must be used.

The role of genetic factors can now be studied, because animal strains susceptible and resistant to seizures, even AWS, have been developed.[10] Methods are also available to explore whether certain receptors, for example benzodiazepine receptors, are involved in the development of susceptibility to AWS.[45]

SUMMARY

The abrupt cessation of prolonged heavy drinking frequently precipitates cerebral seizures. However, these seizures do not affect all persons who drink heavily, and a particular person may not always develop seizures during alcohol withdrawal. Susceptibility to seizures, intensity and duration of the preceding intoxication, simultaneous drug abuse, erratic drug taking, and drinking habits all influence the occurrence of AWS. Weekend drinking has long been considered less harmful than prolonged consumption of large doses of alcohol. However, both experimental and clinical observations suggest that this is not true. Using animal models of physical dependence on alcohol, seizures were provoked after short periods (2-4 days) of continuous heavy intoxication. Furthermore, if such periods repeatedly occur, resulting in multiple intoxication and withdrawal episodes, there is a decrease in seizure threshold, supporting the kindling hypothesis of AWS. These findings are compatible with clinical data. Subjects who develop acute seizure problems after short episodes (1-3 days) of intoxication are frequently seen in emergency wards. Some are binge drinkers, but others have known epilepsy or are occasional drinkers who have alcohol-provoked seizures because their seizure threshold is lowered by yet undiagnosed mechanisms.

References

1. Aminoff, MJ and Simon, RP: Status epilepticus: Causes, clnical, features and consequences in 98 patients. Am J Med 69:657, 1980.
2. Arfken, CL: Temporal pattern of alcohol consumption in the United States. Alcoholism: Clinical Experimental Research 12:137, 1988.
3. Avdaloff, W: Alcoholism, seizures and cerebral atrophy. Advances in Biological Psychiatry 3:20, 1979.
4. Ballenger, JG and Post, RM: Kindling as a model for alcohol withdrawal syndrome. Br J Psychiatry 133:1, 1978.
5. Brown, ME, et al: Alcohol detoxification and withdrawal seizures: Clinical support for a kindling hypothesis. Biol Psychiatry 23:507, 1988.
6. Cannon DS, et al: A rapid technique for producing ethanol dependence in the rat. Pharmacol Biochem Behav 2:831, 1974.

7. Carrington, CD, Ellinwood, EH, Jr, and Krishnan, RR: Effects of single and repeated alcohol withdrawal on kindling. Biol Psychiatry 19:525, 1984.
8. Chan, AWK: Alcoholism and epilepsy. Epilepsia 26:323, 1985.
9. Clemmesen, L and Hemmingsen, R: Physical dependence on ethanol during multiple intoxication and withdrawal episodes in the rat: Evidence of a potentiation. Acta Pharmacologica et Toxicologica 55:345, 1984.
10. Crabbe, JC and Kosobud, A: Sensitivity and tolerance to ethanol in mice bred to be genetically prone or resistant to ethanol withdrawal seizures. J Pharmacol Exp Ther 239:327, 1986.
11. Dickinson, ES: Seizure disorders in the elderly. Primary Care 9:135, 1982.
12. Earnest, MP and Yarnell, PR: Seizure admissions to a city hospital: The role of alcohol. Epilepsia 17:387, 1975.
13. Feussner, JR, et al: Computed tomography brain scanning in alcohol withdrawal seizures: Value of the neurologic examination. Ann Intern Med 94:519, 1981.
14. Freer, DE and Statland, BE: Effects of ethanol (0.75 g/kg body weight) on the activities of selected enzymes in sera of healthy young adults. 2. Interindividual variations in response of gamma-glutamyltransferase to repeated ethanol challenges. Clin Chem 23:2099, 1977.
15. Gallenkamp, U: Cerebrale anfalle, alkoholkrankheit und delir. Archiv fuer Psychiatrie und Nervenkrankheiten 227:135, 1979.
16. Goldstein, DB: Rates of onset and decay of alcohol physical dependence in mice. J Pharmacol Exp Ther 190:377, 1974.
17. Goldstein, DB: Relationship of alcohol dose to intensity of withdrawal signs in mice. J Pharmacol Exp Ther 180:203, 1972.
18. Gross, MM, et al: A daily clinical course rating scale for the evaluation of the acute alcoholic psychoses and related states. Quarterly Journal of the Study of Alcohol 32:611, 1971.
19. Hillbom, ME: Alcohol withdrawal seizures: Alternatives for treatment and prevention. Nord Psykiatr Tidsskr 41 (Suppl 17):45, 1987.
20. Hillbom, ME: Occurrence of cerebral seizures provoked by alcohol abuse. Epilepsia 21:459, 1980.
21. Hillbom, ME and Hjelm-Jäger, M: Should alcohol withdrawal seizures be treated with antiepileptic drugs? Acta Neurol Scand 69:39, 1984.
22. Hopen, G, Nesthus, I, and Laerun, OD: Fatal carbamazepine-associated hepatitis: Report of two cases. Acta Med Scand 210:333, 1981.
23. Hopkins, A, Garman, A, and Clarke, C: The first seizure in adult life: Value of clinical features, electroencephalography, and computerized tomographic scanning in prediction of seizure recurrence. Lancet 1:721, 1988.
24. Isbell, H, et al: An experimental study of the etiology of "rum-fits" and delirium tremens. Quarterly Journal of Studies on Alcohol 16:1, 1955.
25. Israel, Y, et al: Monoclonal and polyclonal antibodies against acetaldehyde-containing epitopes in acetaldehyde-protein adducts. Proc Natl Acad Sci USA 83:7923, 1986.
26. Kater, RMH, et al: Increased rate of clearance of drugs from the circulation of alcoholics. Am J Med Sci 258:35, 1969.
27. Lennox, WG: Alcohol and epilepsy. Quart J Stud Alcohol 2:1, 1941.
28. Lipowski, ZJ: Delirium updated. Compr Psychiatry 21:190, 1980.
29. Majchrowicz, E: Induction of physical dependence upon ethanol and the associated behavioral changes in rats. Psychopharmacologia (Berlin) 43:245, 1975
30. Majchrowicz, E and Hunt, WA: Temporal relationship of the induction of tolerance and physical dependence after continuous intoxication with maximum tolerable doses of ethanol in rats. Psychopharmacology 50:107, 1976.
31. Majchrowicz, E and Mendelson, JH: Blood methanol concentrations during experimentally induced ethanol intoxication in alcoholics. J Pharmacol Exp Ther 179:293, 1971.
32. Mucha, RF and Pinel, PJ: Increased susceptibility to kindled seizures in rats following a single injection of alcohol. J Stud Alcohol 40:258, 1979.
33. Newsom, JA: Withdrawal seizures in an in-patient alcoholism program. In Galanter, M (ed): Currents in Alcoholism, Vol 6, Treatment and Rehabilitation and Epidemiology. Grune & Stratton, New York, 1979, p 11.
34. Orringer, CE, et al: Natural history of lactic acidosis after grand-mal seizures: A model for the study of an anion-gap acidosis associated with hyperkalemia. N Engl J Med 297:796, 1977.
35. Pilke, A, Partinen, M, and Kovanen, J: Status epilepticus and alcohol abuse: An analysis of 82 status epilepticus admissions. Acta Neurol Scand 70:443, 1984.
36. Pinel, JP: Alcohol withdrawal seizures: Implications of kindling. Pharmacol Biochem Behav 13 (Suppl 1):225, 1980.
37. Pinel, JP, Van Oot, PH, and Mucha, RF: Intensification of the alcohol withdrawal syndrome by repeated brain stimulation. Nature 254:510, 1975.
38. Sanders, B: Withdrawal-like signs induced by a single administration of ethanol in mice that differ in ethanol sensitivity. Psychopharmacology (Berlin) 68:109, 1980.
39. Simpura, J: Decomposition of changes in aggregate consumption of alcohol: Finland, 1968, 1969 and 1975. J Stud Alcohol 41:572, 1980.
40. Simpura, J: Drinking: An ignored leisure activity. Journal of Leisure Research 17:200, 1985.
41. Skinner, HAS, et al: Clinical versus laboratory detection of alcohol abuse: The alcohol clinical index. Br Med J 292:1703, 1986.
42. Stibler, H, Borg, S, and Allgulander, C: Abnormal heterogeneity of serum transferrin: A new diagnostic marker of alcoholism? Acta Psychiatr Scand 62 (Suppl 286):189, 1980.
43. Storey, EL, et al: Desialylated transferrin as a serological marker of chronic exessive alcohol ingestion. Lancet 1:1292, 1987.
44. Storey, EL, et al: Use of chromatofocusing to detect a transferrin variant in serum of alcoholic subjects. Clin Chem 31:1543, 1985.

45. Syapin, PJ and Alkana, RL: Chronic ethanol exposure increases peripheral-type benzodiazepine receptors in brain (EJP 50144) Eur J Pharmacol 147:101, 1988.
46. Wadstein, J and Skude, G: Does hypokalemia precede delirium tremens? Lancet 2:549, 1978.
47. Weill, J, et al: The decrease of low serum gamma glutamyl transferase during short-term abstinence. Alcohol 5:1, 1988.
48. Vessell, ES, Passananti, GT, and Lee CH: Impairment of drug metabolism by disulfiram in man. Clin Pharmacol Ther 12:785, 1971.
49. Victor, M: The alcohol withdrawal syndrome. Postgrad Med 47:68, 1970.
50. Victor, M and Brausch, C: The role of abstinence in the genesis of alcohol epilepsy. Epilepsia 8:1, 1967.
51. Yamane, H and Katoh, N: Alcoholic epilepsy: A definition and a description of other convulsions related to alcoholism. Eur Neurol 20:17, 1981.

Ilo E. Leppik, M.D.
Margaret P. Jacobs
Ruth B. Loewenson, Ph.D
W. Allen Hauser, M.D.
Martha Micks
Martha Taylor

CHAPTER 20

Alcohol and *Status Epilepticus*

Seizures related to alcohol abuse are common phenomena.[5] In one study in the United States of 472 emergency room visits for seizures, 41 percent involved a history of alcohol abuse.[7] A report from Finland indicated that a history of alcohol intoxication was implicated in 49 percent of 560 consecutive emergency room visits for seizures.[8] The best known syndrome associated with alcohol abuse and seizures is alcohol withdrawal seizures (AWS).[13] These seizures are usually single generalized seizures occurring within a few hours of cessation of alcohol ingestion.

More serious than isolated seizures in the context of alcohol abuse are serial seizures and status epilepticus. Most studies of alcohol and seizures do not address this less common entity in great detail.[3,11] Only a few studies in the last decade have done so.[1,4,12] In this chapter we present recently collected data from the St. Paul Ramsey Medical Center (SPRMC), and review the literature on the relationship of alcohol use to *status epilepticus* and serial seizures.

THE ST. PAUL RAMSEY STUDY

Characteristics of Patients

In this study of *status epilepticus* and serial seizures, a prospective registry of patients admitted for seizures to the neurology department at SPRMC was reviewed. Data from a three-year-period were used. This interval began after the implementation of the diagnostically related groups (DRG) rules regarding admission to the hospital. In general, only the most severely affected persons are hospitalized in the adult neurology department; persons with uncomplicated AWS are usually admitted to the detoxification unit, and patients with delirium tremens to the medical department. The registry was reviewed to find patients treated with loading doses of either intravenous (IV)[9] or oral phenytoin. Phenytoin loading is reserved for patients with serial generalized tonic-clonic seizures (defined as three or more convulsions in the last 24 hours) and patients with *status epilepticus*. Patients were given loading doses based on a judgment about the seriousness of their conditions.

Of the 476 persons in the registry, 156 met the criterion of having received a load of 12 or more mg/kg of phenytoin. Seven received loading doses after subarachnoid hemorrhage as prophylaxis against seizures; these persons were excluded from further analysis. The final study population of 149 persons included 86 male and 63 female patients, ranging in age from 17 to 96 years (mean = 54). Two analyses were performed. First, the patients' history of alcohol use was reviewed. Persons with heavy alcohol intake meeting the criteria for the International Classification of Diseases (ICD) diagnosis of alcoholism, past alcohol-related seizures, or notations by staff of heavy alcohol use were categorized as having positive alcohol histories. Second, the etiologic categories developed by Hauser for the University of Minnesota Comprehensive Epilepsy Program by one of the authors (WAH) were used.

Medical records were reviewed by a team of four persons, including a registered nurse. A four-page data form developed for this study was used. Notes by the residents, medical students, nurses, consultants, and attending physicians were reviewed for use classification. Only one primary etiologic classification was permitted for each case. If a significant condition such as acute head trauma or stroke was present in conjunction with alcohol use, alcohol was not considered the primary etiology. A person was considered to have alcohol-related seizures if there was evidence of alcohol abuse but no evidence of other major contributing factors for seizures.

The basis for admission to the neurology department was status epilepticus in 46 cases (30 percent) and serial seizures 103 (70 percent). Of the 46 patients admitted with status epilepticus, 20 had an alcohol history and 26 had no alcohol history. Of the 103 patients admitted with serial seizures, 42 had an alcohol history, 60 had no alcohol history, and one patient's history was unknown. Seizure types and their breakdown into status and serial seizures are given in Table 20–1.

Etiology Analysis

Etiologic analysis revealed that 14 patients (9 percent) suffered alcohol-related seizures with no other significant symptomatic cause. Eight of these patients engaged in both chronic and acute alcohol use, and recent heavy alcohol use was the symptomatic etiology for six patients. Seizure etiologies for all subjects are shown in Table 20–2. It is interesting that vascular etiology (including occlusive, hemorrhagic, and structural) accounted for 26 acute symptomatic and 16 remote symptomatic cases, or 28 percent of cases. Only 18 percent were judged to have had serial seizures or *status epilepticus* resulting from poor compliance with anti-epileptic drug regimens. These persons had pre-existing epilepsy of various causes.

Table 20–1. SEIZURE CLASSIFICATION OF 149 PERSONS ADMITTED FOR PHENYTOIN LOADING

	Status Epilepticus	Serial Seizures	Total
Generalized	37	91	128
Complex	4	4	8
Simple	4	5	9
Absence	1	0	1
Unknown	0	3	3
TOTAL	46	103	149

There was no significant age difference between people who had a history of alcohol abuse, people who had no history of alcohol abuse, and people whose seizures were of alcohol-related etiology. There was, however, a significant difference in sex ratio. Fifty-three women and 33 men had no history of alcohol abuse, whereas only ten women but 52 men had a history of alcohol abuse. With regard to cause, only two women but 12 men had seizures with alcohol abuse as the symptomatic etiology.

There was no overall difference in the outcome of treatment with phenytoin loading followed by benzodiazepine or phenobarbital administration. One hundred twenty-six (85 percent) patients had no further seizures. Nineteen patients had further seizures during the first 24 hours of admission: seven had a single seizure,

Table 20–2. ETIOLOGY OF SERIAL SEIZURES AND *STATUS EPILEPTICUS* IN 149 PATIENTS TREATED WITH PHENYTOIN LOADING

	Total	% of Patients
Alcohol related	14	9
Vascular	42	28
Noncompliance	27	18
Undetermined/idiopathic	24	16
Neoplasm	12	8
Metabolic/degenerative	10	7
Traumatic	8	5
Other	12	8
TOTAL	149	100

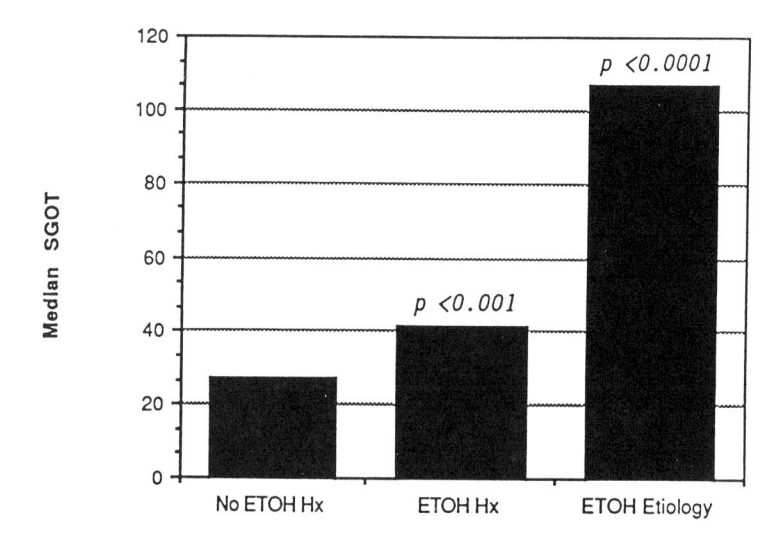

Figure 20–1. SGOT in persons with no alcohol abuse, those with a history of abuse, and those with alcohol as the etiology of serial seizures or *status epilepticus*.

nine had two to five seizures, and three had six or more seizures. In four cases, the information could not be retrieved from the records. Eleven had additional seizures after the first 24 hours of hospitalization.

Twenty-one of 149 patients had a history of drug abuse, primarily of marijuana, but serum or urine screen for drugs was positive in only five. Seventeen had a history of alcohol abuse plus drug abuse. In three for whom alcohol abuse was the primary etiology, drug abuse was also present.

The most useful laboratory test was the SGOT measurement. In persons whose seizures had an alcohol-related etiology, the median SGOT was greater than 100 (significantly higher than that of subjects in the nonalcohol history group) (Fig. 20–1).

Persons who had a history of alcohol abuse had a much greater probability of having had previous seizures (Fig. 20–2). These differences were statistically significant ($p<0.001$) by chi-square.

To determine if alcohol use was overrepresented among persons admitted to

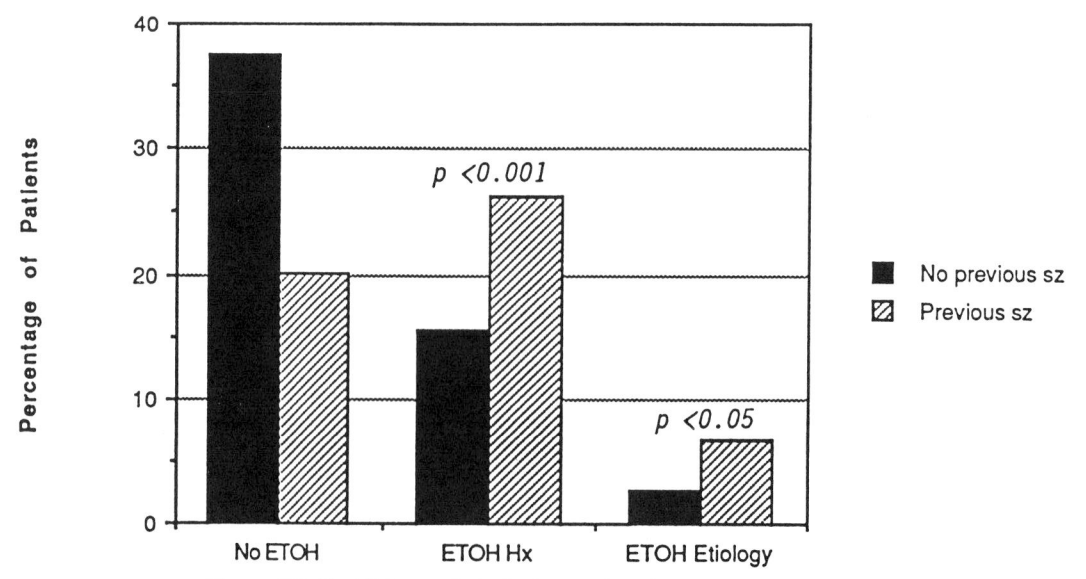

Figure 20–2. History of alcohol use related to previous seizures.

the hospital for seizures, the frequencies of alcohol use as recorded by ICD coding in the status epilepticus and serial seizure groups were compared to the frequency of this code in all adult admissions during the same period. Thirty-six (24 percent) of the 149 seizure patients had an ICD code for alcohol or alcohol syndrome; but only 9 percent of all hospital admissions to SPRMC during this period had this code. Thus, persons admitted for serial seizures and status epilepticus were much more likely to have a history of alcohol use, compared with the overall admission population (p<.001).

The average length of stay in the neurology department for nonalcohol-related serial seizures or *status* was 11 days. For persons with a history of alcohol abuse, length of stay averaged 9 days. However, for the 14 patients whose seizures had alcohol as acute etiology, the length of stay was only 6 days. In part, the short length of stay is attributable to the fact that some of these patients left against medical advice. A total of 8 patients died during hospitalization. In none of these cases was alcohol the primary diagnosis (Table 20–3).

EEGs were performed on 124 patients. Abnormalities were detected in 107; most were nonspecific. CT scans were performed on 124 individuals. Abnormal findings were present in 75. Most of these were nonspecific changes such as atrophy and enlarged ventricles.

Table 20–3. IN-HOSPITAL MORTALITY OF PERSONS WITH SERIAL SEIZURES AND *STATUS EPILEPTICUS*

Age	Sex	Days Hospitalized	Diagnoses
58	F	14	CNS neoplasm
73	M	5	CNS neoplasm
76	F	9	Stroke
79	F	4	Renal failure and congestive heart failure
81	F	7	Stroke
84	F	15	Stroke
85	F	11	Myocardial infarction and chronic renal failure
87	M	11	Stroke

Table 20–4. DISPOSITION OF THE 149 PERSONS ADMITTED FOR TREATMENT OF SERIAL SEIZURES OR *STATUS EPILEPTICUS*

Admitted From	Discharged To	Number
Home	Home	71
Home	Other hospital service/other hospital	23
Home	Care facility	9
Home	ADTP	1
Home	Deceased	5
Care facility	Care facility	23
State hospital	State hospital	1
Care facility	Other hospital service	2
Care facility	Deceased	3
Detoxification facility	VA hospital	1
Halfway house	Care facility	1
Halfway house	Other hospital service	1
Halfway house	Halfway house	3
Jail	Other hospital service	1
Jail	Home	1
Other hospital service	Home	2
Other hospital service	Other hospital service	1
		149

One hundred nine patients were admitted from home but only 74 returned home. Only three people were admitted from another hospital department, but 23 were discharged to another hospital department (Table 20–4).

ROLE OF ALCOHOL IN PRECIPITATING SEIZURES

The role of alcohol in precipitating seizures is not well understood, and alcohol may indeed have multiple mechanisms of action. The best studied relationship is that of alcohol and AWS. These seizures have been ascribed to the excitatory response of the central nervous system (CNS) after chronic depression from alcohol. The majority, however, are single seizures occurring within 48 hours of withdrawal, and only occasionally are multiple.[14] A recent study of the onset of first seizures in 308 alcohol abusers failed to demonstrate a definite withdrawal phenomenon but did find a significant relationship between the amount of alcohol consumed and the probability of having a seizure.[11] *Status* and serial seizures were not described in this report. In one study of adults admitted to a hospital following alcohol-related seizures, *status epilepticus* or serial seizures were not common.[8]

Frequency of *Status Epilepticus*

Data on the prevalence of status epilepticus among alcohol abusers are difficult to obtain. In reports on status epilepticus, alcohol is not often identified as the sole precipitating factor.[1,4] In data presented in this chapter, a clear exclusive relationship between excessive drinking and serial seizures or status epilepticus was demonstrable in only 14 of 149 cases (9 percent). These numbers are similar to those reported by Pilke, Partinen, and Kovanen,[12] who studied 82 cases of "grand mal status epilepticus." They found that excessive use of alcohol was the only precipitating factor in 16 cases (20 percent). In the series reported by Aminoff and Simon,[1] alcohol abuse, although common among patients at San Francisco General Hospital, was not the most common cause of *status epilepticus*. Alcohol abuse was considered the cause of *status epilepticus* in 17.5 percent of cases in a European series.[2] Nevertheless, in 42 percent of persons in the SPRMC study, *status epilepticus* or serial seizures were accompanied by a history of alcohol abuse.

The mechanisms by which alcohol abuse may precipitate *status epilepticus* are not clear. Because *status epilepticus* is a relatively uncommon complication of alcohol use, an interaction between alcohol and other factors that make the individual prone to seizures must exist. Many of the persons who presented with serial seizures or *status epilepticus* in the SPRMC study had previously suffered seizures. Alcohol history was present in 42 percent of persons with serial seizures or *status epilepticus*, and was a probable contributing factor in many of these cases. It may therefore be possible to ascribe to alcohol a facilitating role in lowering the seizure threshold in persons with an underlying propensity for seizures.

Persons with alcohol abuse differed from persons not using or abusing alcohol in the following respects. Although their ages were similar, there was a marked male predominance in the alcohol use groups. Although 38 percent of the persons in the nonalcohol history group were men, 83 percent of the alcohol history and 85 percent of the alcohol-etiology group were men. This finding is most likely related to the higher prevalence of alcohol abuse among men.

Treatment of Alcohol-Related Seizures

Treatment of alcohol-abuse-related seizures usually falls into three areas: prophylactic treatment in order to prevent seizures, treatment after a single seizure, and treatment after serial seizures or *status epilepticus*. Although there is considerable controversy regarding the use of phenytoin and other anti-epileptic medication in the first two areas,[13] the need for treatment of serial seizures and *status epilepticus* seems obvious.[10] Administering loading doses of phenytoin has become the current practice at SPRMC for the treatment of *status epilepticus*.[9] In the present study, the treatment protocol using phenytoin as the initial drug appeared to be effective, since 85 percent of the persons treated had no subsequent seizures. However, the parenteral preparation has some disadvantages, and more work is necessary to define the best treatment in this situation. The success rates in treating conditions in which alcohol was the etiology were not different than success rates in treating conditions with other causes. In some animal studies of AWS, phenytoin has not been effective. In a recent study of phenytoin loading following a single alcohol-related seizure, there was no difference in the effects of placebo and phenytoin. However, the recurrence rate was low in both the treated and the placebo groups, so the power of that study was low.[13] Differences between other investigators' findings (lack of effectiveness of phenytoin in AWS) and Simon's findings (effectiveness of phenytoin) may be due to the differences in the pathophysiology of the conditions. In serial seizures or *status epilepticus* related to alcohol abuse, excitatory mechanisms within the CNS that are responsive to phenytoin may be involved. In addition, persons who develop serial seizures or *status epilepticus* may have as-yet undiagnosed pathology that lowers their seizure threshold.

Usefulness of EEGs

The EEG may be useful in determining the etiology or associated factors. In one study, paroxysmal or focal EEG abnormalities were rarely observed in persons with simple AWS, but were common in persons with epilepsy as a consequence of alcohol use.[6]

SUMMARY

A prospective registry of all persons admitted to the neurology department with a diagnosis of *status epilepticus* or new-onset seizure disorder at SPRMC has been maintained. Of the 476 persons entered into the registry during the last three years, preliminary chart review revealed that 19.5 percent were described as having alcohol-related seizures or *status epilepticus*. Approximately two thirds of the patients in the registry were treated with IV or oral phenytoin using doses of approximately 20 mg/kg regardless of the etiology of the condition. Treatment outcomes for alcohol-related seizures were compared with outcomes of seizures occurring without evidence of substance abuse. In summary, alcohol use is commonly associated with seizures. Results from the SPRMC study and a review of the literature, however, indicate that alcohol abuse commonly associated with single seizures is not a major cause of *status epilepticus* or serial seizures, even in facilities where many alcohol abusers are treated.

ACKNOWLEDGMENTS

This work was supported in part by the NINCDS Grant #P50-NS-16308. These data were presented in part at the First International Symposium on Alcohol and Seizures, Washington, DC, September 29 and 30, 1988.

References

1. Aminoff, MJ and Simon, RP: Status epilepticus: Causes, clinical features and consequences in 98 patients. Am J Med 69:657, 1980.
2. Avdaloff, W: Alcoholism, seizures, and cerebral atrophy. Advances in Biological Psychiatry 3:20, 1979.
3. Chan, AWK: Alcoholism and epilepsy. Epilepsia 26:323, 1985.
4. Cranford, RE, et al: Intravenous phenytoin in acute treatment of seizures. Neurology 29:1474, 1979.
5. Dam, AM, Frederiksen, AF, and Svarre-Olsen, U: Late-onset epilepsy: Etiologies, types of seizure, and value of clinical investigation, EEG, and computerized tomography scan. Epilepsia 25:227, 1985.
6. Deisenhammer, E, Klingler, D, and Tragner, H: Epileptic seizures in alcoholism and diagnostic value of EEG after sleep deprivation. Epilepsia 4:526, 1984.
7. Earnest, MP and Yarnell, PR: Seizure admissions to a city hospital: The role of alcohol. Epilepsia 17:387, 1976.
8. Hillbom, ME: Occurrence of cerebral seizures provoked by alcohol abuse. Epilepsia 21:459, 1980.
9. Leppik, IE: Status epilepticus. Neurol Clin 4:633, 1986.
10. McMicken, D: Seizures in the alcohol-dependent patient: A diagnostic and therapeutic dilemma. J Emerg Med 1:311, 1984.
11. Ng, KCS, et al: Alcohol consumption and withdrawal in new-onset seizures. N Engl J Med 319:666, 1988.
12. Pilke, A, Partinen, M, and Kovanen, J: Status epilepticus and alcohol abuse: An analysis of 82 status epilepticus admissions. Acta Neurol Scand 70:443, 1984.
13. Simon, RP and Aldredge, B: Phenytoin treatment of alcohol withdrawal seizures. In this volume.
14. Victor, M and Brausch, C: The role of abstinence in the genesis of alcoholic epilepsy. Epilepsia 8:1, 1967.

CHAPTER 21

R.J.E.A. Höppener, M.D.

The Effect of Social Alcohol Use on Seizures in Patients with Epilepsy

People suffering from epilepsy often face exclusionary restrictions when considering various professions, driving, swimming, etc., because of their seizures. An important consideration in supporting a person with epilepsy is to help him or her to achieve social integration, and in particular, to minimize the stigma he or she feels. Alcohol use is very common and nearly always present at social events in contemporary Western society; one must be very careful, therefore, when advising patients about using alcohol, because prohibiting or discouraging alcohol use exaggerates the anomalous position in which they find themselves in various social circumstances. Because social use of alcohol is the norm in our society, epileptic patients may feel, rightly or wrongly, excluded if they must refuse when offered alcoholic drinks. The admission that one is not allowed to drink due to epilepsy is often seen by the patient as yet another stigma. (The refusal of alcohol by one who makes a free choice to do so is different in that the abstainer may in fact take some pride in abstinence.)

DRINKING HABITS IN THE 20TH CENTURY

Between 1936 and 1940, Lennox[24] measured the extent of alcohol use of 1,254 male and 92 female nonepileptic hospital patients. Compared with the epileptic patients, the control group contained fewer women and the general economic status was higher. Of the epileptic patients, 864 (69 percent) said they never used alcohol, 330 (26 percent) said that they used it sometimes, and 60 (5 percent) said they used it frequently. Of the control group, 53 percent were drinkers, compared with 31 percent of the patients.

In 1976, at the request of the Health and Social Department, Sylbing[35] examined the drinking habits of Dutch people from 12 to 70 years of age. It appeared that 81 percent drank at least occasionally. When only persons 20 years and older were studied, the level reached 87.5 percent. In 1952, the average Dutch person was found to use the equivalent of 1.7 liters of pure alcohol annually. From 1952 to 1982, alcohol use increased from 1.7 liters to 8.4 liters per person, an increase of 500 percent.[30] In Germany, the consumption of alcohol has been increasing continually, reaching 12.25 liters of alcohol per person annually in 1977.[13] However, the greatest consumers of alcohol are the French, who consume 16.5 liters annually.[30]

THE RELATION OF ALCOHOL USE TO SEIZURES IN EPILEPTIC PATIENTS

From the author's experience in the outpatient treatment of people with epilepsy, abolishing the total prohibition of alcohol use did not affect seizure frequency. This view was supported by Livingstone,[25] who found that permitting moderate alcohol use by more than 5,000 adolescent patients did not adversely influence the frequency of their seizures. In 1927, Kuffner[22] concluded that there was no relationship between alcohol use and seizures in the epileptic patient. On the other hand, Lennox[24] thought that seizures in epileptic patients occurring as a result of alcohol use were sometimes due to alcohol abuse and had occurred in the abstinence period. Therefore, he ascribed the seizures to circumstances surrounding alcohol use rather than to alcohol use itself. After reviewing the literature, Berry[3] decided that alcohol is a narcotic, and thus should have an anticonvulsive action. He found neither pharmacologic nor experimental evidence of a convulsive action for alcohol, and concluded that there was no proof that moderate or even excessive use of alcohol provoked seizures.

Rodin, Frohman, and Gottlieb[31] administered large quantities of alcohol to 25 epileptic patients. They all showed clinical symptoms of intoxication. The blood alcohol levels 1 hour after alcohol ingestion were 125 g/dl on average. There was no appreciable influence of alcohol intake on these patients' seizures. It could not be demonstrated that alcohol predictably produced seizures in the epileptic patient who was maintained on anticonvulsant medication. These investigators concluded that instead of categorically forbidding all epileptics to use moderate amounts of alcohol, it would be advisable to discuss alcohol intake with each patient.

Lund[26] argued that whenever alcohol is used in small quantities it is not seizure provoking. He felt that prohibition of alcohol use is unacceptable intervention in a patient's personal freedom. Paludin[29] found that epileptic patients who ingested large quantities of alcohol usually suffered from seizures the day after the night they used alcohol. However, he concluded that the alcohol itself may not have provoked the seizures, but that intoxication caused them to forget their daily dose of medication, thereby decreasing its serum level and inducing the seizures. Thus, there would be nothing to prevent people with epilepsy from enjoying a beer with a meal or a few drinks on festive occasions, such as two or three glasses of wine at dinner or a corresponding quantity of beer at lunch.

Advice in Textbooks About the Use of Alcohol

It is striking that so many investigators offer dogmatic advice about the use of alcohol by people with epilepsy, seemingly without any scientific foundation and with a total disregard for the published evidence. Rodin, Frohman, and Gottlieb[31] commented that eight textbooks consulted (on neurology, psychiatry, and internal medicine) recommended that alcohol use be discouraged or prohibited. Review of 14 other texts generally yielded the same negative advice.[1,2,4,5,8,12,15,21,23,25,28,32–34]

THE INFLUENCE OF SOCIAL ALCOHOL USE ON EPILEPSY: A STUDY

No well-documented study has proven the provocative effect of social alcohol use on seizures. Therefore, an investigation[17,18] was undertaken with epileptic patients who had never before used alcohol.

Questions Addressed

The following questions were asked:

1. Does social alcohol intake, defined as the consumption twice per week of

one to three average drinks within 2 hours, influence seizure incidence?
2. What is the effect of such alcohol intake on the blood levels of anti-epileptic medications?
3. If clinically there is no change in seizure frequency, are there any indications that the social use of alcohol causes a change in the amount of epileptic electroencephalographic (EEG) activity?
4. What is the general attitude of Dutch neurologists and of attending specialists in other countries with regard to alcohol intake by epileptics?

Participants

Participating patients had to meet the following criteria:

1. During the entire investigation all were inpatients. The clinical setting was necessary to ensure that the quota for alcohol intake would not be exceeded, the number of seizures would be registered correctly, and the intake of medication was reliable.
2. The diagnosis of epilepsy was definite, and based on the clinical picture as well as on EEG findings.
3. There was no functional disorder of the liver or kidneys that would contraindicate participation.
4. There had been no use (or very incidental use) of alcohol in the past, because otherwise the effect of alcohol would be difficult to measure.
5. Other members of the supporting team (e.g., psychologists, social workers, and observers) agreed that there were no contraindications for participation.
6. After explanation of the purpose and plan of the investigation, the patients voluntarily participated and gave written consent.

The participants were selected so that the group using alcohol was completely comparable with the group that did not. Attention was paid to age, sex, type of epilepsy, medication, IQ, and severity of brain damage.

The investigation continued for 2 years. In the first year, 22 persons participated, divided into two groups of 11. When the results of this experiment were studied later, no effect due to alcohol use could be found. In light of these results, in the second year 13 patients were chosen for the control group and 19 patients for the alcohol group; one patient dropped out from each group because of transfer to another hospital.

For both years combined, the alcohol group thus consisted of 29 persons: 20 men ranging in age from 17 to 45 years (average 27.7 ± 7.2 years), and 9 women ranging in age from 18 to 41 years (average 29 ± 8.7 years) (Table 21–1). For this alcohol group, the epilepsies were classified as follows: one (3 percent) primary generalized epilepsy, 14 (48 percent) secondary generalized epilepsy, and 14 (48 percent) partial epilepsy.

The control group included 23 persons: 13 men ranging in age from 18 to 41 years (average 28.8 ± 6.4 years), and 10 women ranging in age from 21 to 46 years (average 35 years ± 7.9 years). The epilepsies of the control group were classified as follows: one (4 percent) primary generalized epilepsy, 12 (52 percent) secondary generalized epilepsy, and 10 (44 percent) partial epilepsy.

Table 21–2 shows the distribution of medication in both groups. The alcohol and control groups were compared statistically with respect to age, sex, type of epilepsy, and medication. There were no significant differences between the two groups for any of these items.

Plan of Investigation

The investigation was double blind. During the investigation, alcoholic drinks were provided on Monday and Thursday evenings between 8 PM and 10 PM. For this purpose, orangeade with or without vodka was used. The alcoholic drinks provided 9.85 g of alcohol, comparable with the alcohol content of a glass of beer, in 200 ml of orangeade. Vodka was used because it does not have a recognizable smell; orangeade was chosen after an investigation in which it was found that 80 percent to 90 percent of healthy volun-

Table 21-1. AGE DISTRIBUTION IN BOTH GROUPS

Group	15-19	20-24	25-29	30-34	35-39	40-44	45-49	Total
Alcohol	4 (14%)	7 (24%)	6 (21%)	7 (24%)	2 (7%)	2 (7%)	1 (3%)	29 (56%)
Control	1 (4%)	3 (13%)	6 (26%)	5 (22%)	4 (17%)	3 (13%)	1 (4%)	23 (44%)
Total	5 (10%)	10 (19%)	12 (23%)	12 (23%)	6 (12%)	5 (10%)	2 (4%)	52 (100%)

teers could detect vodka in cola, tonic, or orange juice, but only 40 percent could distinguish orangeade with vodka from orangeade without it. The maximum number of drinks allowed per evening was three. Throughout the study, medication was unchanged and seizure frequency was recorded by experienced observers.

At the beginning of the experiment, the head of the catering department decided which patients were to use orangeade bottles with lemon-lime stoppers and which were to use orangeade bottles with cola stoppers. Once a patient was assigned to a particular stopper, the assignment was maintained throughout the experiment. The stoppers were codes identifying the vodka-containing bottles for the head of the catering department. Because generally the alcohol could not be tasted or smelled by the participants or nursing staff, it was undetectable.

Stages of the Investigation

The investigation was divided into four stages (Table 21-3):

Table 21-2. DISTRIBUTION OF MEDICATION IN BOTH GROUPS

Generic Name of Antiepileptic Drug	Alcohol Group (n = 29)	Control Group (n = 23)
Carbamazepine	21 (72%)	18 (78%)
Phenobarbital	20 (69%)	17 (74%)
Phenytoin	17 (59%)	14 (61%)
Valproic acid	10 (34%)	8 (35%)
Primidone	4 (14%)	1 (4%)
Clonazepam	3 (10%)	1 (4%)
Ethosuximide	5 (17%)	3 (13%)
Sulthiame	1 (3%)	1 (4%)

BASIC PERIOD (P-I): TWENTY-TWO WEEKS

During the five months before the active investigation (the basic period), the patients' medication doses were held constant and their seizure frequencies were carefully monitored by experienced observers. Because all participants continued to be inpatients of the clinic, seizure frequencies under unchanged medical conditions could be compared with frequencies in the later stages of the study.

PRELIMINARY STAGE (P-II): SIX WEEKS

In the preliminary stage, drinks without vodka were given to all participants twice a week. Neither observers nor participants were informed how long this stage would last. Each patient retained his or her own bottle-stopper code throughout the rest of the investigation. For purposes of comparison with values in the period of alcohol use, the following laboratory tests were performed at 10 PM and 8 AM three times during this six-week period, unless otherwise noted:

— Determination of serum levels of antiepileptic drugs, tested in each patient at the same time on two different days
— Measurement of urea concentration
— Comprehensive determination of liver and kidney functions
— Tests of enzyme functions of the liver
— Routine EEG registration, performed only once, in the morning after beverage use.

ALCOHOL STAGE (P-III): SIXTEEN WEEKS

During the alcohol stage, drinks with and without vodka were given to the participants each Monday and Thursday eve-

Table 21–3. PLAN OF INVESTIGATION

Periods of Investigation	Time in Weeks	Medication	EEG	Laboratory Tests: Blood Levels Anti-epileptic Drugs 8 AM and 10 PM	Liver Function 8 AM and 10 PM	Kidney Function 8 AM and 10 PM	Serum Alcohol in mg/dl	Seizure Registration	Beverage Use/Week * = with Alcohol † = without Alcohol
Basic period P-I	22	Unchanged						Monitored by observers	
Preliminary stage P-II	6	Unchanged	EEG	Blood levels Blood levels	Liver function Liver function Liver function	Kidney function Kidney function Kidney function		Monitoring unchanged	† † † †
Alcohol stage P-III	16	Unchanged	EEG	Blood levels Blood levels Blood levels Blood levels Blood levels	Liver function Liver function Liver function Liver function Liver function	Kidney function Kidney function Kidney function Kidney function Kidney function	0/00 0/00 0/00 0/00 0/00	Monitoring unchanged	* * † *
Final stage P-IV	5	Unchanged	EEG	Blood levels	Liver function	Kidney function		Monitoring unchanged	† † † †

ning. Blood levels of anti-epileptic medication, urea concentration, and liver enzyme functions were determined at 10 PM and 8 AM on five occasions during the 16-week period. Blood alcohol concentration was determined at 10 PM on five occasions after beverages were consumed, and the EEG was recorded twice, on mornings after beverage use.

FINAL STAGE (P-IV): FIVE WEEKS

During the final stage, beverages without alcohol were given to all the participants twice a week. Blood levels of anti-epileptic medications were determined and chemical blood examination was conducted at 10 PM and 8 AM on one occasion, and the EEG was registered once, the morning after consumption.

Test Methods

LABORATORY TESTS

Serum levels of phenobarbital, phenytoin, carbamazepine, and primidone were determined by gas chromatography using the method described by Cramers and associates[7] and Driessen and Edmonds.[11] Valproic acid level was determined quantitatively by gas chromatography according to the method of Dijkhuis and Vervloet.[10] Ethanol was measured using the method of Buecher and Redetzik.[6]

EEG EXAMINATION

EEGs were recorded with a 16-channel apparatus and routine procedure was followed; five minutes of hyperventilation and a period of stroboscopy were included. The four EEGs were made at the same hour of the day to eliminate as many variations due to differences in physiologic state during the day as possible. The EEGs were inspected visually by a skilled electroencephalographer. This part of the experiment was also double blind; neither the technician nor the electroencephalographer knew whether the patient belonged to the alcohol group or the control group. In addition, when reading and scoring the EEGs, the electroencephalographer did not know their sequence.

Results

ALCOHOL INTAKE AND SERUM ALCOHOL CONCENTRATION

Each evening when beverages were served, the participants in the study could determine their intake themselves during a two-hour period, within the limits of a minimum of one drink and a maximum of three. Average beverage intake during the 16-week alcohol stage was 2.16 glasses/patient/evening in the control group, and 2.14 glasses/patient/evening in the alcohol group. In the alcohol group, the measured serum alcohol concentration was 5 mg/dl to 33 mg/dl.

SEIZURE FREQUENCY

Fluctuations in a Steady State

Seizures often occur at irregular intervals. In cases of partial epilepsy, they often occur in clusters. Spontaneous fluctuations in seizure frequency also occur when there are no changes of medication, as during the 22-week basic period. This period was divided into two stages of 11 weeks each, and the number of seizures during these two stages was compared for each of the 52 patients completing the study. For 17 (33 percent) persons there were no changes in the frequency of seizures; for 21 (40 percent) there was an increase; and in 14 (27 percent) the number of seizures decreased. These results illustrate the spontaneous fluctuations in seizure frequency in a steady state.

Influence of Social Alcohol Use

To study the influence of alcohol use on seizure frequency, the total number of seizures per person during the last 16 weeks of the basic period (P-I) was compared with the total number of seizures during the 16 weeks of the alcohol stage (P-III). Table 21-4 provides a summary of changes in seizure frequency between patients in the alcohol and control groups during these two periods. Alcohol intake did not affect seizure frequency. The reproducibility of these findings was checked when the frequencies recorded during 16 weeks of the alcohol period were compared with frequencies recorded

Table 21–4. CHANGES IN SEIZURE FREQUENCY P-1–P-III

Number of Seizures	Alcohol Group (n = 29)	Control Group (n = 23)	Total (n = 52)
Unchanged	8	6	14
Increased	10	10	20
Decreased	11	7	18

Chi-square = 0.48

during 16 other weeks when no alcohol was taken (Table 21–5). This nonalcohol period consisted of the last 5 weeks of the basic period (P-I), the 6 weeks of the preliminary stage (P-II), and the 5 weeks of the final stage (P-IV).

A variety of other analyses and statistical tests failed to demonstrate an effect of alcohol use on seizure frequency. In addition, the influence of alcohol on the frequency of generalized tonic-clonic convulsions and partial complex seizures was examined; alcohol did not affect either type of seizure.

INFLUENCE OF ALCOHOL USE ON BLOOD LEVELS OF MEDICATION

The patients participating were taking carbamazepine, phenobarbital, phenytoin, valproic acid, ethosuximide, primidone, clonazepam, and sulthiame for their seizures. The number of patients using primidone, clonazepam, and sulthiame was too small for statistical analysis.

The blood levels of medication were determined in the evening (10 PM) and morning (8 AM) after beverage use, four times during the nonalcohol stages (P-II and P-IV) and five times during the alcohol stage (P-III). The two-tailed t-test[9] was used to determine whether there were significant differences at each time of day between blood levels of an anti-epileptic drug tested during the alcohol stage and the nonalcohol stages, in the control and alcohol groups (Table 21–6).

No significant differences in either morning or evening levels of carbamazepine, ethosuximide, or phenytoin were found. For subjects taking phenobarbital, there was a marginal significant difference in the morning for the control group. The reason for this result is not evident.

Valproic acid levels showed significant differences, probably as a result of the ethanol intake. However, valproic acid concentration fluctuated greatly throughout the day; differences between two serum levels of valproic acid in one patient on the same day varied by as much as 200 percent. Moreover, there is very poor reproducibility for the measured valproic acid serum level.[16] Therefore, the increase in valproic acid concentration could be caused by coincidence as well as by the ethanol.

INFLUENCE OF ALCOHOL USE ON EEG

The frequency of background rhythms was not altered following alcohol use. The amount of alpha, beta, and theta activity did not change the number of EEGs with only a bilateral spike-and-wave complex. There were too few EEGs with focal spikes to group statistically. When changes of "total epileptic activity" were compared in both groups, such activity was not found to be affected.

SURVEY OF PHYSICIANS' ATTITUDES ON ALCOHOL USE BY EPILEPTIC PATIENTS IN 25 COUNTRIES

At the time of the above-mentioned study, 519 multiple-choice survey forms were mailed to neurologists in Holland, of which 328 were returned (a response rate

Table 21–5. CHANGES IN SEIZURE FREQUENCY: 5 w. P-1 + P-II + P-IV VERSUS P-III

Number of Seizures	Alcohol Group (n = 29)	Control Group (n = 23)	Total (n = 52)
Unchanged	7	7	14
Increased	11	10	21
Decreased	11	6	17

Chi-square = 0.83, no significant differences between the two groups.

Table 21-6. INFLUENCE OF ALCOHOL USE ON BLOOD LEVELS OF ANTI-EPILEPTIC DRUGS

	Control Group		Alcohol Group	
Medication	8 AM	10 PM	8 AM	10 PM
Carbamazepine	ns	ns	ns	ns
Ethosuximide	ns	ns	ns	ns
Phenytoin	ns	ns	ns	ns
Phenobarbital	p=0.049	ns	ns	ns
Valproic acid	p=0.005	ns	p=0.02	p=0.004

ns = not significant

of 63.2 percent). One thousand, one hundred eighty questionnaires were sent to 26 other countries. The response from two countries was so inadequate that they were excluded from further consideration. For the other 24 countries, a total of 478 out of the 1,120 forms were completed and returned, yielding a response rate of 42.7 percent.

Gadourek[14] mentioned that a response rate of 40 percent to 50 percent to mailed questionnaires was high and that 50 percent or more could be considered very high. House, Gerber, and McMichael[19] stated that a response of 53 percent to 60 percent was very high. Kerlinger[20] found that the response rate for mailed questionnaires is usually poor, with a return of 40 percent to 50 percent being average and higher percentages very rarely obtained. He considered 50 percent to 60 percent to be a better response rate. For Mooy,[27] the average response for mailed questionnaires was 40 percent to 50 percent. Therefore, the response rate of this survey (63.2 percent in Holland and 42.7 percent elsewhere) was deemed normal to high.

Advice on Alcohol Use

Since opinions about alcohol use by epileptic patients are not based on scientific investigations, one could expect a great variety of advice within each country as well as among countries. The 25 countries participating in the investigation were divided into three categories with regard to the reported advice given (Table 21-7). The categories were:
1. Permissive: 40 percent or more of the respondents allow social use of alcohol (nine countries).
2. Moderate: 10 percent to 39 percent of the respondents allow social use of alcohol (eight countries).

Table 21-7. CLASSIFICATION OF COUNTRIES ACCORDING TO PHYSICIANS' ATTITUDES ABOUT SOCIAL DRINKING BY EPILEPTICS

Permissive		Moderate		Strict	
Denmark	80.0%*	Japan	32.8%	Yugoslavia	7.1%
United Kingdom	61.9%	Australia	30.0%	Germany	6.5%
Ireland	60.0%	Finland	27.3%	Hungary	0.0%
India	57.1%	Holland	25.0%	Austria	0.0%
South Africa	52.4%	Switzerland	17.6%	Poland	0.0%
France	50.0%	Italy	16.7%	Spain	0.0%
Canada	48.1%	Chile	15.0%	Czechoslovakia	0.0%
Norway	46.2%	China	10.0%	Belgium	0.0%
United States	44.3%				

*Percentage of responding neurologists from each country who allow social use of alcohol by epileptic patients.

3. Strict: 0 percent to 9 percent of the respondents allow social use of alcohol (eight countries).

The factors determining attitudes are not immediately obvious. Countries with high social alcohol consumption are found in all three categories. Ireland and France—*permissive*; Australia, Japan—*moderate*; Hungary, Poland, and Spain—*strict*. The four socialist countries are all in the *strict* group. This association is highly significant (p<0.01, Fischer's exact probability two-tailed test), but since Germany and Austria are in the same category, the effect may be geographic rather than political. A striking effect more readily acceptable at face value is the association of permissive attitudes with former membership in the British Empire (p<0.01 by Fischer's exact probability two-tailed test).

Alcohol Use and Provocation of Seizures

Opinion about whether alcohol provokes seizures varies widely among the different countries (Table 21–8). In Denmark, only 5 percent of the respondents ascribed a provocative action to alcohol (lowest score), while in Hungary 83 percent felt that alcohol use does cause seizures (highest score). Note that Denmark was in the *permissive* category with regard to advice on alcohol use, while Hungary was in the *strict* category. Such associations did not always hold true,

Table 21–8. RANKING OF COUNTRIES ACCORDING TO WHETHER PHYSICIANS BELIEVE THAT ALCOHOL USE PROVOKES SEIZURES

Rank Not Sharing Belief	Rank on Table 21–7	Country	Percentage of Physicians Who Report This Belief*
1	1	Denmark	5
2	4	India	7
3	10	Japan	16
4	15	Italy	17
5	2	United Kingdom	19
6	17	China	20
7	5	South Africa	25
8	22.5	Poland	36
9	13	Holland	36
10	9	United States	38
11	7	Canada	41
12	14	Switzerland	41
13	11	Australia	50
14	18	Yugoslavia	50
15	8	Norway	54
16	12	Finland	55
17	6	France	58
18	22.5	Czechoslovakia	60
19	16	Chile	60
20	22.5	Austria	67
21	22.5	Spain	67
22	19	Germany	72
23	22.5	Belgium	74
24	3	Ireland	80
25	22.5	Hungary	83

*Proportion of respondents from each country who believe that alcohol use provokes seizures in epileptic patients.
Spearman test quantity r = 1.247.
Rank correlation coefficient of Spearman rs = 0.52.
Significance p < 0.02.

however; although Ireland was in the *permissive* category with 60 percent of the respondents allowing social drinking, 80 percent of Irish respondents believed that alcohol provokes seizures. Similarly, although Poland was in the *strict* category, only 36 percent of Polish respondents ascribed a provocative action to alcohol. Nevertheless, there was a positive correlation between advice on alcohol use and opinions on the provocation of seizures by alcohol (Table 21-8).

HOW TO ADVISE IN PRACTICE

On the basis of the above study, an absolute alcohol prohibition for epileptic patients can no longer be justified. Although the number of seizures often fluctuates (thus increasing in some patients), no connection can be proven between moderate alcohol consumption and seizures. Some apparent connections may be the result of poor medication compliance or sleep deprivation linked with alcohol use.

However, in each case contraindications to incidental and social alcohol use should be considered. Contraindications include:
1. The patient does not follow prescribed advice, or follows it only partly as indicated by inadequate compliance with regard to antiepileptic medication.
2. There is a possibility of alcohol abuse in the history.
3. There is an "individual sensitiveness" for alcohol. Although this problem did not occur in our investigation, it cannot be excluded with certainty.

The attitude of the attending specialist should not play a part in the advice.[17]

SUMMARY

People suffering from epileptic seizures are often excluded from certain professions and sports, not allowed to drive a car, and prohibited from drinking alcohol. Consultation of manuals to trace studies on which the alcohol prohibition was based was unsuccessful; there was no mention of the original research demonstrating that alcohol provoked seizures. To determine the influence of social alcohol intake on epilepsy, a double-blind study was undertaken with epileptic patients who had never before or very sporadically used alcohol. During 16 weeks, twice a week, one to three glasses of an alcoholic beverage were consumed within a two-hour period, in a clinical setting. We concluded the following:
1. Social alcohol use did not affect tonic-clonic seizures or partial complex seizures.
2. Blood levels of carbamazepine, phenobarbital, and phenytoin were not influenced by alcohol intake.
3. Alcohol use did not change either frequency bands or amount of epileptic activity.

A survey was conducted among neurologists in 25 countries to determine their attitudes regarding alcohol intake by epileptic patients and provocation of seizures by alcohol. The results differed widely among countries. In one country, 90 percent of the respondents favored an absolute alcohol prohibition, while in another country, 80 percent felt social alcohol use was acceptable. Such discrepant attitudes cannot be supported by scientific investigations and probably are determined by cultural or social factors.

References

1. Berg, JH van de: Kleine Psychiatrie. GF Callenbach, Nijkerk, The Netherlands 1966, p 84.
2. Bergh, R van de and Folkerts, JF: Neurologie van de algemene praktijk. Agon Elsevier, Amsterdam, 1972, p 279.
3. Berry, RG: The role of alcohol in convulsive seizures. Epilepsia 1:21, 1952.
4. Biemond, A: Hersenziekten, diagnostiek en therapie. De Erven F Bohn NV, Haarlem, The Netherlands, 1972, p 220.
5. Brain, L and Walton JN: Brain's Diseases of the Nervous System. Oxford University Press, London, 1969, p 939.
6. Buecher, TH and Redetzik, H: Eine spezifische photometrische Bestimmung von Aethylalkohol auf fermentatieven Wege. Klinische Wochenschrift 29:615, 616, 1951.
7. Cramers, C, et al: Quantitative determination of underivatized anticonvulsant drugs by high res-

olution gaschromatography with support-coated open tubular columns. Clinical Chemistry Acta 73:97, 1976.
8. Davidson, S: Principles and Practice of Medicine. E and S Livingstone Ltd, Edinburgh, 1965, p 1090.
9. Davies, OL: Statistical Methods in Research and Production. Oliver and Boyd, Edinburgh, 1947, p 57.
10. Dijkhuis, IC and Vervloet, E: Rapid determination of the antiepileptic drug di-n-propylacetic acid in serum. Pharm Weekbl 109:42, 1974.
11. Driessen, O and Emonds, A: Simultaneous determination of antiepileptic drugs in small samples of blood plasma by gas chromatography. K Ned Akad Wet 77:171, 1974.
12. Epen, JH van de: Drugverslaving en Alcoholisme. Agon Elsevier, Amsterdam, 1974, p 150.
13. Feuerlein, W: Zur Frage des Alkohol-Entzugssyndroms. Nervenartz 43:247, 253, 1972.
14. Gadourek, J: Sociologische onderzoekstechnieken. Van Loghum Slaterus, Deventer, 1976, p 204.
15. Gibbs, FA: Epilepsy Handbook. Charles C Thomas, Springfield, IL, 1958, p 80.
16. Höppener, RJ: Unpublished material, 1979.
17. Höppener, RJ: Epilepsy and alcohol. BDU BV, Barneveld, The Netherlands, 1981, thesis.
18. Höppener, RJ, et al: Epilepsy and alcohol: The influence of social alcohol intake on seizures and treatment in epilepsy. Epilepsia 24:459, 1983.
19. House, JS, Gerber, W, and McMichael, W: Increasing mail questionnaire response: A controlled replication and extension. Public Opinion 41:95, 1977.
20. Kerlinger, FN: Foundations of Behavioural Research. Holt, Rinehart and Winston, London, 1970.
21. Kraus, G: Leerboek der Psychiatrie. HE Stenfert Kroese NV, Leiden, 1964, p 351.
22. Kuffner, W: Epilepsie and alcohol. Zeitschrift fuer die Gesamte Neurologie und Psychiatrie 11:145, 1927.
23. Laidlaw, J and Richens, A: Textbook of Epilepsy. Churchill Livingstone, Edinburgh, 1976, p 172.
24. Lennox, WG: Alcohol and epilepsy. Quarterly Journal of Studies on Alcohol, 2:1, 1941.
25. Livingstone, S: Comprehensive Management of Epilepsy in Infancy, Childhood and Adolescence. Charles C Thomas, Springfield, IL, 1972, p 117.
26. Lund, M: Epilepsy and driving licence. Hexagon Roche 2:19, 1974.
27. Mooy, AJ: Responssnelheid in een postenquete. Tijdschr Onderzoek Res 3:187, 1978.
28. Mumenthaler, M: Neurology. Georg Thieme Publishers, Stuttgart, 1977, p 254.
29. Paludin, J: Alcohol and epilepsy. Epilepsy International Newsletter 47:6, 1976.
30. Philipsen, H, Knibbe, R, and van Reek, G: Alcohol gebruik in Nederland als sociaal verschignsel. Vocding 15:10, 1984.
31. Rodin, EA, Frohman, CE, and Gottlieb, S: Effect of acute alcohol intoxication on epileptic patients. Arch Neurol 4:115, 1961.
32. Scheid, W: Lehrbuch der Neurologie. Georg Thieme Verlag, Stuttgart, 1966, p 379.
33. Schultz, W: Epilepsie und ihre Randgebiete in Klinik und Praxis. JE Lehmans Verlag, München, 1964, p 102.
34. Scott, D: About Epilepsy. Cox and Wymon Ltd, London, 1973, p 19.
35. Sylbing, G: Drinkgewoonten van de Nederlanders. Tijdschr Alc Drugs 4:109, 114, 1978.

CHAPTER 22

Richard H. Mattson, M.D.
M. Linda Fay
John K. Sturman, M.D.
Joyce A. Cramer
Jan D. Wallace, M.D.
Elena M. Mattson

The Effect of Various Patterns of Alcohol Use on Seizures in Patients with Epilepsy

The effect of alcohol intake on epilepsy patients has not been investigated thoroughly. An adverse effect on seizure frequency has been assumed, in part because of the well-known association of alcoholism and seizures,[5,14] In a survey of 390 epileptic patients who used alcohol, Lennox[8] reported that 79 percent detected no increase in seizures, 16 percent noted an occasional facilitation, and only 5 percent reported frequent association with alcohol use. There was some relationship between precipitation of seizures and quantity and frequency of alcohol intake, but the relationship was not fully evaluated. No electroencephalography (EEG) was performed or anti-epileptic drug serum concentrations measured and no validation of the results of the survey was possible. Giove and Gastaut[2] reported that only seven of the 317 epileptics they surveyed who used alcohol noted an associated increase in seizures. In a carefully controlled clinical trial, Höppener, Juyer, and van der Lugt[4] administered small amounts of alcohol to patients with epilepsy, and found that "social" quantities of alcohol had no effect on epileptic seizures.

Several neurophysiology studies have examined the clinical and EEG effects of alcohol intake, but the results have been contradictory. Kaufman, Marshall, and Walker[6] reported that the "alpha rhythm became more prominent and the amplitude of previous abnormal activity decreased" following 40 to 150 ml of alcohol rapidly administered intravenously (IV). Kershman,[7] describing an opposite effect, found that a spike wave focus was activated following oral alcohol intake in one case. A more detailed study was performed by Rodin, Frohman, and Gottlieb[13] who gave 6 ounces of 50 percent ethanol orally to 25 epilepsy patients. Although clinical intoxication was common, blood alcohol levels varied greatly among subjects. Although EEG activity slowed, no epileptiform activity was elicited and no seizures were precipitated. These investigators concluded that alcohol intake had little effect on seizure activity. In none of these studies was continuous long-term EEG recording correlated with clinical status, blood electrolytes, and alcohol or anti-epileptic drug serum concentrations.

Although some reports have suggested that modest alcohol use has little effect on seizure occurrence, total abstinence from alcohol is often advised for patients with epilepsy.[4] It remains to be clearly defined whether a specific quantity of alcohol is likely to significantly alter brain excitability and elicit seizure recurrence. For this reason, we studied the effect of alcohol use in nonalcoholic patients with epilepsy.

PATIENT SELECTION AND STUDY METHODS

The study was designed in two parts. The first section consisted of a detailed survey of the effects of alcohol use as part of an investigation of seizure precipitation and inhibiting factors in epilepsy patients. The second part tested the effects of administering low to moderate alcohol intake in nonalcoholic epilepsy patients in an EEG laboratory equipped and staffed for intensive neurodiagnostic (CCTV/EEG) monitoring.

Clinical Survey

One hundred seventy seven cases were studied in a clinical survey of the possible association of various factors with seizure occurrence.[11] Patients were selected from the seizure clinics at the West Haven, Connecticut Veterans Administration Medical Center and Yale-New Haven Hospital. One hundred twelve patients who reported using alcohol in the preceding two years were interviewed about the frequency, quantity, and effect of their alcohol use. This information was obtained in part from the patient, but was always supplemented by interviews with family and friends, and validated by long-term clinical follow-up and medical record review. Cases were divided into three categories according to frequency and quantity of intake. Frequency of use was designated occasional, moderate, or frequent, as follows:

Occasional: Alcohol used less than once monthly
Moderate: Alcohol used more than once monthly but less than twice weekly
Frequent: Alcohol used more than twice weekly.

Quantity of intake was defined as light, moderate, or heavy, as follows:

Light: One or two drinks in an evening or on a single occasion
Moderate: Three or four drinks per occasion
Heavy: Five or more drinks per occasion.

The alcohol content of each drink was calculated as equivalent to 1¼ oz of distilled spirits (whiskey, vodka, for example), 6 oz of 12 percent wine, or a 12-oz bottle of beer. The relationship of frequency or quantity of alcohol use to seizure exacerbation was tabulated for each category. In addition, one group of patients was identified who drank heavily but infrequently, and another group was identified whose intake was light but frequent. This grouping enabled us to test whether the quantity or frequency of intake was selectively important in seizure occurrence.

Clinical Neurophysiologic Study

The clinical survey results led to a study of the neurophysiologic effects of light and moderate amounts of alcohol intake in nonalcoholic epilepsy patients. Twenty-four patients and ten normal controls volunteered to participate in the study with full understanding of the purposes and possible side-effects. The control group consisted of three female and seven male volunteers ranging in age from 19 to 35. The epilepsy patients were all men ages 20 to 55, having either partial or generalized seizure types (simple and complex partial, tonic-clonic, absence, and myoclonic). Patients with other significant medical and neurologic diseases were excluded. Participants were accustomed to using some alcoholic beverages in everyday life, at least occasionally.

The patients and controls drank either a single or double dose (0.5 or 1 ml/kg of body weight) of 95 percent ethanol diluted in fruit juice (for the average 70-kg male this amount was approximately equivalent to one or two drinks containing 2 oz of 80-proof vodka). The alcohol was consumed in 15 minutes for the single dose and 30 minutes for the double dose. Continuous EEG and clinical videotape monitoring were conducted before and during the test. Baseline blood alcohol, glucose, and electrolyte (sodium, potassium, calcium, magnesium, chloride, phosphate, and bicarbonate) levels were measured. These tests and anti-epileptic drug serum concentration measurements were repeated initially at 15-minute and at subsequent half hour intervals for 3 hours. Thereafter, samples were obtained and analyzed at 6, 12, and 24 hours. Clinical examinations were also performed at these times to identify the presence of intoxication as manifested by dysarthria, nystagmus, sleepiness, ataxia, and change in mental status. EEG recordings were performed in both control and epileptic subjects with eyes open and closed for half of each 15-minute period prior to and for the first 3 hours of the study and repeated again at 6 and 12 hours. The baseline number of spike and spike-wave discharges was counted. Each subsequent 15-minute count was expressed as a percent of this baseline rate. The background was examined simultaneously, and EEG recordings were taped for frequency power spectral analysis. All electrographic analyses were made without knowledge of whether a baseline or post-alcohol sample was being analyzed.

RESULTS

Survey Findings

The clinical survey revealed a positive association between alcohol intake and exacerbation of seizures. Of the 112 patients who had consumed alcohol in the preceding 2 years, 20 (18 percent) reported seizures more often in association with greater frequency of alcohol intake (Table 22–1). Similarly, seizure occurrence varied directly with quantity of intake (Table 22–2). When alcohol-related seizure exacerbation was noted, it occurred 6 to 24 hours after drinking in 95 percent of patients. A group of 12 patients could be identified whose drinking fell into one of the two categories: light but frequent (three patients), or heavy but infrequent (nine patients). Patients who drank frequently, but in light quantity, had no associated increase in seizures. On the other hand, eight of nine (88 percent) patients who drank moderate to large quantities of alcohol on infrequent occasions experienced seizures more often than otherwise would have occurred. The numbers are small, but using Fisher's exact test, the difference is significant ($p \leq .05$) (Table 22–3).

Table 22–1. ASSOCIATION OF SEIZURE EXACERBATIONS WITH FREQUENCY OF ALCOHOL USE

Frequency of Use	Number of Cases	Increased Seizures, Number (%)
Infrequent	82	11 (13%)
Moderate	17	7 (18%)
Frequent	13	6 (46%)
Total	112	20 (18%)

Neurophysiologic Findings

Following alcohol intake, there was a prompt rise in blood concentration, varying with the amount consumed. We found that mean peak alcohol levels were 54 mg/dl 45 minutes after the 0.5 ml/kg dose and 101 mg/dl 60 minutes after the 1 ml/kg dose. Thereafter, the alcohol concentration decreased at a rate of 18 mg/dl per hour.

No patient experienced seizures while alcohol was present in the blood. Two pa-

Table 22–2. ASSOCIATION OF SEIZURE EXACERBATIONS WITH QUANTITY OF ALCOHOL INTAKE

Quantity	Number of Cases	Increased Seizures, Number (%)
Light	72	2 (3%)
Moderate	18	3 (17%)
Heavy	22	15 (60%)
Total	112	20 (18%)

Table 22–3. RELATIONSHIP OF QUANTITY VS. FREQUENCY TO SEIZURE EXACERBATION

Intake	Number of Cases	Increased Seizures, Number (%)
Light and Frequent	3	0 (0%)
Heavy and Infrequent	9	8 (89%)

tients had myoclonic seizures while EEGs were being recorded the morning after the intake of alcohol. Both had frequently noticed this association in the past. Another patient had two focal seizures 12 hours after ingesting the alcohol. Although 20 of the 24 patients had had abnormal EEGs in the past, only 11 had a clear epileptiform EEG abnormality at the beginning of the procedure: six had focal sharp waves or spikes, and five had generalized spike-wave discharges. No activation of abnormalities occurred during alcohol intake. Rather, a prompt suppression of the interictal abnormality in both focal and generalized epileptiform patterns was observed in six patients (Fig. 22-1 and Fig. 22-2).

The suppression of paroxysmal activity was concurrent with the rise in blood alcohol level, and activity returned as the blood alcohol level declined. In three patients, epileptiform activity was suppressed initially, but increased above baseline after 12 and 24 hours (Fig. 22-3). Blood glucose, electrolyte, (including calcium and magnesium), and anti-epileptic drug serum concentrations remained unchanged throughout the 24-hour study. A modest rise in glucose level followed intake of fruit juice containing alcohol.

Background EEG changes were minimal. When alertness was maintained, no theta or delta frequencies appeared in the EEG, but frequency power spectral analysis in both normals and controls sometimes revealed a downward frequency shift in the alpha background of 1 to 2 Hz. During the second and third hour, patients tended to become sleepy, and if they were not alerted by the investigator, their EEGs demonstrated slower frequencies and patterns consistent with sleep.

Seventy-five percent of the patients and control subjects experienced a subjective "high" or awareness of the effect of the alcohol intake. Mild nystagmus, conjuncti-

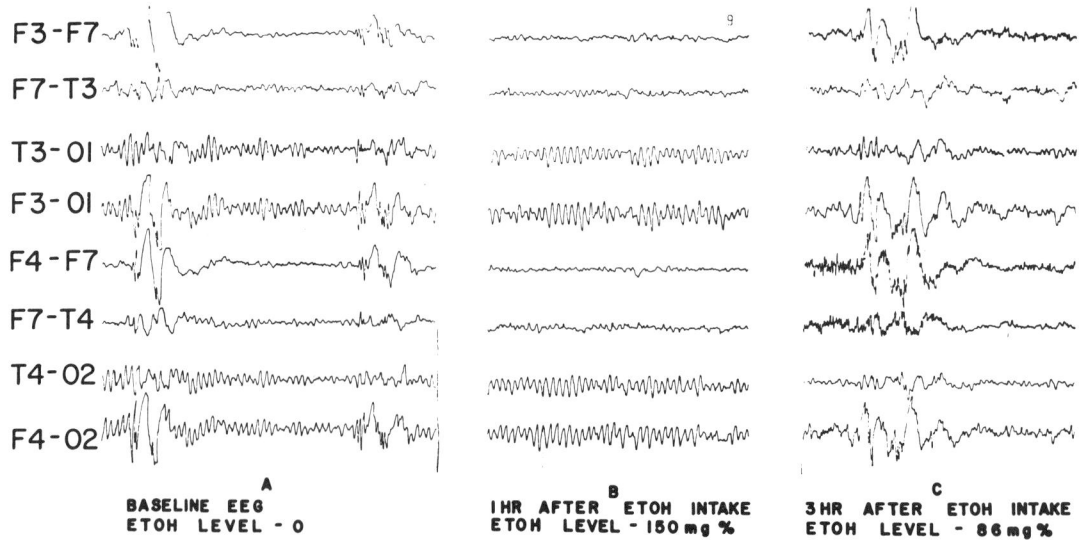

Figure 22–1. Paroxysmal spike and wave discharge (A) is transiently suppressed, (B) in a 40-year-old white male with generalized idiopathic epilepsy and tonic clonic seizures following intake of 1 ml/kg of 95% alcohol in fruit juice. (C) Abnormal discharges returned after 3 hr.

SPIKE SUPPRESSION FOLLOWING ALCOHOL INTAKE

A	B	C
BASELINE EEG BLOOD ALCOHOL LEVEL - 0	1/2 HOUR AFTER ALCOHOL INGESTED BLOOD ALCOHOL LEVEL - 65 mg%	ONE HOUR AFTER ALCOHOL INTAKE BLOOD ALCOHOL LEVEL - 49 mg%

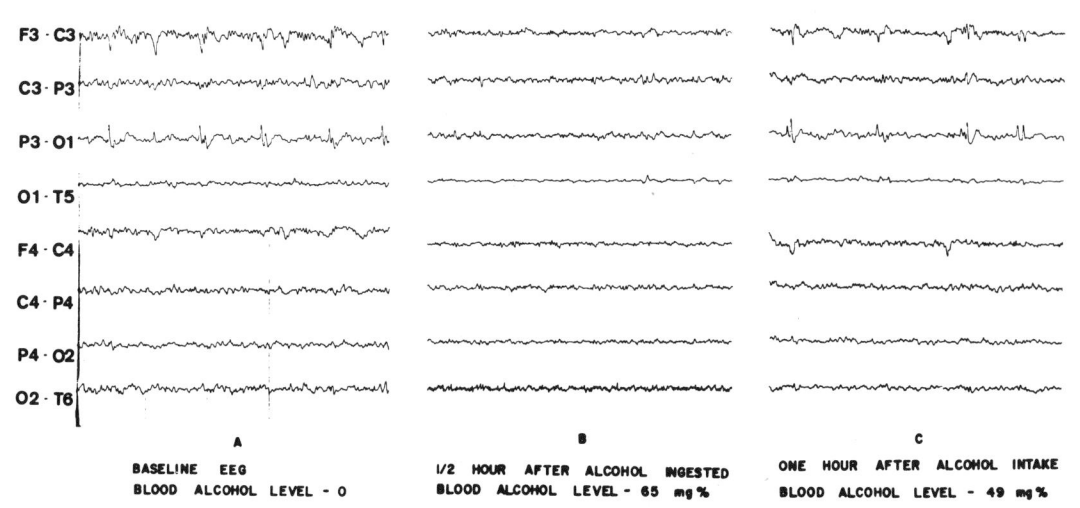

Figure 22–2. (A) Left central spikes became markedly attenuated (B) in a 50-year-old white male with partial seizures after intake of 0.5 ml/kg of alcohol. (C) Spikes returned 1 hr later with decreasing alcohol levels.

val redness, and dysarthria were also observed. These clinical signs and symptoms often appeared 15 minutes after beginning alcohol intake and were most prominent 30 to 45 minutes later, often before blood level reached its peak. The clinical effects disappeared or almost cleared 1½ to 2 hours later, despite the fact that blood alcohol levels were often still as high at that time as when signs and symptoms were first noted. These clinical effects were less apparent in patients accustomed to frequent, moderate intake of alcohol than in patients who drank only occasionally, even though blood alcohol levels were similar in the two groups.

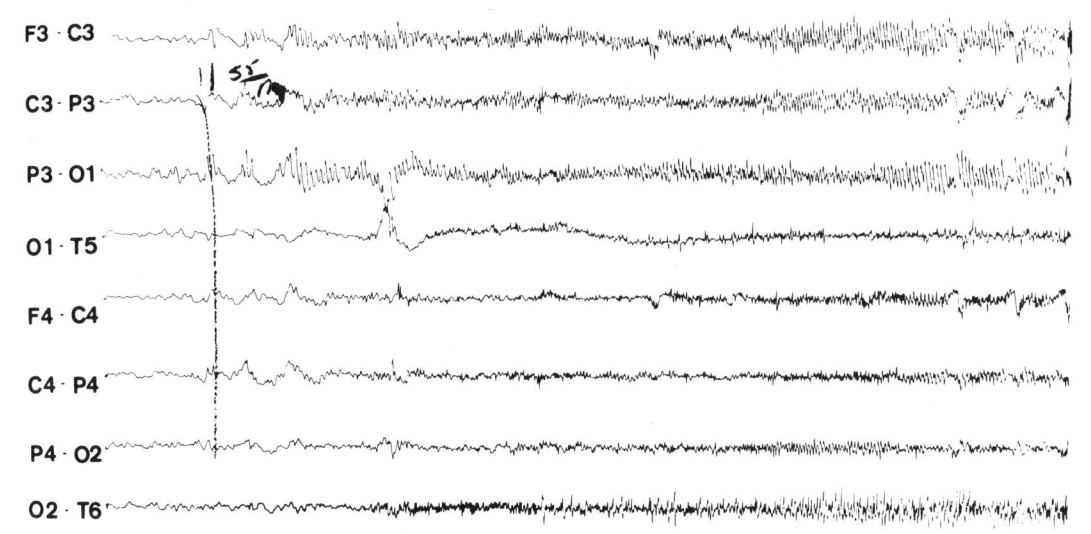

Figure 22–3. The EEG of the same patient depicted in Figure 22–2 demonstrates a partial seizure arising in the left central area 12 hr after alcohol intake.

DISCUSSION

Our clinical survey of 177 patients with epilepsy suggests that patients who consume a large quantity of alcohol on a single occasion, even if infrequently, are much more likely to have an exacerbation of seizures than would otherwise be expected. This increased risk of seizure occurrence affected 88 percent of the subgroup who drank a large amount on infrequent occasions. This finding appears to conflict with the reports of Lennox[8] and Giove and Gastaut,[2] who found infrequent seizure exacerbation with alcohol use. The different results are best explained by examining the overall pattern of seizure occurrence in patients during alcohol use. Although we found that seizures frequently occur at times of heavy alcohol intake, the overall frequency of exacerbation associated with alcohol use in our 177 patients was 12%. Of the 177 patients surveyed, 112 had used alcohol in the 2 years preceding the survey. Thus, some did not drink at all, and the majority only drank small or occasionally moderate quantities. Little relationship could be detected between drinking and seizure behavior in patients who drank only small quantities of alcohol on any given occasion, even if they drank frequently (Table 22-1, Table 22-3). Thus, the overall frequency of seizure exacerbation associated with alcohol use is quite low. On the other hand, if the quantity of alcohol taken on a specific occasion falls into the category of heavy intake, seizure exacerbation is common. The conclusion that can be drawn from our survey as well as those of other investigators[2,8] suggests that light intake of one or even two drinks on a "social" occasion will probably not precipitate seizures. This conclusion also agrees with the careful study of Höppener, Juyer, and van der Lugt.[4] These investigators conducted a long-term controlled trial with a group of inpatients with epilepsy to determine the effect of light amounts of alcohol on seizures and the EEG. Twice weekly the test subjects were given the equivalent of one or two glasses of "beer" provided as vodka disguised in orangeade. The results were assessed in a double-blind fashion so that neither the patients nor the evaluators knew when or if they received alcohol. The investigators found that light "social" alcohol intake had no effect on seizure frequency.

Our clinical neurophysiologic study of patients with epilepsy who consumed either a light or moderate amount of alcohol during intensive clinical and EEG monitoring and laboratory surveillance showed clear evidence of a transient anti-epileptic effect of alcohol during the rising and peak blood levels (Figs. 22-2 and 22-3). The changes are probably a direct alcohol effect, because no significant changes were observed in blood levels of anti-epileptic drugs, chemicals, or electrolytes. In the 11 patients who had abnormalities present at the start of the study, epileptiform EEG activity returned to baseline while blood alcohol decreased. In three subjects, the abnormality increased the morning after alcohol intake to above that recorded at the beginning of the test. The absence of a control group with epileptiform abnormalities who were given a placebo rather than alcohol, as well as the small number of patients, makes this only an anecdotal observation. However, the study does suggest that the increased excitability represents a rebound phenomenon, because such a phenomenon has also been observed in animal experimental models. Using a focal spike model, Baker and Benedict[1] found suppression with alcohol administration, and increased spike frequency with decreasing alcohol levels. Similarly, McQuarrie and Fingl[12] noted that the seizure threshold to pentylenetetrazol (PTZ) administration initially increased during alcohol administration and subsequently decreased during the withdrawal period. The suppression and rebound exacerbation of clinical and EEG epileptiform activity occurred in patients with both partial and generalized seizures. This finding suggests that the anti-epileptic effect of alcohol is exerted through a broad spectrum of action and may not affect a single neurotransmitter, receptor site, or ion channel. However, Marinacci[9] reported the activation of epileptiform activity in a large number of patients with "pathologic intoxication" after alcohol administration. Although the abnormalities were well illustrated in several of his cases, the patients clearly were awake in the baseline recording, and asleep after alcohol administration. The activation may have been due to the sleep induced by drinking rather than by the alcohol itself. In our study, patients were kept awake, and minimal changes in background frequencies were observed, in contrast to the slowing reported by Holmberg and Martens[3] and Rodin, Frohman, and Gottlieb.[13] This contrast may be explained by the forced arousal and lower dose of alcohol administered in our study.

The reason seizure exacerbation is associated with heavy alcohol consumption is not entirely clear. Our clinical neurophysiologic data suggest along with animal experimental data that alcohol has a biphasic action with an initial anti-epileptic effect, followed by a transient effect producing increased excitability. In our survey, patients who reported an association between alcohol use and exacerbation of seizures almost always indicated that their seizures usually occurred 6 to 24 hours after drinking and not while drinking. This clinical history strongly suggests a rebound effect consistent with a pattern seen during withdrawal in patients with alcohol withdrawal seizures (AWS).[5,14] Rodin, Frohman, and Gottlieb[13] postulated that the reported exacerbation of seizures in patients with epilepsy who use alcohol may be explained by the accompanying circumstances. When patients drink heavily they are often up late and become sleep deprived. They may fail to take their anti-epileptic medication, either accidentally or even intentionally. Emotional stress may also be present. All these factors together with alcohol intake can contribute to lowering the seizure threshold in these patients.[10] We found no evidence that alcohol exerted an effect on seizure exacerbation by changing anti-epileptic drug, chemical, or electrolyte levels.

In conclusion, our own and others' clinical survey and laboratory findings suggest that light alcohol intake by patients with epilepsy will only infrequently affect the frequency of seizure occurrence, and that epilepsy itself need not be the reason to prohibit all intake of alcoholic beverages. Whether the use of alcohol is otherwise an appropriate activity is beyond the scope of this study. On the other hand, the risk of seizure exacerbation steadily increases with the quantity of alcohol consumed, so that heavy intake, even if infrequent, places the patient at considerable risk of having seizures. Such alcohol use should therefore be avoided.

SUMMARY

A survey of 112 nonalcoholic epileptic patients indicated that using alcohol exacerbates seizure occurrence primarily in patients who drink moderate to heavy quantities. Attacks characteristically occurred the morning after alcohol use. We found no evidence to support the belief that light alcohol intake has any influence on seizures in nonalcoholic epileptic patients. The neurophysiologic data on 24 nonalcoholic epileptics showed that acute alcohol intake produced a transient but distinct anti-epileptic effect and did not activate EEG abnormalities. Three cases suggested that some rebound may follow 12 to 24 hours later. The suppression of EEG epileptiform activity produced by alcohol intake appeared to be a direct pharmacodynamic effect on the brain, because no changes in blood electrolyte, chemical, or anti-epileptic drug concentrations were observed.

ACKNOWLEDGMENT

Supported by the Veterans Administration Medical Research Service and NINDS Grant No. 5PONSO6208-22.

References

1. Baker, WW and Benedict, F: Effects of ethanol on chemically-induced hippocampal foci. Arch Int Pharmacodyn Ther 162:170, 1966.
2. Giove, G and Gastaut, H: Epilepsie alcoolique et d'enclenchement alcoolidesque crises chez les epileptiques. Rev Neurol 113:347, 1965.
3. Holmberg, G and Martens, S: Electroencephalographic changes in man correlated with blood alcohol concentration and some other conditions following standardized ingestion of alcohol. Quarterly Journal of Studies on Alcohol 16:411, 1955.

4. Höppener, RJ, Juyer, A, and van der Lugt, PJM: Epilepsy and alcohol: The influence of social alcohol intake on seizures and treatment in epilepsy. Epilepsia 24:459, 1983.
5. Isbell, H, et al: An experimental study of the etiology of "rumfits" and delerium tremens. Quarterly Journal of Studies on Alcohol 16:1, 1955.
6. Kaufman, IC, Marshall, C, and Walker, AE: Activated electroencephalography. Arch Neurol Psychiatr 58:533, 1947.
7. Kershman, J: The borderland of epilepsy. Arch Neurol Psychiatry 62:551, 1949.
8. Lennox, WG: Alcohol and epilepsy. Quarterly Journal of Studies on Alcohol 2:1, 1941.
9. Marinacci, AA: A special type of temporal lobe (psychomotor) seizures following ingestion of alcohol. Bull LA Neurol Soc 28:241, 1963.
10. Mattson, RH: Seizures associated with alcohol use and alcohol withdrawal. In Browne, TR and Feldman, RG (eds): Epilepsy: Diagnosis and Management. Little, Brown, & Co, Boston, 1983, p 325.
11. Mattson, R, Lerner, E, and Dix, G: Precipitating and inhibiting factors in epilepsy: A statistical study. Epilepsia 15:271, 1974.
12. McQuarrie, DG and Fingl, E: Effects of single doses and chronic administration of ethanol on experimental seizures in mice. J Pharmacol 124:264, 1958.
13. Rodin, EA, Frohman, CE, and Gottlieb, JS: Effects of acute alcohol intoxication on epileptic patients. Arch Neurol 4:103, 1961.
14. Victor, M and Brausch, J: The role of abstinence in the genesis of alcoholic epilepsy. Epilepsia 8:1, 1967.

CHAPTER 23

Joyce A. Cramer, B.S.
Richard D. Scheyer, M.D.

The Effect of Alcohol Use on Anti-Epileptic Drugs

Ethanol is the most widely used self-prescribed chemical in the world, with a history of use for medicinal and other purposes for millenia. In a teleologic sense, we can guess that the ingestion of ethanol was anticipated because of the presence of enzyme systems specifically created to metabolize this chemical. Although Adam and Eve were prohibited from eating the fruits of the garden of Eden, they were endowed with the alcohol dehydrogenase enzyme to allow enjoyment of products of fermentation! A more realistic interpretation of the presence of alcohol dehydrogenase can be explained by the need to metabolize alcohols that are byproducts of bacterial fermentation processes in the intestine. The widespread sporadic and chronic use of various quantities of ethanol places an extreme burden on the gastrointestinal system at times and affects the metabolic capacity of the liver to eliminate ethanol and numerous other endogenous and exogenous compounds. A brief overview follows of ethanol metabolism, the acute and chronic effects of ethanol use, and the interactions between ethanol and anti-epileptic drugs.

ETHANOL METABOLISM

Absorption and Distribution

Ethanol is absorbed from the small intestine, more rapidly when taken without food. The presence of food that delays gastric emptying delays the absorption of ethanol. Once absorbed, ethanol is distributed to total body water. The partition between serum and cerebrospinal fluid (CSF) is 0.9, suggesting no binding to plasma proteins.[8]

Elimination

Ethanol elimination follows a mixed-order elimination model. Stated simply, elimination is rapid when ethanol concentrations are very high, moderate and linear at moderate concentrations, and slow at low concentrations. This model is explained in part by the capacity of enzymes to transform ethanol into acetaldehyde.

The Michaelis constant (K_M) is the ethanol concentration in blood at which metabolism proceeds at 50 percent of enzyme capacity. Thus the extremes of

241

blood ethanol levels clearly affect the rate of ethanol metabolism. When ethanol levels are very high relative to K_M (enzyme capacity), metabolic conversion is near its maximum elimination rate (V_{max}). Thus, the rate of ethanol conversion is constant and independent of blood level, providing a nonlinear elimination, as in zero-order kinetics. As ethanol concentrations fall below the K_M, first-order kinetics take over. The amount of ethanol transformed is proportional to the concentration, and elimination follows a monoexponential decline. The common experience of saturating metabolism at very high ethanol levels differs from typical drug metabolism where dosage is monitored clinically and an effective, therapeutic range is anticipated. An uncontrolled, large bolus dose of ethanol produces extraordinarily high blood levels that saturate the metabolic process. Thereafter, the kinetic pattern between zero-order and first-order kinetics is affected. This effect can be described in the Michaelis-Menten equation. Use of a mixed order elimination rate model is based on the presence of two types of ethanol-metabolizing enzymes. The high-K_M system is active at higher ethanol levels and the low-K_M system is active at lower levels.[5]

Wilkinson and associates[49] studied the elimination of ethanol after four doses ranging from 10 to 40 g/70 kg. Maximal concentrations reached 160 to 770 mg/liter. They found that elimination capacity averaged 7.5 g/hour (V_{max}) and that the concentration at 50 percent of V_{max} was 82 mg/liter (K_M). The half-life of ethanol elimination after overdosage has been calculated at 4 hours[34] to 4.5 hours.[14] In these cases, intoxicating blood ethanol concentrations were 15 g/liter and 7.8 g/liter, respectively, and were cleared at 6 liters/hour/70 kg in predominantly first-order elimination. These reports confirm that an enhanced elimination rate results at very high blood ethanol levels.

Biotransformation

Ethanol is converted to acetaldehyde by two enzyme systems. Alcohol dehydrogenase (ADH) is the major pathway for oxidation of ethanol. ADH transfers hydrogen from ethanol to nicotinamide adenine dinucleotide (NAD), thereby reducing it to NADH and producing acetaldehyde. The second enzyme system for ethanol metabolism is the microsomal ethanol oxidizing system (MEOS). ADH is not an inducible system whereas MEOS is. This inducibility is similar to that seen in its related hepatic microsomal drug-metabolizing enzymes.

The presence of MEOS was first noticed 20 years ago by Lieber and DeCarli,[28] who reported that chronic ethanol feeding of rats caused proliferation of the smooth endoplasmic reticulum. They also found a cytochrome-P450-dependent system that also oxidizes ethanol to acetaldehyde. In this system, nicotinamide adenine dinucleotide phosphate (NADP) contributes hydrogen during reduction to NADPH, cytochrome P450-reductase, and cytochrome P450. A water molecule is produced during the oxidation of ethanol to acetaldehyde.[48] Thus, MEOS is similar to other drug-metabolizing (mixed-function oxidase system) enzymes in its requirement for cytochrome P450, NADPH, and oxygen.

Induction of MEOS is similar to the known effect of drugs such as phenobarbital on drug-metabolizing enzymes.[44] Brodie and associates[2] described the role of the hepatic microsomal system in the oxidation of many drugs. Gillette, Davis, and Sasame[12] defined the role of cytochrome P450 in the oxidation of drugs. Nine forms of cytochrome P450 have been identified in animals treated with drugs.[29] Chronic ethanol administration was shown to induce cytochrome P450 in the same manner as some drugs.[44] The duration of ethanol use has been shown to affect induction. Morgan, Devine, and Skett[33] demonstrated that a unique isoenzyme of cytochrome P450 develops during ethanol treatment. This reaction differs from the relatively nonspecific induction produced by drugs such as phenobarbital.

Cytochrome P450 is necessary in the oxidative metabolism of numerous compounds. The fact that drugs, steroids, and alcohol all serve as substrates for cytochrome P450 suggests that interactions may occur among these compounds. Estabrook and associates[11] showed that cytochrome P450 from three sources (liver and adrenal cortex microsomes and adrenal mitochondria) reacts to the addition of drugs, steroids, and alcohol.

Thus, the differences between ADH and MEOS include the microsomal presence of MEOS, its activity at pH 7.4, its requirement for oxygen and NADPH as a cofactor, and its inhibition by carbon dioxide. In addition, MEOS is induced during chronic ethanol intake to 2 to 3 times its normal state. ADH is present in hepatic cytosol, and is optimal at pH 10 or 11, and requires NAD as a cofactor. Greater MEOS activity can account for half to two thirds of the increase of ethanol clearance. The remainder is probably due to ADH enhanced activity.

Metabolism of Acetaldehyde

Ethanol is metabolized to acetaldehyde by ADH and MEOS, which is oxidized to acetate by aldehyde dehydrogenase (ALDH). The conversion of the acetaldehyde metabolite is not a rate-limiting factor in the normal ethanol oxidation system. The active site of ALDH is a sulfhydryl. Disulfiram (Antabuse) utilizes this sulfhydryl group to form disulfide bridges, thereby irreversibly inhibiting the enzyme. Thereafter, elevated acetaldehyde levels cause severe side-effects that reinforce the prohibition against ethanol ingestion. The genetic variant in ALDH that causes approximately 50 percent of Asian people to be intolerant to alchol is related to an ALDH isoenzyme that limits the rate of conversion to acetaldehyde.[15]

Metabolic Differences and Other Factors

Skett and Paterson[45] described sex differences in the effects of phenobarbital and ethanol on hepatic metabolism of drugs. The actions of these drugs were shown to be related to sex-specific induction, inhibition, and repression of enzymes. The animals' hormonal status were shown to influence ethanol metabolism. The interaction of ethanol and sex steroid hormones is well known, and ethanol treatment of animals has been shown to reduce testosterone levels.[1]

Sturtevant and Sturtevant[47] described the chronopharmacokinetics of ethanol. Their work followed Saar and Paulus'[40] 1941 finding that ethanol elimination is slower during sleep. In a study of five male volunteers assessed over a 30-hour period and administered ethanol every 4 hours, Sturtevant and associates[46] discovered significant differences in the rate of ethanol elimination according to time of day. During late evening hours, from approximately 10 PM to 4 AM, ethanol elimination is slowest. More rapid rate of elimination occurs mid-morning, late afternoon, and early evening. Their calculations were based on linear, zero-order decay, because they restricted their attention to the linear portion of the curve above 10 mg/dl to 20 mg/dl.

The effect of food on ethanol metabolism is important. As mentioned, absorption is slowed in the presence of food. Brown, Forrest, and Roscoe[3] demonstrated a 25 percent increase in ethanol elimination when fructose was infused into intoxicated patients. Heavy cigarette smoking almost doubled the rate of ethanol elimination in chronic drinkers.[24] Dietary changes affect the quality and quantity of hepatic cytochrome P450 stimulation during ethanol use. Sitar and Gordon[44] showed that no differences result from lipid and carbohydrate dietary changes, but demonstrated that the duration of alcohol use influences cytochrome P450 induction.

The presence of severe liver disease compromises ethanol metabolism after excessive drinking because of reduced hepatic ADH content. An inadequate amount of this major enzyme decreases ethanol clearance. However, metabolism and clearance are not affected by cirrhosis. Similarly, alcoholic fatty liver and alcoholic hepatitis do not alter ethanol metabolism or clearance. Nevertheless, Hall[13] indicated that ADH activity may decrease with chronic alcohol use, even without liver damage.

ACUTE EFFECTS OF ETHANOL

Ingesting a large quantity of ethanol over a short period of time produces an extreme condition in the body. Blood ethanol levels often exceed 100 mg/dl to 200 mg/dl. The overload of substrate on both the ADH and MEOS enzyme systems is overwhelming, leading to inhibition of the microsomal enzyme system. Cytochrome P450 is blocked during ethanol binding to its heme ring.[18] The microsomal electron transport system involved in drug metabolism is slowed during the acute phase of ethanol overload.[39] Not only is ethanol metabolism decreased because of blockage of the MEOS system, but other drugs that use the same microsomal monooxygenase system also are metabolized more slowly, partly because of competitive inhibition. This acute action enhances the pharmacodynamic effect of drugs and prolongs their half-lives. For example, barbiturate elimination is slowed, thereby extending the duration of effect of these hypnosedative drugs. Ethanol intoxication is exacerbated by the potential for increased toxicity from drugs and alcohol used concomitantly (Table 23-1).

A convenient nomogram used in emergency departments is to expect clearance of approximately 20 mg% of ethanol/hour. This formula assumes a linear, zero-order elimination ($K_M = 10$) from an intoxicating concentration of ethanol.

CHRONIC EFFECTS OF ETHANOL

The initial effect of inhibition of microsomal enzyme activity is transient, lasting no longer than 6 hours.[36] As the competitive binding to cytochrome P450 diminishes after approximately 12 hours, induction develops with a slow rise in activity. Chronic ethanol use results in hypertrophy of the smooth endoplasmic reticulum, with increased cytochrome P450 isozyme production. MEOS and other monooygenase enzymes capable of metabolizing drugs are also increased. Thus, ethanol intake prepares the liver to increase its capacity for both ethanol and drug metabolism. Hoensch[18] demonstrated that induction depends on sex, duration and amount of ethanol, diet, the extent of liver damage, and genetic factors. Studies of endoplasmic reticulum have shown that induction is reversible on abstinence from ethanol for at least 2 or 3 weeks.[18]

ANTI-EPILEPTIC DRUG ENZYME INDUCTION

Anti-epileptic drugs, including carbamazepine, phenobarbital, phenytoin, and primidone, are potent enzyme inducers. These drugs are metabolized by the monooxygenase system in which cytochrome P450, NADPH, and molecular oxygen requirements are shared with the MEOS system. The relative enzyme-inducing potencies of these drugs were described by Perucca and associates,[35] in comparison with antipyrine clearance and urinary excretion of D-glucaric acid (D-GA). In this study, patients had used carbamazepine, phenobarbital, phenytoin, and primidone on a long-term basis, and were found to have significantly higher antipyrine clearance levels and increased D-GA excretion compared with untreated control subjects. A dose-dependent effect was found within the therapeutic dose range. In contrast, no enzyme-inducing effect was found for valproate in either index measured. Phenobarbital caused the greatest change in both measures, suggesting that it has the highest potency of these four drugs, although carbamazepine, phenytoin, and primidone were not significantly less effective. These four drugs were approximately equipotent inducers. The lack of additive and synergistic effects when drugs were administered in combination suggests that maximal induction occurs within the usual therapeutic dose range. Although valproate can inhibit the oxidative metabolism of ethosuximide, phenobarbital, and phenytoin,[25] it has not

TABLE 23–1. EFFECTS OF ETHANOL ON METABOLISM

	Acute	Chronic
ETOH Metabolism	Inhibit	Induce
Drug Metabolism	Inhibit	Induce
Pharmacodynamics	↑ effect	↑ tolerance
Action on P450	Reversible binding	Competing substrate
Reversibility	P450 binding ↓ as ETOH level ↑	↓ Smooth endoplasmic reticulum if abstinent

been shown to stimulate enzymes to the degree demonstrated for other major anti-epileptic drugs.

INTERACTIONS BETWEEN ETHANOL AND ANTI-EPILEPTIC DRUGS

Mechanism

Ethanol and anti-epileptic drugs are metabolized by the mixed-function oxygenase enzyme system located in liver microsomes. The function of the enzyme system is to convert fat-soluble (lipophilic) compounds into water-soluble (hydrophilic) compounds, which are readily excreted in urine. The major processes by which this conversion takes place include hydroxylation, demethylation, and glucuronidation. During acute administration of ethanol, these metabolic processes are inhibited, thereby retarding drug elimination. During chronic ethanol use, the general increase in microsomal enzyme systems enhances the metabolism of both ethanol and other molecules, including anti-epileptic drugs. Thus, interactions occur at the microsomal level.

The relative enzyme-inducing properties of various drugs depend on lipid solubility; affinity for cytochrome P450 binding; long duration of reaction with the enzyme system; and high concentration in the liver or high affinity for the enzyme.[37,38] Drugs with short half-lives are oxidized rapidly and detached from the enzyme after conversion. This mechanism suggests a reason phenobarbital might be a better inducer than short-acting barbiturates, even though phenobarbital has lower lipid solubility. It is estimated that phenobarbital pretreatment of animals enhances synthesis of microsomal enzymes within 3 to 5 hours.[36] Primary induction is in the mitochondria where gamma-ALA (amino levulinic acid) synthetase levels increase either by enhanced synthesis, or in some cases, by decreased degradation. Proliferation of the smooth endoplasmic reticulum and hepatic microsomal enzymes increases affect processes other than alcohol and drug metabolism. For example, thyroid function, calcium metabolism, regulation of sex hormone, folate, and bilirubin levels, and omega oxidation of fatty acids are all affected by either stimulation or inhibition at this locus of action. Any drug or molecule that acts as a substrate to bind with the oxidized form of cytochrome P450 hemoprotein can affect the metabolism of numerous compounds. Molecules that increase or decrease microsomal and cytochrome P450 activity similarly affect overall drug metabolism (Table 23–1).

Concomitant Treatment

Conney and associates[4] presented preliminary evidence that pretreatment of animals with drugs such as phenobarbital stimulates liver microsomal enzymes. They concluded that accelerated drug metabolism caused a corresponding diminution in drug action by stimulating liver protein synthesis. These experiments suggested that pretreatment with any drug that is an enzyme inducer affects the pharmacologic activity of other drugs administered concomitantly. Mezey and Robles[31] showed that the enhanced ethanol clearance after pretreatment with phenobarbital is not accompanied by enhanced activity of ADH or MEOS or by increased liver size. Neither phenobarbital pretreatment nor alcohol use affect the quantity of ADH available to metabolize ethanol.[43] However, ADH may be inhibited by high acetaldehyde levels if ALDH is inhibited by phenobarbital.[17] Acetaldehyde can bind to serum proteins, thereby affecting attachment of anti-epileptic drugs that bind to the same site on albumin. Conversely, the inhibitory effect of comparative enzyme saturation was demonstrated by Curry and Scales,[7] who found that when phenobarbital was administered with ethanol, phenobarbital peak concentrations were reached earlier and were higher than when phenobarbital was administered alone.

Pharmacodynamic Effects

The pharmacodynamic effects of enhanced metabolism include increased tolerance (e.g., to barbiturate sedation) and dose-related side-effects of other drugs. Drug clearance is affected when multiple compounds are administered concomitantly, thus increasing morbidity and mortality. The combination of phenobarbital and alcohol has lethal effects. Mean blood ethanol level in patients consuming both phenobarbital and ethanol before death has been shown to be 175 mg/dl, far lower than lethal levels of ethanol used alone (500–800 mg/dl).[9] Although drug-metabolizing capacity is increased after ethanol pretreatment, actual clearance rates of drugs may not be enhanced because ethanol is a competing substrate for the monooxygenase system. As alcohol use is discontinued, drug metabolism may then increase (because no competing substrate is present), an effect that can alter the pharmacodynamic effect of the drug until disinduction occurs. These effects can be alleviated by continuing to consume ethanol or by carefully adjusting drug dose during the discontinuation, disinduction phase. An example is the 25 percent decrease in half-life of pentobarbital after ethanol feeding for four weeks in animals.[23,32]

Pharmacokinetic Factors

Decreases in liver blood flow because of alcoholic liver disease diminish the first-pass effect of drugs with high intrinsic clearance, such as oral diazepam and chlordiazepoxide.[27]

Although ethanol is not protein bound, in the presence of liver disease it can affect the pharmacokinetics of anti-epileptic drugs, because liver disease causes albumin changes. In patients with cirrhosis, hypoalbuminemia causes reduction in protein binding of most anti-epileptic drugs. Phenobarbital (50 percent bound) is least affected by this problem, but carbamazepine (75 percent), phenytoin (90 percent), and valproate (80–95 percent) are highly bound to albumin and have lower total steady-state serum concentrations when serum protein is reduced. The higher free-drug fraction results in increased hepatic clearance for phenytoin, carbamazepine, and valproate because these drugs have low extraction ratios. Interpretation of drug serum concentrations are problematic in hypoalbuminemia. Phenytoin dosing increases could saturate metabolism and produce excessive side-effects. Lower carbamazepine serum concentrations should be interpreted in relation to possible autoinduction during this stage of enhanced clearance. Valproate has variable binding to serum albumin and its clearance is associated with free rather than total valproate levels.[6] Enzyme induction as well as protein binding must be considered when serum concentrations are interpreted.

Clinical Aspects

Lieber[26] stated that it is essential to know a patient's history of alcohol use and abuse when prescribing drugs because "even abstaining alcoholics need doses different from that required by nondrinkers to achieve therapeutic levels of certain drugs." Differences in drug metabolizing capacity were studied by Kater and associates,[22] who compared groups of abstinent control subjects and alcoholic patients. Total phenytoin serum concentrations were almost 50 percent lower in the alcoholic than the control group, when tested 24 hours after the last dose. The dimension of enhanced drug metabolism was commensurate with the similarly doubled rate of elimination of ethanol in alcoholic patients demonstrated by Kater, Carulli, and Iber.[23] The comparison of abstinent control subjects who had slow ethanol clearance with alcoholics studied after several months of abstinence who also had normal clearance rates, indicated that rapid ethanol clearance in actively alcoholic patients is directly attributable to recent alcohol consumption and its inducing capacity. The duration of effect was estimated to be one or two months.[21] Iber and associates[20] evaluated four alcoholic patients while the patients were drinking and a month after they stopped. In two subjects, the nine-day course of phenytoin yielded significantly lower phenytoin serum concentrations during the initial period than during the later abstinent phase. Hooper and associates[19] evaluated the effects of liver disease on phenytoin binding in 13 patients finding a mean 15.9 percent free fraction. Review of these data, however, suggested that only six patients definitely had alcohol-related liver disease, and in these patients mean 12.7 percent free phenytoin fraction were found. Normal patients had 10.8 percent free phenytoin fraction. Much of the increase in the free fraction could have been attributable to lower plasma albumin levels in these patients.

A study of the effects of brief and chronic alcohol use on phenytoin kinetics showed that phenytoin clearance is the same as that reported for nonalcoholic, normal subjects.[41] Thus, at the end of ethanol use, phenytoin clearance appeared similar to that in nondrinkers (as reported in the literature), but rose during the alcohol withdrawal period to a significantly higher clearance rate (0.023 vs. 0.033 liter/kg/hour, $p<.05$). Median phenytoin serum concentrations were 7 μg/ml during ethanol ingestion, 5.6 μg/ml during early withdrawal ($p<.05$, 4–6 days after alcohol use), and 4.7 μg/ml during late withdrawal ($p<.05$, 14–16 days after use). Free phenytoin levels corresponded closely with changes in total drug serum concentrations. Sandor and associates[41] attributed the higher phenytoin level prior to ethanol withdrawal to acute enzyme inhibition. Clearance increased by 50 percent six days after discontinuing alcohol administration. Review of Sandor's data suggests that phenytoin clearance increased after ethanol was removed as a competitive substrate. If so, the previously enhanced enzyme system was fully accessible for phenytoin metabolism during partial disinduction after ethanol administration was discontinued. These data differ from Schmidt's[42] data. Schmidt assessed phenytoin clearance during acute co-administration of phenytoin and ethanol *versus* administration of phenytoin alone. He found no difference in phenytoin half-life in five normal subjects; however, the opportunity for enzyme induction was not available in this study of acute administration. DeLeacy and associates[10] also saw no statistically significant effect of alcohol use on phenytoin serum concentrations. However, only 2 percent of their subjects were heavy drinkers, 13 percent were light drinkers, and the remainder were abstinent or irregular, light drinkers.

The benzodiazepines (diazepam, chlordiazepoxide, and oxazepam) are widely prescribed so that enormous potential for interactions with ethanol exists. Hayes and associates[16] found that diazepam levels were significantly higher for one to four hours post-dose when administered with ethanol instead of water. It was not clear whether enhanced absorption or inhibited metabolism was the mechanism. Lucas and associates[30] demonstrated that acetaldehyde adducts enhanced the binding capacity of albumin for diazepam but not for phenytoin. Thus, increased diazepam binding can be observed when acetaldehyde levels are high, as they are in chronic alcoholics.

TREATMENT OF EPILEPTIC ALCOHOLIC PATIENTS WITH ANTI-EPILEPTIC DRUGS

Prescribing patterns for epileptic patients must be based on the aforementioned enhanced enzyme capacities for drug metabolism. If acute therapy to prevent or control withdrawal seizures (AWS) is necessary, the dose must be adjusted to allow for acute inhibition of metabolism during intoxication, in order to avoid adverse pharmacodynamic effects. Particular caution is necessary if phenobarbital is used because of its long (96 hour) half-life. Excessive quantities of phenobarbital administered as acute therapy remain in the body for many days. Some physicians prefer to use a large loading dose with no follow-up treatment, allowing the drug to self-taper. A drug with a short half-life given in multiple, smaller-than-usual dosages may be a better choice for careful titration for the patient facing AWS. Dosages prescribed for long-term therapy should not be based on those prescribed for acute therapy. A low dose that is adequate for treatment of acute problems during enzyme inhibition may be inadequate for long-term use. Later chapters describe specific treatment plans for benzodiazepines, phenytoin, phenobarbital, carbamazepine, valproate, and paraldehyde. All these drugs are commonly used for acute treatment, and each compound has advantages and disadvantages.

If a patient is susceptible to further seizures after ethanol withdrawal, long-term use of an anti-epileptic drug may be advisable. As I have described, the concurrent chronic use of ethanol stimulates the microsomal enzyme system so that metabolism of anti-epileptic drugs is enhanced. Thus, larger than usual doses of any anti-epileptic drug selected for chronic therapy may be necessary. For example, 600 mg per day of phenytoin may be necessary in order to establish drug serum concentrations in the range of 10 to 20 μg/ml. Similarly, the shortened half-life of drugs suggests a need for multiple daily doses instead of single daily doses. Dividing the daily dose into two or three aliquots will reduce interdose fluctuations in serum concentrations and provide an approximate steady-state drug level.

To conclude, the multiple metabolic pathways and rates of elimination of ethanol produce significant variability in metabolism and pharmacodynamic effects on other drugs. Understanding the metabolism and interactions between ethanol and anti-epileptic drugs allows the physician to select appropriate drugs and doses to treat alcoholic epileptic patients.

SUMMARY

Ethanol is a self-administered chemical that is widely used as a social drug and that can affect the metabolism of prescribed drugs. Elimination is nonlinear and zero order when blood ethanol levels are high, changing to first-order as levels fall. Ethanol is metabolized to acetaldehyde by two enzyme systems. The primary pathway for biotransformation is the ADH system. The secondary pathway is MEOS. This oxidative system is similar to that operative in anti-epileptic drug metabolism and uses cytochrome P450, NADPH, and oxygen. MEOS is inducible with chronic ethanol use, as the monooxygenase system is inducible by anti-epileptic drugs: carbamazepine, phenobarbital, and phenytoin. The acute effect of ethanol is to inhibit oxidative systems during competitive binding to cytochrome P450. Induction develops later, leading to enhanced oxidative capacity of ethanol and anti-epileptic drugs. Pharmacodynamic drug effects are enhanced with acute and diminished with chronic ethanol use. The dose of barbiturate that produces little effect in routine use can cause lethal sedation in an intoxicated person. Rapid phenytoin clearance in chronic alcoholics provides subtherapeutic serum concentrations at standard doses.

ACKNOWLEDGMENT

Supported by the Veterans Administration Medical Research Service.

References

1. Badr, FM and Bartke, A: Effects of ethyl alcohol on plasma testosterone level in mice. Steroids 23:921, 1974.
2. Brodie, BB, et al: Detoxification of drugs and other foreign compounds by liver microsomes. Science 121:603, 1955.
3. Brown, SS, Forrest, JAH, and Roscoe, P: A controlled trial of fructose in the treatment of acute alcoholic intoxication. Lancet 2:898, 1972.

4. Conney, AH, et al: Adaptive increases in drug-metabolizing enzymes induced by phenobarbital and other drugs. J Pharmacol Exp Ther 130:1, 1960.
5. Crabb, DW, Bosron WF, and Li, TK: Ethanol metabolism. Pharmacol Ther 34:59, 1987.
6. Cramer, JA, et al: Variable free and total valproic acid concentrations in sole and multidrug therapy. In Levy, RH, et al (eds): Metabolism of Antiepileptic Drugs. Raven Press, New York, 1984, p 105.
7. Curry, SH and Scales, AH: Interaction of phenobarbitone and ethanol studied from dose-response curves and drug concentrations in blood. J Pharm Pharmacol 25:142, 1973.
8. Danhof, M, Hisaoka, M, and Levy, G: Effect of experimental liver diseases on the pharmacodynamics of phenobarbital and ethanol in rats. J Pharm Sci 74:321, 1985.
9. Deitrich, RA and Petersen, DR: Interaction of ethanol with other drugs. In Majchrowicz, E and Noble, EP (eds): Biochemistry and Pharmacology of Ethanol. Plenum Press, New York, 1979, p 283.
10. DeLeacy, EA, et al: Effects of subject's sex, and intake of tobacco, alcohol and oral contraceptives on plasma phenytoin levels. Br J Clin Pharmacol 17:33, 1979.
11. Estabrook, RW, et al: Drugs, alcohol and sex hormones: A molecular perspective of the receptivity of cytochrome P-450. Ann NY Acad Sci 312:27, 1973.
12. Gillette, JR, Davis, DC, and Sasame, HA: Cytochrome P-450 and its role in drug metabolism. Ann Rev Pharmacol 12:57, 1972.
13. Hall, P: Alcoholic Liver Disease: Pathology, Epidemiology and Clinical Aspects. John Wiley & Sons, New York, 1985.
14. Hammond, KB, Rumack, B, and Rodgerson, DO: Blood ethanol: A report of unusually high levels in a living patient. JAMA 226:63, 1973.
15. Harada, S, Agarwal, DP, and Goedde, HW: Electrophoretic and biochemical studies of human aldehyde dehydrogenase isozymes in various tissues. Life Sci 26:1773, 1980.
16. Hayes, SL, et al: Ethanol and oral diazepam absorption. N Engl J Med 296:186, 1977.
17. Hobara, N, Watanabe, A, and Nagashima, H: Effect of various central nervous system-acting drugs on ethanol and acetaldehyde metabolism in rats. Pharmacology 30:333, 1985.
18. Hoensch, H: Ethanol as enzyme inducer and inhibitor. Pharmacol Ther 33:121, 1987.
19. Hooper, WD, et al: Plasma protein binding of diphenylhydantoin effects of sex hormones, renal and hepatic disease. Clin Pharmacol Ther 15:276, 1974.
20. Iber, FL, et al: Comparison of steady state phenytoin metabolism in alcoholics immediately after drinking ceases and three weeks later. Currents in Alcoholism 7:109, 1979.
21. Iber, FL: Drug metabolism in heavy consumers of ethyl alcohol. Clin Pharmacol Ther 22:735, 1977.
22. Kater, RMH, et al: Increased rate of clearance of drugs from the circulation of alcoholics. Am J Med Sci 258:35, 1969.
23. Kater, RMH, Carulli, N, and Iber, FL: Differences in the rate of ethanol metabolism in recently drinking alcoholic and nondrinking subjects. Am J Clin Nutr 22:1608, 1969.
24. Kopun, M and Popping, P: The kinetics of ethanol absorption and elimination in twins and supplementary repetitive experiments in singleton subjects. Eur J Clin Pharmacol 11:337, 1977.
25. Levy, RH: Drug absorption, distribution, and elimination. In Woodbury, DM, Penry, JK, and Pippenger, CE (eds): Antiepileptic Drugs. Raven Press, New York, 1982.
26. Lieber, C: Interaction of ethanol with drug toxicity. Am J Gastroenterol 74:313, 1980.
27. Lieber, CS: Medical Disorders of Alcoholism: Pathogenesis and Treatment. WB Saunders, Philadelphia, 1982.
28. Lieber, CS and DeCarli, LM: Ethanol oxidation by hepatic microsomes: Adaptive increase after ethanol feeding. Science 162:917, 1968.
29. Lu, AY and West, SB: Multiplicity of mammalian microsomal cytochromes. Pharmacol Rev 31:277, 1980.
30. Lucas, D, et al: Acetaldehyde adducts with serum proteins: Effect on diazepam and phenytoin binding. Pharmacology 32:134, 1986.
31. Mezey, E and Robles, EA: Effects of phenobarbital administration on rates of ethanol clearance and on ethanol-oxidizing enzymes in man. Gastroenterology 66:248, 1974.
32. Misra, PS, et al: Increase of ethanol, meprobamate and pentobarbital metabolism after chronic ethanol administration in man and in rats. Am J Med Sci 51:346, 1971.
33. Morgan, ET, Devine, M, and Skett, P: Changes in the rat hepatic mixed function oxidase system associated with chronic ethanol vapor inhalation. Biochem Pharmacol 30:595, 1981.
34. O'Neill J, et al: Survival after high blood alcohol levels. Arch Intern Med 144:641, 1984.
35. Perucca, E, et al: A comparative study of the relative enzyme inducing properties of anticonvulsant drugs in epileptic patients. Br J Clin Pharmacol 18:401, 1984.
36. Pirola, RC: Drug Metabolism and Alcohol, pp. 31–54. University Park Press, Baltimore, 1978.
37. Remmer, H, et al: Drug interaction with hepatic microsomal cytochrome. Mol Pharmacol 2:187, 1966.
38. Remmer, H, and Merker, HJ: Drug-induced changes in the liver endoplasmic reticulum: Association with drug-metabolizing enzymes. Science 152:1657, 1963.
39. Rubin, E, et al: Induction and inhibition of hepatic microsomal and mitochondrial enzymes by ethanol. Lab Invest 22:569, 1970.
40. Saar, H and Paulus, W: Experimentelle untersuchunger uber die ausscheidung des alkohols im schlaf. Deutsche Zeitschrift Gesamte Gerichtliche Medizin 35:28, 1941.
41. Sandor, P, et al: Effect of short- and long-term alcohol use on phenytoin kinetics in chronic alcoholics. Clin Pharmacol Ther 30:390, 1981.
42. Schmidt, D: Effect of ethanol intake on phenytoin metabolism in volunteers. Experientia 31:1313, 1975.
43. Schwarzmann, V and Berthaux, N: The action of

barbiturates upon liver alcohol dehydrogenase: Their interference with alcohol metabolism. Biomedicine 21:26, 1974.
44. Sitar, DS and Gordon, ER: Effect of diet and drugs on the qualitative and quantitative distribution of cytochrome P-450 in rat liver. Can J Physiol Pharmacol 58:331, 1980.
45. Skett, P and Paterson, P: Sex differences in the effects of microsomal enzyme inducers on hepatic phase I drug metabolism in the rat. Biochem Pharmacol 34:3533, 1985.
46. Sturtevant, FM, et al: Chronopharmacokinetics of ethanol II: Circadian rhythm in rate of blood level decline in a single subject. Naunyn Schmiedebergs Arch Pharmacol 293:203, 1976.
47. Sturtevant, FM and Sturtevant, R: Chronopharmacokinetics of ethanol. In Majchrowicz, E and Noble, EP (eds): Biochemisry and Pharmacology of Ethanol. Plenum Press, New York, 1979, p 27.
48. Teschke, R and Gellert, J: Hepatic microsomal ethanol-oxidizing systems (MEOS): Metabolic aspects and clinical implications. Alcoholism: Clinical and Experimental Research 10:20S, 1986.
49. Wilkinson, PK, et al: Pharmacokinetics of ethanol after oral administration in the fasting state. J Pharmacokinet Biopharm 5:207, 1977.

PART IV

Prevention and Treatment of Alcohol-Related Seizures

CHAPTER 24

Orrin Devinsky, M.D.
Roger J. Porter, M.D.

Alcohol and Seizures: Principles of Treatment

Seizures associated with alcoholism are common and necessitate a systematic approach to evaluation and treatment. The vast majority of seizures in alcoholic patients are caused by withdrawal and occur 7 to 48 hours after cessation of drinking. Other causes of seizures may be important during either intoxication or withdrawal states and include head trauma (*e.g.*, subdural hematoma), drug ingestion (*e.g.*, cocaine), drug withdrawal (*e.g.*, barbiturates), meningitis, and metabolic disorders (*e.g.*, hypomagnesemia) (Table 24-1). Alcohol withdrawal seizures (AWS) usually occur in chronic alcoholics between the ages of 30 and 60. Alcoholic patients under the age of 25 often have idiopathic or post-traumatic seizure disorders.[26] There are also nonalcoholic patients with seizure disorders for whom consumption of alcohol over an evening or weekend leads to mild withdrawal—often resulting in noncompliance with antiepileptic drug regimens—and an exacerbation of seizures.[14]

The initial management of seizures in an alcoholic should focus on stabilizing vital signs and determining the cause of the seizures. Because alcohol withdrawal is the most common etiology, especially in patients with severe ethanol abuse, the physician should explore symptoms and signs of chronic alcoholism during the history and physical and laboratory examinations (Table 24-2). A thorough history of ethanol, sedative/hypnotic, and central nervous system (CNS) stimulant use should be obtained for all patients who have had a seizure of unknown cause, including the employed and affluent. If possible, both the patient and available witnesses should be questioned about the seizure to determine if there was: a change in the patient's medical or neurologic status prior to the seizure; a precipitant; an aura or focal motor onset; loss of consciousness or automatism; head trauma during the ictus; or focal weakness or other deficit after the seizure. The medical and neurologic examinations should be as complete as possible, and include inspection of the skull for signs of head trauma, and evaluation of focal neurologic abnormalities that suggest a treatable CNS disorder. Because the initial evaluation is often performed during the postictal period and serves to exlude life-threatening disorders, a follow-up history and examination may reveal important new findings.

INTOXICATION

Alcohol is not a convulsant. Therefore, seizures during acute intoxication are not

Table 24–1. CAUSES OF SEIZURES IN PATIENTS WITH ALCOHOLISM

Alcohol withdrawal

Withdrawal from other sedative/hypnotic drugs
    Barbiturates
    Benzodiazepines

Drug intoxication
    Cocaine
    Amphetamines
    Phencyclidine

Head trauma
    Contusion
    Intracerebral hematoma
    Subdural hematoma

Stroke

Infections
    Meningitis
    Cerebral abscess

Metabolic
    Hypomagnesemia
    Hyponatremia
    Hypoglycemia

caused directly by alcohol but by other mechanisms (Table 24–1). In addition, relative alcohol withdrawal may occur despite continued drinking if there has been a substantial reduction in total intake. Thus, the smell of liquor on the breath and a history of recent moderate ethanol consumption do not exclude alcohol withdrawal. The clinical features, evaluation, and treatment of acute alcohol intoxication are relevant to the problem of seizures in alcoholic patients because seizures may occur in inebriated patients.

The signs and symptoms of acute intoxication depend on the amount and rate of consumption, rate of absorption, tolerance, whether the patient has ingested other drugs, and the coexistence of systemic and CNS disorders. Cognitive impairment and emotional lability, nystagmus, dysarthria, and ataxia may result from acute ethanol toxicity. Focal neurologic findings suggest that intoxication coexists with structural brain disease. Also, symmetric neurologic abnormalities may result from diffuse or bilateral CNS lesions (e.g., subdural hematomas or fat emboli after fracture of long bones). The triad of acute confusion, memory deficits, and nystagmus (often associated with ophthalmoplegia) suggests Wernicke's encephalopathy and should be treated with 50 to 100 mg of intravenous (IV) thiamine.

The most dangerous complication of ethanol intoxication is coma with respiratory depression. A blood level of 500 mg/dl is lethal in approximately 50 percent of patients.[13] In chronic abusers, alcoholic coma is uncommon with blood levels less than 400 mg%, and should raise the suspicion that there is another cause of impaired consciousness.[23] The treatment of alcoholic coma includes ventilatory support, correction of metabolic and temperature abnormalities as needed, and administration of parenteral thiamine and glucose. Gastric lavage and activated charcoal are only helpful if performed within 1 to 2 hours of consumption, or if other drugs were ingested. Hemodialysis or peritoneal dialysis are indicated only in the presence of extremely high blood levels (>600 mg/dl) of alcohol, or of lower levels (>400 mg/dl) if they are associated with severe acidosis, ingestion of methanol, ethylene glycol, or another dialyzable drug or occur in children with severe poisoning.[23] Analeptics such as caffeine and amphetamine are not recommended to reverse intoxication because they may lower the threshold for seizures and cardiac arrhythmias.

WITHDRAWAL

Clinical Features

Chronic alcohol intoxication results in tolerance, meaning ever larger doses are necessary to produce the same physiologic effects. A physical dependence develops, so that when alcohol is abruptly discontinued or rapidly decreased, a withdrawal reaction occurs. In many patients, withdrawal is caused by the presence of an associated illness such as pneumonia or gastrointestinal bleeding that prevents the continued ingestion of alcohol. The manifestations of alcohol withdrawal vary, but may be divided into three important groups based on severity: simple withdrawal, seizures (rum fits), and delirium

Table 24-2. SIGNS AND SYMPTOMS OF CHRONIC ALCOHOLISM

Hematologic
  Anemia (folate and other nutritional deficiencies)
  Leukopenia and impaired granulocyte function; increased incidence of infection
  Thrombocytopenia
  Decreased clotting factors due to liver disease

Cardiovascular
  Cardiomyopathy
  Arrhythmias

Gastrointestinal
  Esophagitis
  Gastritis
  Mallory-Weiss tear
  Esophageal varices
  Acute and chronic pancreatitis
  Hepatic: fatty accumulation, hepatitis, cirrhosis with portal hypertension and encephalopathy

Genitourinary
  Testicular atrophy
  Impotence
  Amenorrhea

Oncologic
  Increased incidence of carcinomas of the head, neck, and GI tract

Metabolic
  Ketoacidosis
  Hyponatremia
  Hypoglycemia
  Hypomagnesemia
  Thiamine and other vitamin deficiencies

Neurologic
  Psychiatric disorders: pathologic intoxication, personality disorders, depression, psychosis, paranoia
  Wernicke's syndrome: delirium, ataxia, dysarthria, ophthalmoplegia, nystagmus
  Korsakoff's syndrome: severe anterograde and moderate retrograde amnesia
  Cerebellar degeneration
  Dementia
  Polyneuropathy
  Amblyopia
  Myopathy

tremens. The intensity of withdrawal reactions depends on the amount and duration of ethanol ingestion and the rapidity of taper. Mild tremor, irritability, and sleeplessness may occur within hours of the last drink; these symptoms are common upon awakening. As withdrawal progresses, there may be fine lateral nystagmus (in the opposite direction of the nystagmus during intoxication), sensory illusions that may progress to hallucinations in all sensory modalities (especially visual, auditory, and tactile), tremulousness, anorexia, nausea, vomiting, anxiety, tachycardia, and diaphoresis.[24]

Alcohol withdrawal seizures (AWS) occur most commonly in middle-aged men with a long history of alcohol abuse. When seizures are associated with reduced ethanol intake in patients less than 25 years old, post-traumatic and idiopathic seizure disorders are often present. Generalized tonic-clonic seizures (GTSCs) are most common, with focal features (usually motor) in approximately 5 percent of seizures. A single seizure occurs in 40 percent of patients. Of the remaining 60 percent, most have two to four seizures; 4 percent have seven to twelve seizures, and 3 percent progress to *status epilepticus*.[26] Half the patients with *status epilepticus* have focal seizure symptoms.[26] *Status epilepticus* suggests the possibility of withdrawal from short-acting sedative/hypnotic agents or antiepileptic medications, or the presence of a coexisting, treatable CNS insult such as subdural hematoma or meningitis.[2,24] More than 90 percent of AWS occur between 7 and 48 hours after the cessation of drinking. Peak incidence is between 13 and 24 hours after the last drink; almost 50 percent of seizures begin during this interval.[26]

Delirium tremens, which occur in 5 percent of hospitalized alcoholics, is the most serious alcohol withdrawal syndrome. Mortality from delirium tremens is approximately 10 percent even with aggressive treatment.[14,25] Delirium tremens is a distinctive syndrome and should be diagnosed only if the following complex of clinical features is present: autonomic hyperactivity (fever, tachycardia, diaphoresis), severe agitated delirium, tremor, illusions, and hallucinations. Delirium tremens usually begins two to four days after the last drink, has an acute or subacute onset, and lasts an average of 56 hours.[25] Patients at increased risk of developing delirium tremens include those who have had seizures during the same withdrawal episode. If both occur, AWS vitually always precede delirium tremens. In some patients, however, especially those with repetitive seizures and associated medical illness, postictal confusion may overlap with the onset of delirium tremens. Because AWS are distinctly uncommon after the onset of delirium, another cause for seizures should be considered in such a case. Morbidity and mortality from delirium tremens are highest in patients with high fever, tachycardia, dehydration, and concomitant illness such as pneumonia, pancreatitis, or hepatitis.[25]

Evaluation and Differential Diagnosis

A history obtained from the patient, friends or relatives, and witnesses of the seizure is invaluable. Patients undergoing alcohol withdrawal must be carefully examined and evaluated for the medical and neurologic complications of alcoholism (Table 24-2). In particular, infection, cranial or other trauma, gastrointestinal hemorrhage (which may precipitate hepatic encephalopathy), liver disease, pancreatitis, and malnutrition must be considered. Fever is often associated with infections such as pneumonia or peritonitis, and a source for the fever should be aggressively sought. Chest x-rays should be performed in all cases. Hematologic and metabolic abnormalities are also common in patients suffering alcohol withdrawal and necessitate investigation with appropriate laboratory screening tests. Toxicology screens for other drugs should be performed if there is any suspicion of drug abuse or if the presentation is atypical for alcohol withdrawal. Blood alcohol level measurements are usually not helpful in assessing alcohol withdrawal. There is often a significant delay in obtaining results; patients in whom tolerance has developed may have moderate blood levels of ethanol despite a significant reduction in intake and despite clinical withdrawal.

Patients with AWS and delirium tremens should have a cerebrospinal fluid (CSF) examination performed if there is no evidence of increased intracranial pressure, especially because some patients have meningitis without nuchal rigidity. In addition, initial CSF examination may reveal bacteria only in the centrifuged sediment or culture, with delayed appearance of leukocytes.[24] The diagnosis of tuberculous meningitis should be considered and a Venereal Disease Research Laboratories (VDRL) test should be performed on all CSF samples. Patients with AWS and patients undergoing alcohol withdrawal in whom there is evidence of new focal signs or symptoms should undergo computerized tomographic (CT) or magnetic resonance imaging (MRI) scans of the head. These radiologic studies are especially important in cases involving a history or signs of head trauma. An electroencephalogram (EEG) may be helpful in identifying focal brain abnormalities, which are often due to trauma. In addition, interictal epileptiform abnormalities suggest that an underlying seizure disorder may be present. Approximately half the patients who have symptoms of abstinence such as tremulousness, hallucinations, and seizures have abnormal photic responses. However, with progression to delirium tremens, the paroxysmal photic responses are usually absent.[26] The differential diagnosis of AWS includes all the disorders listed in Table 24-1. In many patients, more than one of these etiologic factors are present. Withdrawal seizures may be the *only* or the most prominent feature of alcohol withdrawal, so that the presence of other characteristic signs and symptoms does not determine diagnosis. Withdrawal or sedative/hypnotic drugs may produce manifestations identical to those of alcohol withdrawal. Patients with chronic seizure disorders often have interictal epileptiform discharges in their EEGs, in contrast to patients with seizures caused solely by abstinence, in whom this abnormality is rarely present. Hepatic encephalopathy is an important consideration in alcoholic patients with mental status changes. Features of hepatic encephalopathy rarely seen in alcohol withdrawal include slow tremor, asterixis, and lethargy; characteristic signs of abstinence, on the other hand, include fast tremor, agitation, and the autonomic features associated with alcohol withdrawal.

The prominent autonomic manifestations attributable to alcohol withdrawal may obscure the presentation of myocardial ischemia, hypoglycemia, and panic attacks. All these disorders may cause anxiety, tachycardia, diaphoresis, and tremor. Also, symptoms of psychiatric disorders (e.g., major depression or psychosis) may be incorrectly attributed to alcohol withdrawal, and important therapeutic opportunities may be missed.

Treatment

GENERAL MEASURES

Therapy for alcohol withdrawal depends on the intensity of symptoms and the presence of concomitant medical and neurologic disorders. All alcohol withdrawal patients with seizures should be admitted to the hospital in order to prevent recurrent seizures and delirium tremens, and to further investigate the etiology of the seizures. Principles of treating AWS include: stabilization of vital signs and immediate treatment of life-threatening disorders such as *status epilepticus* and myocardial infarction; diagnosis and treatment of associated disorders (Table 24-2); provision of a supportive and calming environment for the patient; administration of a cross-tolerant drug such as a benzodiazepine to reduce the severity of withdrawal; and prevention of excessive treatment and iatrogenic complications.[14]

All patients with acute AWS should receive 50 to 100 mg of thiamine, parenterally. Glucose must never be administered before thiamine because doing so could further deplete thiamine reserves and precipitate Wernicke's disease. Multivitamins are often given but are of no proven benefit. Fluid replacement is essential for patients with recurrent seizures, high fever, and myoglobinuria. However, care must be exercised not to overhydrate, especially in patients with head trauma and elevated intracranial pressure. Metabolic abnormalities should be corrected. Potassium replacement is especially important in hypokalemic patients with arrhythmias (common when IV glucose is given in large amounts to malnourished patients), and in patients receiving digitalis or digoxin. Hyponatremia necessitates therapy only when symptomatic or severe; if needed, correction must be gradual in order to prevent rapid changes in serum sodium levels, which can cause central pontine myelinolysis.[15] Hypomagnesemia is common in acute withdrawal and replacement therapy may help prevent or treat seizures, tremor, and arrhythmias. Magnesium replacement should not involve administering a dose greater than 1 g $MgSO_4$ IV every six hours for patients with normal renal function.

BENZODIAZEPINES

The benzodiazepines represent the cornerstone of drug therapy for alcohol withdrawal. Benzodiazepines are cross-tolerant with alcohol and have proven to be an efficacious replacement therapy for ethanol. Both the sedative/hypnotic and antiepileptic activities of these agents are important in treating alcohol withdrawal. Diazepam and chlordiazepoxide have been the most extensively studied and utilized. Both drugs are effective when given orally or IV but are erratically absorbed after intramuscular administration. The half-lives of diazepam and chlordiazepoxide are approximately 45 and 10 hours, respectively.[3] Diazepam is more potent, more rapidly absorbed after oral administration, and better tolerated IV than chlordiazepoxide.[3,11] For these reasons diazepam is the benzodiazepine most often used to treat acute alcohol withdrawal. A newer benzodiazepine, lorazepam, may prove to be the best drug to treat withdrawal. It is predictably absorbed after intramuscular injection,[10] it is effective for *status epilepticus*,[7] and its excretion is less affected by age or renal and hepatic dysfunction than is the excretion of diazepam.[20]

Parenteral administration of diazepam or another benzodiazepine is recommended for patients with agitation, *status epilepticus*, or severe withdrawal reactions. The most serious side-effects of IV diazepam are respiratory depression and hypotension. These complications most often affect patients who are older than 65, who have advanced cardiac, pulmonary, or hepatic disease, or who have previously received sedative drug treatment or a rapid bolus injection.[22] The rate of IV infusion must not exceed 2 mg/minute and should probably be slower in patients with cardiopulmonary disease. IV diazepam has a short duration of action (15–20 minutes) due to tissue distribution. Therefore, additional doses are almost always necessary to control repetitive seizures and to maintain a calm state. The total dose necessary is highly variable, but is greatest in patients with delirium tremens. After the agitation, seizures, and other acute withdrawal symptoms have been controlled, oral medication should be administered at regular intervals, and later tapered gradually.

Anti-epileptic Drugs

Anti-epileptic drugs other than benzodiazepines have a limited role in the treatment of AWS. When *status epilepticus* or life-threatening repeated seizures occur, using an anti-epileptic drug with a serum half-life longer than diazepam is warranted. In this setting, phenytoin or phenobarbital in combination with diazepam, may be most effective in controlling seizures. When an anti-epileptic drug is necessary for emergency treatment of seizures, it should be administered parenterally (phenytoin, however, should not be given intramuscularly because it is poorly absorbed) with an initial loading dose. Because of their sedative effect, barbiturates are less optimal than phenytoin because impairment of consciousness makes it more difficult to recognize associated neurologic disease.

The routine use of phenytoin and barbiturates for treatment or prevention of AWS is not recommended. Less than ten percent of patients have more than five seizures during alcohol withdrawal. In addition, parenteral anti-epileptic medications may cause toxic reactions such as hypotension and arrhythmias when co-administered with benzodiazepines. Oral phenytoin (100 mg tid.) was reported to be helpful for withdrawal seizures.[21] However, the failure to achieve steady-state plasma phenytoin levels until at least seven days after onset of therapy and the inclusion of patients with epilepsy in Sampliner and Iber's[21] study weaken their case for oral phenytoin. Long-term use of anti-epileptic drugs is unwarranted for patients with AWS. Abstinence from drinking will prevent further seizures unless there is pre-existing epilepsy, and continued drinking ensures noncompliance.

Other Agents

Paraldehyde, a polymer of acetaldehyde that shows cross-tolerance with alcohol, was once the drug of choice for treating the alcohol withdrawal syndrome. It is now a second-line agent after the safer benzodiazepines. Paraldehyde is effective for alcohol withdrawal symptoms, including seizures, but is difficult to administer safely: oral therapy irritates the gastric mucosa; rectal absorption is erratic and irritates the rectal mucosa; intramuscular administration can cause sterile abscesses; and IV injection may cause fatal paraldehyde emboli. Also, paraldehyde must be stored away from light in nonplastic containers (usually glass) and prepared shortly before use.

Antipsychotic drugs are indicated only to counteract refractory hallucinosis. Although effective against agitation, antipsychotics may aggravate withdrawal—

they lower the seizure threshold and increase the incidence of delirium tremens and seizures.[24] Aliphatic phenothiazines such as chlorpromazine are potent sedatives, but may cause profound hyptotension due to alpha-adrenergic blocking activity. Butyrophenones have moderate sedative activity but cause greater extrapyramidal toxicity than aliphatic phenothiazines.

Pathophysiology

The pathogenesis of seizures and other components of alcohol withdrawal is only partially understood. Alcohol has the properties of a general anesthetic,[18] and therefore has anti-epileptic activity. The exposure of a tolerant and dependent CNS to reduced concentrations of ethanol is probably the critical factor in the etiology of alcohol withdrawal symptoms such as tremor, autonomic hyperactivity, seizures, and delirium. Decreased serum magnesium concentration and respiratory alkalosis may also contribute to withdrawal symptoms.[27] The role of sleep deprivation, head trauma, and cerebral atrophy in the pathogenesis of withdrawal seizures is less certain.[5]

SPECIAL PROBLEMS

The Single Seizure

The single seizure presents a controversial dilemma for the treating physician. The single seizure can be divided into two fundamental categories: the first, unprovoked seizure, and the single, provoked seizure in a patient who has had previous attacks. These types will be discussed separately.

The first, unprovoked seizure, in a patient with no history of epilepsy is a problem that is usually, although not always, unrelated to alcohol-induced seizures. The fundamental question is not how to treat the seizure that has already occurred, but whether the seizure is likely to recur, and whether medication is indicated to prevent recurrence. Although much has been written about whether to prescribe anti-epileptic drugs for patients who have had only one seizure, these considerations are unfortunately based on the erroneous assumption that the disorder is homogeneous in all such patients. Most physicians would not prescribe drugs for a patient who presents with a single, unprovoked, generalized tonic-clonic seizure, unless other evidence suggested the possibility of repetitive seizures. On the other hand, what approach should be taken to treating a single partial seizure? Since a single partial seizure is much less common than a single generalized tonic-clonic seizure, is a single partial seizure likely to recur? Do patients ever *present* with a single absence seizures or single myoclonic seizures? The problems of interpreting single seizures are obviously more complex than they would at first appear.[17]

In reviewing the thoughts of most epileptologists about the presentation of a single seizure, an important underlying assumption becomes apparent. This precept is that generalized tonic-clonic seizures, even when uncommon in a particular patient, are usually detected either by the patient or by someone else, but virtually all other seizures may—especially if they are low frequency—easily go undetected. The first generalized tonic-clonic seizure may properly be left untreated; however, when other seizure types are diagnosed, one frequently assumes (and very often correctly) that the detected event is not the first such occurrence. Such seizures are likely to recur and treatment is necessary. The reason for not treating single generalized tonic-clonic attacks is that a significant percentage of patients (albeit determined by many risk factors) never have another seizure and have only toxicity to gain from taking medication.[16] Neurologic concomitants such as an obvious focal brain lesion or prominent epileptiform EEG findings may affect the decision to treat single seizures. Social factors must also be taken into account. Factors determining treatment of children and elderly persons may be different from those determining treatment of a working adult.[17]

More difficult and more relevant to the present volume is the single seizure in a patient who is withdrawing from ethanol. The problem is heterogeneous and necessitates considerable individualization of therapy among various population groups. For patients in whom the single seizure is their *first* seizure, the above-mentioned criteria are appropriate for consideration. Each of the remaining groups will be considered separately below.

It is important to emphasize that single-seizure cases have a relatively benign prognosis with regard to seizure recurrence—benign at least in terms of *status epilepticus*, which I will describe in the following section. In the following discussion seizures are assumed to be generalized tonic-clonic in type. Patients can usually be categorized into one of the four groups below; if a patient cannot be categorized, either the patient is unusual or diagnosis and therapy should be reconsidered. An underlying assumption in this categorization is the lack of enthusiasm for chronic treatment of patients whose seizures occur only on ethanol withdrawal.

1. Patients in whom the single seizure is a rare occurrence, associated only with ethanol withdrawal: the seizures are not treated chronically.

> The patient with a rare single withdrawal seizure, even in the acute medical setting, almost never requires therapy for the attack. The patient continues through the withdrawal phase and even if a second seizure occurs, the likelihood of further problems is not great. Exceptions might include special cases in which a second seizure would be particularly undesirable, for example, if other medical problems complicate management. Such treatment, however, has its own attendant risks. The use of benzodiazepines to suppress the seizures, for example, will probably worsen the patient's state of consciousness and may create problems more severe than another seizure.

2. Patients in whom the single seizure is a common occurrence, but only in conjunction with ethanol withdrawal: the seizures are not treated chronically.

> These patients are the most difficult to treat. The risk of a second seizure may be relatively high, but the physician does not wish to sedate the patient with benzodiazepines or to institute chronic phenytoin therapy; in the latter case, the physician would later have to address problems of withdrawal from the anti-epileptic drug. One usually waits until the second seizure before initiating treatment with anti-epileptic drugs. Patients who are known to have severe bouts of seizures during withdrawal or who are very ill are prominent exceptions; these cases may necessitate intervention after one seizure, or even before the first attack. Because therapy is necessary for a few days at the very least, the drug of choice is usually IV phenytoin; its use has been reviewed.[16] Phenobarbital is also effective and useful if phenytoin fails, but its sedative properties are usually a drawback.

3. Patients in whom the single seizure is a rare occurrence, but in whom nonwithdrawal seizures also occasionally occur: the seizures are treated chronically.

> These cases usually necessitate some intervention at the time of the seizure, but the degree of intervention is determined by circumstances. At one end of the spectrum is the patient who is known to be in compliance with an anti-epileptic drug regimen—a rare patient in this population—and in whom blood levels of appropriate drugs (such as phenytoin or carbamazepine) are in the therapeutic range. Little intervention is required; perhaps an extra dose of medication may be necessary for medication levels to reach the upper portion of the therapeutic range. More often, the patient is suspected of noncompliance and blood level data are "not yet available" for urgent decisions. If it is determined that the patient takes the usual chronic medications, and if either phenytoin or phenobarbital are among them, an extra dose may be considered—either orally or IV. Carbamazepine and pri-

midone can only be administered orally and are therefore appropriate only for patients who are alert and not particularly ill. If the patient's condition is stable, the physician may consider waiting for the second seizure before instituting any therapy; however, one must be prepared to vigorously intervene if the patient's condition deteriorates.

4. Patients in whom the single seizure is a common occurrence, and in whom nonwithdrawal seizures are frequent: the seizures are treated chronically.

During ethanol withdrawal, even a single seizure places a patient with chronic, severe epilepsy at considerable risk for repeat seizures. Especially if the patient seems ill, chronic therapy should be considered early and the patient's condition monitored carefully for possible progression to serial seizures and *status epilepticus*. Measurement of drug blood levels may be very useful, but adequate doses of drugs such as phenytoin should be administered even when measurements cannot be obtained, because morbidity associated with drug toxicity is less than that associated with *status*.

Certain other principles apply. Patients with repeat bouts of ethanol withdrawal become known to the medical staff of the hospital, and the tendency of each patient to have seizures becomes evident. Such anticipation may be very useful to tailoring the regimen. Finally, of course, many factors other than just the seizures and their frequency must be considered in these cases.

Status Epilepticus

Diagnosis

In convulsive (tonic-clonic) *status epilepticus*, a patient has generalized tonic-clonic seizures so frequently that another seizure occurs before he or she returns to normal consciousness from the postictal state; *status* is a medical emergency with an associated mortality of approximately 10 percent. It is essential that convulsive *status* be stopped as quickly as possible because the molecular events leading to selective cell death are already in place during the first two to three convulsions.[8] According to Gastaut,[9] tonic-clonic *status* is characterized by two types of seizures: primary generalized tonic-clonic attacks or, more frequently, secondarily generalized tonic-clonic seizures following a partial onset. The seizures themselves are typical generalized tonic-clonic seizures, and in patients withdrawing from ethanol, a greater number of seizures are primarily generalized than is the case among patients with epilepsy—most epileptic patients with *status* have partial seizures progressing to generalized tonic-clonic attacks.

In a study of 98 urban patients with generalized tonic-clonic status, Aminoff and Simon[2] noted that alcohol withdrawal was a major factor in 21 percent of cases; a similar number involved cerebrovascular disease as the cause of *status epilepticus*. Other causes included intracranial infection, metabolic disorders, drug overdose, and cardiac arrest. In 15 percent of patients, no specific cause could be found. Poor outcome correlated primarily with long-lasting *status epilepticus*. These investigators also noted that *status epilepticus* was usually accompanied by hyperthermia, and that the leukocyte count increased not only in the peripheral circulation but also in the CSF in 18 percent of patients.

Status epilepticus with localizing features suggestive of partial seizures does not always indicate localized pathologic lesions. The phenomenon of partial or lateralized attacks has been associated in some patients with such diffuse cerebral insults as drug overdose or metabolic disturbance.[2] Similar observations have been made in patients with hepatic encephalopathy; localized epileptic seizures do not necessarily mean localized pathologic change.[1]

Therapy

The treatment of generalized tonic-clonic (grand mal) *status epilepticus* depends on the severity of the presentation.

Occasionally, patients present with persistent, or nearly persistent, tonic-clonic activity that is bilateral and severe. Control of such seizure activity demands minute-to-minute emergency efforts. More often, the patient presents with a short history involving a series of tonic-clonic seizures; perhaps one attack has been observed by the emergency physician. The seizures are separated by prolonged stuporous periods. These periods may be the predominant clinical presentation when the seizures are separated by intervals of 20 to 30 minutes or more.[16] In either case, certain life support measures are necessary, including maintaining satisfactory cardiorespiratory function and monitoring respiration, blood pressure, and EEG readings. An IV catheter should be inserted, and blood samples should be obtained for chemistry tests, including blood urea nitrogen, electrolyte, calcium, magnesium, and glucose level measurements, as well as complete blood cell counts and plasma anti-epileptic drug level measurement. Arterial blood gases should also be monitored.[8] Thiamine should be given IV, followed by glucose, if alcoholism or hypoglycemia is suspected. Appropriate efforts should be made to determine the etiology of the *status epilepticus*.[16]

In patients who are having continuous generalized tonic-clonic seizures, the therapy of choice is immediate IV administration of diazepam, beginning with 5 to 10 mg given at a maximum rate of 2 mg/minute, with the objective of stopping the attacks. Up to 20 mg can be given to an adult. Simultaneously loading with an IV injection of phenytoin should begin. The anticonvulsant effect of IV diazepam is relatively short—usually only 20 to 30 minutes—but highly effective in most cases. The drug does have a sedative effect, like other benzodiazepines, and this effect long outlasts the anticonvulsant activity. Respiratory depression occurs, especially if the patient has taken barbiturates. Bradycardia and hypotension may also complicate therapy. Diazepam is indicated only as long as there are active seizures. A newer benzodiazepine, lorazepam, may be more effective than diazepam. Studies suggest that lorazepam causes less cardiorespiratory depression and has a longer duration of action.[7,10]

When it appears that the attacks have temporarily ceased, or if the patient is having *status epilepticus* with prolonged stuporous periods between attacks, IV injection of phenytoin should be started immediately.[4,6,8] In patients who are having *status epilepticus* with prolonged periods between attacks (sometimes called "serial seizures"), diazepam may thus be avoided entirely. The patient's already depressed consciousness will not thereby be further depressed by a sedative anti-epileptic drug. IV administration of phenytoin involves special precautions.[16] Phenytoin has the outstanding advantage of being nonsedative in a setting where depression of consciousness may greatly decrease the opportunity to obtain information from the neurologic examination.

If the patient does not respond to diazepam and phenytoin, phenobarbital should be given IV. Doses as high as 18 mg/kg (1,000–1,500 mg in adults) may be required. Respiratory depression and hypotension are common, especially at high doses, and endotracheal intubation should usually be accomplished at or before this step in therapy.

Some patients simply do not respond to IV doses of diazepam, phenytoin, or phenobarbital; other drugs such as paraldehyde or lidocaine may be tried. Although paraldehyde and lidocaine are occasionally effective, many physicians prefer next to administer general anesthesia if phenytoin and phenobarbital fail to control the attacks. General anesthesia stops brain function, and treatment of *status epilepticus* may occasionally necessitate its use. Anesthesia is usually maintained for several hours.

Alcoholism and Alcohol-Related Seizures in Patients with Epilepsy

Epilepsy and alcoholism are common disorders and may coexist. When alcoholism precedes the onset of a seizure disorder, the epilepsy is often post-traumatic. In contrast, when alcoholism complicates the course of epilepsy, the etiology of seizures is often unknown. Regardless of which disorder develops first, the concomitance of epilepsy and alcoholism creates a therapeutic dilemma. The alcoholic patient is often subject to mild withdrawal syndromes that facilitate seizures. Other problems that may increase seizure frequency in the alcoholic patient include poor nutrition, metabolic disorders, head trauma, sleep deprivation, and most important, noncompliance with anti-epileptic medications.[19] When patients with epilepsy and alcoholism undergo withdrawal, they should be treated with anti-epileptic drugs such as phenytoin in addition to benzodiazepines. Rapid determination of serum anti-epileptic drug level is critical because loading doses are required if a therapeutic level is not present.

Nonalcoholic patients with epilepsy may also suffer an increase in seizures in association with excessive drinking. Mattson and associates[12] found that consumption of one to two alcoholic drinks had no significant effect on seizure frequency. However, more than 75 percent of patients who consumed five to six drinks suffered an exacerbation of their seizure disorder. The increased seizure frequency occurred during the period when blood alcohol levels were declining. These findings agree with Victor and Brausch's[26] observation that in patients with idiopathic epilepsy, cessation of drinking had a close temporal relation with seizure occurrence. Brief discontinuation of anti-epileptic drug administration during acute intoxication exposes these patients to withdrawal of both alcohol and anti-epileptic drugs. Teaching them to either abstain from alcohol or moderate their future drinking is vital if recurrences are to be prevented. Finally, does acute ethanol intoxication increase the frequency of seizures in some patients? There is no convincing evidence to support such a claim.

SUMMARY

Seizures in alcoholic patients are common and necessitate a systematic approach to evaluation and treatment. Initial management should focus on stabilization of vital signs and determination of the cause of the seizure. History from an informant, inspection of the skull for signs of head trauma, and careful medical and neurologic examinations are mandatory. Laboratory investigations should rule out possible metabolic and infectious disorders. The vast majority of seizures in alcoholics occur during withdrawal, usually 7 to 48 hours after cessation of drinking. *Status epilepticus* and focal seizures are uncommon and suggest withdrawal from short-acting sedatives or a treatable CNS disorder such as subdural hematoma or meningitis. All patients with AWS should be admitted to the hsopital so as to prevent recurrent seizures and delirium tremens (which may occur in up to one third of these patients) and further to investigate the etiology of the seizures. Benzodiazepines should be administered to patients withdrawing from alcohol; patients with recurrent seizures and delirium tremens usually need higher doses. All patients should receive thiamine, and metabolic disorders such as hypoglycemia or hypomagnesemia should be corrected. Chronic anti-epileptic therapy has a very limited role in preventing AWS because abstinence from drinking prevents seizures, and continued drinking ensures medication noncompliance. There are also patients with idiopathic seizure disorders in whom consumption of alcohol is followed by an exacerbation of their seizures. Abstinence is again the treatment of choice.

References

1. Adams, RD and Foley, JM: The neurological disorder associated with liver disease. Research Publication for the Association of Nervous and Mental Disorders 32:198, 1953.
2. Aminoff, MJ and Simon, RP: Status epilepticus: Causes, clinical features, and consequences in 98 patients. Am J Med 69:657, 1980.
3. Baldessarini, RJ: Drugs and the treatment of psychiatric disorders. In Gilman, AG, et al (eds): The Pharmacologic Basis of Therapeutics. Macmillan, New York, 1985, p 387.
4. Browne, TR: Drug therapy reviews: Drug therapy of status epilepticus. Am J Hosp Pharm 35:915, 1978.

5. Chan, AWK: Alcoholism and epilepsy. Epilepsia 26:323, 1985.
6. Cloyd, JC, Gumnit, RJ, and McLain, LW, Jr: Status epilepticus: The role of intravenous phenytoin. JAMA 244:1479, 1980.
7. Crawford, TO, Mitchell, WG, and Snodgrass, SR: Lorazepam in childhood status epilepticus and serial seizures: Effectiveness and tachyphylaxis. Neurology 37:190, 1987.
8. Delgado-Escueta, AV, et al: Current concepts in neurology: Management of status epilepticus. N Engl J Med 306:1337, 1982.
9. Gastaut, H: Classification of status epilepticus. In Delgado-Escueta, AV, et al (eds): Advances in Neurology, Vol 34, p. 15 Status Epilepticus: Mechanisms of Brain Damage and Treatment. Raven Press, New York, 1983.
10. Greenblatt, DJ, et al: Clinical pharmacokinetics of the newer benzodiazepines. Clin Pharmacokinet 8:233, 1983.
11. Harvey, SC: Hypnotics and sedatives. In Gilman, AG, et al (eds): The Pharmacologic Basis of Therapeutics. Macmillan, New York, 1985, p 339.
12. Mattson, RH, et al: Effect of alcohol intake in nonalcoholic epileptics. Neurology 25:361, 1975.
13. Morgan, R and Cagan, EJ: Acute alcohol intoxication, the disulfiram reaction, and methyl alcohol intoxication. In Kissin, B and Begleiter, H (eds): The Biology of Alcoholism. Vol 3, Clinical Pathology. Plenum Press, New York, 1974, p 163.
14. Morris, JC and Victor, M: Alcohol withdrawal seizures. Emerg Med Clin North Am 5:827, 1987.
15. Norenberg, MD, Leslie, KO, and Robertson, AS: Association between rise in serum sodium and central pontine myelinolysis. Ann Neurol 11:128 1982.
16. Porter, RJ: Epilepsy: 100 Elementary Principles. WB Saunders, London, 1984.
17. Porter, RJ: How to use antiepileptic drugs. In Leny, RH, et al (eds): Antiepileptic Drugs, Ed 3. Raven Press, New York, 1989 (in press).
18. Ritchie, JM: The aliphatic alcohols. In Gilman, AG, et al (eds): The Pharmacologic Basis of Therapeutics. Macmillan, New York, 1985, p 372.
19. Rodin, EA, Frohman, CE, and Gottlieb, JS: Effect of acute alcohol intoxication on epileptic patients. Arch Neurol 4:115, 1961.
20. Rosenbloom, AJ: Optimizing drug treatment of alcohol withdrawal. Am J Med 81:901, 1986.
21. Sampliner, R and Iber, FL: Diphenylhydantoin control of alcohol withdrawal seizures: Results of a controlled study. JAMA 230:1430, 1974.
22. Schmidt, D: Benzodiazepines: Diazepam. In Woodbury, DM, Penry, JK, and Pippenger, CE (eds): Antiepileptic Drugs. Raven Press, New York, 1982, p 711.
23. Sellers, EM and Kalant, H: Alcohol intoxication and withdrawal. N Engl J Med 294:757, 1976.
24. Thompson, WL: Management of alcohol withdrawal syndromes. Arch Intern Med 138:278, 1978.
25. Thompson, WL, Johnson, AD, and Maddrey, WL: Diazepam and paraldehyde for treatment of severe delirium tremens. Ann Intern Med 82:175, 1975.
26. Victor, M and Brausch, C: The role of abstinence in the genesis of alcoholic epilepsy. Epilepsia 8:1, 1967.
27. Wolfe, SM and Victor, M: The relationship of hypomagnesemia and alkalosis to alcohol withdrawal symptoms. Ann NY Acad Sci 162:973, 1969.

CHAPTER 25

Arthur W. K. Chan, Ph.D.

Treatment of Alcohol Withdrawal Seizures with Benzodiazepines: Neurochemical Basis

The primary objectives of drug treatment of the alcohol withdrawal syndrome are to relieve symptoms and prevent or treat serious complications of withdrawal, such as seizures, hallucinations, and cardiac arrhythmias.[72] Drug treatment also allows a smooth transition to other treatment programs and ultimately to long-term rehabilitation.[72] For these purposes, the benzodiazepines (BZD), such as chlordiazepoxide (CDP) (Fig. 25-1) and diazepam (DZP) (see Fig. 1-3), are considered the drugs of choice.[51] The pharmacologic actions of BZD, namely sedative, anxiolytic, muscle-relaxant, and anticonvulsant effects, are well suited for relieving and preventing some symptoms of alcohol withdrawal. Other properties of BZD such as cross-tolerance[20] and cross-dependence[21] with ethanol also account for their efficacy in treating alcohol withdrawal.

The availability of a variety of animal models has greatly facilitated investigation of the many biochemical, neurochemical, and endocrinologic changes associated with the alcohol withdrawal syndrome.[46] Some of these changes may trigger seizure activity in susceptible persons. About 2 percent to 15 percent of alcoholics in withdrawal develop seizures, and the percentage may be higher in alcoholics who have a history of withdrawal seizures or who develop delirium tremens.[19,87] It is difficult to determine whether the neurochemical changes associated with alcohol withdrawal are the result or the cause of withdrawal hyperexcitability. Several central nervous system (CNS) models of alcohol withdrawal have been reviewed.[123] The basic premise of CNS models is that during chronic alcohol exposure the CNS compensates for the imbalance of biologic systems produced by the depressant actions of ethanol; when alcohol is withdrawn abruptly, the overcompensation is unmasked and a hyperexcitable state is evident. According to these models, the biologic systems affected are the neurotransmitter synthetic machinery, postsynaptic receptor sites, neural activity, and neuronal membrane. Drugs that have neurochemical effects opposite to those occurring during withdrawal are therefore expected to be useful in treating alcohol withdrawal reactions, irrespective of whether the neurochemical changes are the cause or the result of the withdrawal signs.

In this chapter I review the neurochemical changes associated with alcohol withdrawal and compare them with the neu-

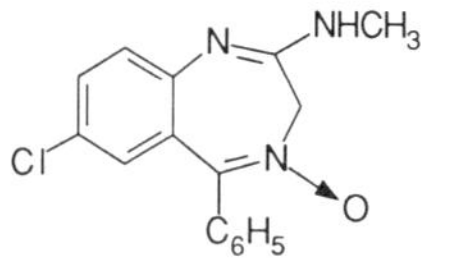

Figure 25–1. The structure of chlordiazepoxide (CDP).

rochemical actions of BZD. I summarize briefly the acute and chronic effects of ethanol on each neurochemical parameter because they are relevant to alcohol withdrawal. However, because the literature on the acute and chronic neurochemical effects of ethanol has been thoroughly reviewed elsewhere, I refer the reader to these articles.[57,60,96,116,117] Therefore, only references not included in these review articles are cited in this chapter.

METHODOLOGIC ISSUES

Several investigators have critically evaluated animal models of alcohol withdrawal reactions.[23,41,47] For practical and economic reasons, virtually all neurochemical studies of alcohol withdrawal have involved rats or mice, whereas studies of biochemical correlates of alcohol withdrawal in humans have usually involved analyses of blood, or under special circumstances, cerebrospinal fluid (CSF) samples.[123] Because many alcoholics undergo some form of pharmacologic treatment during alcohol withdrawal, some biochemical findings may be confounded by the CNS actions of medications the patient is taking concurrently. Methodologic issues relating to the neurochemical aspects of alcohol withdrawal seizures (AWS) are summarized below.

1. Although animal models offer researchers the advantage of studying the effects of alcohol *per se* under controlled conditions, alcohol withdrawal reactions in humans generally include other interacting factors such as trauma, infection, malnutrition, polydrug use, duration of alcohol abuse, smoking, and impaired liver function. Therefore, the neurochemical changes associated with alcohol withdrawal in animals are not necessarily the same as those in humans.

2. In general, the time course of withdrawal reactions is shorter in rodents than in humans. Rodents undergoing alcohol withdrawal also do not experience all the symptoms humans do.[41] In humans, seizures during alcohol withdrawal are primarily of the generalized tonic-clonic type (grand mal). Although spontaneous tonic-clonic seizures have been reported in rodents undergoing alcohol withdrawal, these seizures were often induced by audiogenic stimuli or by handling, for instance, lifting the animal by the tail.[46]

3. In some studies of neurochemical changes associated with alcohol withdrawal, information is lacking concerning when the samples were taken relative to the time of the last dose of alcohol.[116] Therefore, it is difficult to interpret whether the neurochemical changes are due to the acute, chronic, or withdrawal effects of alcohol.

4. The time courses used in neurochemical studies often have not paralleled the time course of withdrawal seizures, because many investigations have addressed withdrawal phenomena as a whole rather than specifically examining the neurochemical correlates of withdrawal seizures. Also, it is often difficult to determine whether an observed neurochemical change is the result or the cause of the withdrawal seizure. Primary neurochemical changes can also lead to secondary neurochemical alterations; the latter could be interpreted erroneously as primary effects.

5. It is often difficult to compare data from various investigations of neurochemical changes associated with alcohol withdrawal because of differences in duration and method of alcohol administration. Many *in vitro* studies have utilized very high ethanol concentrations (>100 mM or >400 mg/dl). The physiologic significance of data from such investigations is questionable.

6. In most studies only one neurochemical parameter is investigated. It should be emphasized that there are complex interactions among the various neurotransmitters and neuromodulators.

NEUROPHARMACOLOGY OF ALCOHOL WITHDRAWAL AND BZD ACTIONS

Gamma-aminobutyric Acid Systems

Numerous studies have linked impaired gamma-aminobutyric acid (GABA) functions to seizure susceptibility.[22,40,91] Therefore, it is logical to expect that during the onset of AWS impairment of some aspects of the GABA systems must occur. Because GABAergic mechanisms in withdrawal seizures, GABAergic mechanisms of ethanol, and the GABA/BZD receptor complex have been discussed in detail in Chapters 10 and 11, only a cursory summary of these areas will be presented here.

GABA Levels

Most animal studies have shown that acute administration of ethanol causes an increase in brain GABA levels, but the opposite effect has also been reported.[57,71,96] Conflicting results have also been reported on the chronic effects of ethanol. Some studies have shown elevated GABA levels and others have found GABA levels unaltered. These discrepancies may be due in part to the biphasic effect of ethanol on GABA synthesis and metabolism.[57] Another difficulty in interpreting data is that measurements of GABA levels do not distinguish the metabolic from the neurotransmitter pools of GABA in the CNS. The same inconsistencies also prevail in measurements of brain GABA levels during or after alcohol withdrawal; there are reports of both increased and decreased levels.[57] For example, a maximal decrease in GABA levels in mouse brain eight hours after alcohol withdrawal reportedly coincided with the occurrence of peak withdrawal symptoms. Mice treated chronically with ethanol via their drinking water did not have withdrawal seizures; their brain GABA levels were unchanged, but there was a persistent increase in GABA turnover during withdrawal.[110] Another study found no changes in synaptosomal GABA concentrations after both acute and chronic treatment with ethanol.[43]

Injections of the GABA inhibitor picrotoxin exacerbate AWS scores, but injections of the GABA agonist aminooxyacetic acid attenuate seizure scores.[57,60,96,117] Intracisternal and intraperitoneal injections of GABA and GABA agonists such as muscimol, progabide, and beta-guanidinoacetic acid also antagonize seizures during alcohol withdrawal in the rat.[39,57,96,123] Likewise, compounds that elevate GABA levels, such as sodium valproate, a commonly used anti-epileptic drug, have the same effect on AWS. The fall of GABA levels (18 percent) in the brain stem during withdrawal may be antagonized by ethanol.[96,123]

Alcoholics who have seizures during withdrawal have lower GABA levels in the CSF than those who do not have seizures.[96] However, in one study, control subjects who did not have seizures also had low CSF GABA levels; in another study, GABA levels in CSF were not changed in alcohol withdrawal.[96] Other investigators have reported that alcoholics had lower plasma GABA levels than control subjects.[25] The plasma samples were obtained 24 to 48 hours after admission. Thus, the alcoholic subjects were still undergoing withdrawal. These investigators assumed that plasma GABA levels reflected brain GABA activity, but such an assumption may not be justified.

GABA/BZD/Chloride Ionophore Receptor Complex

The receptor complex is thought to be a tetrameric protein complex with each subunit having three distinct areas, namely the BZD receptor, the GABA receptor, and the chloride ionophore, which in turn contains one or more binding sites for agents such as picrotoxinin and barbiturates.[15,52] The effects of acute and chronic alcohol intake as well as alcohol withdrawal on individual components of the complex have been thoroughly reviewed.[57,60,96]

GABA Receptors

When [³H]GABA is used as the radioligand, and if an endogenous inhibitor of binding is removed, two binding sites are apparent in the receptor, a low-affinity and a high-affinity site.[60] An apparent increase in the number of low-affinity binding sites was observed 30 minutes after an acute injection of ethanol (4 g/kg) in mice and rats.[57,60] However, conflicting results have also been reported. For instance, one study found that acute ethanol administration reduced specific GABA binding in the cerebellum, but caused no changes in striatum, cortex, or substantia nigra.[57,60,96] Another study found that an acute injection of ethanol (5 g/kg) in rats increased the binding capacity (B_{max}) of the high-affinity sites and decreased the B_{max} of the low-affinity sites in the cerebellum; but in the hypothalamus the opposite effect was observed, with a decreased B_{max} at the high-affinity sites and increased B_{max} at the low-affinity sites.[96] Using the same dose of ethanol, another group of investigators did not find any change in GABA receptors in the rat forebrain or cerebellum. However, no distinction was made between high- and low-affinity binding sites in this study.[57] The addition of ethanol to brain membranes *in vitro* had no effect on [³H]muscimol binding to the GABA receptors.[113]

More consistent findings have been reported regarding changes in GABA receptor binding after chronic ethanol treatment. Nearly all studies reveal a decrease in number or affinity of GABA receptors in selective brain areas after chronic alcohol treatment or withdrawal.[57,60] The greatest decrease in binding appeared to coincide with the maximal severity of withdrawal symptoms. These changes could lead to a decrease in efficacy of GABA transmission. Only one study reported an increased number of high- and low-affinity GABA binding sites in several brain areas after chronic ethanol treatment for three weeks.[57]

Recent experimental evidence indicates that at concentrations present during acute intoxication, ethanol stimulates GABA-receptor-mediated chloride transport in brain preparations and spinal cord cultured neurons.[4,5,112,113] The potentiation of GABA-mediated chloride influx by ethanol was not observed in mice that had developed acute or chronic tolerance to ethanol,[4] but there has been no study of the same phenomenon during ethanol withdrawal.

BZD Receptors

Benzodiazepine binding is not affected by acute injection of ethanol or by 10 to 100 mM or 46 to 460 mg/dl ethanol added to *in vitro* preparations of either unwashed brain tissue or tissue washed in Triton X-100.[33,57,60] However, if the tissue is solubilized with one percent Lubrol-PX, ethanol (20–100 mM) enhances BZD binding in a dose-dependent manner.[60] This effect is probably due to the ability of ethanol to modify binding allosterically via the chloride channel,[57] but the details of the molecular mechanisms involved remain to be elucidated. The relevance of findings based on extensively washed or solubilized brain preparations to *in vivo* situations has been questioned.[57,60]

Conflicting data have been reported about the effect of chronic ethanol treatment on BZD binding in the *central type* BZD receptors. Several studies reported no change in BZD binding after rats were administered ethanol (19–22 days) by inhalation or liquid diet.[33,57,60] However, a slight reduction of BZD binding was observed after long-term ethanol treatment (nine months) and after daily multiple intubations of ethanol for five days. In one study, chronic ethanol inhalation produced a significant decrease in the capacity of GABA to enhance BZD binding,[33] but no information was provided concerning whether the mice were tolerant to or dependent on ethanol, or whether the brain preparations were obtained when the mice were having withdrawal reactions. There are no systematic studies of BZD binding during ethanol withdrawal, or in particular, during AWS. A study of currently drinking alcoholics showed that these subjects had a significant reduction in the density of peripheral BZD binding sites in platelets, as measured by the ligand PK 11195.[111] This effect disappeared following abstention from alcohol, but no information was available on the same parameter in alcoholics undergoing alcohol withdrawal. Nevertheless, mice and rats that had developed physical dependence on ethanol showed increases in the binding of the *peripheral type* BZD receptors in different brain regions;[115,118] these increases also occurred during withdrawal, and in one report the effects persisted for 3 days after cessation of ethanol intake.[118] These studies revealed no changes in the binding of *central type* BZD receptors. The increase in *peripheral type* receptor binding was due to an increase in the number of binding sites but not to a change in the affinity.[115,118]

An increase in BZD receptor binding material was found in the urine of alcoholics undergoing withdrawal.[104] This finding led investigators to suggest that the substance may be an endogenous BZD inverse agonist whose action could account for the alcohol withdrawal syndrome. If this were true, the BZD antagonist Ro15-1788 would be expected to decrease the severity of alcohol withdrawal reactions. However, investigators were unable to demonstrate an effect of Ro15-1788 on AWS.[1,74] Thus, it appears that the therapeutic effects of BZD in alcohol withdrawal are not due to a competitive antagonism of a putative endogenous inverse agonist. The ability of Ro15-1788 to antagonize the ameliorating effect of DZP on ethanol withdrawal demonstrates that DZP's efficacy against alcohol withdrawal is due in part to its interaction at the central BZD receptor site.[1] This theory is indirectly supported by data showing that the putative alcohol antagonist Ro15-4513, which binds to BZD receptors, induces seizures in mice undergoing alcohol withdrawal.[73]

BZD ACTIONS

Although the precise mechanism of the CNS actions of BZD remains to be identified, electrophysiologic and biochemical evidence supports the hypothesis that the anticonvulsant activity of BZD is mediated by an enhancement of GABAergic synaptic transmission.[52,62,105] In general, BZD reduce brain GABA turnover, but are without effect on GABA levels, uptake, and release, or on activities of enzymes controlling the synthesis and degradation of GABA.[105] In humans, IV injection of DZP increases CSF GABA levels.[77] BZD enhance GABA receptor binding and vice versa. A positive correlation has been demonstrated between the degree of GABA enhancement of [^{3}H]flunitrazepam binding and resistance to the seizure-inducing properties of 3-mercaptopropionic acid, an agent that reduces GABA activity.[82] Recently Morrow and Paul[86] reported that BZD enhance the GABA-receptor-mediated chloride flux in rat brain synaptoneurosomes in a manner similar to that of ethanol. Genetic strains of mice that differ in their sensitivity to BZD also have a corresponding difference in the GABA-receptor-operated chloride channel function.[3] Together these data support the notion that the efficacy of BZD in preventing and alleviating alcohol withdrawal symptoms may be related to their ability to counteract the decrease in GABAergic activity that occurs during alcohol withdrawal.

Glutamate

Acute injection of ethanol has been shown to decrease cerebellar and cortical levels of glutamate.[57] After chronic ethanol treatment in rats, glutamate levels are increased in the cortex, hippocampus, and substantia nigra, but remain low in the cerebellum.[57] The response to glutamate of developing Purkinje neurons in culture is reduced after chronic ethanol (19.5 mM) exposure.[125] Whether the same phenomenon occurs in adult neurons under *in vivo* conditions remains to be determined. Binding to glutamate receptors is stimulated by low and physiologically relevant concentrations (<50 mM) of ethanol, but is inhibited by higher concentrations.[57,60] Chronic exposure to ethanol also causes enhanced glutamate binding, whether measured before or one day after withdrawal.[60] Glutamate diethyl ester, the glutamate receptor antagonist, was found to attenuate handling-induced seizures during alcohol withdrawal in mice. During withdrawal, the mice were more sensitive to kainic acid- (a glutamate agonist) induced seizures than to seizures induced by pentylenetetrazole (PTZ).[60] These data suggest that chronic ethanol treatment caused the mice to develop supersensitivity to glutamate.[60]

BZD ACTIONS

It has been suggested that BZD augmentation of GABA function can lead to reduced glutamate release.[122] However, a study indicated that the potassium-induced release of glutamate from rat cortical slices is little affected by DZP in concentrations up to 10 μM.[52] Flurazepam does not affect glutamate-induced neuronal responses.[119] If BZD can decrease glutamate release, then they are probably able to counteract the supersensitivity to glutamate observed in mice during alcohol withdrawal. Schwarz and Freed[106] reported that at a dose that produced marked sedation in mice, DZP only slightly decreases the incidence of seizures induced by quisqualate, an activator of a subtype of glutamate receptors.

Catecholamine Systems

DOPAMINE

In general, low ethanol levels inhibit dopaminergic activity and high ethanol levels stimulate it. Release and turnover of dopamine (DA) are increased by acute ethanol, but DA turnover is decreased after chronic ethanol treatment.[57,96] Ethanol has no effect on *in vitro* DA receptor binding unless the concentration administered is well above that normally causing intoxication.[57,60] Likewise, an acute dose of ethanol has no effect on DA receptors. Varying results have been reported on DA receptor binding following chronic ethanol administration. Some investigators have reported no change, others have reported increases and decreases.[57,60] Differences in the duration of ethanol treatment could have contributed to these discrepancies in the data. Thus, in one study, chronic ethanol treatment for 21 days caused a significant increase in density of both D_1 and D_2 DA receptors but did not cause a change in either of their affinities, but the same treatment for 14 days caused none of these changes. The changes in DA binding did not appear to correlate with tolerance development, and they were not reversed 24 hours after alcohol withdrawal. The relevance of this finding to the neurochemical basis of AWS remains to be determined.

Several studies have suggested that dopaminergic subsensitivity develops after chronic ethanol treatment and withdrawal because affected animals have decreased responses to both DA agonists and antagonists.[30,57,60] However, increased DA turnover and supersensitivity have also been reported. Human alcoholics showing withdrawal symptoms have lower CSF levels of homovanillic acid (HVA), the major metabolite of DA, than alcoholics not showing symptoms.[57] However, alcoholics having delirium tremens have increased CSF levels of HVA.[10] Although a correlation between CSF levels of HVA and clinical symptoms of alcohol withdrawal in humans has been reported,[13] HVA levels in alcoholics are not different from levels in control subjects between days two and eight of alcohol withdrawal. The authors suggested that medical treatment might have masked differences. In testing whether decreased DA activity contributes to withdrawal symptoms, investigators administered the DA agonist bromocriptine to alcoholics during withdrawal. One report showed amelioration of certain withdrawal signs by the agonist but another study did not.[16,57,60,96] There was no correlation between serum dopamine-beta-hydroxylase activity and the severity of withdrawal symptoms.[7]

NOREPINEPHRINE

Chronic ethanol treatment increases the turnover of norepinephrine (NE) in both brain and peripheral tissues.[57,96] An overall state of hyperexcitability exists during alcohol withdrawal. In humans, CSF levels of NE and 3-methoxy-4-hydroxyphenyl glycol (MHPG), a primary metabolite of NE, are elevated in alcoholics during alcohol withdrawal.[55,96,123] The increased plasma MHPG levels are considered an indication of increased NE turnover in the brain.[90] Whether the adrenergic hyperactivity occurring during alcohol withdrawal is a determinant of severity of withdrawal or simply a reflection of the stress of withdrawal remains to be determined. The former possibility is favored by some investigators.[2] However, pharmacologic studies in animals have shown that the severity of handling seizures during withdrawal is increased by drugs that decrease noradrenergic function (e.g., propranolol). In contrast, propranolol and atenolol decrease some but not all withdrawal symptoms in alcoholics.[50,70,96] Similarly, the alpha$_2$-adrenoceptor agonist clonidine has been proven efficacious in treating some symptoms of alcohol withdrawal in humans[11,26,81,96,124] and animals.[92,123] Data conflict on the effect of lesions of the noradrenergic system on the severity of AWS: some researchers report no effect and others report increased seizure activity.[24]

The increase of NE turnover after chronic ethanol ingestion can affect NE receptors. Thus, decreased numbers of beta-adrenergic antagonist binding sites in mouse and rat brains have been reported.[57,60] In one study only a decrease in beta-adrenergic receptors was observed. Valverius, Hoffman, and Tabakoff[21] stressed that ethanol may produce changes in beta-adrenergic receptor number by a mechanism other than increasing NE turnover; the effect of ethanol on the interaction of guanine nucleotide-binding protein (Gs) with the beta-adrenergic receptor[103] should be considered. These investigators found that after chronic ethanol diet treatment and at the time of ethanol withdrawal the beta-adrenergic receptors were "uncoupled" from Gs. After seven days of chronic ethanol intake, mice showed a small but significant decrease in the number of agonist binding sites without a concomitant change in the number of antagonist binding sites.

BZD Actions

Few studies have examined the effects of BZD on catecholamine systems. BZD decreases DA turnover and reduces HVA levels in the striatum.[52,62,88] It is possible that stress-induced increase of brain DA and NE turnover in the frontal cortex is blocked by BZD.[61] It is not known whether BZD have any effect on CSF levels of HVA, which are decreased during alcohol withdrawal (see previous section). Both the DA and NE systems have been implicated in some aspects of anxiety expression, one of the symptoms of alcohol withdrawal.[62,88] Investigators have also suggested that the depressant action of BZD may be mediated in part by reduced noradrenergic activity. BZD lower NA turnover and inhibit *locus coeruleus* activity. The latter effect may involve GABA as the intermediating neurotransmitter.[62] This action of BZD may be capable of counteracting the increase in brain NE turnover during alcohol withdrawal.

Serotonin Systems

Although there have been a large number of animal studies on the acute and chronic effects of ethanol on serotonin (5-HT), no coherent picture has emerged.[60,96] Nor has chronic ethanol treatment been shown to have any significant direct effects on 5-HT receptors; one study showed a slight reduction in the number of receptors in the hippocampus but not in the number of other brain regions.[60] Hunt[60] investigated this possibility because behavioral hyperactivity has been associated with stimulation of 5-HT$_2$ receptors, and because the signs of hyperactivity, such as tremor and aberrant head movements, are similar to those observed in animals during ethanol withdrawal. Supersensitivity of this receptor subtype may occur after chronic ethanol treatment. This hypothesis remains to be tested. Pharmacologic manipulations of the 5-HT system have also produced conflicting results regarding such effects on ethanol withdrawal. For instance, in one study methysergide, a 5-HT antagonist, increased the number of handling-induced seizures during alcohol withdrawal, but in others it did not.[60] Another study reported that head twitches occurring during withdrawal were antagonized by 5-HT antagonists.[60,96] In humans, disorientation and hallucination during delirium tremens seem to be caused mostly by elevation of CSF 5-hydroxyindoleacetic acid (5-HIAA) levels,[10] but it is not clear whether CSF 5-HIAA levels correlate with the occurrence of withdrawal seizures.

BZD Actions

Most studies of the effects of BZD on 5-HT indicate that BZD increase brain 5-HT levels and reduce 5-HT turnover and activity.[63,88,90,108] However, these actions of BZD appear to be irrelevant to their anxiolytic properties, despite the fact that 5-HT hypersensitivity has been hypothesized to be one of the mechanisms of anxiety.[63,108]

Adenosine

Adenosine decreases the spontaneous activity of central neurons, probably by inhibiting synaptic transmission.[29] The CNS-depressant effects of adenosine are mediated via selective adenosine receptors located on extracellular neural membranes.[29] Only a few studies have investigated a possible role of adenosine in the CNS actions of ethanol. One study showed that the adenosine-receptor-stimulated cAMP levels in cultured neuroblastoma-glioma hybrid cells are increased by acute ethanol exposure. With chronic ethanol treatment, these cells developed tolerance to this effect, and "physical dependence" was evident by reduced adenosine-stimulated cAMP levels in the absence of ethanol.[49] The same two phenomena were also demonstrated in lymphocytes from alcoholic patients.[34] In mice undergoing acute ethanol administration, pretreatment with theophylline (the specific adenosine antagonist) substantially reduced the duration of ethanol sleep time and also decreased the intensity and duration of motor incoordination.[29] Similar results were obtained with dipyridamole, a blocker of adenosine reuptake. However, neither agent had any effect on ethanol-induced hypothermia. After chronic ethanol treatment (10 days) there was an apparent increase (28 percent) in the number of brain adenosine receptors, but this result was not statistically significant. The number of adenosine receptors and the dissociation constant were reduced 40 percent 24 and 48 hours after withdrawal, and returned to prewithdrawal levels after 72 hours.[29] It is not clear whether these changes were partly responsible for causing the hyperexcitable state during alcohol withdrawal.

BZD Actions

Adenosine may act as an endogenous anticonvulsant.[6] Phillis and O'Regan[94] have recently reviewed the literature on the role of adenosine in the central actions of BZD. They hypothesized that, besides their action at the GABA/BZD/Cl$^-$ ionophore complex, BZD may act by inhibiting adenosine uptake. Evidence supporting this hypothesis includes the following: 1) at therapeutically and pharmacologically relevant concentrations in the brain, BZD potentiate the depressant actions of adenosine on the spontaneous firing of cerebral cortical neurons, and theophylline blocks the depressant action of BZD; 2) BZD inhibit adenosine uptake by rat brain cerebral cortical synaptosomes, and there is a strong correlation between therapeutic potencies of BZD and their potencies in inhibiting adenosine uptake; 3) intraperitoneal administration of DZP enhances the rate of efflux of [^{3}H]adenosine from the cortex; 4) coadministration of DZP and adenosine at doses that have no significant effect on locomotor activity when given separately, produce a significant depression of locomotor activity; and 5) several beta-carbolines, which are non-BZD ligands for BZD receptors and which have pharmacologic effects opposite to those of BZD, are potent antagonists of the depressant actions of adenosine.

Calcium Metabolism

In general, acute ethanol treatment increases resting intraneuronal Ca^{2+}, decreases Ca^{2+} in the synaptic membrane fraction, and increases Ca^{2+} uptake or binding in brain preparations. The increase in intraneuronal Ca^{2+} probably enhances neurotransmitter release, an effect that may vary both in different parts of the brain and in neurotransmitter systems.[27,57,76] The effect of neurotransmitter release probably depends on the balance between the stimulatory and inhibitory actions of ethanol on processes regulating Ca^{2+}.[27] The ethanol-induced increases in resting intracellular Ca^{2+} may lead to a reduction of depolarization-induced Ca^{2+} uptake,[27,28] an effect that was observed in a number of studies. In animals treated chronically with ethanol, the in vitro effects of ethanol on Ca^{2+} uptake and binding are reduced.[28,57] These data suggest a biochemical basis for the development of tolerance and physical dependence. Thus, an increase in the sensitivity of the neurotransmitter release process to Ca^{2+} opposing the inhibitory effect of ethanol on Ca^{2+} entry, would be an adaptive change.[59,79] An increase in the number of voltage-operated Ca^{2+} channels (see Chapter 6) would also be adaptive. These adaptations would tend to decrease extracellular Ca^{2+} levels when ethanol is suddenly withdrawn, and may trigger seizures, perhaps because decreases in extracellular Ca^{2+} precipitate epileptic seizures.[56] A similar cellular adaptation to ethanol was demonstrated in clonal neural cells (PC12) in which acute exposure to ethanol produced a concentration-dependent decrease in depolarization-evoked $[^{45}Ca]^{2+}$ uptake; prolonged (2 to 10 days) exposure to ethanol led to a reciprocal increase in $[^{45}Ca]^{2+}$ uptake and in the number of Ca^{2+}-channel binding sites labeled by the dihydropyridine Ca^{2+}-channel antagonist $[^3H]$nitrendipine.[84]

Rats that were made physically dependent on ethanol by the inhalation technique showed increased functional activity of the dihydropyridine-sensitive subtype of voltage-operated Ca^{2+} channels on neuronal membranes.[36] This effect may alter the intraneuronal sensitivity to Ca^{2+}, possibly by modulating the inositol lipid signaling system.[75] Little, Dolin, and Halsey[75] reported that Ca^{2+}-channel antagonists (verapamil, flunarizine, nimodipine and nitrendipine) significantly attenuate withdrawal seizures in rats. These compounds had no sedative effects in normal animals. These results confirm the suggestion that some Ca^{2+} antagonists may be useful in treating seizures.[32] A randomized double-blind study indicated that caroverine, a group-B Ca^{2+} channel blocker, is as effective as meprobamate in treating acute alcohol withdrawal.[66] Caroverine is reputed to be effective against some forms of epileptic seizures.[66]

BZD Actions

A possible role for BZD as regulators of Ca^{2+} channel activity has been suggested for both centrally and peripherally acting BZD ligands.[93,99] Most studies have shown that at micromolar concentrations BZD stereoselectively inhibit depolarization-induced Ca^{2+} uptake into synaptosomes.[98,99] The resulting increase in extracellular Ca^{2+} may lead to suppression of seizures.[56] One study reported the opposite effect, however.[96] Carlen, Gurevich, and Polc[18] found that when applied in low nanomolar concentrations to CA1 hippocampal neurons in vitro, the BZD midazolam causes neuronal inhibition; they suggested that the BZD caused neuronal inhibition by increasing transmembrane inward Ca^{2+} currents, thereby raising intracellular Ca^{2+}, which in turn increased K^+ conductance. Further investigations are needed to determine the exact nature of the interaction of BZD with Ca^{2+} channels.

Acetylcholine

Acute exposure to ethanol depresses the cholinergic neuronal system because it decreases acetylcholine (ACh) release, elevates brain ACh levels, and decreases choline uptake.[57,96] There appears to be a differential sensitivity to the acute effects of ethanol in different brain regions.[57,96] In contrast, during chronic ethanol treatment the cholinergic system is activated, presumably due to an adaptive response to the actions of ethanol.[57,96] Thus, rats that are behaviorally tolerant to ethanol show an increase in stimulated ACh release, a decreased inhibitory response to ethanol, and reduced brain ACh levels at the time of ethanol withdrawal.[57,96] Increases in mouse striatal and hippocampal choline acetyltransferase (ChAT), the enzyme for ACh synthesis, occur about one hour after an acute dose of ethanol. However, after chronic ethanol treatment ChAT activity is decreased in rat hippocampus, but increased in the striatum.[57] Postmortem hippocampal ChAT activity is lower in chronic alcoholics than in controls.[57,96]

There appears to be no direct effect of acute ethanol on ACh receptors. However, changes in muscarinic ACh receptors have been reported to occur after chronic ethanol administration, although the data are conflicting.[57,60,96] There is a significant increase in the binding of quinuclidinyl benzylate (QNB), an antagonist to muscarinic ACh receptors, in the hippocampus and cortex but not in the striatum of ethanol-treated mice at the time of withdrawal and eight hours after withdrawal.[57] The time course of these changes appears to parallel the disappearance of overt withdrawal symptoms. Other studies did not report any change in QNB binding after chronic treatment; the length of ethanol exposure might have been a determining factor.[60] In one study where an increase in striatal ACh receptors was observed during ethanol withdrawal, rats that had withdrawal seizures showed less of an increase than rats that did not have seizures.[57] Rats that had been exposed to low levels of ethanol vapor for 14 days exhibited mild withdrawal signs; intrahippocampal injection of physostigmine, the cholinesterase inhibitor, elicited hippocampal seizure activity in 80 percent of the ethanol-dependent animals tested during withdrawal. Seizure activity was elicited in only 30 percent of control animals.[48] These results suggest that some of the symptoms of ethanol withdrawal may be related to an increase in sensitivity of hippocampal neurons to cholinergic stimulation.[48] Nicotinic receptors were also affected by long-term ethanol treatment (5 months of 8 to 12 percent ethanol solution), with a decrease in high affinity binding of [³H]nicotine in the hippocampus and an increase in similar bindings in hypothalamus and thalamus.[57,96] The significance of these changes needs further investigation. Rats with AWS are very sensitive to nicotine tremor.[2] In postmortem brain samples from alcoholics there was no change in the number of nicotinic receptors, but there was a decline in the number of muscarinic receptors, compared with control samples.[96]

BZD Actions

There have been suggestions that cholinergic neurotransmission participates in the mechanism of action of BZD and that there are relationships (direct or indirect) between central BZD effects and muscarinic receptor functions.[97] Some reports indicate that BZD reduce ACh turnover,[78] depress ACh release,[95,97] and increase endogenous brain level of ACh.[65,78] The reduction in ACh release caused by DZP is reversed by theophylline; this finding prompted Phillis, Siemens, and Wu[95] to hypothesize that this effect of DZP may be a result of preventing adenosine uptake, thereby enhancing the levels of extracellular adenosine. Conflicting results have been reported by Metlas and associates[85] who found no effect of DZP on synthesis and release of ACh in synaptosomal preparations. The K^+-induced release of ACh from rat cortical slices is also barely affected by DZP in concentrations up to 10 μM.[52]

Although BZD do not bind to muscarinic receptors, chronic treatment with DZP and medazepam in rats causes an overall decrease in muscarinic receptor binding affinity and an increase in the number of receptors in the cerebral cortex and hypothalamus, but a decrease in the number of receptors in the hippocampus and striatum.[97] The investigators suggested that the actions of BZD on the GABA/BZD/Cl⁻ ionophore receptor complex may provoke conformational changes in muscarinic receptors.

Opiates

Opioid peptides may play a role in epileptic seizures.[3] Acute ethanol treatment in animals increases striatal levels of methionine enkephalin[57] and beta-endorphin in hypothalamus and plasma.[64] However, one study found that a high dose of ethanol did not alter levels of leucine enkephalin.[57] Responses to ethanol also vary among different genetic strains of mice.[45] In rats, simultaneous administration of ethanol and beta-endorphin causes a greater impairment of the aerial righting reflex than administration of ethanol alone.[43] Beta-endorphin alone has no effect on this behavioral measure. In humans, acute alcohol intake increases plasma opioid-like activity but does not change beta-endorphin concentrations.[14] Data on the chronic effects of ethanol on endogenous "opiate" peptides are conflicting. Discrepancies may reflect the fact that different means of ethanol administration impart different levels of stress to the animals, or they may reflect inconsistencies of analytic methods and limitations imposed by *in vitro* studies of endorphin biosynthesis.[57] One research group reported an increase in the synthesis and release of beta-endorphin-like peptides from the pituitary, while another group found a decrease.[57] Methionine enkephalin levels in the rat brain were decreased after chronic ethanol treatment.[14,57,69] Conflicting results have also been reported for plasma levels of beta-endorphins in chronic alcoholics; some data reveal normal levels, some high, and some low.[14] Reduced CSF levels of beta-endorphin and a possible trend toward lower CSF levels of enkephalin have been reported in chronic alcoholics, but Hoffman and Tabakoff[57] cautioned that these studies might suffer from methodologic problems similar to those discussed above for animal studies.

Some studies have reported that the opioid antagonists naloxone or naltrexone can block the effects of ethanol on locomotor activity and duration of loss of righting reflex, but not other ethanol-induced behavioral decrements.[57,60] However, these results were not confirmed in other investigations.[54] In human studies, these opiate antagonists have been reported to be effective in reversing ethanol-induced coma and in preventing the symptoms of ethanol intoxications; however, these findings were not confirmed by others.[57,60] Two studies reported that naloxone given during ethanol withdrawal has no effect on the severity of withdrawal reactions, but one study stated that naloxone reduced AWS.[60,68,69] More consistent results were obtained if naloxone was administered daily during the development of ethanol dependence and also at the time of ethanol withdrawal; under these conditions, the number of withdrawal seizures was reduced significantly.[12,68] Audiogenic seizures during ethanol withdrawal could also be blocked by delta-opioid agonists such as synthetic analogues of enkephalins.[69] Delta sleep-inducing peptide (DSIP), a neuropeptide that has been postulated to possess an agonistic activity on opiate receptors, has been shown efficacious in diminishing some clinical signs of opiate and alcohol withdrawal in humans.[35] However, the usefulness of DSIP in preventing seizures is questionable.

Most studies concerning the influence of ethanol on the binding of opiates to the multiple opiate receptors involved very high ethanol concentrations (100–1000 mM). Therefore, the significance of these data for *in vivo* situations remains to be established. Other methodologic issues such as the presence of Na^+ in binding assays, reversibility of the *in vitro* effects of ethanol, and the temperature at which binding assays are performed have been discussed by Hoffman and Tabakoff.[57] In general, *in vitro* ethanol decreased binding to delta receptors (high affinity for enkephalin), increased mu-receptor binding (high affinity for morphine), and did not affect kappa-receptor binding.[57,60,96] One group of investigators attributed the changes in binding to changes in receptor affinity for ligands while another group to changes in the number of receptors.[57] The time course of the changes in mu-receptor affinity and the changes in function of opiate receptors in control of DA release did not correlate well with the time course over which overt withdrawal symptoms occur.[57] It has been suggested that the changes in opiate receptor function after chronic ethanol treatment might be related to the reinforcing effects of ethanol, rather than to its sedative actions.[57]

BZD Actions

Acute treatment of rats with BZD causes a rapid, dose-dependent decrease in striatal enkephalin levels but an increase in hypothalamic enkephalin levels.[37,52] These BZD actions are similar to those of ethanol. The striatal effect appeared to be mediated via a GABAergic mechanism, but the effect in the hypothalamus did not.[37] The release of met[5]-enkephalin elicited by depolarization was inhibited by BZD.[53] This inhibition was also purported to be mediated through the GABA system. Experimental evidence in rats suggests that an interaction exists between a BZD receptor mechanism(s) and regulation of hypothalamic corticotropin-releasing factor(s), which in turn controls the secretion of pituitary beta-endorphin.[80]

Sodium- and Potassium-Activated Adenosine Triphosphatase

The activity of sodium- and potassium-activated adenosine triphosphatase (Na^+/K^+-ATPase) was inhibited by ethanol, especially in the presence of very low concentrations of NE.[57,96] Chronic ethanol reduced the sensitivity of Na^+/K^+-ATPase to NE, possibly as a result of membrane effects of ethanol tolerance.[114] Other factors that may influence the effect of ethanol on ATPase are the person's age and genetic background.[96] Results conflict concerning the effect of chronic ethanol treatment on Na^+/K^+-ATPase; some studies describe no change and other studies reporting increased activity.[96] Enzyme activity is elevated during ethanol withdrawal (12-48 hours after termination of ethanol treatment), with the peak increase occurring after 24 hours.[96] This increase in ATPase activity has been postulated to be secondary to NE release as a result of stress during ethanol withdrawal.[96]

BZD Actions

Several studies have found that DZP inhibits Na^+/K^+-ATPase activity, sometimes only at high concentrations.[31,107,120] However, CDP was virtually ineffective.[109] Another study reported that DZP increased Na^+/K^+-ATPase activity in unstressed mice,[38] but reversed the stress-induced increase in enzyme activity. Injection of DZP (2 mg/kg) in rats with a penicillin-induced epileptogenic focus resulted in a 100 percent increase in Na^+/K^+-ATPase and suppression of seizures, despite increases in the frequency and amplitude variation of interictal discharges.[100]

Cyclic Nucleotide System

Cyclic Adenosine 3', 5'—Monophosphate

Results conflict about the acute effects of ethanol on brain levels of cyclic adenosine 3', 5'— monophosphate (cAMP). There are reports of increases, of decreases, and of no change, depending on the area of the brain studied. Some of these studies might have been confounded with postmortem changes brought about by the activities of adenylate cyclase and phosphodiesterase.[57,60,96] In general, acute ethanol treatment resulted in a dose-dependent decrease in cAMP levels, especially in the cerebellum and cortex.[57] Alcoholics showed a decrease in CSF levels of cAMP after ingestion of 3 g/kg of ethanol.[57] Chronic ethanol treatment resulted in either increased or decreased levels of cAMP, and the same phenomena persisted during ethanol withdrawal.[57,60] These findings may be related to changes of the cAMP system in response to increases in NE turnover during alcohol withdrawal.[123] However, a direct relationship between brain or CSF levels of cAMP and AWS has not been established. Alcoholics undergoing delirium tremens had reduced CSF levels of cAMP.[57] During this phase of alcohol withdrawal seizures are uncommon.[87]

Cyclic Guanosine 3',5'—Monophosphate

Acute ethanol treatment general decreases cyclic guanosine 3',5' — monophosphate (cGMP) levels, particularly in the cerebellum, and the levels remain low during chronic ethanol intake.[57,60,96] Alcoholics undergoing delirium tremens have increased CSF levels of cGMP.[57] When injected into the ventricular system of the brain, dibutyryl cGMP enhances ethanol-withdrawal-induced twitches in mice. On the other hand, a similar injection of dibutyryl cAMP reduces the head twitches.[60]

BZD Actions

In rodents, cerebellar cGMP levels are reduced by BZD in a dose-dependent manner.[52] This effect is blocked by Ro15-1788 and correlates strongly with the sedative and anticonvulsant potency of BZD.[52] BZD inhibit the stimulated cGMP increase in rat cerebellar slices.[52]

Hormones

Changes in blood levels of several hormones often occur in alcoholics undergoing withdrawal.[17,123] Thus, increases have been reported in adrenocorticotropic hormone (ACTH), cortisol, and vasopressin, as well as decreases in prolactin, the thyroid-stimulating hormone (TSH) response to thyrotropin-releasing hormone (TRH), and the growth hormone (GH) response to insulin-induced hypoglycemia.[17,123] The responses of GH to clonidine,[90] apomorphine,[9] and L-tryptophan[89] were also blunted. These changes are probably due to the brain's responses to the chronic effects of ethanol and to the stress of alcohol withdrawal. Some of these changes are long-lasting; for example, the blunted response of TSH to TRH has been reported to be still detectable 2 years after alcohol abstinence.[123] Therefore, hormonal changes are not likely to cause the appearance of withdrawal signs. It should be noted that TRH produces various central actions on neurotransmitters or neuromodulators unrelated to the pituitary-thyroid axis.[83]

BZD Actions

At low doses BZD generally do not affect basal secretion of prolactin, whereas high doses have been shown to lower basal serum prolactin levels in rats. BZD also reduce the prolactin increase produced by various neuroleptics and by stress.[52] DZP does not block the basal secretion of TSH, but BZD do inhibit TRH binding to specific sites in rat pituitary to suppress the release of TSH and growth hormone.[52,102] The interactions of BZD with TRH binding sites in rat amygdala, striatal, and cortical membranes do not appear to be related to their anxiolytic effects.[101]

SUMMARY

It is clear from the foregoing discussion that the neurochemical changes underlying the symptoms (e.g., seizures) of alcohol withdrawal are complex. Interpreting neurochemical correlates of AWS is hampered by our incomplete knowledge of the mechanisms of epileptic seizures and the neurochemical bases of tolerance and physical dependence. It is unlikely that perturbation of any particular neurotransmitter system adequately explains all withdrawal reactions, especially in light of the complex interactions among the neurotransmitter and neuromodulator systems in the brain.[57,96] Much remains to be learned about these complex interactions.

Although the alleviation of alcohol withdrawal reactions by BZD does not necessarily indicate that these drugs act on the neuronal systems that cause the manifestations of physical dependence,[57] it is informative to compare the neuropharmacologic changes induced by BZD with analogous changes associated with alcohol withdrawal. A summary of these changes is provided in Table 25–1. These data indicate that changes induced by BZDs in several neurochemical parame-

Table 25-1. NEUROPHARMACOLOGY OF BENZODIAZEPAM ACTIONS AND ALCOHOL WITHDRAWAL REACTIONS

System	BZD Actions	Withdrawal Reactions
GABA	Enhance GABA transmission ↓turnover ↑CSF GABA levels ↑GABA receptor binding ↑GABA-mediated Cl⁻ flux	Decrease in GABAergic activity ↓CSF GABA levels ↓GABA receptor binding
Glutamate	↓Glutamate release?	Glutamate supersensitivity?
DA	↓DA turnover ↓HVA levels	↓DA activity ↓HVA levels
NE	↓NE turnover	↑NE turnover
5-HT	↓5-HT turnover and activity	Inconsistent information
ACh	↓ACh turnover ↓ACh release ↑ACh levels	↑ACh release ↓ACh levels
Adenosine	↑Adenosine activity ↓Adenosine uptake ↑Release of adenosine	↓Adenosine receptor activity
Calcium	↓Depolarization-induced Ca^{2+} uptake	↑Ca^{2+} channel activity Ca^{2+}-channel antagonists attenuate withdrawal seizures
Opioid	↓Depolarization-induced enkephalin release ↓Striatal enkephalin ↑Hypothalamic enkephalin	Delta-opioid agonist blocked audiogenic seizures Conflicting data on ability of naloxone to block withdrawal seizures

Increase (↑) Decrease (↓)
GABA = γ-aminobutyric acid; DA = dopamine; NE = norepinephrine; 5-HT = serotonin; ACh = acetylcholine.

ters are opposite to those associated with alcohol withdrawal. These changes include changes in the GABA, NE, ACh, adenosine, and calcium systems, and may constitute the neurochemical bases on which BZD are effective in preventing and treating alcohol withdrawal reactions. Because adrenergic hyperactivity and GABAergic hypoactivity are the two neurochemical alterations most consistently associated with alcohol withdrawal, they may be at least partially responsible for the manifestations of withdrawal symptoms. Neurochemical investigations with specially bred strains of mice which differ in severity of alcohol withdrawal seizures[67] and sensitivity to DZP[44] are likely to provide some useful information on the neurochemical mechanisms of alcohol withdrawal and the actions of BZD.

Some of the neurochemical changes associated with ethanol withdrawal are similar to those postulated to be mechanisms of epileptic seizures[6,22,40,56,91] However, whether an alcoholic develops seizures during alcohol withdrawal also depends on a host of other factors such as the person's genetic makeup, seizure threshold, drinking history, infection, malnutrition, health status, and history of drug use or abuse, trauma, epilepsy, and alcohol withdrawal seizures.

ACKNOWLEDGMENTS

Thanks to Carol Tixier for typing and to Donna L. Schanley for proofreading this manuscript.

References

1. Adinoff, B, et al: The benzodiazepine antagonist Ro15-1788 does not antagonize the ethanol withdrawal syndrome. Biol Psychiatry 21:643, 1986.
2. Airaksinen, MM and Peura, P: Mechanisms of alcohol withdrawal syndrome. Medical Biology 65:105, 1987.
3. Allan, AM, et al: Genetic selection for benzodiazepine ataxia produces functional changes in γ-aminobutyric acid receptor chloride channel complex. Brain Res 452:118, 1988.
4. Allan, AM and Harris, RA: Acute and chronic ethanol treatments alter GABA receptor-operated chloride channels. Pharmacol Biochem Behav 27:665, 1987.
5. Allan, AM, Spuhler, KP, and Harris, RA: γ-aminobutyric acid-activated chloride channels: Relationship to genetic differences in ethanol sensitivity. J Pharmacol Exp Ther 244:866, 1988.
6. Ault, B and Wang, CM: Adenosine inhibits epileptiform activity arising in hippocampal area CA3. Br J Pharmacol 87:695, 1986.
7. Bagdy, G and Arato, M: Serum dopamine-β-hydroxylase activity and alcohol withdrawal symptoms. Drug Alcohol Depend 19:45, 1987.
8. Bajorek, JG, Lee, RJ, and Lomax, P: Neuropeptides: A role as endogenous mediators or modulators of epileptic phenomena. Ann Neurol 16(Suppl):S31, 1984.
9. Balldin, J, et al: Changes in dopamine receptor sensitivity in humans after heavy alcohol intake. Psychopharmacology 86:142, 1985.
10. Banki, CM and Molnar, G: Cerebrospinal fluid amine metabolites in delirium tremens. Psychiatria Clinica 14:167, 1981.
11. Baumgartner, GR and Rowen, RC: Clonidine vs chlordiazepoxide in the management of acute alcohol withdrawal syndrome. Arch Intern Med 147:1223, 1987.
12. Berman, RF, et al: Effects of naloxone on ethanol dependence in rats. Drug Alcohol Depend 13:245, 1984.
13. Borg, S, Kvande, H, and Valverius, P: Clinical conditions and central dopamine metabolism in alcoholics during acute withdrawal under treatment with different pharmacological agents. Psychopharmacology 88:12, 1986.
14. Brambilla, F, et al: Plasma opioids in alcoholics after acute alcohol consumption and withdrawal. Acta Psychiatr Scand 77:63, 1988.
15. Bruun-Meyer, SE: The GABA/benzodiazepine receptor-chloride ionophore complex: Nature and modulation. Prog Neuropsychopharmacol Biol Psychiat 11:365, 1987.
16. Burroughs, AK, Morgan, MY, and Sherlock, S: Double-blind controlled trial of bromocriptine, chlordiazepoxide and chlormethiazole for alcohol withdrawal symptoms. Alcohol Alcoholism 20:263, 1985.
17. Camerlingo, M, et al: Neuroendocrinological abnormalities in chronic alcoholic men after withdrawal. Neuroendocrinology (Letters) 8:123, 1986.
18. Carlen, P, Gurevich, N, and Polc, P: Low-dose benzodiazepine neuronal inhibition: Enhanced Ca^{2+}-mediated K^+-conductance. Brain Res 271:358, 1983.
19. Chan, AWK: Alcoholism and epilepsy. Epilepsia 26:323, 1985.
20. Chan, AWK: Effects of combined alcohol and benzodiazepine: A review. Drug Alcohol Depend 13:315, 1984.
21. Chan, AWK: Ethanol and chlordiazepoxide cross-dependence. Alcohol Alcoholism (Suppl)1:423, 1987.
22. Chugani, HJ and Olsen, RW: Benzodiazepine/GABA receptors and chloride channels: Structural and functional properties. In Olsen, RW and Venter, JC (eds): Receptor Biochemistry and Methodology, Vol 5. Alan R Liss, New York, 1986, p 315.
23. Cicero, TJ: Alcohol self-administration, tolerance and withdrawal in humans and animals: Theoretical and methodological issues. In Rigter, H, Crabbe, JC (eds): Alcohol Tolerance and Dependence. Elsevier/North-Holland, New York, 1980, p 1.
24. Clemmesen, L, et al: Convulsive and nonconvulsive ethanol withdrawal behaviour in rats with lesions of the noradrenergic *locus coeruleus* system. Brain Res 346:164, 1985.
25. Coffman, JA and Petty, F: Plasma GABA levels in chronic alcoholics. Am J Psychiatry 142:1204, 1985.
26. Cushman, P, Lerner, W, and Cramer, W: Adrenergic agonist therapy in alcohol withdrawal states in man. Psychopharmacol Bull 21:651, 1985.
27. Daniell, LC, Brass, EP, and Harris, RA: Effect of ethanol on intracellular ionized calcium concentrations in synaptosomes and hepatocytes. Mol Pharmacol 32:831, 1987.
28. Daniell, LC and Harris, A: Effect of chronic ethanol treatment and selective breeding for hypnotic sensitivity to ethanol on intracellular ionized calcium concentrations in synaptosomes. Alcoholism 12:179, 1988.
29. Dar, MS, Mustafa, SJ, and Wooles, WR: Possible role of adenosine in the CNS effects of ethanol. Life Sci 33:1363, 1983.
30. Dar, MS and Wooles, WR: Striatal and hypothalamic neurotransmitter changes during ethanol withdrawal in mice. Alcohol 1:453, 1984.
31. Das, S, et al: Role of imipramine and desipramine in counteracting diazepam induced changes of adenosinetriphosphatase and cholinesterase of human fetal brain. Indian J Exp Biol 19:738, 1981.
32. De Sarro, GB, Meldrum, BS, and Nistico, G: Anticonvulsant effects of some calcium entry blockers in DBA/2 mice. Br J Pharmacol 93:247, 1988.
33. DeVries, DJ, et al: Effects of chronic ethanol inhalation on the enhancement of benzodiazepine binding to mouse brain membranes by GABA. Neurochem Int 10:231, 1987.
34. Diamond, I, et al: Basal and adenosine receptor-stimulated levels of cAMP are reduced in lymphocytes from alcoholic patients. Proc Natl Acad Sci USA 84:1413, 1987.

35. Dick, P, et al: DSIP in the treatment of withdrawal syndromes from alcohol and opiates. Eur Neurol 23:364, 1984.
36. Dolin, S, et al: Increased dihydropyridine-sensitive calcium channels in rat brain may underlie ethanol physical dependence. Neuropharmacology 26:275, 1987.
37. Duka, T, Wuster, M, and Herz, A: Benzodiazepines modulate striatal enkephalin levels via a GABAergic mechanism. Life Sci 26:771, 1980.
38. Eroglu, L, Keyer-Uysal, M, and Baykara, S: Effects of lithium, diazepam and propranolol on brain Na^+/K^+-ATPase activity in stress-exposed mice. Arzneimittel-Forschung 34:762, 1984.
39. Fadda, F, et al: Suppression by progabide of ethanol withdrawal syndrome in rats. Eur J Pharmacol 109:321, 1985.
40. Fariello, RG: Biochemical approaches to seizure mechanisms: The GABA and glutamate systems. In Porter, RJ and Morselli, PL (eds): The Epilepsies. Butterworth & Co, London, 1985, p 1.
41. Friedman, HJ: Assessment of physical dependence on and withdrawal from ethanol in animals. In Rigter, H and Crabbe, JC (eds): Alcohol Tolerance and Dependence. Elsevier/North-Holland, New York, 1980, p 93.
42. Frye, GD, et al: Modification of the actions of ethanol by centrally active peptides. Peptides 2(Suppl)1:99, 1981.
43. Frye, GD and Fincher, AS: Effect of ethanol on γ-vinyl GABA-induced accumulation in the substantia nigra and on synaptosomal GABA content in six rat brain regions. Brain Res 449:71, 1988.
44. Gallaher, EJ, et al: Mouse lines selected for genetic differences in diazepam sensitivity. Psychopharmacology 93:25, 1987.
45. Gianoulakis, C and Gupta, A: Inbred strains of mice with variable sensitivity to ethanol exhibit differences in the content and processing of β-endorphin. Life Sci 39:2315, 1986.
46. Goldstein, DB: The alcohol withdrawal syndrome: A view from the laboratory. In Galanter, M (ed): Recent Developments in Alcoholism, Vol 4. Plenum Press, New York, 1986, p 231.
47. Goldstein, DB: Animal studies of alcohol withdrawal reactions. In Israel, Y, et al (eds): Research Advances in Alcohol and Drug Problems, Vol 4. Plenum Press, New York, 1978, p 77.
48. Gonzalez, LP: Changes in physostigmine-induced hippocampal seizures during ethanol withdrawal. Brain Res 335:384, 1985.
49. Gordon, AS, Collier, K, and Diamond, I: Ethanol regulation of adenosine receptor-stimulated cAMP levels in a clonal neural cell line: An in vitro model of cellular tolerance to ethanol. Proc Natl Acad Sci USA 83:2105, 1986.
50. Gottlieb, LD: The role of beta blockers in alcohol withdrawal syndrome. Postgrad Med Special No:169, 1988.
51. Greenblatt, DJ, Shader, RI, and Abernethy, DR: Current status of benzodiazepines. N Engl J Med 309:354, 1983.
52. Haefely, W: Tranquilizers. In Grahame-Smith, DG (ed): Psychopharmacology 2, Part 1: Preclinical Psychopharmacology. Elsevier Science Publishers BV, 1985, p 92.
53. Harsing, LG, Yang, HYT, and Costa, E: Evidence for a γ-aminobutyric acid (GABA) mediation in the benzodiazepine inhibition of the release of met[5]-enkephalin elicited by depolarization. J Pharmacol Exp Ther 220:616, 1982.
54. Hatch, RC and Jernigan, AD: Effect of intravenously-administered putative and potential antagonists of ethanol on sleep time in ethanol-narcotized mice. Life Sci 42:11, 1988.
55. Hawley, RJ, et al: Cerebrospinal fluid 3-methoxy-4-hydroxyphenylglycol and norepinephrine levels in alcohol withdrawal. Arch Gen Psychiatry 42:1056, 1985.
56. Heinemann, U and Hamon, B: Calcium and epileptogenesis. Exp Brain Res 65:1, 1986.
57. Hoffman, PL and Tabakoff, B: Ethanol's action on brain biochemistry. In Tarter, RE and Van Thiel, DH (eds): Alcohol and the brain: Chronic effects. Plenum Press, New York, 1985, p 19.
58. Hruska, RE: Effect of ethanol administration on striatal D_1 and D_2 dopamine receptors. J Neurochem 50:1929, 1988.
59. Hudspith, MJ, et al: Dihydropyridine-sensitive Ca^{2+} channels and inositol phospholipid metabolism in ethanol physical dependence. Ann NY Acad Sci 492:156, 1987.
60. Hunt, WA: Alcohol and Biological Membranes. The Guilford Press, New York, 1985.
61. Ida, Y, et al: Attenuating effect of diazepam on stress-induced increases in noradrenaline turnover in specific brain regions of rats: Antagonism by Ro15-1788. Life Sci 37:2491, 1985.
62. Iversen, S: Where in the brain do benzodiazepines act? In Trimble, MR (ed): Benzodiazepines Divided. John Wiley & Sons, New York, 1983, p 167.
63. Kahn, RS, et al: Serotonin and anxiety revisited. Biol Psychiatry 23:189, 1988.
64. Keith, LD, et al: Ethanol stimulates endorphin and corticotropin secretion in vitro. Brain Res 367:222, 1986.
65. Kolasa, K, et al: Blockade of the diazepam-induced increase in rat striatal acetylcholine content by the specific benzodiazepine antagonists ethyl-β-carboline-3-carboxylate and Ro15-1788. Brain Res 336:342, 1985.
66. Koppi, S, et al: Calcium-channel-blocking agent in the treatment of acute alcohol withdrawal: Caroverine versus meprobamate in a randomized double-blind study. Neuropsychobiology 17:49, 1987.
67. Kosobud, A and Crabbe, JC: Ethanol withdrawal in mice bred to be genetically prone or resistant to ethanol withdrawal seizures. J Pharmacol Exp Ther 238:170, 1986.
68. Kotlinska, J and Langwinski, R: Does the blockade of opioid receptors influence the development of ethanol dependence? Alcohol Alcoholism 22:117, 1987.
69. Kotlinska, J and Langwinski, R: Audiogenic seizures during ethanol withdrawal can be blocked by a delta opioid agonist. Drug Alcohol Depend 18:361, 1986.

70. Kraus, ML, et al: Randomized clinical trial of atenolol in patients with alcohol withdrawal. New Engl J Med 313:905, 1985.
71. Kulonen, E: Ethanol and GABA. Medical Biology 61:147, 1983.
72. Linnoila, M: Benzodiazepines and alcoholism. In Trimble, MR (ed): Benzodiazepines Divided. John Wiley & Sons, New York, 1983, p 291.
73. Lister, RG and Karanian, JW: Ro15-4513 induces seizures in DBA/2 mice undergoing alcohol withdrawal. Alcohol 4:409, 1987.
74. Little, HJ, et al: The benzodiazepine antagonist Ro15-1788 does not decrease ethanol withdrawal convulsions in rats. Eur J Pharmacol 107:375, 1985.
75. Little, HJ, Dolin, SJ, and Halsey, MJ: Calcium channel antagonists decrease the ethanol withdrawal syndrome. Life Sci 39:2059, 1986.
76. Littleton, JM: Biochemical pharmacology of ethanol tolerance and dependence. In Edwards, G and Littleton, J (eds): Pharmacological Treatment for Alcoholism. Methuen & Co, New York, 1984, p 119.
77. Loscher, W and Schmidt, D: Diazepam increases γ-aminobutyric acid in human cerebrospinal fluid. J Neurochem 49:152, 1987.
78. Lundgren, G, et al: Effects of diazepam on blood choline and acetylcholine turnover in brain of mice. Pharmacol Toxicol 60:96, 1987.
79. Lynch, MA, Archer, ER, and Littleton, JM: Increased sensitivity of transmitter release to calcium in ethanol tolerance. Biochem Pharmacol 35:1207, 1986.
80. Maiewski, SF, et al: Evidence that a benzodiazepine receptor mechanism regulates the secretion of pituitary β-endorphin in rats. Endocrinology 117:474, 1985.
81. Manhem, P, et al: Alcohol withdrawal: Effect of clonidine treatment on sympathetic activity, the renin-aldosterone system, and clinical symptoms. Alcoholism 9:238, 1985.
82. Marley, RJ and Wehner, JM: Correlation between the enhancement of flunitrazepam binding by GABA and seizure susceptibility in mice. Life Sci 40:2215, 1987.
83. Matsumoto, A, et al: Clinical effects of TRH for severe epilepsy in childhood. A comparative study with ACTH therapy. Epilepsia 28:49, 1987.
84. Messing, RO, et al: Ethanol regulates calcium channels in clonal neural cells. Proc Natl Acad Sci USA 83:6213, 1986.
85. Metlas, R, et al: Acetylcholine synthesis and release by brain cortex synaptosomes of rats treated with diazepam. Iugoslavica Physiologica et Pharmacologica Acta 20:213, 1984.
86. Morrow, AL and Paul, SM: Benzodiazepine enhancement of γ-aminobutyric acid-mediated chloride ion flux in rat brain synaptoneurosomes. J Neurochem 50:302, 1988.
87. Naranjo, CA and Sellers, EM: Clinical assessment and pharmacotherapy of the alcohol withdrawal syndrome. In Galanter, M (ed): Recent Developments in Alcoholism, Vol 4. Plenum Press, New York, 1986, p 265.
88. Norman, TR and Burrows, GD: Anxiety and the benzodiazepine receptor. Prog Brain Res 65:73, 1986.
89. Nutt, D, et al: α-2-Adrenoceptor function in alcohol withdrawal: A pilot study of the effects of IV clonidine in alcoholics and normals. Alcoholism 12:14, 1988.
90. Nutt, DJ and Cowen, PJ: Diazepam alters brain 5-HT function in man: Implications for the acute and chronic effects of benzodiazepines. Psychol Med 17:601, 1987.
91. Olsen, RW, et al: Role of the γ-aminobutyric acid receptor-ionophore complex in seizure disorders. Ann Neurol 16(Suppl):S90, 1984.
92. Parale, MP and Kulkarni, SK: Studies with α2-adrenoceptor agonists and alcohol abstinence syndrome in rats. Psychopharmacology 88:237, 1986.
93. Paul, SM, Luu, MD, and Skolnick, P: The Effects of benzodiazepines on presynaptic calcium transport. In Usdin, E, et al (eds): Pharmacology of Benzodiazepines. Verlag Chemie, Weinheim, 1983, p 87.
94. Phillis, JW and O'Regan, MH: The role of adenosine in the central actions of the benzodiazepines. Prog Neuropsychopharmacol Biol Psychiatry 12:389, 1988.
95. Phillis, JW, Siemens, RK, and Wu, PH: Effects of diazepam on adenosine and acetylcholine release from rat cerebral cortex: Further evidence for a purinergic mechanism in action of diazepam. Br J Pharmacol 70:341, 1980.
96. Pohorecky, LA and Brick, J: Pharmacology of ethanol. Pharmacol Ther 36:335, 1988.
97. Popova, J, Petkov, VV, and Tokuschieva, L: The effect of chronic diazepam and medazepam treatment on the number and affinity of muscarinic receptors in different rat brain structures. Gen Pharmacol 19:227, 1988.
98. Rampe, D and Triggle, DJ: Benzodiazepine interactions at neuronal and smooth muscle Ca^{2+} channels. Eur J Pharmacol 134:189, 1987.
99. Rampe, D and Triggle, DJ: Benzodiazepines and calcium channel function. Trends in Pharmacological Sciences 7:461, 1986.
100. Rekhtman, MB, Samsonov, NA, and Kryzhanovsky, GN: Electrical activity and sodium-potassium ATPase level in penicillin-induced epileptogenic focus in the rat brain cortex and diazepam effect on them. Neirofiziologiia 12:349, 1980.
101. Rinehart, RK, et al: Benzodiazepine interactions with central thyroid-releasing hormone binding sites: Characterization and physiological significance. J Pharmacol Exp Ther 238:178, 1986.
102. Roussel, JP, Astier, H, and Tapia-Arancibia, L: Benzodiazepines inhibit thyrotropin-releasing hormone-induced TSH and growth hormone release from perfused rat pituitaries. Endocrinology 119:2519, 1986.
103. Saito, T, et al: Effects of chronic ethanol treatment on the β-adrenergic receptor-coupled adenylate cyclase system of mouse cerebral cortex. J Neurochem 48:1817, 1987.
104. Sandler, M, et al: Ethanol and endogenous ligands in humans. Psychopharmacol Bull 27:485, 1984.
105. Schmutz, M: Benzodiazepines, GABA, and ep-

ilepsy: The animal evidence. In Trimble, MR (ed): Benzodiazepine Divided. John Wiley & Sons, New York, 1983, p 149.
106. Schwarz, SS and Freed, WJ: Inhibition of quisqualate-induced seizures by glutamic acid diethyl ester and antiepileptic drugs. J Neural Transm 67:191, 1986.
107. Sethi, JS and Tanwar, RK: The effect of diazepam and chlorpromazine on the activity of ATPase in mice neocortex and hippocampal formation. Z Mikrosk Anat Forsch 100:913, 1986.
108. Shephard, RA: Neurotransmitters, anxiety and benzodiazepines: A behaivoral review. Neurosci Biobehav Rev 10:449, 1986.
109. Sikora, J and Krulik, R: Psychotropic drugs and differently stimulated ATPase in CNS. Activitas Nervosa Superior (Praha) 16:222, 1974.
110. Simler, S, et al: Brain γ-aminobutyric acid turnover rates after spontaneous chronic ethanol intake and withdrawal in discrete brain areas of C57 mice. J Neurochem 47:1942, 1986.
111. Suranyi-Cadotte, B, et al: Decreased density of peripheral benzodiazepine binding sites on platelets of currently drinking, but not abstinent alcoholics. Neuropharmacology 27:443, 1988.
112. Suzdak, PD, et al: Alcohols stimulate γ-aminobutyric acid receptor-mediated chloride uptake in brain vesicles: Correlation with intoxication potency. Brain Res 444:340, 1988.
113. Suzdak, PD and Paul, SM: Ethanol stimulates GABA receptor-mediated Cl^- ion flux in vitro: Possible relationships to the anxiolytic and intoxicating actions of alcohol. Psychopharmacol Bull 23:445, 1987.
114. Swann, AC: (Na^+, K^+)-ATPase and noradrenergic function: Effects of chronic ethanol. Eur J Pharmacol 134:145, 1987.
115. Syapin, PJ and Alkana, RL: Chronic ethanol exposure increases peripheral-type benzodiazepine receptors in brain. Eur J Pharmacol 147:101, 1988.
116. Tabakoff, B and Hoffman, PL: Alcohol and neurotransmitters. In Rigter, H and Crabbe, JC (eds): Alcohol Tolerance and Dependence. Elsevier/North-Holland, New York, 1980, p 201.
117. Tabakoff, B and Hoffman, P: Neurochemical aspects of tolerance to and physical dependence on alcohol. In Kissin, B and Begleiter, H (eds): The Biology of Alcoholism, Vol 7. Plenum Press, New York, 1983, p 199.
118. Tamborska, E and Marangos, PJ: Brain benzodiazepine binding sites in ethanol dependent and withdrawal states. Life Sci 38:465, 1986.
119. Tancredi, V, et al: Interactions between amino acid neurotransmitters and flurazepam in the neocortex of unanesthetized rats. Journal of Neuroscience Research 9:159, 1983.
120. Ueda, I, Wada, T, and Ballinger, CM: Sodium and potassium-activated ATPase of beef brain: Effect of some tranquilizers. Biochem Pharmacol 20:1697, 1971.
121. Valverius, P, Hoffman, PL, and Tabakoff, B: Effect on mouse cerebral cortical β-adrenergic receptors. Mol Pharmacol 32:217, 1987.
122. Vellucci, SV and Webster, RA: GABA and benzodiazepine-induced modification of $[^{14}C]$L-glutamic acid release from rat spinal cord slices. Brain Res 330:201, 1985.
123. Wilkins, JN and Gorelick, DA: Clinical neuroendocrinology and neuropharmacology of alcohol withdrawal. In Galanter, M (ed): Recent Developments in Alcoholism, Vol 4. Plenum Press, New York, 1986, p 241.
124. Wilkins, AJ, Jenkins, WJ, and Steiner, JA: Efficacy of clonidine in treatment of alcohol withdrawal state. Psychopharmacology 81:78, 1983.
125. Yool, AJ and Gruol, DL: Development of spontaneous and glutamate-evoked activity is altered by chronic ethanol in cultured cerebellar Purkinje neurons. Brain Res 420:205, 1987.

CHAPTER 26

David M. Treiman, M.D.

Treatment of Alcohol Withdrawal Seizures with Benzodiazepines: Clinical Applications

A wide variety of drugs has been used to manage alcohol withdrawal (Table 26-1), and many clinicians hold strong opinions about the best regimen for treating this condition. Unfortunately, few data exist to document the efficacy of most drugs used for the alcohol withdrawal syndrome. In considering the optimal management of both the alcohol withdrawal syndrome and alcohol withdrawal seizures (AWS), two questions must be addressed. What is the evidence that any drugs are effective in treating alcohol withdrawal? Do data show that one drug or class of drugs is more effective than any other?

CLINICIAL TRIALS

In order to answer these qustions, Moskowitz and associates,[16] analyzed the results of 81 clinical trials of drugs used to treat the alcohol withdrawal syndrome, involving 6,808 patients and published in English between 1954 and 1983. In 29 of the trials, patients were randomly assigned to a treatment category; in 19, patients were alternately assigned treatment categories; 3 used historical controls; and 13 employed other treatment assignment methods. Thirty-five of the 48 randomized and alternate trials were conducted in a double-blind fashion.

Of the 29 randomized controlled trials, placebo controls were used in 17 and active controls in the remaining 12. Table 26-2 shows the various treatments compared in the 29 randomized controlled trials. The quality of the protocol was graded using a system developed by Chalmers and associates,[5] for evaluating adequacy of descriptions, blinding procedures, and essential measurements in the design of a clinical trial. Table 26-3 lists the percentage of the 29 randomized controlled trials that fulfilled each of a series of criteria for quality of experimental design. Only 72 percent of the trials were double blind, and 55 percent listed specific selection criteria. The mean protocol quality for the 29 randomized controlled trials, using the Chalmers rating system, was 0.49 ± 0.03 (using this scale, a perfect study would score 1.00). Data presentation and statistical analysis in these trials were similarly rated and had a mean score of 0.18 ± 0.03. Many investigators did not report confidence intervals, handle dropouts properly, or provide adequate details about side-effects.

Table 26–1. DRUGS USED TO MANAGE ALCOHOL WITHDRAWAL

α-adrenergic agonists
    Clonidine
    Lofexidine
Anticonvulsants
    Carbamazepine
    Phenytoin
Antihistamines
    Diphenhydramine
    Hydroxyzine
Barbiturates
    Pentobarbital
    Phenobarbital
    Secobarbitol
Benzodiazepines
    Alprazolam
    Chlordiazepoxide
    Clobazam
    Diazepam
    Halazepam
    Lorazepam
    Oxazepam
β-adrenergic blockers
    Atenolol
    Propanolol
    Timolol
Neuroleptics
    Chlorpromazine
    Haloperidol
    Perphenazine
    Promazine
Sedative/hypnotics
    Chlomethiazole
    Chloral hydrate
    Paraldehyde
Vitamins, *etc.*
    Magnesium
    Nicotinamide
    Thiamine

Table 26–2. ALCOHOL WITHDRAWAL THERAPIES IN 29 RANDOMIZED CONTROLLED TRIALS

Drug Type	Number of Times Tested*
Antipsychotics	24
Placebo	17
Benzodiazepines	15
Anticonvulsants	6
β-blockers	4
Hormones	4
Sedative/hypnotics	3
Vitamins	3
Barbiturates	2
Other minor tranquilizers	1
Other drugs	1

*The number of times each drug category was noted was tested in 29 randomized controlled trials of treatment of alcohol withdrawal. The total numbers are higher than the number of papers because many trials compared more than the minimum of two drug regimens.
Adapted from Moskowitz et al.[16]

Benzodiazepines

Thirteen of the 29 randomized controlled trials included testing at least one benzodiazepine. In ten, at least one antipsychotic drug was tested, and in 14 a placebo was included. Most often antipsychotics were compared with other antipsychotics, but the same drugs were not consistently compared. Although Moskowitz and her associates[16] attempted to compare, in a variety of ways, the 80 treatment and placebo regimens used in the 29 randomized controlled trials, the only conclusion they reached was that benzodiazepines are clearly superior to placebos. Six benzodiazepines were compared with placebos in randomized controlled trials, and in five of the comparisons benzodiazepines were judged significantly better in treating alcohol withdrawal.[9,10,22,23,29] One study found that chlordiazepoxide was superior to chlorpromazine, hydroxyzine, thiamine, and placebos in preventing delirium tremens and seizures.[10] By combining the results (using the Mantel-Haenszel technique[14]), Moskowitz and associates[16] determined

Table 26–3. QUALITY OF PROTOCOL: PERCENTAGE OF STUDIES WITH DESIRABLE EXPERIMENTAL DESIGN FEATURES

Characteristics of 29 Randomized Controlled Trials	Percentage
Selection criteria	55
Number of patients seen and rejection log	3
Withdrawals: number and reason	34
Blinding of patients and physicians	72
Prior estimate of sample size	0
Placebo	
Appearance	52
Taste	24
Testing	
Randomization	34
Compliance	0
Biological equipment	17

Adapted from Moskowitz et al.[16]

that benzodiazepines are much better than placebos ($\chi^2 = 40.43$, $p > 0.001$) to treat the alcohol withdrawal syndrome.

Moskowitz and associates[16] realized that the studies they had reviewed had substantial limitations. Even when all the data were analyzed together it was impossible to determine which benzodiazepine was most effective in treating the alcohol withdrawal syndrome. It was also impossible to compare the efficacy and toxicity of other classes of drugs used in treating alcohol withdrawal. In addition, none of the side-effects of the drugs studied could be compared. Furthermore, it was impossible to determine the prevalence of either AWS or delirium tremens. One study, not reviewed by Moskowitz, compared the efficacy of rectal paraldehyde and intravenous (IV) diazepam in treating 34 patients with severe delirium tremens.[26] Diazepam calmed patients significantly faster than paraldehyde.

Since publication of Moskowitz and associates'[16] analysis, only one additional study comparing benzodiazepine with placebos has been published.[4] This report demonstrated the superiority of chlordiazepoxide (and chlormethiazole but not bromocriptine) over placebos in managing the alcohol withdrawal syndrome. Nine other randomized double-blind controlled studies (involving 526 patients) published since 1983 demonstrated no difference in effectiveness for treating the alcohol withdrawal syndrome between chlordiazepoxide and clobazam,[17] lorazepam,[25] halazepam,[15] alprazolam,[31] or clonidine,[1] between diazepam and lorazepam,[18,21] and no difference in efficacy between alprazolam and chlormethiazole.[28]

Unfortunately, no new conclusions can be drawn from these studies; although they support the observation that benzodiazepines are effective in managing the alcohol withdrawal syndrome. Few data adequately support the efficacy of benzodiazepines or any other drug in preventing or managing AWS.

TREATMENT OF AWS

Table 26-4 describes the characteristics of an ideal drug for managing AWS. Be-

Table 26–4. CHARACTERISTICS OF AN "IDEAL" DRUG TO TREAT ALCOHOL WITHDRAWAL SEIZURES

A drug that:
  has both sedative and anticonvulsant properties
  is rapidly effective against ongoing seizures
  is available for either IV or intramuscular administration
  is potent, so small volumes can be given rapidly
  is "safe"—i.e., does not depress either cardiorespiratory function or consciousness, and has no systemic effect(s)
  has a long, effective half-life, preventing additional seizures as well as controlling ongoing seizures
  has a relatively short elimination half-life, so the drug can be readily tapered and discontinued.

cause the efficacy of benzodiazepines in handling the alcohol withdrawal syndrome has been clearly demonstrated, and at least one study has shown chlordiazepoxide's efficacy against AWS,[10] it is worthwhile to consider how well benzodiazepines fulfill the characteristics of an ideal drug for managing AWS. Benzodiazepines have both sedative and anticonvulsant properties,[6] and are rapidly effective against ongoing seizures.[27] They are available for rapid IV administration and quickly enter the brain. Most benzodiazepines have relatively long half-lives, so they can used used to prevent further seizures as well as to stop ongoing seizures. Some benzodiazepines have a relatively short elimination half-life and thus can be rapidly tapered and discontinued after acute administration. However, there is a potential for withdrawal reactions if benzodiazepines are administered after the acute phase of an alcohol withdrawal syndrome. There is risk of respiratory decompensation, especially in patients with chronic obstructive pulmonary disease and patients simultaneously receiving barbiturates. Because other benzodiazepines have longer elimination half-lives, discontinuation is more difficult. There is also the potential for accumulation of benzodiazepines when multiple doses are given over a short period during the acute phase of alcohol withdrawal; such a regimen may result in prolonged sedation of the patient. Chlordiazepoxide has been shown to have a prolonged half-life and decreased clearance during acute intoxication[30] and during early withdrawal from alcohol,[19] characteristics that may also cause drug accumulation. However, diazepam and its N-demethyl metabolite are more rapidly eliminated after chronic alcohol intake.[24]

Although no data from controlled clinical trials suggest the superiority of one benzodiazepine over another in the management of the alcohol withdrawal syndrome or AWS, clinical experience suggests the relative advantages and disadvantages of a number of benzodiazepine compounds;[8,12] these are listed in Table 26-5. Table 26-6 shows the pharmacokinetic parameters of benzodiazepines used in managing alcohol withdrawal. There are significant differences among benzodiazepines in half-lives, lipid solubility, and degree of protein binding. In the absence of data clearly supporting the choice of one benzodiazepine over another in treating both the alcohol withdrawal syndrome and AWS, the choice of drug should be influenced by the relative pharmacokinetic properties of the various benzodiazepines.

General Principles

Whichever benzodiazepine is chosen, general principles apply to their use in managing the alcohol withdrawal syndrome. It is important to avoid doses that result in accumulation of the drug or an active metabolite and thus cause drowsiness, ataxia, lethargy, diplopia, confusion, and respiratory depression. A progressive dose reduction schedule can be used in which the initial dose is reduced by 25% on each successive day of treatment. In general, benzodiazepines should be given IV or orally, because intramuscular injection results in erratic and sometimes poor absorption.[6,13] Lorazepam, however, is rapidly and completely absorbed after intramuscular injection, and reaches peak plasma concentrations 1.5 hours after injection.[2] Heavy smokers may need higher doses of benzodiazepines because nicotine induces hepatic microsomal enzyme activity. On the other hand, lower doses of benzodiazepines should be used to treat patients with liver failure because drug clearance may be impaired in these patients; also, in liver failure patients free drug concentrations may be higher be-

Table 26–5. ADVANTAGES AND DISADVANTAGES OF BENZODIAZEPINES IN TREATING ALCOHOL WITHDRAWAL

Drug	Clinical Experience	Half-Life (hr)	Active Metabolite	Reduced Clearance with Liver Disease	Intramuscular Bioavailability	Comments
Chlordiazepoxide	+++	10	Desmethylchlordiazepoxide;* demoxepam; oxazepam; desmethyldiazepam	Yes	Poor	Inexpensive; parenteral formulation inconvenient
Clorazepate	+	Very short	Desmethyldiazepam,* oxazepam	Yes	—	Expensive; no advantage over diazepam
(= Desmethyldiazepam)	+	51	Oxazepam	Yes	—	
Diazepam	+++	31	Desmethyldiazepam;* temazepam; oxazepam	Yes	Poor	Inexpensive; easy parenteral formulation
Lorazepam	++	14	Inactive glucuronide	No	Good	Expensive; IV formulation; most potent
Oxazepam	++	12	Inactive glucuronide	No	—	Expensive; no parenteral formulation

*Major active metabolite in blood; prolongs biological half-life and causes drug accumulation.
Adapted from Linnoila.[12]

Table 26–6. PHARMACOKINETIC PARAMETERS OF BENZODIAZEPINES USED IN MANAGING ALCOHOL WITHDRAWAL

Drug	Half-Life	% Protein Binding	V_d	Octanol/Water Partition Coefficient
Alprazolam	12–15	68		19
Chlordiazepoxide	6–30	94–97	0.26–0.58	171
Clobazam	9–55	87–90		9
Clorazepate	24–60	82		
Diazepam	20–70	96.8–98.6	0.95–2	309
Lorazepam	10–22	85–93	0.7–1.0	73
Oxazepam	4–15	87–90	0.6	97

cause lower serum protein concentrations result in relatively less binding of the drug. Fixed-dose regimens should be avoided. Small frequent doses of the benzodiazepine of choice should be administered and the dose individually adjusted, according to the clinical presentation of the patient, to maintain a calm but awake state.

If a generalized tonic-clonic seizure occurs during alcohol withdrawal, the patient can be given lorazepam 0.1 mg/kg IV or diazepam, 0.15 mg/kg IV at the time of the seizure. Both drugs should be administered no faster than 2 mg/minute and the patient watched closely for respiratory depression. Lorazepam and diazepam are equally effective in treating *status epilepticus*[11] and presumably are equally useful in managing acute seizures. However, lorazepam has the advantage of having a much smaller volume of distribution of unbound drug and thus has a considerably longer duration of action. Greenblatt and Divoll[7] have reported that the volume of distribution of unbound diazepam is 132.7 liter/kg, whereas the volume of distribution for unbound lorazepam is 12 liter/kg. This difference is a reflection of diazepam's greater lipid sol-

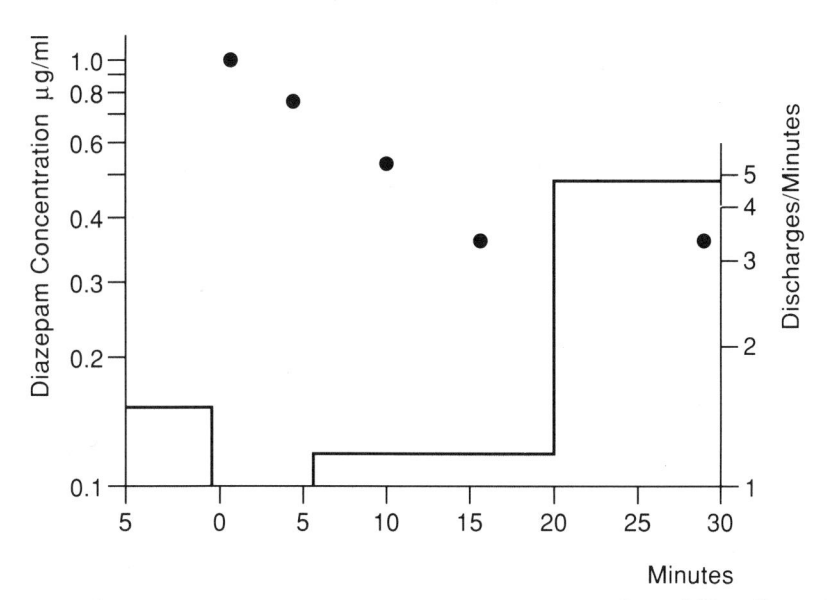

Figure 26–1. The effect of intravenous administration of diazepam on 3- to 4-Hz spike-and-wave complexes during *status epilepticus*. Discharges are suppressed at peak concentrations of about 1,000 ng/ml. Discharge frequency is indicated by a bar graph, scale on right. Diazepam concentrations are indicated by filled circles, scale on left. (Adapted from Booker and Celesia,[3] p. 191.)

ubility. In one study, the octanol/water partition coefficient in a normal volunteer was 820 for diazepam and 240 for lorazepam.[7] These data are consistent with results reported by Ritchel and Hammer.[20] The net result of the difference in lipid solubility is that although diazepam may enter the brain slightly faster than lorazepam,[27] it redistributes more rapidly and completely to other body lipid stores, and thus brain levels rapidly fall. When this happens, the patient may begin seizing again; this phenomenon[3] is illustrated in Figure 26-1. Because of its much smaller volume of distribution, however, lorazepam remains in the brain considerably longer than diazepam. Because of this pharmacokinetic difference between diazepam and lorazepam, the latter may be preferable in managing acute seizures, including AWS and *status epilepticus.*

SUMMARY

Evidence from a number of clinical trials clearly indicates that the benzodiazepines are better than placebos in managing the alcohol withdrawal syndrome. There are no adequate data comparing benzodiazepines with other drugs or indicating superiority of one benzodiazepine over another in treating alcohol withdrawal; IV diazepam or lorazepam is effective in controlling seizures during alcohol withdrawal. Because it has a much smaller volume of distribution, lorazepam is likely to have a longer effective duration of action.

References

1. Baumgartner, GR and Rowen, RC: Clonidine vs chlordiazepoxide in the management of acute alcohol withdrawal syndrome. Arch Intern Med 147:1223, 1987.
2. Bellantuono, C, et al: Benzodiazepines: Clinical pharmacology and therapeutic use. Drugs 19:195, 1980.
3. Booker, HE and Celesia, GG: Serum concentrations of diazepam in subjects with epilepsy. Arch Neurol 29:191, 1973.
4. Burroughs, AK, Morgan, MY, and Sherlock, S: Double-blind controlled trial of bromocriptine, chlordiazepoxide and chlormethiazole for alcohol withdrawal symptoms. Alcohol Alcohol 20:263, 1985.
5. Chalmers, TC, et al: A method for assessing the quality of a randomized control trial. Controlled Clin Trials 2:31, 1981.
6. Greenblatt, DS, et al: Clinical pharmacokinetics of chlordiazepoxide. Clin Pharmacokinet 3:381, 1978.
7. Greenblatt, DJ and Divoll, M: Diazepam versus lorazepam: Relationship of drug distribution to duration of clinical action. In Delgado-Escueta, AV, et al (eds): Advances in Neurology, Vol 34, Status Epilepticus: Mechanisms of Brain Damage and Treatment. Raven Press, New York, 1983, p 487.
8. Greenblatt, DJ and Shader, RI: Benzodiazepines. N Engl J Med 291:1011, and 1239, 1974.
9. Hekimian, LJ, Friedhoff, AJ, and Alpert, M: Treatment of acute brain syndrome from alcohol with nicotinamide adenine dinucleotide and methaminodiazepoxide. Quarterly Journal of Studies on Alcohol 27:214, 1966.
10. Kaim, SC, Klett, CJ, and Rothfeld, B: Treatment of acute alcohol withdrawal state: A comparison of four drugs. Am J Psychiatry 125:1640, 1969.
11. Leppick, IE, et al: Double-blind study of lorazepam and diazepam in status epilepticus. JAMA 249:1452, 1983.
12. Linnoila, M: Benzodiazepines and alcoholism. In Trimble, MR (ed): Benzodiazepines Divided. John Wiley & Sons, New York, 1983, p 291.
13. Mandelli, M, Tognoni, M, and Garattini, S: Clinical pharmacokinetics of diazepam. Clin Pharmacokinet 3:71, 1978.
14. Mantel, N and Haenszel, W: Statistical aspects of the analysis of data from retrospective studies of disease. J Natl Cancer Inst 22:719, 1981.
15. Mendels, J, et al: Halazepam in the management of acute alcohol withdrawal syndrome. J Clin Psychiatry 46:172, 1985.
16. Moskowitz, SB, et al: Deficiencies of clinical trials of alcohol withdrawal. Clinical Trials 7:42, 1983.
17. Mukherjee, PK: A comparison of the efficacy and tolerability of clobazam and chlordiazepoxide in the treatment of acute withdrawal from alcohol in patients with primary alcoholism. J Int Med Res 11:205, 1983.
18. O'Brien, JE, Meyer, RE, and Thomas, DC: Double-blind comparison of lorazepam and diazepam in the treatment of the acute alcohol abstinence syndrome. Current Therapeutic Research 34:825, 1983.
19. Perry, PJ, et al: Absorption of oral and intramuscular chlordiazepoxide by alcoholics. Clin Pharmacol Ther 23:535, 1987.
20. Ritchel, WA and Hammer, GV: Prediction of the volume of distribution from in vitro data and use for estimating the absolute extent of absorbtion. International Journal of Clinical Pharmacology, Therapy and Toxicology 18:298, 1980.
21. Ritson, B and Chick, J: Comparison of two benzodiazepines in the treatment of alcohol withdrawal: Effects on symptoms and cognitive recovery. Drug and Alcohol Depend 18:329, 1986.

22. Rosenfeld, JE and Bizzoco, DH: A controlled study of alcohol withdrawal. Quarterly Journal of Studies on Alcohol Suppl 1:77, 1961.
23. Sellers, EM: Comparative efficacy of propranolol and diazepoxide in alcohol withdrawal. J Stud Alcohol 38:2096, 1977.
24. Sellman, R, et al: Human and animal study on elimination from plasma and metabolism of diazepam after chronic alcohol intake. Acta Pharmacology et Toxicologica 36:33, 1975.
25. Solomon, J, Rouck, LA, and Koepke, HH: Double-blind comparison of lorazepam and chlordiazepoxide in the treatment of acute alcohol abstinence syndrome. Clin Ther 6:52, 1983.
26. Thompson, WL, et al: Diazepam and paraldehyde for treatment of severe delirium tremens. Ann Intern Med 82:175, 1975.
27. Treiman, DM: Pharmacokinetics and clinical use of benzodiazepines in the management of status epilepticus. Epilepsia 30 (Suppl 2): S4, 1989 (in press).
28. Tubridy, P: Alprazolam versus chlormethiazole in acute alcohol withdrawal. Br J Addict 83:581, 1988.
29. Wegner, ME and Fink, DW: Chlordiazepoxide compared with meprobamate and promazine (prozine) for the withdrawal symptoms of acute alcoholism. Wis Med J 64:436, 1965.
30. Whiting, B, et al: Effect of acute alcohol intoxication on the metabolism and plasma kinetics of chlordiazepoxide. Br J Clin Pharmacol 7:95, 1979.
31. Wilson, A and Vulcano, BA: Double-blind trial of alprazolam and chlordiazepoxide in the management of the acute ethanol withdrawal syndrome. Alcoholism: Clinical and Experimental Research 9:23, 1985.

CHAPTER 27

Brian K. Alldredge, Pharm. D.
Roger P. Simon, M.D.

Treatment of Alcohol Withdrawal Seizures with Phenytoin

Although many different therapeutic regimens have been advocated for treating alcohol withdrawal seizures (AWS), the optimal drug and the optimal administration schedule for alcoholics at risk for seizures during acute withdrawal remain to be determined. The importance of effective seizure treatment is underscored by Aminoff and Simon's[1] review of 98 cases of *status epilepticus* treated at the San Francisco General Hospital. Fifteen of the patients in this study had conditions related to alcohol use, and most were treated within 48 hours of alcohol withdrawal. This finding suggests that the AWS population may be at significant risk for central nervous system (CNS) damage. Prompt, rational treatment of AWS is therefore critical in preventing neurologic sequelae.

RATIONALE FOR TREATMENT OF AWS WITH PHENYTOIN

History

Phenytoin (5, 5-diphenylhydantoin) treatment of AWS is standard in many emergency departments and alcohol detoxification centers. It is presumably the effectiveness of this drug in the treatment of primary and secondary convulsive disorders that led many researchers to advocate its use in suppressing AWS. However, it should not be assumed that the anti-epileptic effect of phenytoin guarantees its usefulness against AWS. Although they are clinically indistinguishable from epileptic seizures, AWS are self limited and therefore not indicative of epilepsy. It is well known that clinical and electroencephalographic (EEG) similarities between seizures of different etiology do not ensure similar responses to therapeutic intervention. Early studies also demonstrated the failure of phenytoin to prevent chemically induced seizures in animals.[5] For these reasons, assessment of phenytoin's role in the prevention or termination of AWS should involve carefully controlled trials optimally designed to provide clinically useful conclusions. Unfortunately, existing studies of phenytoin treatment of AWS do not meet these criteria, and the role of this drug remains controversial.[16,26,38] Nevertheless, many investigators recommend its use[3,13,22,23,27,30–32,40] and phenytoin probably remains the most commonly used anticonvulsant drug for treating AWS.[41]

Alcohol Cross-Tolerance

Administering a drug that demonstrates cross-tolerance with alcohol is a pharmacologically sound way to treat

AWS.[18,19,34,37,38,42] Barbiturates and alcohol have shown cross-tolerance in dogs[12] and humans[14,21,33] (they have been shown to suppress specific abstinence symptoms). With careful dose titration, chemically distinct drugs such as barbiturates, paraldehyde, and benzodiazepines can be used to reduce or abolish alcohol withdrawal symptoms, with minimal adverse effects. Phenytoin and alcohol are not cross tolerant. Phenytoin has also been shown to be ineffective in suppressing barbiturate withdrawal seizures in dogs.[11]

Animal Studies

Animal studies assessing the efficacy of phenytoin in AWS treatment have used mouse or rat models (Table 27–1). The results of these studies are equivocal. Gessner[15] demonstrated the failure of phenytoin (12–50 mg/kg) to control AWS in mice when administered orally or by intraperitoneal (IP) injection. In this study, phenytoin administered in a dosage of 100 mg/kg increased seizure scores, probably by causing paradoxical intoxication.[24] Although phenytoin levels were not measured in this study, previous data have shown that phenytoin doses between 9 and 20 mg/kg are effective in preventing maximal electroshock seizures in mice.[4,10,36] Chloral hydrate, an agent adjunctively effective in suppressing withdrawal symptoms in humans,[18] successfully prevented AWS in this study.

Using handling-induced convulsions as a measure of abstinence severity in mice, Sprague and Craigmill[35] found that phenytoin (10–20 mg/kg IP) effectively suppressed alcohol withdrawal symptoms.

Table 27–1. PHENYTOIN TREATMENT OF ALCOHOL WITHDRAWAL SEIZURES IN ANIMALS

Investigators	Animal Model	Treatment	Control	Results	Comments
Gessner,[15] 1974	Mouse	a) PHT 12,20,50 mg/kg b) PHT 100 mg/kg c) Chloral hydrate 175–350 mg/kg		a) PHT ineffective b) Increase in seizure scores c) Dose-dependent reduction in seizure scores	PHT levels not measured
Gessner and Hu,[17] 1976	Mouse	PHT 20 mg/kg + CDZP 1–10 mg/kg	CDZP 1–10 mg/kg	No reduction in seizure scores in PHT-treated mice compared with control	Full report not published
Sprague and Craigmill,[35] 1976	Mouse	a) PHT 5–20 mg/kg b) PHT vehicle (PG/E) c) Ethanol 2–4 gm/kg	a) PHT vehicle (PG/E) b) Isotonic saline c) Isotonic saline	a) Dose-dependent reduction in seizure scores compared with control b) Reduction in seizure scores compared with control c) Dose-dependent reduction in seizure compared with control	
Chu,[6] 1981	Rat	PHT 50, 250 mg/kg	No treatment	Dose-dependent reduction in seizure scores compared with control	Effect not noted at PHT serum levels <8 mcg/ml

PHT = phenytoin; CDZP = chlordiazepoxide; PG/E = propylene glycol (40%)/ethanol (10%)

This dose-dependent effect was at least partially mediated by the propylene glycol (40 percent):ethanol (10 percent) vehicle used for phenytoin injection; this vehicle by itself was shown to reduce seizure scores more than isotonic saline.

Chu[6] used a rat model to evaluate the effectiveness of phenytoin in preventing AWS. Administration of phenytoin 50 and 250 mg/kg via nasogastric tube protected animals against AWS when phenytoin serum levels were above 8 mcg/ml; seizure protection was not evident at serum concentrations below this level. Because animals were not matched according to withdrawal sign scores before treatment group assignment, equivalence in withdrawal seizure susceptibility between control, low-, and high-dose phenytoin-treated rats cannot be assessed. Genotypic correlation of withdrawal seizure susceptibility and resistance has been reported and selectively exploited in subsequent animal studies.[7-9]

Human Trials

PROTOCOL DESIGN

Treatment of humans for AWS is, of course, more complex than treatment of animals in a controlled environment. First, patients with pre-existing epilepsy should be distinguished if possible from patients with recurrent AWS, in order to ensure proper subject selection and data interpretation. Unfortunately this distinction is often unclear and cannot be made using objective diagnostic tests. Postictal and interictal monitoring of the EEG has been used to make this distinction, but this technique lacks precision and may not be helpful. A careful medical history is often the most useful tool for assessing the contribution of other "epileptogenic" factors (e.g., head trauma, genetic susceptibility) that may coexist in patients with a history of withdrawal seizures.

Second, therapeutic trials should be performed under circumstances that optimize the clinical utility of the result. Patients at highest risk for AWS (e.g., those with a history of AWS and those who have had a seizure during the current withdrawal episode) should be enrolled during periods of peak susceptibility. This setting mimics the clinical circumstances under which the drug is most likely to be used. Like animal studies of alcohol withdrawal, human trials of phenytoin treatment are also subject to deficiencies in protocol design and data presentation. A recent evaluation of therapeutic trials in alcohol withdrawal demonstrated this point quite dramatically. A data analysis scoring system unfavorably compared the literature on alcohol withdrawal with literature on other therapeutic topics subjected to the same grading standards.[28] Papers on alcohol withdrawal received low scores in the areas of statistical analyses, handling of dropouts, and discussion of type II error for negative clinical trials.

Review and Interpretation of Previously Published Data

Finer[13] and Smith[34] independently reported their retrospective observations on the prophylactic use of phenytoin in patients detoxifying from alcohol and reached different conclusions regarding the relative efficacy of this agent. In both treatment centers, phenytoin was administered for a limited time during the detoxification period when the risk of seizures is highest. Finer found that phenytoin 400 mg daily for two days followed by one or more intramuscular injections was effective is seizure suppression when administered to withdrawing alcoholics "who appear(ed) to be likely to convulse or enter the state of delirium tremens." Although the number of patients treated in this manner was not specified, Finer reported that no phenytoin-treated patients experienced convulsions during alcohol withdrawal. Smith reported the results of a random medical record survey of 6500 patients treated in an alcohol and drug detoxification program. He found the combination of primidone and chlordiazepoxide to be more effective than phenytoin with chlordiazepoxide in preventing alcohol and sedative withdrawal seizures. The retrospective design and lack of clear inclusion criteria are obvious limitations of this report.

Rothstein[30] conducted the first study in which patients were randomly assigned to receive phenytoin during alcohol withdrawal. Two hundred patients received either chlordiazepoxide, 50 to 100 mg as needed for withdrawal symptom suppression, or chlordiazepoxide with phenytoin, 200 mg orally twice daily for five days. Both treatment groups also received thiamine supplementation. No seizures were reported in either treatment group. Rothstein concluded that additional anticonvulsant therapy is unnecessary when chlordiazepoxide is administered in doses adequate to produce a somnolent state (approximately 360 mg over the first 24 hours in each group). Although this conclusion is partly supported by the data, the effectiveness of phenytoin in the treatment of AWS remains unresolved. The outcome of the 200 cases in this study is not unexpected when one considers that chlordiazepoxide has proven quite effective in suppressing AWS, with a post-treatment seizure rate near one percent.[38] Furthermore, 80 percent of patients enrolled in the study had no history of seizures during previous episodes of withdrawal; these patients may have been at lower risk for AWS than patients with a history of withdrawal seizure.[29,31] In a study exploring the possibility of synergism between phenytoin and chlordiazepoxide for treating AWS, Gessner and Hu[17] compared the combination with chlordiazepoxide alone and found no difference in withdrawal seizure scores between groups.

Using a study design virtually identical to Rothstein's Sampliner and Iber[31] reached a different conclusion about the effectiveness of phenytoin in the treatment of AWS. All 136 subjects in this study received chlordiazepoxide as needed for sedation; concomitant therapy with phenytoin 100 mg thrice daily, or placebo, was also administered during a 5-day period. All subjects had a history of seizures in adulthood, but no attempt was made to exclude persons with prior seizures unrelated to alcohol withdrawal. Seizures occurred in 13 patients during the 10-day observation period—in 11 patients in the placebo-treated group and in 2 patients in the phenytoin-treated group. Review of the histories of the 13 patients in whom a seizure occurred revealed that each of five patients without a close association between previous seizures and alcohol withdrawal were assigned to the placebo group. Also, it is not known whether equivalent doses of chlordiazepoxide were used in both groups. Finally, phenytoin blood levels averaged less than 4 mcg/ml on the first day of therapy, when most seizures occurred. It would be difficult to ascribe a significant anticonvulsant effect to such low serum concentration of phenytoin.

THE SAN FRANCISCO GENERAL HOSPITAL STUDY

Because of the methodologic problems and conflicting results of existing human trials, we investigated the effectiveness of IV phenytoin in the acute treatment of AWS, using a randomized, placebo-controlled, double-blind study design. The investigation was conducted at the San Francisco General Hospital (SFGH) from October, 1982 through June, 1988.

Methods

Patients were eligible for study entry at the time of emergency department admission for at least one witnessed seizure. A clinical diagnosis of AWS was required from both the admitting neurologist and one of the study investigators. If phenytoin administration could not be completed within 6 hours of the first AWS in the current withdrawal episode, patients were not included, because they were believed to be at a significantly reduced risk for subsequent seizures whether they were effectively treated or not. Patients with a history of seizures unrelated to alcohol use were excluded from the study, as were patients whose seizures may have had other secondary causes (e.g., significant head trauma, electrolyte abnormalities, epileptogenic drug ingestion). Patients who had received magnesium supplementation, benzodiazepines, other sedative drugs, or any anti-epileptic drug in the emergency department, or within

14 days of study entry, were also excluded.

All subjects were examined by a neurologist. IV fluids with normal saline (0.9 percent sodium chloride) were administered and phlebotomy was performed to measure serum electrolyte, glucose, osmolality, blood urea nitrogen, serum creatinine, and anti-epileptic drug concentrations, and blood alcohol level. Liver function tests, complete blood count, and electrocardiogram (ECG) were also performed. Patients were then blindly and randomly assigned to receive 100 mg of phenytoin sodium injection (50 mg/ml) (Dilantin) IV over 20 minutes or an equivalent infusion of 0.9 percent sodium chloride. During the infusion, the ECG was continuously monitored, and supine blood pressure was checked every 3 to 5 minutes.

Subjects were then admitted for observation and received standard care during the study period. The investigators, patients, nursing staff, and neurology department personnel were blinded with regard to the study treatment. Sixteen subjects received either atenolol 50 to 100 mg daily or clonidine 0.1 to 0.2 mg BID-TID for treatment of alcohol withdrawal symptoms; sedative drugs (e.g., benzodiazepines, barbiturates, and other related compounds) were not administered during the observation period. Postinfusion phenytoin levels were also measured in each patient. The result was not reported until the observation period had ended. The endpoint of the study was considered to have been reached after a seizure-free observation period of at least 12 hours, or when the subject experienced a single postinfusion seizure. If the subject experienced a subsequent seizure, the treating physician had the option of unblinding the patient's treatment to assess whether further anticonvulsant therapy was necessary.

Results

Ninety patients completed the study; the average age of the 85 men and 5 women was 40.1 ± 9.8 years (range 24–75 years). Of the 72 patients with a history of seizures, all reported a close association between seizures and alcohol withdrawal (a range of 2–72 hours after the last drink). Approximately half these patients reported having had more than five AWS during their lifetime. The remaining 19 patients were admitted to the study after their first seizure; the clinical diagnosis of AWS was made in each case.

Forty-five subjects received phenytoin and 45 received placebo. Table 27–2 compares the two groups with regard to age, sex, and seizure history. The number of patients reaching the study endpoint by having another AWS was equal in the two groups. Six placebo-treated patients and six phenytoin-treated patients experienced at least one recurrent seizure during the postinfusion observation period. Seizures occurred an average of 3.2 ± 4.5 and 2.7 ± 1.4 hours (mean ± SD) after the end of the phenytoin and placebo infusions respectively. No subsequent seizures occurred in the remaining 78 patients. Table 27–3 compares patients'

Table 27–2. SAN FRANCISCO GENERAL HOSPITAL STUDY: PATIENT CHARACTERISTICS

Characteristic	Phenytoin	Placebo
Number of patients (M/F)	45 (42/3)	45 (43/2)
Age (years)*	39.7 ± 9.3	40.6 ± 10.3
History of AWS prior to entry	37	35
History of minor head injury	11	13
Number of AWS in current episode prior to entry:		
1	30	28
2–3	14	15
4–5	1	2

*Mean ± standard deviation.

Table 27-3. SAN FRANCISCO GENERAL HOSPITAL STUDY: PATIENT LABORATORY DATA

	Total Patients (n = 91)			
	No Seizure (79)		Recurrent AWS (12)	
	PHT (41)	Placebo (38)	PHT (6)	Placebo (6)
Calcium (mg/dl)	9.1 ± 0.8	8.9 ± 0.7	8.8 ± 0.7	9.0 ± 0.2
Magnesium (mg/dl)	1.7 ± 0.4	1.6 ± 0.5	1.5 ± 0.4	1.5 ± 0.4
Glucose (mg/dl)	122 ± 42	130 ± 44	131 ± 44	120 ± 14
Postinfusion (PHT) (mcg/ml)	13.6 ± 3.0	0.0	16.2 ± 5.0	0.0

PHT = phenytoin concentration; all values expressed as mean ± SD.

prestudy calcium, magnesium, and glucose concentrations as well as postinfusion phenytoin levels.

Discussion

Based on these data, it cannot be proven that phenytoin is effective in treating AWS when administered in the period immediately following a withdrawal seizure. Therapeutic phenytoin levels were found both in patients with subsequent seizures and those without; therefore one would expect any benefit from this treatment to be evident immediately after administration of the IV loading dose. Most patients were observed for 24 hours after the first seizure in the withdrawal period studied. Based on the experience of Victor and Brausch,[39] one expects nearly 100 percent of patients with more than one AWS during a given withdrawal episode to have all seizures within 20 hours of the first convulsion.

We did not assess the effectiveness of phenytoin for chronic maintenance therapy in patients with recurrent AWS. However, it is generally believed that long-term anticonvulsant therapy is not necessary, and may increase the risk of subsequent seizures.[2,29,38] Further, anti-epileptic drug noncompliance is known to increase the risk of seizures, and alcoholic patients have a poor record of adherence to prescribed regimens.[25] Moreover, some patients' alcohol binges coincide with medication noncompliance. Hillbom and Hjelm-Jager[20] emphasized the risk of seizures in alcoholics for whom chronic anticonvulsant treatment has been prescribed. They also noted that because most AWS occur before hospital or detoxification center admission, effective therapy should be started on an outpatient basis while the patient is still intoxicated. The logistic problems inherent in such an approach are obvious.

SUMMARY

Clinician's beliefs about the usefulness of phenytoin in treating AWS have been based on the drug's activity against epileptic seizures and on a long history of anecdotal experience in emergency departments and alcohol detoxification centers. Review of animal and human studies addressing this issue yields conflicting results. Deficiencies in protocol design (e.g., subject selection and control treatment) and data presentation (e.g., statistical analysis) may explain the divergent conclusions.

We evaluated phenytoin treatment of AWS using a randomized, double-blind, placebo-controlled study design. Strict patient selection criteria were established to mimic acute clinical situations in which this drug would be appropriately used. Control treatment, inclusion, and exclusion criteria were also designed to minimize ambiguous conclusions. We were not able to demonstrate a beneficial effect of phenytoin therapy in AWS. Based on the current AWS treatment literature and data from our study, we cannot support the use of phenytoin for preventing or initially treating AWS in patients without other risk factors for a seizure. Furthermore, we do not recommend long-term phenytoin treatment for patients with recurrent AWS. The drug's efficacy for treating these patients has not been proven, and previous observations suggest that patients so treated may be at increased risk for seizures.

Note: The complete manuscript of the San Francisco General Hospital Study summarized here has been recently published: (Alldredge, BK, Lowenstein, DH, Simon, RP: A placebo-controlled trial of intravenous diphenylhydantoin for the short-term treatment of alcohol withdrawal seizures. Am J Med 87:645, 1989.)

References

1. Aminoff, MJ and Simon, RP: Status epilepticus: Causes, clinical features and consequences in 98 patients. Am J Med 69:657, 1980.
2. Ashley, MJ, et al: "Mixed" (drug abusing) and "pure" alcoholics: A socio-medical comparison. Br J Addict 73:19, 1978.
3. Chafetz, M: Alcohol withdrawal and seizures. JAMA 200:195, 1967.
4. Chen, G and Ensor, CR: Evaluation of antiepileptic drugs. Archives of Neurologic Psychiatry 63:56, 1950.
5. Chen, G and Ensor, CR: A study of the anticonvulsant properties of phenobarbital and Dilantin. Arch Int Pharmacodyn Ther 100:234, 1954.
6. Chu, NS: Prevention of alcohol withdrawal seizures with phenytoin in rats. Epilepsia 22:179, 1981.
7. Crabbe, JC, et al: Bidirectional selection for susceptibility to ethanol withdrawal seizures in Mus musculus. Behav Genet 15:521, 1985.
8. Crabbe, JC, et al: Genetic differences in anticonvulsant sensitivity in mouse lines selectively bred for ethanol withdrawal severity. J Pharmacol Exp Ther 239:154, 1986.
9. Crabbe, JC, Kosobud, A, and Young, ER: Genetic selection for ethanol withdrawal severity: Differences in replicate mouse lines. Life Sci 33:955, 1983.
10. Cucinell, SA, et al: Stimulatory effect of phenobarbital on the metabolism of diphenylhydantoin. J Pharmacol Exp Ther 141:157, 1963.
11. Essig, CF and Carter, WW: Failure of diphenylhydantoin in preventing barbiturate withdrawal convulsions in the dog. Neurology 12:481, 1962.
12. Essig, CF, Jones, BE, and Lam, RC: The effect of pentobarbital on alcohol withdrawal in dogs. Arch Neurol 20:554, 1969.
13. Finer, MJ: Diphenylhydantoin for treatment of alcohol withdrawal syndromes. JAMA 215:119, 1971.
14. Fraser, HF, et al: Partial equivalence of chronic alcohol and barbiturate intoxications. Quarterly Journal of Studies on Alcohol 18:541, 1957.
15. Gessner, PK: Failure of diphenylhydantoin to prevent alcohol withdrawal convulsions in mice. Eur J Pharmacol 27:120, 1974.
16. Gessner, PK: Is diphenylhydantoin effective in the treatment of alcohol withdrawal? JAMA 219:1072, 1972.
17. Gessner, PK and Hu, EH: Chlordiazepoxide and diphenylhydantoin in the control of alcohol withdrawal syndrome in mice. Absence of synergism. Pharmacologist 18:237, 1976.
18. Golbert, TM, et al: Comparative evaluation of treatments of alcohol withdrawal syndromes. JAMA 201:113, 1967.
19. Haddox, VG, et al: Clorazepate use may prevent alcohol withdrawal convulsions. West J Med 146:695, 1987.
20. Hillbom, ME and Hjelm-Jager, M: Should alcohol withdrawal seizures be treated with anti-epileptic drugs? Acta Neurol Scand 69:39, 1984.
21. Isbell, H, et al: An experimental study of the etiology of "rum fits" and delirium tremens. Quarterly Journal of Studies on Alcohol 16:1, 1955.
22. Khoury, N: When alcoholics stop drinking. Postgrad Med 43:119, 1968.
23. Knott, DH, Beard, JD, and Wallace, JA: Acute withdrawal from alcohol. Postgrad Med 42:A109, 1967.
24. Levy, LL and Fenichel, GM: Diphenylhydantoin activated seizures. Neurology 15:716, 1965.
25. Little, RE and Gayle, JL: Epilepsy and alcoholism. Alcohol Health and Research World 5:31, 1980.
26. McMicken, D: Seizures in the alcohol-dependent patient: A diagnostic and therapeutic dilemma. J Emerg Med 1:311, 1984.
27. McNichol, R, Cirksena, WJ, and Glasgow, MC: Management of withdrawal from alcohol (including delirium tremens). South Med J 60:7, 1967.
28. Moskowitz, G, et al: Deficiencies of clinical trials of alcohol withdrawal. Alcoholism: Clinical and Experimental Research 7:42, 1983.
29. Newsom, JA: Withdrawal seizures in an in-patient alcoholism program. In Currents in Alcoholism, Vol 6: In Seixas, F, (ed.): Treatment and Rehabilitation and Epidemiology. Grune and Stratton, New York, 1979, p 11.
30. Rothstein, E: Prevention of alcohol withdrawal seizures: The roles of diphenylhydantoin and chlordiazepoxide. Am J Psychiatry 130:1381, 1973.
31. Sampliner, R and Iber, FL: Diphenylhydantoin control of alcohol withdrawal seizures. JAMA 230:1430, 1974.
32. Sellars, EM and Kalant, H: Alcohol intoxication and withdrawal. N Engl J Med 294:757, 1976.
33. Smith, DE and Wesson, DR: Phenobarbital technique for treatment of barbiturate dependence. Arch Gen Psychiatry 24:56, 1971.
34. Smith, RF: Relative effectiveness of primidone (Mysoline) and diphenylhydantoin (Dilantin) in the management of sedative withdrawal seizures. Ann NY Acad Sci 273:378, 1976.
35. Sprague, GL and Craigmill, AL: Control of eth-

anol withdrawal symptoms in mice by phenytoin. Res Commun Chem Pathol Pharmacol 15:721, 1976.
36. Swinyard, EA, Brown, WC, and Goodman, LS: Comparative assays of antiepileptic drugs in mice and rats. J Pharmacol Exp Ther 106:319, 1952.
37. Thomas, DW and Freedman, DX: Treatment of alcohol withdrawal syndrome: Comparison of promazine and paraldehyde. JAMA 188:316, 1964.
38. Thompson, WL: Management of alcohol withdrawal syndromes. Arch Intern Med 138:278, 1978.
39. Victor, M and Brausch, C: The role of abstinence in the genesis of alcoholic epilepsy. Epilepsia 8:1, 1967.
40. Walsh, PJF: Prophylaxis in alcoholics in the withdrawal period. Am J Psychiatry 119:262, 1962.
41. Wilbur, R and Kulik, FA: Anticonvulsant drugs in alcohol withdrawal: Use of phenytoin, primidone, carbamazepine, valproic acid, and the sedative anticonvulsants. Am J Hosp Pharm 38:1138, 1981.
42. Young, GP, et al: Intravenous phenobarbital for alcohol withdrawal and convulsions. Ann Emerg Med 16:847, 1987.

CHAPTER 28

Gary P. Young, M.D.
Robert H. Dailey, M.D.

Treatment of Alcohol Withdrawal Seizures with Intravenous Phenobarbital

Many pharmacologic agents have been used to treat acute alcohol withdrawal and to prevent alcohol withdrawal seizures (AWS). The benzodiazepines have become the drugs of choice during the past 10 years, although "the benzodiazepines are by no means ideal . . . agents in (the) treatment of most of the symptoms" of alcohol withdrawal.[14] Intravenous (IV) diazepam requires close monitoring and frequent redosing. Because it is loosely bound to brain tissue its anticonvulsant effect is maintained for only approximately 20 minutes.[4] On the other hand, diazepam accumulates when used for its sedative effect in chronic therapy, especially in patients with liver disease.[6] And if the unpleasant symptoms of alcohol withdrawal recur because of diazepam's short half-life, patients treated with this drug often prematurely return to alcohol consumption. Thus, large, frequent oral dosing on an outpatient basis may be necessary, but can be harmful, in alcoholic patients.

For several reasons, we thought that IV phenobarbital (IV–PB) might be an excellent drug to treat alcohol withdrawal and prevent AWS. First, cross-tolerance exists between barbiturates and ethanol.[16] Second, PB has a wide margin of safety when used for hypnosedative withdrawal: doses efficacious for treating withdrawal symptoms do not produce significant central nervous system (CNS) depression.[13] Third, because of its long duration of action (its half-life is approximately 90 hours),[1] serum PB concentrations remain stable for long periods after single loading doses; therefore, patients do not need to take oral PB for alcohol withdrawal after discharge. Fourth, IV–PB has a rapid onset of action (approximately 15 minutes),[7] so clinical monitoring of the effects of PB loading doses is practical. Finally, at therapeutic serum concentrations, PB has an anticonvulsant efficacy similar to that of both diazepam and phenytoin.[3]

We have previously demonstrated the efficacy and safety of IV–PB in suppressing the manifestations of acute alcohol withdrawal.[20] In this chapter we stress both the benefits of IV–PB in preventing AWS and the relationship between the dose of IV–PB administered and the resultant serum PB level in alcoholic patients and in patients on chronic PB therapy.

METHODS

We conducted a prospective, uncontrolled clinical trial to address the objectives listed above. We randomly enrolled in our study patients who presented in acute alcohol withdrawal with or without seizures and patients on chronic PB anticonvulsant therapy whose blood levels were subtherapeutic. Acute alcohol withdrawal was defined as a condition involving one or more of the following symptoms: seizures, tremulousness, agitation, diaphoresis, and tachycardia not due to any other reason.

We excluded from our study patients with PB allergies; patients older than 60; pregnant and breast-feeding women; patients with CNS disease; and patients with moderately severe cardiac, pulmonary, renal, or hepatic disease. We did not exclude patients with documented alcoholic liver disease (ALD) unless their condition was complicated by acute alcoholic hepatitis or hepatic encephalopathy. We also excluded or withdrew patients with signs of acute drug intoxication (including blood alcohol levels [BALs] above 100 mg/dl) and patients who were concurrently receiving diazepam or phenytoin to treat their alcohol withdrawal or convulsion.

We also collected data on level of consciousness, weight, and orthostatic vital signs. Blood pressure, pulse, and respiratory rate were recorded before and after each dose of IV-PB. An IV line was started with normal saline, and blood samples were obtained for measuring baseline PB and BALs, glucose, electrolytes, creatinine, blood urea nitrogen, total bilirubin, aspartate aminotransferase (SGOT), alkaline phosphatase, and prothrombin time. All patients were placed on an electrocardiogram (ECG) monitor.

All patients received an initial infusion of 260 mg of IV-PB (two 130-mg ampules administered over about 5 minutes) while we awaited information on baseline PB levels. If the initial PB level was above 10 mcg/ml, the patient received no more than this initial 260 mg of IV-PB, and a final PB level was subsequently measured. If the baseline PB level was subtherapeutic (<10 µg/ml), the patient received additional 130-mg boluses of IV-PB until the clinical endpoint of light sedation was reached or some adverse effect was noted, such as worsening of the baseline of CNS status (e.g., a convulsion, worsening agitation, disorientation, confusion, or dysarthria), respiratory depression, hypotension, or a dysrhythmia. A final PB level was drawn 30 minutes after the last IV-PB dose was administered. All patients were observed in the emergency department for a minimum of 1 hour after receiving the last IV-PB dose. Data were recorded on the patient's final level of consciousness, changes in the signs of alcohol withdrawal, side-effects, complications, and any other drugs administered.

We then reviewed each patient's emergency department charts and old medical records. We received approval for this research from our county's human subjects protection committee.

RESULTS

One hundred ten patients received IV-PB. Eighty-eight patients qualified for the first part of the study on the efficacy of IV-PB in treating alcohol withdrawal or preventing seizures: 62 for the treatment of alcohol withdrawal, and 26 for postictal PB therapy. Of the 62 patients in alcohol withdrawal, 38 presented with an AWS. Twenty-two of the 110 patients were excluded from the first part of the study because they had BALs above 100 mg/dl or because they were concurrently receiving diazepam or phenytoin; the changes in these patients' serum PB levels made their cases still useful for the second part of the study on the relationship between the dose of IV-PB administered and the resultant serum PB level.

The 110 patients consisted of 90 men and 20 women with a mean age of 40 years and a mean weight of 70 kg. For all 110 patients, a mean loading dose of 542 ($\pm$194) mg or 7.7 mg/kg of IV-PB was administered. The mean increase in the serum PB level was 12.9 ($\pm$4.8) µg/ml, or 1.67 µg/ml for each mg/kg of IV-PB administered. The 62 patients undergoing alcohol withdrawal consisted of 55 men and 7 women, whose mean age was 42 years and mean weight was 70 kg. The mean loading dose of IV-PB given these patients was 598 mg or 8.4 mg/kg, and the mean final serum PB level in this group was 13.9 µg/ml. Thus, the serum PB level rose approximately 1.65 µg/ml for

Table 28–1. INTRAVENOUS PB DOSAGES AND CHANGES IN SERUM PB LEVEL

Patient Subgroups (No. of Patients)		IV–PB Dosage mg	IV–PB Dosage mg/kg	Change in Serum PB Level (µg/ml)
Total IV–PB	(110)	542	7.7	12.9
Total AW	(62)	598	8.4	13.9
Tremulousness	(48)	624	8.5	14.0
Seizures	(38)	576	8.3	13.8
ALD	(21)	561	8.2	13.7
Chronic oral PB	(26)	420	6.3	10.1

each mg/kg of IV–PB administered to the patients in alcohol withdrawal with or without seizures.

The 38 patients presenting with AWS received a mean dose of 576 mg of IV–PB or 8.3 mg/kg; this group had a mean serum PB level of 13.8 µg/ml. Comparing our data on each of the different subgroups of alcohol withdrawal patients (i.e., the 38 patients presenting with AWS, patients with tremulousness, and patients with ALD) revealed no appreciable difference in effects on serum PB concentrations (Table 28–1).

The 26 patients who presented with nonalcohol withdrawal seizures while receiving chronic PB therapy included 18 men and 8 women. Their mean age was 39 years and mean weight 64 kg. The mean loading dose of IV–PB administered to these patients was 420 mg (6.6 mg/kg), and the final mean serum PB level 20.6 µg/ml. The mean increase in the serum PB level in this group was 10.1 µg/ml above the mean baseline serum PB concentration of 10.5 mg/ml. Thus, for every mg/kg of IV–PB administered to an adult patient on chronic PB therapy, serum PB level rose approximately 1.53 µg/ml.

Our clinical goal was safe discharge of the patient from the emergency department after the IV–PB experiments. Fifty-seven of our 62 alcohol withdrawal patients (92 percent) were discharged, after an average emergency department stay of 3 hours and 47 minutes. All 26 patients receiving chronic PB therapy were discharged. Additionally, all 22 patients excluded from the first part of the study because of concurrent ethanol, diazepam, or phenytoin use were discharged after receiving IV–PB. Review of their medical charts revealed that none of these discharged patients returned to our emergency department for alcohol withdrawal or convulsions within the week following treatment. Of the five alcohol withdrawal patients requiring admission to the hospital, four developed overt delirium tremens. These four patients (6.5 percent) were the only alcohol withdrawal patients who failed to respond adequately to IV–PB. One patient was admitted with pneumonia.

Forty-eight (77 percent) of the 62 alcohol withdrawal patients were markedly tremulous, 38 (61 percent) had convulsed, and 24 (39 percent) had both tremulousness and seizures. The condition of 46 of the 48 (96 percent) tremulous patients was improved upon discharge, and 23 (48 percent) had no detectable tremor upon discharge. None of the 38 patients presenting with AWS and none of the 26 patients on chronic PB therapy presenting with seizures were observed to convulse after they received IV–PB; the average emergency department stay of both groups was almost 4 hours.

Adverse reactions ascribed to IV–PB were documented in 4 (6 percent) of the 62 alcohol withdrawal patients and none of the patients already receiving chronic PB therapy. After this last bolus of IV–PB (total dose of 520 mg), one patient had an asymptomatic blood pressure fall to 90/60 but his blood pressure rose without intervention within 30 minutes. Three patients were kept in the emergency department 1 to 3 hours after their last IV–PB bolus: one was ataxic (total dose of 650 mg) and two were lethargic (doses of 390 and 780 mg). Ataxia was a common clinical feature in patients (6 of 17) excluded from the study because they had also received diazepam or phenytoin in the emergency department. However, none of these 17 patients and none of the five patients excluded from the study with elevated BALs required admission after receiving IV-PB.

DISCUSSION

Relationship of Initial PB Dosing and Blood Levels

Few studies have addressed the dosage of IV-PB necessary to achieve a therapeutic serum PB concentration in humans. In one study,[12] neonates suffering *status epilepticus* received IV-PB loading doses of 15 to 20 mg/kg; mean peak serum PB concentrations were 19.4 µg/ml. Thus, the ratio of serum PB level (µg/ml) to dose of IV-PB (mg/kg) approximated unity in these neonates receiving a continuous rapid-rate infusion. In another study,[10] seven adult inpatients undergoing barbiturate withdrawal received a slow continuous IV-PB infusion at a rate of more than 2 mg/kg/hour until they slept but were easily arouseable. The mean peak serum PB level was 26 µg/ml after the patients received nearly 1 g of IV-PB over a mean duration of 8 hours. The investigators found the total PB dosage to be predictive of the peak serum PB level. The ratio of peak serum PB concentration (µg/ml) to dose (mg/kg) of PB following the infusion was 1.5 in the seven barbiturate-dependent patients and in one control patient. This control patient required less than half as much IV-PB (7.8 mg/kg) to achieve sedation (at a serum PB level of 11.7 µg/ml).[10] This finding is consistent with an earlier finding that in an equivalent state of sedation, epileptics on chronic PB therapy had 1.5 to 2 times the serum PB level of patients admitted for acute barbiturate intoxication.[18] The rate of IV-PB infusion (2 mg/kg/hour) in this study was much slower than the rate of IV-PB boluses administered in our study (*i.e.*, a total of 520 mg over the first hour or 7.4 mg/kg/hour).

A recent study of the treatment of *status epilepticus*[15] found a dose of almost 12 mg/kg of IV-PB efficacious in stopping convulsions in 16 of 18 patients. This dose resulted in a mean serum level of 18.3 µg/ml. In this study, the resultant serum level of PB was expressed as 1.2x + 3, where x is the dose of IV-PB administered. Another study reported the use of oral PB to treat hypnosedative withdrawal.[13] Oral PB was given to 21 patients at 120 mg/hour or 2 mg/kg/hour. The mean total PB loading dose was 23.4 mg/kg (or 1440 mg) and the mean peak PB level was 35.9 µg/ml. The serum PB level (µg/ml) to oral dose (mg/kg) ratio was again 1.5. We observed a similar blood-level-to-dose ratio (1.53 to 1.67) in patients in our study receiving IV-PB.

Phenobarbital Therapy for Sedative Withdrawal

For the treatment of "life-threatening" barbiturate withdrawal, one investigator recommends that patients receive an initial loading dose of 1.75 mg/kg of IV-PB over 5 minutes.[3] But a dose of 1.75 mg/kg in a 70-kg patient would be only about 130 mg, a dose that would result in a very low serum PB level (2–3 µg/ml). We recommend the IV-PB regimen used in our study as a minimum dosage. We also recommend rapid administration for the patient whose condition is stable and who can tolerate receiving an IV-PB load over 1 to 2 hours.

In the study mentioned above of oral PB therapy for hypnosedative withdrawal,[13] patients requiring less than 7 mg/kg or 500 mg were thought not to be physically dependent on barbiturates. Most of our 62 alcohol withdrawal patients (45 or 73 percent) required at least 520 mg of IV-PB to suppress their symptoms. This dose was administered by the end of the first hour (260 mg initially, then 130 mg at 30 and 60 minutes). More IV-PB can be administered if necessary for acute alcohol withdrawal: three such patients received 910 mg, and two required 1040 mg. The investigators who conducted the oral PB study[13] concluded that because virtually all patients improve without supplemental dosing, blood level measurements are not essential to determine loading doses of oral PB. To guide the administration of IV–PB, we recommend measuring an initial baseline serum PB level only in patients already receiving chronic PB therapy. We do not suggest that the administration of at least the initial 260 mg of IV–PB must wait for the initial serum PB level result. We also suggest measuring another serum PB level only in patients who do not appear to be responding to an adequate dosage of IV–PB (10–20 mg/kg). We measured an initial and a final serum PB level on every patient for study purposes only.

Barbiturates are probably effective in treating alcohol withdrawal. Pentobarbital prevents the convulsions and death that occurred in a control group of untreated dogs undergoing delirium tremens.[5] There are few published comparisons of barbiturates with other drug therapies for acute alcohol withdrawal in humans. Kaim and Klett[9] reported that chlordiazepoxide, paraldehyde, perphenazine, and pentobarbital all produced favorable results in the treatment of "uncomplicated" delirium tremens. Only one of the 41 patients receiving pentobarbital "failed to respond adequately." These patients were the only ones who did not experience a convulsion during the study. In another study, Smith[17] retrospectively analyzed the medical records of 2000 patients in alcohol withdrawal and determined that oral primidone (Mysoline), which is metabolized to phenobarbital, was superior to phenytoin, chlordiazepoxide, and phenothiazines in the prevention of AWS. Again, the patients receiving primidone were the only ones who did not experience convulsions during the study.

Phenobarbital Therapy for Convulsions

None of our patients had a seizure if they had recieved at least 260 mg of IV–PB. Thus, considering the results of the studies cited above, barbiturates seem to be effective in preventing AWS. In addition, barbiturates are effective chronic therapy for idiopathic epilepsy.[3] But the literature on parenteral PB for the treatment of *status epilepticus* is conflicting. For the treatment of *status epilepticus*, intramuscular (IM) doses as low as 90 to 120 mg every 4 to 6 hours have been recommended;[19] however, the ratio of peak serum PB concentration (μg/ml) to single oral or IM dose (mg/kg) of PB is also approximately 1.5 to 1.[2,8] Thus, 90 to 120 mg of IM–PB would result in very low serum PB levels (2–3 μg/ml). Furthermore, therapeutic serum PB levels are not reached for at least 1 hour following administration of IM–PB doses of over 10 mg/kg.[2,8]

Recommendations for the dosage of IV–PB effective in treating *status epilepticus* range from a maximum dose of 1000 mg at a rate of 60 mg/minute[11] to a dose of 20 mg/kg at a rate of 100 mg/minute.[4,12] A recent prospective comparison of diazepam plus phenytoin versus PB plus optional phenytoin found PB monotherapy to be more rapidly effective and more effective overall, comparable in safety, and easier to administer.[15] These investigators began with an IV–PB dose of 10 mg/kg at 100 mg/minute, which they then increased to as much as 20 to 30 mg/kg at 50 mg/minute until the convulsions stopped. Patients responding to PB monotherapy did so at relatively low therapeutic levels, ranging from 15 to 27 μg/ml (mean 18.3 μg/ml).[15] According to our data, only larger doses (10–20 mg/kg) of IV–PB would guarantee the therapeutic serum PB levels (a predicted range from 15–30 μg/ml) necessary to treat *status epilepticus*. Although none of our patients on chronic PB anticonvulsant therapy had a seizure if they had received at least 260 mg of IV–PB, it should be noted that none of our patients presented in *status epilepticus*.

Study Design

There are limitations to our study design: First, there were no placebo controls. Second, there was no comparison with a standard agent for the treatment of alcohol withdrawal, such as a benzodiazepine. Third, the assignment of patients to be given IV–PB was not random. Fourth, many patients were excluded or withdrawn from the study because of inadequate physician compliance with the study protocol. Finally, it is possible that some patients in our study relapsed after treatment with IV–PB, and either resorted to ethanol or required further care at another emergency department.

SUMMARY

This prospective, uncontrolled study of 110 emergency department patients addressed the use of IV–PB for the treatment of convulsions and other manifestations of alcohol withdrawal. Every patient received an initial dose of 260 mg of IV–PB and then 130 mg every 30 minutes until light sedation was achieved. A mean loading dose of 542 (± 194) mg of IV–PB resulted in a mean increase in the serum PB level of 12.9 (± 4.8) μg/ml. The serum PB level rose about 1.67 μg/ml for each mg/kg of IV–PB administered. Analysis of the subgroup with previous usage of PB revealed no significant difference in the increase in their serum PB level after IV–PB (the serum PB level rose about 1.53 μg/ml for each mg/kg of IV–PB in this group). None of the patients who presented with AWS or with seizures due to noncompliance with chronic PB therapy had another convulsion during a mean observation period of nearly 4 hours after receiving IV–PB. Alcohol withdrawal tremors were almost universally ameliorated, except in patients requiring admission for acute delirium tremens. Adverse effects of PB therapy were minor and frequent only in patients who were ethanol-intoxicated or receiving concurrent IV phenytoin or diazepam. We conclude that IV–PB may prevent AWS, and is safe and effective therapy for mild to moderate alcohol withdrawal.

References

1. Alvin, J, et al: The effect of liver disease in man on the disposition of phenobarbital. J Pharmacol Exp Ther 192:224, 1975.
2. Brachet-Liermain, A, Goutieres, F, and Aicardi, J: Absorption of phenobarbital after the intramuscular administration of single doses in infants. J Pediatr 87:624, 1975.
3. Buchtal, F and Lennox-Buchtal, MA: Phenobarbital: Relation of serum concentration to control of seizures. In Woodbury, DM, Penry, JK, and Schmidt, RP (eds): Antiepileptic Drugs. Raven Press, New York, 1971, p 335.
4. Delago-Escueta, AV, et al: Management of status epilepticus. N Engl J Med 306:1337, 1982.
5. Essig, CF, Jones, E, and Lam, RC: The effect of pentobarbital on alcohol withdrawal in dogs. Arch Neurol 20:554, 1969.
6. Harvey, SC: Hypnotics and sedatives: Benzodiazepines. In Gilman, AG, Goodman, LS, and Gilman, A (eds): The Pharmacologic Basis of Therapeutics. Macmillan, New York, 1980, p 339.
7. Harvey, SC: Sedatives and hypnotics: barbiturates. In Gilman, AG, Goodman, LS, and Gilman, A (eds): The Pharmacologic Basis of Therapeutics. Macmillan, New York, 1980, p 349.
8. Jalling, B: Plasma and cerebrospinal fluid concentrations of phenobarbital in infants given single doses. Dev Med Child Neurol 16:781, 1974.
9. Kaim, SC and Klett, CJ: Treatment of delirium tremens: A comparative evaluation of four drugs. Quarterly Journal of the Study of Alcohol 33:1065, 1972.
10. Martin, PR, et al: Intravenous phenobarbital therapy in barbiturate and other hypnosedative withdrawal reactions. Clin Pharmacol Ther 26:256, 1979.
11. Nicol, CF: Status epilepticus. JAMA 234:419, 1975.
12. Painter, MJ, et al: Metabolism of phenobarbital and diphenylhydantoin by neonates with seizures. Neurology 27:376, 1977.
13. Robinson, GM, Sellers, EM, and Janacek, E: Barbiturate and hypnosedative withdrawal by a multiple oral phenobarbital loading dose technique. Clin Pharmacol Ther 30:71, 1981.
14. Sellers, EM and Kalant, H: Alcohol intoxication and withdrawal. N Engl J Med 294:757, 1976.
15. Shaner, DM, et al: Treatment of status epilepticus: A prospective comparison of diazepam and phenytoin versus phenobarbital and optional phenytoin. Neurology 38:202, 1988.
16. Smith, DE and Wesson, DR: Phenobarbital technique for treatment of barbiturate dependence. Arch Gen Psychiatry 24:56, 1971.
17. Smith, RF: Relative effectiveness of primidone (Mysoline) and diphenylhydantoin (Dilantin) in the management of sedative withdrawal seizures. Ann NY Acad Sci 273:378, 1976.
18. Sunshine, I: Chemical evidence of tolerance to phenobarbital. J Lab Clin Med 50:127, 1957.
19. Tintinalli, JE: Status epilepticus. J Amer Coll Emerg Phys 5:896, 1976.
20. Young, GP, et al: Intravenous phenobarbital for alcohol withdrawal and convulsions. Ann Emerg Med 16:847, 1987.

CHAPTER 29

Susanna. A. Mathé, M.D.
Robert. J. DeLorenzo, M.D., PhD., M.P.H.

Treatment of Alcohol Withdrawal with Paraldehyde

Paraldehyde, a cyclic polymer of acetaldehyde, is one of the most effective and safe treatments for alcohol withdrawal (Fig. 29–1). Unfortunately, because of the unusual chemical properties and odors associated with this compound, it has become unpopular and has often been overlooked as an effective treatment. In this chapter we discuss the chemical properties of paraldehyde and its oral, intravenous (IV), and rectal administration in the treatment of alcohol withdrawal and delirium tremens. Paraldehyde can quickly reach effective therapeutic concentrations in the blood when administered by any of these routes. We also compare the effectiveness and practicality of paraldehyde in treating alcohol withdrawal with other well-known therapies. We conclude that paraldehyde is as effective if not more so in treating alcohol withdrawal than other treatments such as the benzodiazepines, and involves less acute monitoring and expensive intensive care unit (ICU) care.

HISTORICAL CONSIDERATIONS

First discovered in 1820 by Weidenbusch, paraldehyde was initially used in Italy by Cervello in 1882 as a hypnotic.[8] In 1885, Strahan had reported great success in utilizing paraldehyde as an effective and safe sedative and hypnotic agent in a wide variety of disorders presenting with accompanying agitation.[24] Strahan praised its rapid onset of action, and found that paraldehyde had no serious side-effects, no adverse effects on the cardiorespiratory system, and quickly produced a light, natural sleep without causing excessive somnolence or headache upon awakening. Enthusiastic reports continued,[16] and it was used to treat a wide range of diseases in which restlessness, delirium, or agitation was present.

In 1912, IV use of paraldehyde (as a hypnotic) was recommended by Noel and Souttar.[21] Paraldehyde (10 ml) and 10 ml of ether were described as adequate dental analgesia prior to extensive dental extractions. It was also found that a patient with incipient alcohol withdrawal slept peacefully following paraldehyde injection while a scalp wound was sutured. The recommended dose to achieve sedation was 5 to 15 ml of paraldehyde with an equal amount of ether mixed in 150 ml of 1 percent sodium chloride injected via a long rubber tube and fine metal hypodermic needle. This IV therapy proved beneficial in treating all forms of agitation and delirium. Paraldehyde was also identified as an effective anticonvulsant. Atkey described the successful use of paraldehyde to treat a patient with tetanus and convulsions.[3]

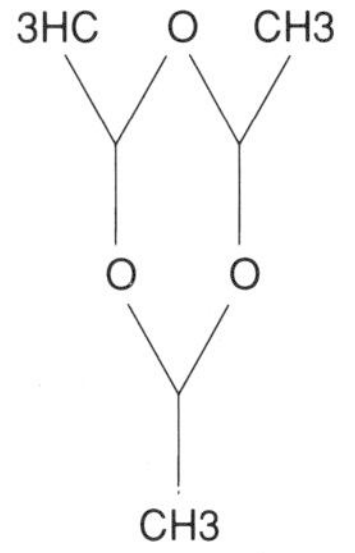

Figure 29–1. Chemical structure of paraldehyde.

In 1940, Weschler[29] published an account of the exceptional efficacy of IV paraldehyde in calming an agitated and delirious patient. With the injection of only 1 ml of paraldehyde IV, the patient calmed and fell asleep immediately. Weschler also reported excellent results using IV paraldehyde to control convulsions of prolonged duration and to combat *status epilepticus.* Although its sedative effects in such patients were well known, the IV administration of paraldehyde had been reported only infrequently and was not commonly utilized. Other reports both preceded and followed this account, documenting paraldehyde as a promptly effective sedative and hypnotic, and this method subsequently became widely used because of its easy utilization.

Paraldehyde continued to grow in popularity, even becoming the subject of periodic enthusiasm as a pre-anesthetic agent and analgesic. Rosenfield and Davidoff[22] reported favorably on its use as an obstetrical analgesic in 1932. In their series of 50 deliveries, no adverse effects were reported using as much as 4 to 10 drams in conjunction with nembutal or sodium amytal. The drug was believed to represent no danger to the mother or fetus. In 1934, Johnson[14] reported more than 20 occasions in which the intramuscular (IM) route was used with impunity to relieve pain no longer controlled with morphine, to treat mania following herniorrhaphy, and to control convulsions in vascular hypertension. Accepted as "state of the art" treatment in a number of conditions, paraldehyde was used widely and successfully.[5]

First Reports of Side-Effects

In 1890, the first report of death following paraldehyde administration was published. A delirious typhoid patient became comatose five minutes after the oral 247administration of six teaspoons of paraldehyde, and died four hours later of "failure of the heart's action."[16] Other paraldehyde-associated deaths followed sporadically in subsequent years, appearing in isolated case reports. In 1925, MacFall[17] reported on a 41-year-old man who had ingested approximately 75 ml of paraldehyde. The patient had been using paraldehyde chronically for some months; however, the source of his supply was unknown, as were the exact doses he habitually ingested. Severe congestion of both lungs was revealed by autopsy. In 1932, McDougall and Wyllie[18] reported on a 44-year-old psychotic woman who lapsed into deep coma and cardiac failure a few minutes after ingesting 120 ml of paraldehyde. Both lungs were severely congested at autopsy. In 1938, Kotz, Roth and Ryon[15] reported the death of a previously healthy 31-year-old woman eight hours following the rectal administration of 31 ml paraldehyde for obstetric analgesia. Right-sided cardiac dilatation and pulmonary edema were revealed by autopsy. Shoor[23] reported a similar case in 1941, in which 12 ml rectal paraldehyde was administered to a healthy obstetric patient. Three-and-a-half hours later the patient was comatose; 21½ hours later she died. Again, autopsy revealed pulmonary edema. In 1943, Burstein[7] reported two cases of autopsy-documented pulmonary edema following administration of 35 ml IV and 45 ml orally of paraldehyde respectively. He then reported on the administration of IV paraldehyde 0.5 ml/kg, undiluted at a rate of 1 ml in 5 seconds to 24 dogs. Eight deaths occurred within 5 minutes and 11 deaths occurred within 6 to 24 hours of induction of anesthesia. The remaining five animals survived but were said to be anorexic, and three of these died within two weeks, with autopsy revealing pulmonary hemorrhages. He concluded that IV paraldehyde administration is extremely hazardous, with a very narrow margin between the minimal anesthetic and minimal lethal dose.

Rapid infusion caused the symptoms described above, but it was also found that slow infusion caused apnea for seconds. By the 1940s, the number of side-effects reported to be associated with paraldehyde administration had grown and by the 1950s, approximately 93 deaths had been attributed to its use.[19] Although the causes of a number of these deaths were unclear, and the deaths were reported briefly and without great detail, paraldehyde subsequently fell into disfavor and its role as a drug of first choice diminished rapidly. When administration of paraldehyde became widespread in a greater variety of clinical settings, more and more side-effects were reported. In 1943, Woodson[30] reported the first three cases of sciatic nerve damage occurring after administration of IM paraldehyde. However, he described a 12-ml injection in one buttock in one patient and a 20-ml injection in another, doses that exceeded current recommendations of only 5 ml per injection.

As late as the 1950s, a number of current and authoritative forsenic medicine textbooks did not mention that paraldehyde may deteriorate to acetic acid. In the 1930s, Hutchinson[12] described severe pain and considerable sloughing of the rectal mucosa occurring after the administration of rectal paraldehyde. The paraldehyde later proved to have decomposed to 75 percent acetic acid. This 1930 report had been followed only infrequently by articles stressing the dangers of paraldehyde stored incorrectly or used more than 24 hours after opening the bottle. In 1955 Agranat and Trubshaw[2] noted that, although it appeared unlikely that acetic acid's pungent and characteristic odor could go unrecognized, a trial in which bottles of paraldehyde and bottles of paraldehyde mixed with various strengths of acetic acid were submitted for identification by smell resulted in confusion. It was not possible to recognize decomposed paraldehyde by smell alone. Pharmacologic specifications were held to only erratically. In 1937 Toal,[28] a pharmacist, examined samples of paraldehyde marketed by seven different manufacturers, and found only one sample that did not contain acetic acid after a few months of storage.

As use of paraldehyde became more widespread, cases of intoxication due to chronic habituation to paraldehyde became more common and deaths due to accidental overdose or suicide were also reported. Doses resulting in intoxication or death were often unknown or varied considerably, making paraldehyde's index of safety a subject of speculation. Hayward and Boshell,[11] reported two, and Beier, Pitts and Gonick[4] reported one case of metabolic acidosis occurring during paraldehyde intoxication.

Reports of deaths or serious side-effects rarely mentioned the purity of the paraldehyde used, total dose administered, dilution, rapidity of administration, or presence of hepatic insufficiency, so the reports were difficult to place in appropriate context. The percentages of patients receiving paraldehyde without benefit or with side-effect versus the percentage suffering no adverse reactions were not reported, and controlled studies were virtually nonexistent. However, with the advent of other, newer drugs, paraldehyde was used less and less frequently, and became neglected as an effective treatment. Contrary to these reports of the drug's toxicity and frequent side-effects, upon review there still appears to be many situations where its use may be indicated, and indeed, situations where paraldehyde may still be the drug chosen for treatment.

CLINICAL PHARMACOLOGY AND MECHANISMS OF ACTION

Paraldehyde is primarily metabolized in the liver. Seventy to 80 percent is depolymerized to acetaldehyde, which is then oxidized by aldehyde dehydrogenase to acetic acid and then further metabolized via the Krebs cycle to CO_2 and H_2O; 20 to 30 percent of paraldehyde is exhaled unchanged by the lungs and residual small amounts are excreted unchanged by the kidneys. Paraldehyde is rapidly distributed to the brain, where its concentration in cerebrospinal fluid (CSF) is approximately 20 to 30 percent lower than plasma concentrations. Although the precise mechanism of action of paraldehyde is not known, it is believed to depress many levels of the central nervous system (CNS), including the ascending reticular activating system, causing an imbalance between inhibitory and facilitory mechanisms. Paraldehyde exhibits anticonvulsant activity in subhypnotic doses. However, the margin between the anticonvulsant and hypnotic dose is small. It readily crosses the placental barrier. The mean elimination half-life of paraldehyde is 7.5 hours.

Because of the depolymerization of paraldehyde to acetaldehyde, and the oxidation of acetaldehyde to acetic acid in the presence of air, improper storage of paraldehyde had resulted in some samples containing *up* to 98 percent acetic acid, as little as 7 ml of which has proven fatal. For this reason, present United States Pharmacopeia specifications state that paraldehyde must be preserved in well-filled, tight, light-resistant containers not exceeding 30 ml, and that the user should discard the unused portion in any container that has been open for more than 24 hours. The water solubility of paraldehyde is poor—only 12.8 percent at 12°C—and decreases as the temperature rises above or falls below this point; at 37°C, its water solubility is 7.8 percent. Administration of IV paraldehyde in its pure form or even in a 10% solution may result in exceeding the solubility of paraldehyde at 37°C, and droplets of pure paraldehyde may be formed in the bloodstream, causing small paraldehyde pulmonary embolisms. Paraldehyde is incompatible with most plastics, because it can dissolve some types of plastic tubing and syringes, therefore, glass syringes must always be used.

INDICATIONS FOR TREATMENT

Alcohol Withdrawal Syndromes

Delirium tremens was first described in 1787 and named in 1838. However, it was not until 1953 that Adams and Victor[1] identified the causal relationship between delirium tremens and alcohol withdrawal and subsequently described the clinical symptoms in vivid and eloquent summary. Following a period of alcoholic intoxication, a decrease in or termination of alcoholic consumption is associated with tremulousness, generalized irritability, alteration in mentation, and seizures. These findings were confirmed by Isbell and associates,[13] who studied withdrawal in well-nourished, healthy volunteers. On sudden abstinence of alcohol, all subjects experienced weakness, anorexia, diaphoresis, and tremulousness, as well as insomnia, nausea, vomiting, diarrhea, hypertension, hyperreflexia, and fever. Of ten patients studied, five developed hallucinations, two developed seizures, and three had florid delirium tremens.

Classically seen in the "holiday" or episodic drinker, the earliest symptom of alcoholic withdrawal is tremulousness, which, though generalized, is most severe in the hands. This first appears the morning following the diminution or cessation of a period of excessive drinking, and is combined with a sensation of malaise, nausea, and vomiting as well as irritability. If alcoholic consumption then resumes, these symptoms abate, only to recur with further abstinence.

If the patient is unable to continue drinking, the symptoms increase in severity and tachycardia, tremor, and anorexia due to gastrointestinal distress become marked. The patient may appear irritable and inattentive as well as somewhat disoriented, but severe confusion is not present, though visual, auditory, olfactory, or tactile hallucinoses may occur. Hospitalization is advisable at this point as the patient will either attempt to obtain alcohol or, if abstinence persists, progress to delirium tremens. Alcohol withdrawal signs first peak within 36 hours following abstinence, and earlier symptoms may be mild.

Paraldehyde is particularly helpful at this stage of alcohol withdrawal in sedating the patient and alleviating these symptoms. In later studies, paraldehyde was found by many to be beneficial in preventing and treating early alcohol withdrawal. Paraldehyde was reported adequately to calm patients suffering from delirium tremens by shortening the duration of delirium. Subsequent studies showed that the adverse consequences of delirium tremens are also diminished in severity in patients treated with paraldehyde. Paraldehyde was found to be cross-tolerant with alcohol, and as such was effective in the replacement of alcohol in alcohol withdrawal syndromes. Because patients in withdrawal are usually significantly dehydrated, they often welcome and tolerate oral paraldehyde mixed with orange or other fruit juices.

Alcohol Withdrawal Seizures

Periodic or chronic intoxication followed by abstinence may result in alcoholic withdrawal seizures in some patients. Such seizures show a peak incidence between 13 and 24 hours in the overwhelming majority of cases, and are generalized and associated with loss of consciousness. Unusual response to photic stimulation may be seen on electroencephalography, with the patient exhibiting photomyoclonic or photoconvulsive responses, but the EEG may be entirely normal if not obtained in the ictal or immediate postictal states. Withdrawal seizures may be solitary or multiple, and on occasion patients may proceed to develop *status epilepticus.* The treatment of such seizure activity often proves difficult with conventional anticonvulsant therapy.

Although EEG recordings may be abnormal in alcohol withdrawal seizure patients, the incidence of EEG abnormalities in these patients does not exceed that of the general population. Alcohol withdrawal seizures are not felt to represent the clinical manifestation of a previously quiescent seizure disorder, but rather are a result of cerebral changes induced by alcohol itself. Focal seizures or focal findings should never be attributed to uncomplicated alcoholic withdrawal, but should prompt a thorough investigation of underlying focal cerebral pathology. Such lesions are commonly the result of multiple falls and head trauma with resultant acute or chronic gliotic scar tissue formation, contusion injury, or extra-axial fluid collections such as subdural hematomas.

Up to one-third of patients proceed to develop delirium tremens following alcoholic withdrawal seizure activity.[1] Such delirium may develop insidiously in the wake of postictal confusion or may develop hours or even days later.

Many investigators have found paraldehyde beneficial in treating seizures associated with alcohol, and some choose it for treatment. In *status epilepticus* induced in rats by lithium and pilocarpine, Morrisett, Jope, and Snead[20] found that conventional anticonvulsants did not interrupt seizure activity that had been continuous for 60 minutes. However, paraldehyde was rapidly effective in terminating these seizures. In a recent study of 13 pediatric patients with *status epilepticus* resistant to phenobarbital and phenytoin, six patients became seizure-free within one hour of paraldehyde administration, and three attained seizure control in one to eight hours.[9] No correlation was found between seizure type and control with therapy.

Delirium Tremens

Delirium tremens is the most serious and dangerous complication of alcoholism and is marked by greatly altered mentation, agitation and extreme confusion, as well as delusions and terrifying hallucinations. Autonomic hyperactivity is present and the patients are flushed, exhibiting tachycardia, tachypnea, papillary dilatation, excessive perspiration, and marked tremor. The patient is irritable and restless and can neither eat nor sleep. The sensorium is clouded and familiar objects or family members are not recognized, and the patient may proceed to incoherence. Symptoms may follow a hospitalization for unrelated illness necessitating abstinence and usually develop over a period of two or three days. On occasion, symptoms may subside gradually or appear limited in duration, ending as abruptly as they presented, but relapses of delirium may occur, sometimes with periods of complete lucidity between episodes.[1]

A 5 to 15 percent mortality rate has been associated with delirium tremens.

Patients may die of apparent peripheral circulatory collapse or hyperthermia, but in some cases, death occurs so suddenly that a clear cause of death cannot be established. Though many cases are associated with infection, injury, or other pre-existing medical conditions, delirium tremens remained the only apparent etiology in some cases in which other complicating illness was not identified.[1]

In a series of 106 alcohol withdrawal patients studied by Thomas and Freedman,[25] paraldehyde was found to be more effective than promazine in treating patients with significant withdrawal symptoms and delirium tremens. Another study, comparing the effects of promazine, chlordiazepoxide, and paraldehyde administered with chloral hydrate found paraldehyde treatment to be the most effective and best tolerated.[10] Although paraldehyde is a highly effective mode of treatment in alcohol withdrawal and delirium tremens, its unpleasant odor made it unpopular among hospital staff and it became relegated to a second-line therapy when medications such as chlordiazepoxide became available. However, even with the new medications available, Golbert and associates[10] found that oral or intramuscular (IM) paraldehyde used alone or in conjunction with chloral hydrate was significantly more effective than promazine or chlordiazepoxide in preventing the occurrence of AWS and delirium tremens and in reducing the complications of delirium tremens already in progress.

Thompson, Johnson, and Maddrey[27] found that IV diazepam has a shorter induction time and causes a smaller incidence of adverse reactions than rectal paraldehyde when used to treat patients with alcohol withdrawal and severe delirium tremens, but their study has been criticized. Patients who received paraldehyde and suffered adverse reactions had greater degrees of fever, tachypnea, and tachycardia, and may well have had graver prognoses because of the severity of their delirium tremens. The validity of this study has also been disputed because of the high dosages of paraldehyde administered. Because rectal paraldehyde is more slowly absorbed than IV diazepam, these two modes of administration are incomparable. A controlled study comparing these two drugs has not been performed.

Many other studies have verified the efficacy of paraldehyde in treating alcohol withdrawal. Withdrawal can be prevented and in most cases arrested by the prompt replacement of alcohol with paraldehyde. Best results have been obtained in early withdrawal when delirium tremens has not yet ensued. Larger doses of paraldehyde are necessary to control agitation, and agitated patients have a larger percentage of morbidity and mortality than do patients in early withdrawal. Although such increased risk may pertain in part to the toxicity of higher doses of paraldehyde, florid delirium tremens is well known to cause high morbidity and mortality when left untreated.

Several investigators have concluded that as an effective sedative and anticonvulsant in treating AWS and *status epilepticus*, paraldehyde is the classic therapy with which other and newer drugs must be compared.[6] Unfortunately, studies comparing paraldehyde with other agents for treating AWS and *status epilepticus* have never been performed using controlled trials with human subjects.

ADMINISTRATION

Recommended dosages of paraldehyde for various routes of administration are presented in Table 29–1. Contraindications and side-effects are listed in Table 29–2.

Oral Administration

Oral administration of paraldehyde is effective for patients in alcohol withdrawal. These patients are frequently quite dehydrated and willingly swallow offered drinks. Although paraldehyde has a strong, penetrating odor, mixed with orange or other fruit juices it is not altogether disagreeable and patients usually drink it voluntarily assuming it is an alcoholic beverage. It must be well diluted before oral administration. Usually 10 ml of paraldehyde mixed with 6 to 10 ounces of juice is adequate. Paraldehyde is rapidly absorbed from the gastrointestinal

Table 29-1. RECOMMENDED DOSES OF PARALDEHYDE*

Route	Initial Dose	Frequency	Max Dose 1st 24 hr	Max Dose/Day in Following Days	Mode
Oral	5–10 ml	4–6 hr prn agitation	60 ml	40 ml	Well diluted in orange juice
IM	5 ml	4–6 hr prn	30 ml	20 ml	Avoid sciatic nerve; inject deep
Rectal	10 ml 1 ml in children†	30 min until calm then 4–6 hr prn agitation† 1 hr to max 5 ml	60 ml 5 ml† in children	40 ml	
IV	5 ml, 0.2–0.4/kg† in adults 0.1–0.15 ml/kg† in children	NA	NA	NA	Infuse slowly

*Dilution to a 4% solution is recommended in all modes of administration.
†In *status epilepticus*.

(GI) tract. Maximal serum concentrations are reached within 20 to 60 minutes of oral administration of 10 ml.

ADVERSE EFFECTS

Oral administration of decomposed paraldehyde has produced a few cases of severe corrosion of the stomach with ulceration. Therefore, appropriate caution must be taken that fresh, sterile paraldehyde is used, and bottles open more than 24 hours discarded. Oral ulceration and gastric irritation have been reported with unusually large doses of paraldehyde, and therefore should not be used in patients with active peptic ulcerative disease or active mouth ulcers or erosions. Oral paraldehyde should be administered in glass cups, taking care to avoid plastic stirrers and other plastic.

Table 29-2. SIDE-EFFECTS OF PARALDEHYDE

General
    Gastric irritation
    Erythematous rash
    Toxic hepatitis
Oral
    Oral ulceration
    Gastric ulceration
    Unpleasant taste and odor
    Contraindicated in active peptic ulcer disease and active mouth ulcers or erosions
Intramuscular
    Skin sloughing
    Sterile abscesses
    Sciatic nerve damage
    Superficial injection contraindicated; injection near sciatic nerve contraindicated
Rectal
    Rectal erosion, ulceration
    Avoid in rectal ulcerative disease
Intravenous
    Coughing, tachypnea, respiratory distress, pulmonary hemorrhage, pulmonary edema
    Avoid in asthma or pulmonary disease

DOSAGE

Dosage of oral paraldehyde in alcohol withdrawal syndromes is 5 to 10 ml every 4 to 6 hours for the first 24 hours, then every 6 hours on the following days, with a maximum dose of 60 ml on the first day and 40 ml on the following days.

Rectal Administration

Following rectal administration, peak plasma concentrations of paraldehyde are attained in 2 to 4 hours. It must be diluted in mineral oil, olive oil, or cottonseen oil or 9% sodium chloride to a 4% solution. Benzyl alcohol (1 ml) added to this mixture can reduce local irritation and prevent reflex expulsion of the drug. In the unruly, agitated patient, rectal administration is easily accomplished because the patient can struggle only ineffectively when brought to a prone position. Administration should be accomplished using a glass syringe and a Foley catheter, with the balloon inflated following administration to prevent reflex expulsion. The rubber catheter should be left in place for only a few hours if possible, because extended inflation of the balloon can cause mucosal irritation and corrosion. This treatment is useful to treat the uncooperative patient.

ADVERSE EFFECTS

Rectal administration of decomposed paraldehyde has produced a few cases of severe corrosion and ulceration of the rectum. For this reason, only fresh, sterile paraldehyde must be used. Paraldehyde must be well diluted to a 4 percent solution prior to rectal administration, and rectal tubing removed after administration as rapidly as possible to prevent pressure ulceration. This mode of administration should be avoided in patients with irritative bowel disease or known previous ulcerative GI disease. Rectal paraldehyde is an effective and rather safe form of administration if used properly and for only short periods.

DOSAGE

Dosing schedules for rectal administration have varied widely. Efficacy has been reported with doses ranging from 10 ml every 30 minutes until the patient is calm, to 10 ml every 4 to 6 hours, to a maximum of 60 ml in the first 24 hours and 40 ml/day in the following days. The least amount of paraledhyde effective in obtaining reasonable sedation is recommended.

IM Administration

Paraldehyde may be administered IM undiluted deep into the buttocks, taking care to avoid the vicinity of nerve trunks. No more than 5 ml should be given per injection site. Absorption from IM sites is somewhat slow, with peak plasma concentrations attained in 2 to 4 hours according to some reports, although other sources have reported hypnotic effects within 15 minutes of injection. Sleep, when attained, lasts up to eight hours, although in some patients with hepatic disease, the drug is metabolized slowly and the hypnotic effects are prolonged.

ADVERSE EFFECTS

Skin sloughing and sterile abscesses have been reported with superficial IM injections. Care must be taken to avoid the sciatic nerve, because injections can cause permanent damage. For this reason, IM administration is contraindicated unless other means of administration are unavailable.

DOSAGE

IM administration should involve 5 ml every 4 to 6 hours for the first 24 hours, then every 6 hours on the following days, with a maximum dose of 30 ml on the first day and 20 ml on the following days.

IV Administration

Peak plasma concentrations are reached immediately after IV injection of paraldehyde. IV paraldehyde must be diluted to a 4 percent solution prior to administration because undiluted IV paraldehyde has been reported to form pulmonary embolisms. IV injection of paraldehyde has been effective in the control of alcohol withdrawal as well as *status epilepticus*, particularly in cases where the cause of *status* was thought to be alcohol associated. However, due to its potential reported side-effects, this mode of administration is only advocated for emergencies.

ADVERSE EFFECTS

IV administration of paraldehyde has been associated with coughing, tachypnea, respiratory distress, pulmonary edema, pulmonary hemorrhage, right-sided cardiac dilatation, and circulatory collapse. Case reports describing the above complications do not specify whether decomposed paraldehyde was administered, or if it was adequately diluted. In many cases, dosages exceeding current USP specifications were administered. A careful toxicity study is definitely indicated. Paraldehyde should be used with caution, if at all, in patients with asthma or pulmonary disease.

DOSAGE

The usual hypnotic dose of IV paraldehyde is 10 ml, and the sedative dose is 5 ml. In the treatment of *status epilepticus*, 0.2 to 0.4 ml/kg diluted to a 4 percent solution in 0.9 percent sodium chloride may be administered to adults. In pediatric cases of *status epilepticus*, 0.1 to 0.15 ml/kg is appropriate with the same dilution. Given the potential adverse effects, oral and rectal rather than IV administration should be used in treating alcohol withdrawal.

Recommended Protocol

At the Medical College of Virginia (MCV) the experience with oral paraldehyde has been highly favorable. Utilized early in alcohol withdrawal, it is highly effective in calming and sedating the patient. Five to 10 ml are well-diluted with orange juice and offered to the patient in beverage form in a glass (not plastic) container. Since these patients are frequently quite dehydrated, they usually drink eagerly, particularly because they often desire an alcoholic beverage and paraldehyde appears to them an effective substitute. The initial 5- to 10-ml dose is repeated as needed to attain sedation but actual sleep is not an imperative goal. A dose of 60 ml should not be exceeded on the first day. The degree of hepatic dysfunction must be taken into consideration, and the minimum dose adequate to attain a quiet, noncombative state is recommended. Paraldehyde should be discontinued as soon as the patient's condition stabilizes, because tolerance may develop, and oral diazepam or chlordiazepoxide can then be substituted.

In agitated patients who refuse oral paraldehyde, rectal paraldehyde has proven effective. The agitated patient is easily brought to the prone position, where he or she has difficulty striking out at restraining personnel. A Foley catheter is then inserted rectally and 10 ml of paraldehyde, diluted to a 4 percent solution with mineral oil, is injected via a glass syringe. This procedure may be repeated every 30 minutes until the patient is calm and then every 4 to 6 hours if needed to maintain a sedated, calm state. Care must be taken not to exceed 30 ml of paraldehyde in the first 24 hours and 20 ml/day on the following days. To avoid compressive irritation of the rectal mucosa, the rectal tubing should be withdrawn as soon as paraldehyde effects become apparent.

Because of the potential side-effects, IM and IV paraldehyde are not routine modes of administration in the MCV alcohol withdrawal syndrome protocol (Table 29–3). IV diazepam is the best treatment to choose if oral or rectal paraldehyde cannot be given.

Other Precautions

Because impaired hepatic function may result in unpredictable rates of paraldehyde metabolism, the drug should be administered very cautiously in the lowest

Table 29–3. MEDICAL COLLEGE OF VIRGINIA NEUROLOGIC TREATMENT PROTOCOL FOR ALCOHOL WITHDRAWAL

Patient with agitation, mild withdrawal, or delirium		
Will drink PO →	Yes →	Oral paraldehyde
↓ No ↓		
Can be brought to lateral or prone position →	Yes →	Rectal paraldehyde
Paraldehyde contraindicated →	Yes →	IV diazepam (Valium)

possible doses in patients with heptatic insufficiency. Toxic hepatitis has been reported in some instances in patients without a history of hepatic disease.

Although paraldehyde has been used as an effective obstetric anesthetic, it readily crosses the placental barrier and has been reported to cause neonatal respiratory depression. Thus, it is not recommended for such use.

Metabolic acidosis, toxic hepatitis, and toxic nephritis have been reported to occur after chronic administration of paraldehyde. In many of these cases, excessive, toxic doses had been ingested. Prolonged use of paraldehyde may produce tolerance and physical as well as psychological dependence. Sudden withdrawal from chronic paraldehyde may produce a withdrawal syndrome with hallucinations and delirium and thus should be avoided.

SUMMARY

Despite its frequent use as a highly effective sedative and hypnotic in the latter part of the 19th and first half of the 20th century, paraldehyde has been neglected in the primary treatment of alcohol withdrawal in the second half of this century. However, it remains highly effective in treating this syndrome, and has been shown in numerous studies to be beneficial both in the prevention and frequently in the early termination of withdrawal as well as in the management of delirium tremens. It has also been effective in the treatment of seizures and *status epilepticus*, often when other, more conventionally used drugs have failed. Its decline in recent years is due predominantly to isolated case reports of side-effects. Controlled population series to substantiate such findings have not been conducted. Cases documenting the use of decomposed paraldehyde have led to more stringent standards of preparation and storage, making the use of such deteriorated preparations far less likely. Further well-structured studies are needed to document the side-effects of paraldehyde and compare its efficacy with that of other drugs, given proper dilution, administration, and dosage.

Although paraldehyde has an acceptable margin of safety, improper use has led to its present decline in popularity. We believe it is as effective as other medications presently advocated in the treatment of AWS, and that given its prompt onset and ease of administration, it should be reevaluated as a primary drug in the choice of treatment of alcohol withdrawal syndromes.

References

1. Adams, RD and Victor, M: Alcohol and alcoholism. In Adams, RD and Victor, M (eds): Principles of Neurology. McGraw-Hill, New York, 1981.
2. Agranat, AL and Trubshaw, WHD: The danger of decomposed paraldehyde. South African Medical Journal 29:1021, 1955.
3. Atkey, O: Tetanus treated by intravenous injections of paraldehyde and copious injections of normal saline resulting in cure. Lancet 1:168, 1913.
4. Beier, LS, Pitts, WH, and Gonick, HC: Metabolic acidosis occurring during paraldehyde intoxication. Ann Intern Med 58:155, 1963.
5. Bodansky, M, Jinkins, J, and Levine, H: Clinical and experimental studies on paraldehyde. Anesthesiology 2:20, 1941.
6. Browne, TR: Paraldehyde, chlormethiazole and lidocaine for treatment of status epilepticus. In Delgado-Escueta, AV, et al (eds): Status Epilepticus: Mechanisms of Brain Damage and Treatment. Advances in Neurology, Vol 34. Raven Press, New York, 1982, p 509.
7. Burstein, CL: The hazard of paraldehyde administration. JAMA 121:3, 187, 1943.
8. Cervello, V: Recherches cliniques et physiologiques sur la paraldehyde. Arch Ital Biol 6:113, 1884.
9. Curless, RG, Holzman, BH, and Ramsey, RE: Paraldehyde therapy in childhood status epilepticus. Arch Neurol 40:477, 1983.
10. Golbert, TM, et al: Comparative evaluation of treatments of alcohol withdrawal syndromes. JAMA 201:99, 1967.
11. Hayward, JN and Boshell, BR: Paraldehyde intoxication with metabolic acidosis. Am J Med 23:965, 1957.
12. Hutchinson, R: A danger from paraldehyde. Br Med J 1:718, 1930.
13. Isbell, H, et al: Experimental study of the etiology of "rum fits" and DT's. Quarterly Journal of Studies on Alcohol 16:1, 1955.
14. Johnson, AS: The parenteral use of paraldehyde for control of pain and convulsive states. N Engl J Med 210:1065, 1934.

15. Kotz, J, Roth, GB, and Ryon, WA: Idiosyncrasy to paraldehyde. JAMA 110:2145, 1938.
16. Lancet, 2:423, 1890.
17. MacFall, JEW: Paraldehyde poisoning. Br Med J 2:255, 1925.
18. McDougall, J and Wylie, AM: Fatal case of paraldehyde poisoning with postmortem findings. Journal Mental Science 78:374, 1932.
19. Moore, M, Alexander, L, and Ipsen, J: Death from poisoning. N Engl J Med 246:46, 1952.
20. Morrisett, R, Jope, R, and Snead, OC: Effects of drugs on the initiation and maintenance of status epilepticus. Experimental Neurology 97:193, 1987.
21. Noel, HCL and Souttar, HS: The intravenous injection of paraldehyde. Lancet 2:818, 1912.
22. Rosenfield, HH and Davidoff, R: A new procedure for obstetrical analgesia. N Engl J Med 207:366, 1932.
23. Shorr, M: Paraldehyde poisoning. JAMA 117:1534, 1941.
24. Strahan, SAK: Action of paraldehyde, the new hypnotic. Lancet 1:201, 1885.
25. Thomas, D and Freedman, D: Treatment of the alcohol withdrawal syndrome. JAMA 3:188, 1964.
26. Thompson, WL: Management of alcohol withdrawal syndromes. Arch Intern Med 138:278, 1978.
27. Thompson, WL, Johnson, AD, and Maddrey, WL: Diazepam and paraldehyde for treatment of severe delirium tremens: A controlled trial. Ann Intern Med 82:175, 1975.
28. Toal, JS: The decomposition of paraldehyde on storage. J Pharm Pharmacol 10:439, 1937.
29. Weschler, IS: Intravenous injection of paraldehyde for the control of seizures. JAMA 114:2198, 1940.
30. Woodson, FG: Sciatic nerve injury due to the intramuscular injection of paraldehyde. JAMA 121:1343, 1943.

CHAPTER 30

Bengt Sternebring, M.D.

Treatment of Alcohol Withdrawal Seizures with Carbamazepine and Valproate

Anticonvulsive treatment is generally recommended to prevent the development of withdrawal seizures occurring as a consequence of heavy and, in most cases, daily alcohol consumption during a long period in alcoholics (according to the *Diagnostic and Statistical Manual of Mental Disorders, Third Edition* [*DSM III*]).[1,8,33,34,35] Prophylactic treatment with anticonvulsants seems to be especially appropriate for alcoholics who in a previous withdrawal phase developed alcohol withdrawal seizures (AWS) or were nutritionally deficient.[17,31,35] Patients who exhibit heavy mixed misuse of alcohol and drugs (*e.g.*, barbiturates or benzodiazepines) are also candidates for prophylactic anticonvulsant therapy.[35]

Carbamazepine (CBZ) and valproate (VPA) (Fig. 30–1) are anticonvulsants. CBZ is mainly used to control grand mal seizures and psychomotor epilepsy.[26] VPA is prescribed for simple and complex absence seizures.[26,30,40] Neither CBZ nor VPA are effective in treating a progressive withdrawal seizure.

In Scandinavia and other parts of Europe, CBZ has been used clinically for many years to prevent AWS.[21,29] Many animal and human studies have confirmed its effectiveness and suggested treatment schedules. The results with CBZ were somewhat more positive than results with phenytoin using the same treatment model.[38]

Because VPA was recently introduced as an anticonvulsant in the withdrawal phase, there is limited literature on its usefulness.[26] A therapeutic tradition does not exist and therefore the appropriate dosage schedule is unconfirmed.[14] Studies confirm the efficacy of VPA in preventing withdrawal seizures[14,16,26] and there are suggestions that the drug acts by the same membrane-disordering mechanism as ethanol both *in vivo* and *in vitro*.[24] Most studies confirm VPA's activity, but the results are clouded by the fact that the alcoholics in published studies also received neuroleptics and sedatives.[40]

CBZ has other advantages in the withdrawal phase. For example, it inhibits the reuptake of epinephrine, an effect that is favorable in the withdrawal phase because investigators believe that catecholamines or their metabolites play an important part in aggravating withdrawal symptoms, including seizures.[9] In this respect CBZ is also useful in treating predelirious and delirious patients.[21,27,29] Also, it has been hypothesized that AWS are part of a kindling process. This possibility suggests

315

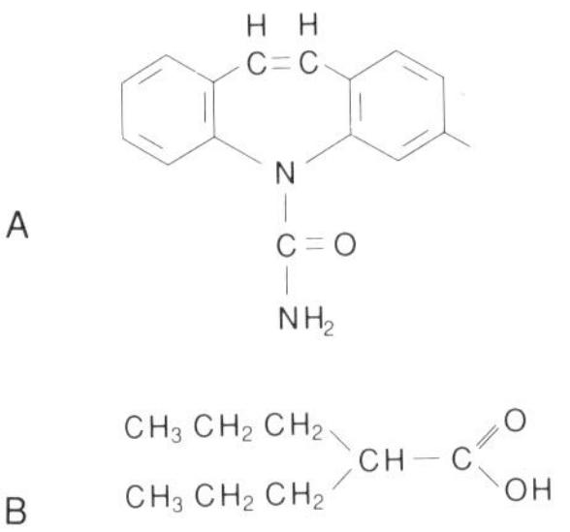

Figure 30–1. Chemical structures of (A) carbamazepine and (B) valproic acid.

another advantage of CBZ—it inhibits development of seizures from the limbic system.[2,3] Other studies concluded that sleep disturbances subsided faster in CBZ-treated patients than in a placebo group.[11] During withdrawal, CBZ is therapeutic for the often-noticed heart arrythmias.[10] This drug belongs to group 1, according to the Vaughan-Williams classification of anti-arrhythmic agents.[20] Several studies have concluded that VPA also has sedative effects.[14,40]

PHARMACOLOGIC ASPECTS

CBZ

CBZ is a lipoid substance that easily passes through all membranes of the body. The protein-binding capacity is between 70% and 80% with albumin.[4,35] In contrast to phenytoin, there is no convincing evidence that there is a specific binding site associated with its anticonvulsant action.[38] Patients with liver disease have a lower protein-binding capacity than controls but the difference is not significant.[25] CBZ is mainly metabolized in two oxidative steps. With regard to this biotransformation, the main metabolite 10,11-epoxycarbamazepine is pharmacologically similar to the original compound.[12,39] The epoxide has a tendency to increase with the number of intakes per day of the drug.[5] The pharmacokinetics are dose dependent,[37] and the elimination of CBZ follows a dose-independent kinetic formula with half-lives that vary approximately four-fold between individuals.[39] The usual half-life in monotherapy is about 15 hours.

Serum levels of CBZ decrease when phenytoin is present in the blood. CBZ is able to induce the metabolism of other drugs such as phenytoin, warfarin, tetracyclines, and contraceptive agents.[4] The elixir form of CBZ is absorbed faster than the tablet form,[23] in alcohol-dependent as well as non–alcohol-dependent patients.[37] There is a significant difference in serum concentrations of CBZ measured in a patient undergoing acute withdrawal and concentrations measured in the same patient after 10 days of alcohol abstinence.[35] The elimination rate is slower during acute withdrawal, which may indicate that ethanol competitively inhibits CBZ metabolism. The total bioavailability is not measurable because CBZ cannot be administered intravenously (IV). Because the treatment period in the withdrawal phase is short, the usual problems of CBZ are negligible, that is, serum concentration fluctuations, the role of the main epoxide, and autometabolism.[18]

VPA

Valproate is a short-chain fatty acid, well-absorbed after oral administration, with almost complete bioavailability. However, measuring anticonvulsant activity using serum levels is difficult, because the time-course of the drug's action is poorly correlated with blood or tissue levels of the drug.[19] The site of action is unknown but there are indications that VPA influences the gamma-aminobutyric acid (GABA) system (increased GABA levels are related to VPA administration). The clearance of VPA is dose dependent, with an increased free fraction of the drug at higher doses. VPA inhibits the metabolism of many drugs,[19] including phenytoin, CBZ, and barbiturates. It therefore achieves a higher steady-state concentration and can cause unexpected side-effects and intoxications. The half-life of VPA is about 16 hours.

The main clinical use of VPA is against absence seizures, but it is not the first choice for treatment because it is associated with a risk for hepatotoxicity.[40] Little is known about the efficacy of VPA therapy in generalized seizures or in AWS.[14,16]

ANTICONVULSIVE TREATMENT MODELS

Convulsive seizures in the withdrawal phase are serious and constitute a withdrawal symptom that cannot be overlooked. The fits are alcohol related and appear only during the first week of abstinence.[17] If the patient has also used barbiturates or benzodiazepines, the risk of seizures lasts an additional 2 weeks, and it is advisable to prolong pharmacologic therapy. Because there is a higher incidence of death among those alcoholics who have had a history of seizures,[36] most investigators believe medication is needed to prevent fits during this short period. Even if the patient has withdrawal fits only relatively infrequently (they affect only 3–7% of alcoholics)[1,8,36] and a long drinking period has preceded the seizures, the administration of anticonvulsants according to certain rules is advisable.

The goal of treatment is to reach therapeutic serum levels as fast as possible and to maintain protection against seizures for as long as the patient is at risk. One should keep in mind that convulsions can appear not only when blood concentrations of alcohol are decreasing or have reached zero (the beginning of the true withdrawal phase), but also when the ethanol concentration is in a steady state or even increasing.[25] The "true" withdrawal phase is the most important therapeutically because most seizures occur during this period. This phase begins as soon as the blood concentration of ethanol begins to decrease. In practice, seizures can be expected from a few hours after the last alcohol intake through 4 or 5 days of abstinence[17,38] unless the patient has also taken other drugs.

CBZ

The basic concepts for testing for anticonvulsant activity have been used since 1952 and some recent studies on animals[38] and humans[37] confirm earlier reports that CBZ has anticonvulsive activity. One animal study showed that CBZ is somewhat more effective than phenytoin in preventing AWS. To establish therapeutic levels of CBZ in a human alcoholic as soon as possible, it is advisable to give the first dose in syrup form: one study showed that during the first 10 hours of abstinence from alcohol, subjects given CBZ in syrup form had a significantly lower rate of withdrawal fits ($p<0.05$) than subjects in a control group given CBZ in tablet form; see Fig. 30–2.[37]

Most of the clinical studies of CBZ come from Scandinavia.[1,6,7,13,17,27,29,37] Together these studies verify that anticonvulsive effects can be achieved with the following regimen: Administration of doses on the first day ranges from 400 to 800 mg (in one study up to 1200 mg; usually 400 mg plus 200 mg administered on day 1). On the following 5 to 7 days of treatment 400 to 600 mg of CBZ are administered. If 400 mg of syrup are given as the first dose, protection against sei-

Figure 30–2. Withdrawal seizures following administration of carbamazepine in tablet and syrup form. The pharmacokinetic differences between the forms are evident in the 2–10 hr. interval, since there is no chance to reach the lower limit of the therapeutic level during the period immediately following administration. (Based on the data of Sternebring[37] et al.)

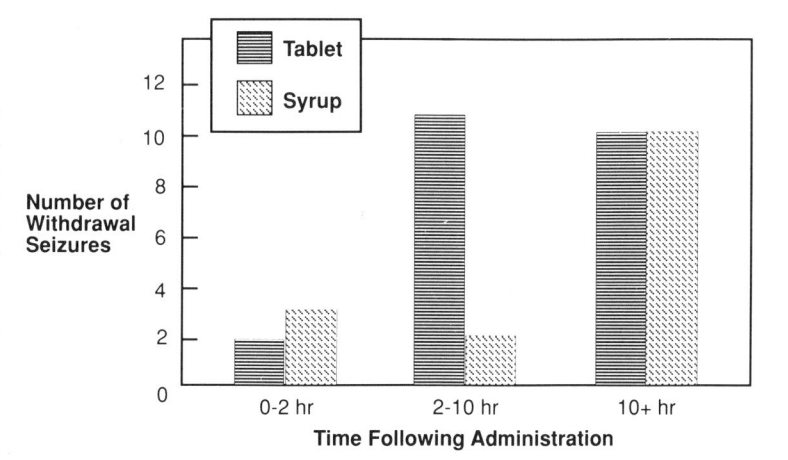

zures is usually achieved within 2 hours.[37] The second dose of CBZ on day 1 is usually 200 mg in tablet form. Thereafter, 200 mg of CBZ in tablet form are given twice a day for another 5 to 7 days.[38] For many years this regimen has been used at most clinics in Scandinavia.[32] Sometimes the daily amount of CBZ administered varies slightly: doses up to 200 mg three times a day have been given without serious side-effects and with effective anticonvulsive activity.[21] With this regimen, CBZ blood levels increase relatively rapidly and may cause mild dose-related side-effects, which are mixed with the usual withdrawal symptoms (dizziness, blurred vision, mild ataxia, etc.) and therefore tolerated by the patient.[36]

It is important to note that even at therapeutic blood concentrations (20–40 μmol/1iter), CBZ does not completely prevent seizures.[35] Because of the interaction between ethanol and CBZ, changes in the protein-binding pattern and changes in the absorption capacity in alcoholics, further investigation is necessary to determine whether recommended doses of CBZ and therapeutic levels are the same for alcoholics and other patients.

VPA

A few studies have used a treatment model of VPA during the withdrawal phase.[40] Unlike CBZ, VPA can be administered parenterally for rapid seizure control.[19] In addition, negative cardiovascular effects are rare.[14] The therapeutic serum level of VPA is 50 to 100 μg/ml, and as with CBZ, dose-related side-effects develop soon after the upper limit is passed. That is, an abrupt start of medication causes side-effects such as abdominal pain, "heartburn," vomiting, and nausea. Unlike CBZ, the neurotoxic effects of VPA usually only occur at levels far beyond therapeutic concentrations.[19] The usual dosage of VPA is 800 to 1200 mg/day administered in tablet form three times a day. Occasionally IV infusion is used.[14,40] However, this medication schedule is not specifically designed for withdrawal seizures.

A Finnish study[16] observed that in rats VPA prevents AWS when the preparation is given immediately after the last alcohol intake but ineffective if administered 12 hours after the beginning of ethanol abstinence. This finding may indicate a therapeutic problem necessitating further investigation in humans.

TREATMENT PROBLEMS

The most striking problem with both CBZ and VPA is a consequence of the drugs' administration. To prevent seizures as soon as possible there is no time to start the medication gradually, but starting it abruptly often causes side-effects. However, alcoholics given CBZ tolerate those side-effects better than nonalcoholics.[36] For patients taking VPA, there is little available literature to evaluate this problem. After 7 seven days of treatment, both CBZ and VPA can be simultaneously discontinued.

CBZ

The effects of CBZ overuse are well known and usually involve the central nervous system (CNS). Problems include nystagmus, diplopia, blurred vision, and ataxia.[21,28] However, only a few cases of severe CBZ intoxication in connection with alcoholism have been reported.[22] A recent study at the Department of Alcohol Diseases in Malmoe, Sweden[35] suggests that CBZ overconsumption leading to severe side-effects and intoxication among alcoholics is much more common than is generally realized. Eighteen consecutive patients were registered. Most of their symptoms originated in the CNS but psychosis was also noted. In most patients intoxication simulated lesions from the cerebellum and the brainstem. No signs of intoxication were encountered in patients with serum concentrations within the therapeutic levels of 20 to 40 μmol/liter. The reason many patients take too much CBZ is unclear. The most probable explanation is exaggerated fear of withdrawal seizures. There is no evidence that the compound has euphoric or anxiolytic effects.

There is also a group of alcoholics that misuses CBZ. They constantly fear seizures and may misjudge symptoms, believing some to be a type of aura. This confusion results in incorrect intake of the drug. Taking CBZ now and then raises the epoxide levels, and taken with ethanol, the serum concentration of CBZ and its epoxide rapidly reach dangerously high levels, producing signs of intoxication (nystagmus, diplopia, blurred vision, etc.).[17] The symptoms of CBZ intoxication are difficult to evaluate because they are nonspecific and very similar to withdrawal symptoms. Serious intoxication symptoms have been noted with serum levels of CBZ just above 100 μmol/liter. Because there is a high risk of developing severe intoxication symptoms when CBZ is mixed with ethanol,[22] and because treatment should be limited to the first week of withdrawal,[2] generous prescription of CBZ to alcoholics has obvious disadvantages. Hypersensitivity reactions (e.g., erythema multiforme, Stevens-Johnson syndrome) are well known but infrequent.[35] Other adverse reactions have been described, but are also infrequent. Most adverse reactions are not dose related.[19] Overall it appears that CBZ is relatively safe when administration is controlled.

VPA

The possibility of hepatotoxicity is a problem when VPA is administered to alcoholics, who often have liver disease.[40] This hepatotoxicity is not dose related. There are also reports of CNS depression when the drug is taken with alcohol.[9] Sedation has been reported,[14] but most patients in that study took sedatives in addition to VPA.[40] In most cases, VPA is fairly safe when administered to nonalcoholics, and only a small number of patients have had severe toxic side-effects.[19]

There are no reports of VPA misuse. However, cross-tolerance with ethanol may be a risk and can result in an abuse of the drug to achieve an euphoric effect.[40]

SUMMARY

Convulsive seizures in alcohol withdrawal are serious, and constitute a withdrawal symptom that cannot be overlooked. Prophylactic treatment with anticonvulsants is therefore appropriate. The goal of treatment is to establish therapeutic serum levels as fast as possible and to maintain protection against seizures as long as the patient is at risk. CBZ and VPA can be used as anticonvulsants; the former is administered in the alcohol withdrawal phase. If CBZ syrup is given immediately as the first dose, seizures are usually prevented within 2 hours. VPA is believed to be effective if administered at the beginning of ethanol abstinence. With this regimen, the blood concentration of the drugs increases relatively quickly and may cause mild to moderate side-effects. However, these effects are usually well tolerated by the patient.

Alcoholics often have an exaggerated fear of developing withdrawal seizures. This fear can result in an overconsumption of anticonvulsants and lead to intoxication. Neither CBZ nor VPA is recommended during pregnancy.

Both drugs have advantages and disadvantages in treating withdrawal seizures. Because CBZ has been more extensively used to prevent withdrawal seizures, a large number of investigations support and advise clinical use of the drug. The benefits of CBZ in treating acute withdrawal symptoms also suggest that this compound is superior to VPA.

References

1. Agricola, R, Mazzarino, M, and Urani, R: Treatment of acute alcohol withdrawal syndrome with carbamazepine: A double-blind comparison with tiapride. Journal of Medical Research 10:160, 1982.
2. Albright, PS and Bruni, J: Effects of carbamazepine and its epoxide metabolite on amygdala-kindled seizures in rats. Neurology 34:1383, 1984.
3. Ballenger, JC and Post, RM: Kindling as a model for the alcohol withdrawal syndromes. Br Journal of Psychiatry 3:234, 1978.
4. Bertilson, L: Clinical pharmacokinetics on carbamazepine. Clin Pharm 3:128, 1978.
5. Bertilsson, L, Tomson, T, and Tybring, G: Pharmacokinetics: Time-dependent changes: Autoinduction of carbamazepine epoxidation. J Clin Pharmacol 26:459, 1986.
6. Björkqvist, SE, et al: Ambulant treatment of alcohol withdrawal symptoms with carbamazepine. Acta Psychiatr Scand 53:333, 1976.

7. Brune, F and Busch, H: Anticonvulsant–sedative treatment of delirium alcoholism. Quarterly Journal of Studies on Alcohol 32:334, 1971.
8. Chan, AWK: Alcoholism and Epilepsy. Epilepsia 26:323, 1985.
9. Chu, NS: Carbamazepine: Prevention of alcohol withdrawal seizures. Neurology 29:1397, 1979.
10. Corday, E, et al: Antiarrhythmic properties of carbamazepine. Geriatrics 10:78, 1971.
11. Elton, M: Carbamazepine in the treatment of alcohol withdrawal symptoms. In Sternebring, B (ed): Carbamazepine in the treatment of alcoholics. Nordic Journal of Psychiatry (Suppl)41:71, 1987.
12. Faigle, JW and Feldmann, KF: Carbamazepine: Biotransformation. In Woodbury, DM, Penry, JK, and Pippenger, CE (eds): Antiepileptic Drugs, ed 2. Raven Press, New York, 1982, p 483.
13. Flygenring, J, et al: Treatment of alcohol withdrawal symptoms in hospitalized patients. Acta Psychiatr Scand 69:398, 1984.
14. Goldstein, DB: Sodium bromide and sodium valproate: Effective suppressants of ethanol withdrawal reactions in mice. J Pharmacol Exp Ther 208:223, 1979.
15. Hillbom, M: Alcohol withdrawal seizures: Alternatives for treatment and prevention. In Sternebring, B (ed): Carbamazepine in the treatment of alcoholics. Nordic Journal of Psychiatry (Suppl)41:45, 1987.
16. Hillbom, ME: The prevention of ethanol withdrawal seizures in rats by dipropylacetate. Neuropharmacology 14:755, 1975.
17. Hillbom, M and Hjelm-Jäger, M: Should alcohol withdrawal seizures be treated with anti-epileptic drugs? Acta Neurol Scand 69:39, 1984.
18. Johannesen, JI, et al: Further observations on carbamazepine and cbz-10,11-epoxide kinetics in epileptic patients. In Gardner-Thorpe, C, et al (eds): Antiepileptic Drugs Monitoring. Beekman Pubs., Woodstock, N.Y. 1977, p 110.
19. Katzung, BG: Basic and Clinical Pharmacology. Lange Medical Publications, Los Altos, 1984, p 276.
20. Kennebäck, G: Cardiac effects of carbamazepine. In Sternebring, B (ed): Carbamazepine in the treatment of alcoholics. Nordic Journal of Psychiatry (Suppl)41:15, 1987.
21. Lier, A and Lier, G: Zur therapie alkoholischer Entzugssyndrome mit carbamazepin. Medizinische Welt 43:1612, 1979.
22. Moore, NC, et al: Three cases of carbamazepine toxicity. Am J Psychiatry 142:8:974, 1985.
23. Morselli, PL, et al: Bioavailability of two carbamazepine preparations during chronic administration to epileptic patients. Epilepsia 16:759, 1975.
24. Perlman, BJ and Goldstein, DB: Genetic influences on the central nervous system depressant and membrane-disordering actions of ethanol and sodium valproate. Mol Pharmacol 26:547,1984.
25. Phillip, M, Seyfeddinipur, N, and Marneros, A: Epileptische Anfälle beim Delirium Tremens. Nervenarzt 47:192, 1976.
26. Pinder, RM, Brogden, RN, and Speight, RM: Sodium valproate: A review of its pharmacological properties and therapeutic efficacy in epilepsy. Drugs 13:81, 1977.
27. Poutanen, P: Experience with carbamazepine in the treatment of withdrawal symptoms in alcohol abusers. Br J Addict 74:201, 1979.
28. Reynolds, EH: Neurotoxicity of carbamazepine. In Daly, P (ed): Advances in Neurology, Vol II. Raven Press, New York. 1975, p 345.
29. Ritola, E and Malinen, L: A double-blind comparison of carbamazepine and clormethiazole in the treatment of alcohol withdrawal syndrome. Acta Psychiatr Scand 64:254, 1981.
30. Sillanpää, M: Treatment of alcohol withdrawal symptoms. Br J Hosp Med 27:4, 1982.
31. Sillanpää, M, Björkqvist, SE, and Alihanka, J: Treatment of convulsions and other alcohol withdrawal symptoms. In Robb, P (ed): Epilepsy Updated: Causes and Treatment. Year Book Medical Publishers, Chicago, 1979, p 243.
32. Sörensen, A, et al: Pharmacological experiences in the treatment of withdrawal syndromes in the Nordic countries. In Sternebring, B (ed): Carbamazepine in the treatment of alcoholics. Nordic Journal of Psychiatry (Suppl)41:49, 1987.
33. Spitzer, R (ed): Diagnostic and Statistical Manual of Mental Disorders, third edition (DSM-III). American Psychiatric Association, Pilgrim Press, Washington DC, 1980.
34. Sternebring, B: Alkoholabstinens: Abstinensepilepsi. Läkartidningen 77:1538, 1980.
35. Sternebring, B: Carbamazepine in the withdrawal phase. In: Pharmacological Treatment of Alcoholism. National Board of Health and Welfare, Drug Information Committee. Stockholm, 1985, p 17.
36. Sternebring, B: Convulsive seizures in the withdrawal phase. In Sternebring, B (ed): Carbamazepine in the treatment of alcoholics. Nordic Journal of Psychiatry (Suppl)41:41, 1987.
37. Sternebring, B, Holm, R, and Wadstein, J: Reduction in early alcohol abstinence fits by administration of carbamazepine syrup instead of tablet. Eur J Clin Pharmacol 24:611, 1983.
38. Wahlström, G: Some aspects of the pharmacology of carbamazepine in relation to ethanol withdrawal. In Sternebring, B (ed): Carbamazepine in the treatment of alcoholics. Nordic Journal of Psychiatry (Suppl)41:7, 1987.
39. Westenberg, H, et al: Kinetics of carbamazepine and carbamazepine epoxide determined by use of plasma and saliva. Clin Pharmacol Ther 23:320, 1978.
40. Wilbur, R and Kulik, FA: Anticonvulsant drugs in alcohol withdrawals: Use of phenytoin, primidone, carbamazepine, valproic acid, and the sedative anticonvulsants. Am J Hosp Pharm 38:1138, 1981.

CHAPTER 31

Charlotte B. McCutchen, M.D.

Treatment of Alcohol Withdrawal Seizures with Other Drugs

Many drugs have been used to treat alcohol withdrawal and alcohol withdrawal seizures (AWS). Opium was used to treat delirium tremens as early as 1854, and many methods, from insulin shock to hypnosis, were tried in the early part of this century.[49] More recently, agents such as magnesium sulfate and chloral hydrate have been shown to have value, but they cannot ameliorate all the symptoms of alcohol withdrawal.[78] This chapter discusses recent attempts to treat this difficult disorder.

NEUROLEPTICS

Chlorpromazine

The modern history of attempts to control alcohol withdrawal begins with the introduction of the neuroleptics in the early 1950s.[49] Initially there was tremendous enthusiasm for chlorpromazine and related drugs because of their sedative, hallucinolytic, and anti-emetic properties, and the fact that they could be administered orally or parenterally.[2,3,57] However, serious side effects were reported. Hypotension due to alpha-adrenergic effects as well as to cardiac arrhythmias (as a result of anticholinergic activity) complicated the care of patients in alcohol withdrawal.[17,42,71] In one study, hepatotoxicity, thought to be due to a hypersensitivity reaction, was reported in 11 out of 1400 mixed neurologic and psychiatric cases, and was responsible for clinical jaundice.[16]

Treatment of alcohol-related seizures with the phenothiazines was strongly criticized as reports were published about seizure exacerbation in epileptics by these drugs.[11,27] Electroencephalographic (EEG) epileptiform activity as well as clinical seizures were reported in these patients.[58,61,63,72,75] Knott and Beard[52] suggested that "some phenothiazines enhance the seizure diathesis in patients suffering acute (alcohol) withdrawal." In alcoholic patients who may already be hypoglycemic and hypomagnesemic, drugs with such an effect may not be therapeutically effective. In addition, comparison of chlorpromazine with older agents such as paraldehyde in treating alcohol withdrawal demonstrated that both were equally effective but that paraldehyde had a slight advantage because it had somewhat less central nervous system (CNS) depressant activity at the doses used than did chlorpromazine.[29]

Haloperidol, Hydroxyzine, Mesoridazine, and Meprobamate

Other neuroleptics have been used to relieve withdrawal symptoms. Haloperidol (Haldol), a butyrophenone with antipsychotic action, was evaluated for use in treating the alcohol withdrawal syndrome and delirium tremens.[67,69] Comparing it with hydroxyzine hydrochloride (Vistaril) and mesoridazine (Serentil), Palestine[67] noted that haloperidol is superior to the other two drugs in controlling alcohol withdrawal symptoms, although it does not protect against convulsions. Moreover, haloperidol, like the phenothiazines, is commonly associated with extrapyramidal symptoms, such as parkinsonism and dystonia.[20] Vistaril, an antihistaminic, is relatively ineffective compared with benzodiazepines in controlling symptoms of alcohol withdrawal.[24,50] Another neuroleptic, meprobamate (Miltown, Equanil) significantly relieved withdrawal symptoms in 58% of 65 alcoholic patients, while 17 percent showed moderate benefits.[79] Unfortunately, the CNS depressant effects of meprobamate are additive with those of alcohol.

BETA-ADRENERGIC BLOCKERS

Propanolol and Atenolol

More recently, the hyperadrenergic symptoms of alcohol withdrawal have stimulated research into the effectiveness of beta-blockers such as propanolol (Inderal) and atenolol (Tenormin). Hunt and Majchrowicz[45] found that chronic ethanol intoxication accelerates brain norepinephrine turnover in alcohol-dependent rats, while Carlsson[13] reported that systemic arterial norepinephrine levels increase after ethanol withdrawal in humans. Earlier studies had shown increases in urine and plasma catecholamines during alcohol withdrawal in humans.[1] After reports that somatically symptomatic anxiety was alleviated by beta-blocking drugs in humans,[84] studies were conducted that showed that these drugs are effective against the tremor, anxiety, agitation, and insomnia associated with alcohol withdrawal.[14,55,94] However, these agents were not shown to have anticonvulsant activity and probably should not be used to treat a patient with a history of AWS.[74] Furthermore, the use of beta-blockers poses a significant risk in alcoholics with hypoglycemia, chronic obstructive pulmonary disease, bronchospasm, and cardiomyopathy,[37,51] in which cases these drugs are contraindicated.

ALPHA-ADRENERGIC RECEPTOR AGONISTS

Clonidine and Lofexidine

With the discovery of alpha-adrenergic receptor agonists, treatment of hypertension changed drastically. These drugs inhibit norepinephrine release, probably by a feedback mechanism by which norepinephrine release from nerve terminals is reduced by stimulation of presynaptic alpha-adrenergic receptors.[12,76,83] It was not long before these drugs were tested in the hyperadrenergic state of alcohol withdrawal.[8,89,92]

In Finland, Bjorkqvist[7] published a report about 60 patients who participated in a double-blind study comparing clonidine with placebos for controlling symptoms of moderately severe alcohol withdrawal. Patients receiving clonidine recovered about 1 day sooner than patients treated with placebos. However, by chance, most of the epileptic patients were treated with placebos and all the patients with a history of seizures received 300 mg of phenytoin daily. Also, all patients received a combination hypnotic (25 mg of diphenhydramine chloride and 250 mg of metaqualone) each night in addition to B vitamins.[8]

In 1981, Wallinder and associates[89] published a brief report on an open trial comparing clonidine (Catapresan) 4 µg/kg twice daily in 11 patients with a combination of carbamazepine (Tegretol) 0.2 g, 3–4/day and a neuroleptic, usually chlorprothixin (Truxal) or dixyrazin (Esucos), in 15 patients. The clonidine-treated group responded as well as the anticonvulsant/neuroleptic-treated group but both groups also received unspecified benzodiazepines (as needed) in unknown amounts. A later double-blind study demonstrated that clonidine was as effective as a combination of chlorprothixen and carbamazepine.[4] However, both treatment groups were given oxazepam (Sobril) or nitrazepam (Mogadon) as needed, although the amounts and frequency of administration were carefully monitored. Seven of the 38 patients in the trial used fairly high doses (200-825 mg/week) of oxazepam, and four of these patients were in the clonidine-treated group. Apparently these patients had been receiving high doses of benzodiazepines before entering the study, and it is not clear whether this affected the study results. In another study of clonidine therapy for alcohol withdrawal, it was apparent that the drug did not relieve all the symptoms of withdrawal, particularly those related to sleep disturbances.[7,90]

Clonidine was compared with various other drugs in further studies. In a trial with chlomethiazole (Hemineurin), a sedative used in Europe, clonidine was found to be equally effective but not to have the abuse potential of chlomethiazole.[88] In a double-blind trial comparing these two drugs, clonidine proved as effective as chlomethiazole, but both treatment groups were also given carbamazepine.[62] Clonidine was found to be as effective as the benzodiazepine chlordiazepoxide (Librium), but patients with a history of seizures were excluded from the study.[5] In another randomized crossover double-blind study comparing clonidine with placebos, clonidine proved more effective in controlling alcohol withdrawal symptoms, but patients with convulsions were excluded from this study too.[92]

Soon after its introduction, reports suggested that withdrawal from clonidine might be associated with a spectrum of symptoms similar to those of alcohol withdrawal.[41] Clonidine withdrawal occurs fairly commonly and consists of rebound hypertension, sweating, palpitations, anxiety, insomnia, nausea, and vomiting.[38,68] The mechanism of this syndrome may be related to adrenergic overactivity, and the syndrome is potentially dangerous.[31] These reports demonstrate that these drugs must be used cautiously in patients who are already experiencing adrenergic overactivity due to alcohol withdrawal.

Of special interest is the finding that the opiate receptor antagonist naloxone can modify the hemodynamic effects of clonidine.[28] Naloxone increased blood pressure and heart rate in 14 of 27 patients treated with clonidine for mild to moderate essential hypertension, but did not have this effect in patients receiving placebos. The authors concluded that "the release of an endogenous opioid" contributes to the antihypertensive action of clonidine, and that this interaction may be responsible for the symptoms of clonidine withdrawal.[28] Other studies have shown clonidine to be effective against the symptoms of opiate withdrawal,[32] and it has been shown to depress morphine withdrawal in the rat.[6,86] However, other studies have failed to confirm the interaction of clonidine with opiate receptors.[35,91]

In a study of 61 alcoholic men admitted to an alcohol detoxification unit, clonidine proved more effective than chlordiazepoxide in reducing the symptoms of alcohol withdrawal. Since none of the patients treated with either drug had seizures, the study did not indicate whether clonidine has any effect on AWS.[5]

Lofexidine, a close analog of clonidine, has also been studied in alcohol withdrawal and found to be effective compared with placebo.[21] However, neither clonidine nor lofexidine modifies the alcohol withdrawal syndrome in rats,[39] and in some doses (0.2 mg/kg) enhances AWS in mice.[10]

ENDOGENOUS OPIATES AND OPIATE RECEPTOR AGONISTS AND ANTAGONISTS

Methionine-Enkephalin and Beta-endorphin

The discovery of endogenously occurring opioid peptides, the enkephalins and endorphins, led to experiments to determine whether release of these agents in the brain occurs during alcohol intoxication. Following reports in 1970[15,22] of a possible link between alcohol and opiate dependence, studies showed that acute alcohol intoxication in the rat increases methionine-enkephalin (met-enkephalin) and beta-endorphin levels.[73] Other studies indicated that alcohol withdrawal is associated with decreased met-enkephalin levels in some brain areas in rats.[43] Naloxone, an opiate receptor antagonist, yielded interesting results in alcoholic humans and animals. Blum and associates[9] reported that naloxone prevents alcohol dependence in mice. Jeffcoate and associates[47] then showed that naloxone prevents the impairment of psychomotor performance associated with low doses of alcohol in nonalcoholic subjects.

Naloxone

A paper describing 100 patients treated with naloxone for suspected ethanol-induced coma reported that coma was completely reversed within 10 minutes of naloxone administration in 20 patients and partially reversed in an additional five. However, alcohol could be confirmed as a cause of the coma in only 12 of these 25 patients.[48] Naloxone also reportedly reduced alcohol withdrawal symptoms in rats in another study, in which the authors hypothesized that the ethanol withdrawal syndrome "may in part be the result of increased sensitivity of mu (opioid) receptors."[54] However, conflicting reports demonstrated that naloxone had no effect on alcohol intoxication or withdrawal in rats,[40] or on acute alcohol intoxication in dogs.[54]

Relevant to the relationship of alcoholism to seizure disorders are studies reporting interactions between opioids and seizures. In one study involving mice, AWS were reduced by beta-endorphin.[30] In other experiments, morphine was shown to have an anticonvulsant effect in rats.[19,85] Other studies have demonstrated that in rabbits naloxone is a gamma-aminobutyric acid (GABA) antagonist that potentiates the convulsant action of other GABA antagonists, such as bicuculline and picrotoxin.[70] In the rat, the convulsant activity of naloxone is thought to be the result of GABA receptor blockade.[25]

Delta Sleep-Inducing Peptide

Tissot[80–82] showed that delta sleep-inducing peptide (DSIP) as well as morphine injected into the bulbomesencephalothalamic recruiting system was associated with the appearance of slow-wave sleep, an effect reversed by naloxone. It was suggested that DSIP is an opiate receptor agonist and may be useful in treating alcohol withdrawal. Tissot tested this hypothesis in a group of 107 patients, 47 with symptoms of alcohol withdrawal and 60 who were withdrawing from opiates. Withdrawal signs and symptoms subsided significantly in 87 percent of the alcohol addicts and in 97 percent of the opiate addicts.[23] These findings suggest that understanding the relationship between alcohol and opiate addiction may be important in developing effective agents to treat alcohol dependence.

GABA AND ALCOHOL

GABA and Alcohol Intoxication and Withdrawal

The relationship between ethanol and GABA, a major inhibitory neurotransmitter, has been reviewed extensively.[56] The consensus appears to be that after a single dose of alcohol a transient increase in brain GABA occurs, but after repeated administration and withdrawal of alcohol, GABA concentrations fall below normal. The suggestion that GABAergic transmission may be reduced during alcohol withdrawal has prompted investigation into the use of drugs that enhance the actions of GABA for treating the alcohol withdrawal syndrome.[44] In a study of alcohol withdrawal in mice, Goldstein[34] found that compounds such as benzodiazepines, barbiturates, and ethanol itself effectively reduced withdrawal signs in the animals, but phenothiazines and chlormethiazole had no beneficial effect.

Muscimol

Goldstein[33] found that the GABA receptor antagonist, muscimol, had no effect on the alcohol withdrawal syndrome when given intraperitoneally to mice rendered physically dependent on alcohol by ethanol inhalation for 3 days. In contrast, Cooper and associates[18] found that in alcohol-dependent rats in withdrawal, audiogenic seizures are reduced by intracisternal injections of muscimol and GABA.

Baclofen

Baclofen (beta(4-chlorophenyl)-gamma-aminobutyric acid), a derivative of GABA, was tested in primates undergoing the alcohol withdrawal syndrome.[77] Baclofen "does not protect against withdrawal-induced tremoring in monkeys." These investigators suggest that baclofen, at least when administered in doses up to 10 mg/kg intramuscularly, has little central GABAergic effect.

CALCIUM CHANNEL BLOCKERS

Recent investigations into the role of calcium in the hyperexcitable state of alcohol withdrawal have suggested that calcium channel blockers may be beneficial in modifying withdrawal phenomena and possibly even in preventing the development of physical dependence.[36] One study in rats demonstrated that nitrendipine and nimodipine abolish spontaneous seizures and prevent audiogenic seizures in rats withdrawing from ethanol.[60] Verapamil was shown to decrease seizure occurrence, and mortality was lowered by both verapamil and flunarizine. In this study, calcium channel blockers compared favorably with diazepam and were nonsedating, suggesting that "alterations in calcium conductance may be involved in the ethanol withdrawal syndrome and offer possibilities for the development of nonsedative therapeutic treatment of this syndrome."[60]

Dolin and associates[26] demonstrated that the number of dihydropyridine (DHP) binding sites is increased in the brains of ethanol-dependent rats. These binding sites represent a subtype of neuronal calcium channel, and these investigators hypothesized that central urons may develop an increased sensitivity to calcium on exposure to alcohol. They believe their results "suggest that an increase in DHP-sensitive calcium channels on central neurons may represent the molecular basis for ethanol physical dependence."[26]

Isaacson and associates conducted a study of effects of nimodipine, the voltage-sensitive calcium channel antagonist, on rats undergoing acute administration of alcohol. Results indicated that inhibition of the voltage-dependent calcium channels enhanced ethanol-induced effects.[46]

Using a clonal cell line (PC12) of neural crest origin, Messing and associates,[64] showed that acute exposure of these cells to ethanol decreased both $^{45}Ca^{2+}$ uptake and the number of binding sites for calcium channels labeled by the DHP calcium antagonist nitrendipine. The authors concluded that "cellular adaptation of ethanol may involve enhanced suppression of dihydropyridine-sensitive, voltage-dependent calcium channels."

An open feasibility study of the use in humans of caroverine, a group B calcium channel blocking agent, demonstrated that this compound may be beneficial in alcohol withdrawal. A randomized, double-blind study was then performed testing caroverine against meprobamate.[53] Nine patients in mild to moderate alcohol withdrawal were treated with caroverine (up to 160 mg/day); ten patients were given meprobamate (up to 3200 mg/day) for five days. On a variety of rating scales, there was no difference in amelioration of withdrawal symptoms, with the exception that less sedative effect was observed in the group treated with caroverine. The authors hypothesized that the effectiveness of caroverine is based on actions proposed after electrophysiologic studies[93] indicated that caroverine "blocks the induction of a nerve action potential by reducing sodium influx" without influencing presynaptic areas or transmitter activity.[66] This reduction in the activity of nerve cells is the proposed mechanism by which the intensity of alcohol withdrawal symptoms is suppressed. Although caroverine is thought (because of the lack of sedative effect) to affect different neuronal systems than meprobamate or diazepam, they noted that it has been reported to suppress epileptic phenomena.[65] The authors proposed that calcium channel blockers should be investigated further because of their effectiveness and lack of sedative and habit-forming properties.

SUMMARY

The investigation of a variety of agents for treating alcohol withdrawal and AWS has led to some interesting findings. It appears that because of their epileptogenicity, neuroleptics must be used cautiously. Beta-blockers may ameliorate some of the symptoms of withdrawal but do not appear to have anti-epileptic activity. Alpha-adrenergic receptor agonists are effective against many adrenergic symptoms of alcohol withdrawal but cause a withdrawal syndrome of their own. Opioid peptides and opiate receptor antagonists are exciting groups to study, and GABAergic compounds hold promise but have been of limited use so far. Finally, calcium channel blockers offer interesting possibilities that need further investigation.

References

1. Anton, AH: Ethanol and urinary catecholamines in man. Clin Pharmacol Therap 6:462, 1965.
2. Anton-Stephens, D: Preliminary observations on the psychiatric uses of chlorpromazine (Largactil). J Ment Sci 100:543, 1954.
3. Azima, H and Ogle, W: Effects of Largactil in mental syndromes. Canad Med Assoc J 71:116, 1954.
4. Balldin, J and Bokstrom, K: Treatment of alcohol abstinence symptoms with the alpha₂ agonist clonidine. Acta Psychiatr Scand (Suppl):327:131, 1986.
5. Baumgartner, GR and Rowen, RC: Clonidine vs chlordiazepoxide in the management of acute alcohol withdrawal syndrome. Arch Intern Med 147:1223, 1987.
6. Bednarczyk, L and Vetulani, B: Antagonism of clonidine shaking behavior in morphine abstinence syndrome and to head twitches produced by serotonergic agents in the rat. Pol J Pharmacol Pharm 30:307, 1978.
7. Bjorkqvist, S-E: Clonidine in alcohol withdrawal. Acta Psychiatr Scand 52:256, 1975.
8. Bjorkqvist, S-E: Clonidine therapy for alcohol withdrawal. Acta Psychiatr Scan Suppl 327:114, 1986.
9. Blum, K, et al: Naloxone induced inhibition of ethanol dependence in mice. Nature 265:49, 1977.
10. Blum, K, Briggs, AH, and Delallo, L: Clonidine enhancement of ethanol withdrawal in mice. Subst Alcohol Actions Misuse 4:59, 1983.
11. Bonafede, VI: Chlorpromazine treatment of disturbed epileptic patients. Arch Neurol Psychiat 74:158, 1955.
12. Brunning, J, Mumford, JP, and Keaney, FP: Lofexidine in alcohol withdrawal states. Alcohol 21:167, 1986.
13. Carlsson, C and Haggendal, J: Arterial noradrenaline levels after ethanol withdrawal. Lancet 2:889, 1967.
14. Carlsson, C and Johansson, T: The psychological effects of propanolol in the abstinence phase of chronic alcoholism. Br J Psychiat 119:605, 1971.
15. Cohen, C and Collins, M: Alkaloids from catecholamines in adrenal tissue: Possible role in alcoholism. Science 167:1749, 1970.
16. Cohen, IM: Complications of chlorpromazine therapy. Am J Psychiat 113:115, 1956.
17. Coleman, JH and Evans, WE: Pharmacotherapy of the acute alcohol withdrawal syndrome. Dis Nerv Syst 36:151, 1975.
18. Cooper, BR, et al: Antagonism of the enhanced susceptibility to audiogenic seizures during alcohol withdrawal in the rat by gamma-aminobutyric acid (GABA) and "GABAmimetic" agents. J Pharmacol Exp Ther 209:396, 1979.
19. Cowan, A, Geller, EG, and Adler, MW: Classification of opioids on the basis of change in seizure threshold in rats. Science 206:465, 1979.
20. Crane, GE: A review of clinical literature on haloperidol. Int J Neuropsychiatry 3:110, 1967.
21. Cushman, P, et al: Alcohol withdrawal syndrome: Clinical management with lofexidine. Alcoholism: Clin Exp Res 9:103, 1985.
22. Davis, VE and Walsh, MJ: Alcohol, amines and alkaloids: A possible biochemical basis for alcohol addiction. Science 167:1005, 1970.
23. Dick, P, Grandjean, ME, and Tissot, R: Successful treatment of withdrawal symptoms with delta sleep-inducing peptide, a neuropeptide with potential agonistic activity on opiate receptors. Neuropsychobiology 10:205, 1983.
24. Dilts, DL, et al: Hydroxyzine in the treatment of alcohol withdrawal. Am J Psychiatry 134:92, 1977.
25. Dingledine, R, Iversen, LL, and Breuker, E: Naloxone as a GABA antagonist: Evidence from iontophoretic, receptor binding and convulsant studies. Eur J Pharmacol 47:19, 1978.
26. Dolin, S, et al: Increased dihydropyridine-sensitive calcium channels in rat brain may underlie ethanol physical dependence. Neuropharmacology 26:275, 1987.
27. Fabisch, W: The effect of intravenous chlorpromazine on the EEG of epileptic patients. Electroenceph Clin Neurophysiol 8:712, 1956.
28. Farsang, C, et al: Possible involvement of an endogenous opioid in the antihypertensive effect of clonidine in patients with essential hypertension. Circulation 66:1268, 1982.

29. Friedhoff, AJ and Zitrin, A: A comparison of the effects of paraldehyde and chlorpromazine in delirium tremens. NY State J Med 59:1060, 1959.
30. Frye, GD, et al: Modification of the actions of ethanol by centrally active peptides. Peptides 2:99, 1981.
31. Geyskes, GG, Boer, P, and Dorhout-Mees, EJ: Clonidine withdrawal mechanism and frequency of rebound hypertension. Br J Clin Pharmacol 7:55, 1979.
32. Gold, MS, et al: Opiate withdrawal using clonidine: A safe, effective and rapid nonopiate treatment. JAMA 243:343, 1980.
33. Goldstein, DB: Sodium bromide and sodium valproate: Effective suppressants of ethanol withdrawal reactions in mice. J Pharmacol Exp Ther 208:223, 1979.
34. Goldstein, DB: An animal model for testing the effects of drugs on alcohol withdrawal reactions. J Pharmacol Exp Ther 183:14, 1972.
35. Golembiowska-Kikitin, K, and Pilc, A: Opiate and specific receptor binding of [^{3}H]clonidine. J Pharm Pharmacol 32:70, 1980.
36. Greenberg, DA, Carpenter, CL, and Messing, RO: Ethanol-induced component of $^{45}Ca^{2+}$ uptake in PC12 cells is sensitive to Ca^{2+} channel modulating drugs. Brain Res 410:143, 1987.
37. Greenblatt, DJ and Koch-Weser, J: Adverse reactions to propanolol in hospitalized medical patients: A report from the Boston Collaborative Drug Surveillance Program. Am Heart J 86:478, 1973.
38. Hansson, L, et al: Blood pressure crisis following withdrawal of clonidine (Catapres, Catapresan), with special reference to arterial and urinary catecholamine levels and suggestions for acute management. Am Heart J 85:605, 1973.
39. Hemmingsen, R, Clemmesen, L, and Barry, DI: Blind study of the effect of the alpha adrenergic agonists clonidine and lofexidine on alcohol withdrawal in the rat. J Stud Alcohol 45:310, 1984.
40. Hemmingsen, R and Sorensen, SC: Absence of an effect of naloxone on ethanol intoxication and withdrawal reactions. Acta Pharmacol Toxicol 46:62, 1980.
41. Hokfelt, B, Hedeland, H, and Dymling, J-F: Studies on catecholamines, renin and aldosterone following catepresan (2-[2, 6 dichlorphenylamine]-2-imidazoline hydrochloride) in hypertensive patients. Eur J Pharmacol 10:389, 1970.
42. Hollister, LE: Clinical use of psychotherapeutic drugs: Current status. Clin Pharmacol Ther 10:170, 1969.
43. Hong, JS, et al: Reduction in cerebral methionine-enkephalin content during the ethanol withdrawal syndrome. Subst Alcohol Actions Misuse 2:233, 1981.
44. Hunt, WA: The effect of ethanol on GABAergic transmission. Neurosci Biobehav Rev 7:87, 1983.
45. Hunt, WA and Majchrowicz, E: Alterations in the turnover of brain norepinephrine and dopamine in alcohol dependent rats. J Neurochem 23:549, 1974.
46. Isaacson, RL, et al: Nimodipine's interactions with other drugs: I: Ethanol. Life Sci 36:2195, 1985.
47. Jeffcoate, WJ, et al: Prevention of effects of alcohol intoxication by naloxone. Lancet 2:1157, 1979.
48. Jefferys, DB, Flanagan, RJ, and Volans, GN: Reversal of ethanol induced coma with naloxone. Lancet 1:308, 1980.
49. Jellinek, EM: Alcohol Addiction and Chronic Alcoholism. New Haven, Yale University Press, 1942.
50. Kaim, SC, Klett, CJ, and Ruthfeld, B: Treatment of the acute alcohol withdrawal state: A comparison of four drugs. Am J Psychiatry 125:1640, 1969.
51. Kallas, P and Sellers, EM: Blood glucose in intoxicated chronic alcoholics. Can Med Assoc J 112:590, 1975.
52. Knott, D and Beard, J: Diagnosis and therapy of acute withdrawal from alcohol. In Masseman, JD (ed): Current Psychiatric Therapies, Vol 10. Grune & Stratton, New York, 1970, p 145.
53. Koppi, S, et al: Calcium channel-blocking agent in the treatment of acute alcohol withdrawal: Caroverine versus meprobamate in a randomized double-blind study. Neuropsychobiology 17:49, 1987.
54. Kotlinski, J and Langwinski, R: Does the blockage of opioid receptors influence the development of ethanol dependence? Alcohol Alcohol 72:117, 1987.
55. Kraus, ML, et al: Randomized clinical trial of atenolol in patients with alcohol withdrawal. N Engl J Med 313:905, 1985.
56. Kulonen, E: Ethanol and GABA. Med Biol 61:147, 1983.
57. Lehmann, HE and Hanrahan, GE: Chlorpromazine: New inhibiting agent for psychomotor excitement and manic states. AMA Arch Neurol Psychiatr 71:227, 1954.
58. Liberson, WT: Effects of chlorpromazine hydrochloride (Thorazine) on EEG and on skin galvanic activity: A preliminary report. Electroencephalogr Clin Neurophysiol 7:474, 1955.
59. Lignian, H, Fontaine, J, and Askenasi, R: Naloxone and alcohol intoxication in the dog. Human Toxicol 2:221, 1983.
60. Little, HJ, Dolin, SI, and Halsey, MJ: Calcium channel antagonists decrease the ethanol withdrawal syndrome. Life Sci 39:2059, 1986.
61. Lomas, J, Boardman, RH, and Markow, M: Complications of chlorpromazine therapy in 800 mental hospital patients. Lancet 1:1144, 1955.
62. Manhem, P, et al: Alcohol withdrawal: Effects of clonidine treatment on sympathetic activity, the renin-aldosterone system, and clinical symptoms. Alcoholism: Clin Exp Res 9:238, 1985.
63. Mauceri, J and Strauss, H: Effects of chlorpromazine on the electroencephalogram, with report of a case of chlorpromazine intoxication. Electroencephalogr Clin Neurophysiol 8:671, 1956.
64. Messing, RO, et al: Ethanol regulates calcium channels in clonal neuronal cells. Proc Natl Acad Sci USA 83:6213, 1986.
65. Moeslinger, D: Ein beitrag zur pruefung der

wirksamkeit und vertraeglichkeit eines neuen spasmolytikums. Subsidia Med 22(3):78, 1970.
66. Nachshen, D and Blaustein, M: The effect of some organic "calcium antagonists" on calcium influx in presynaptic nerve terminals. Mol Pharmacol 16:579, 1979.
67. Palestine, ML: Drug treatment of the alcohol withdrawal syndrome and delirium tremens. Quarterly Journal of Studies on Alcohol 34.185, 1973.
68. Reid, JL, et al: Clonidine withdrawal in hypertension. Lancet 1:1171, 1977.
69. Ritter, RM and Davidson, DE: Haloperidol for acute psychiatric emergencies: A double-blind comparison with periphenazine in acute alcoholic psychosis. South Med J 64:249, 1971.
70. Sagratella, S and Massotti, M: Convulsant and anticonvulsant effects of opioids: Relationship to GABA-mediated transmission. Neuropharmacology 21:991, 1982.
71. Sainz, AA: The management of side effects of chlorpromazine and reserpine. Psychiatr Q 30:647, 1956.
72. Samuels, AS: Acute chlorpromazine poisoning. Am J Psychiatry 113:746, 1957.
73. Schultz, R, et al: Acute and chronic ethanol treatment changes endorphin levels in brain and pituitary. Psychopharmacology 68:221, 1980.
74. Sellers, EM, Zilm, DH, and Degani, NC: Comparative efficacy of propanolol and chlordiazepoxide in alcohol withdrawal. J Stud Alcohol 38:2096, 1977.
75. Shagass, C: Effect of intravenous chlorpromazine on the electroencephalogram. Electroencephalogr Clin Neurophysiol 7:306, 1955.
76. Starke, K and Monte, H: Involvement of alpha receptors in clonidine-induced inhibition of transmitter release from central monoamine neurons. Neuropharmacology 12:1073, 1973.
77. Tarika, JS and Winger, G: The effects of ethanol, phenobarbitol and baclofen on ethanol withdrawal in the rhesus monkey. Psychopharmacology 70:201, 1980.
78. Tavel, ME: A new look at an old syndrome. Delirium tremens. Arch Intern Med 109:129, 1962.
79. Thimann, J: Newer drugs in the treatment of acute alcoholism with special consideration of meprobamate. In Himwich, HE (ed): Alcoholism. American Association for the Advancement of Science, Washington, DC, 1957, p 141.
80. Tissot, R: Recepteurs à opiaces et sommeil I: Effets de microinjections de morphine dans le thalamus median et la substance grise centrale peri-aqueducale du lapin. Neuropsychobiology 6:170, 1980.
81. Tissot, R: Recepteurs de l'opium et sommeil II: Effets de microinjections d'alcohol ethylique et de pentobarbital dans le thalamus median, la substance grise centrale peri-aqueducale et du noyau de tractus solitaire du lapin. Neuropsychobiology 7:74, 1981.
82. Tissot, R: Recepteurs de l'opium et sommeil III: Effets de microinjections de DSID (delta sleep peptide) dans le thalamus median, la substance grise centrale peri-aqueducale et le noyau de tractus solitaire du lapin. Neuropsychobiology 7:321, 1981.
83. Trzaskowska, E and Kostowski, W: Further studies on the role of noradrenergic mechanisms in the ethanol withdrawal syndrome in rats. Pol J Pharmacol Pharm 35:351, 1983.
84. Tyrer, PJ: Use of beta-blocking drugs in psychiatry and neurology. Drugs 20:300, 1980.
85. Urca, G and Frank, H: Pro- and anticonvulsant action of morphine in rats. Pharmacol Biochem Behav 13:343, 1980.
86. Vetulani, L and Bednarczyk, J: Depression by clonidine of shaking behavior elicited by nalorphine in morphine dependent rats. J Pharm Pharmacol 29:567, 1977.
87. Vogel, RA, et al: Differential effects of TRH, amphetamine, naloxone and fenmetozole on ethanol actions: Attenuation of the effects of punishment and impairment of aerial righting reflex. Alcoholism: Clin Exp Res 5:386, 1982.
88. Wadstein, J, et al: Clonidine versus chlomethiazole in alcohol withdrawal. Alcoholism: Clin Exp Res 9:238, 1985.
89. Wallinder, L, et al: Clonidine suppression of the alcohol withdrawal syndrome. Drug Alcohol Depend 8:345, 1981.
90. Washton, MA and Resnick, RB: The clinical use of clonidine in outpatient detoxification from opiates. In Lal, H and Fielding, S (eds): Psychopharmacology of Clonidine. Alan R Liss, New York, 1981, p 277.
91. Watkins, J, et al: Absence of opiate and histamine H_2 receptor-mediated effects of clonidine. Clin Pharmacol Ther 28:605, 1980.
92. Wilkins, AJ, Jenkins, WS, and Steiner, JA: Efficacy of clonidine in treatment of alcohol withdrawal state. Psychopharmacology (Berlin) 8:78, 1983.
93. Yoshihisa, K and Shoji, S: Effects of caroverine and diltiazem on synaptic responses, L-glutamate-induced depolarization and potassium efflux in the frog spinal cord. Br J Pharmacol 83:813, 1984.
94. Zilm, DH: Propanolol effect on tremor in alcoholic withdrawal. Ann Intern Med 83:234, 1975.

CHAPTER 32

Maurice Victor, M.D.

SUMMARY: Questions Answered and Unanswered

In summing up the clinical issues discussed in this volume I will comment on certain selected subjects that I consider particularly interesting and important.

It may be useful to begin with Mattson's introductory chapter. He points out that the majority of seizures in alcoholic adults can be readily related to alcohol withdrawal, but he is quick to add that several other factors may account for seizures in an alcoholic person, for instance, hypoglycemia or electrolyte imbalance, previous head trauma, or a short period of excessive alcohol use and sleep deprivation in a person with idiopathic symptomatic or latent epilepsy. Thus, he identifies the major clinical problem in treating the person with alcoholism and epilepsy—elucidating the factor(s) causing seizures. In Lennox's[3] large series of patients with epilepsy and in our own study of alcoholic patients with idiopathic and post-traumatic epilepsy, sufficient reason (aside from drinking) for the patient to have seizures was always demonstrated, but seizures characteristically occurred not during intoxication but in the "sobering up" period. I would add only that in seeking the reasons for epilepsy in the alcoholic patient, it is not a question of identifying *either* withdrawal *or* some other factor. Usually both are at work. Earnest's data illustrate the same point. In a prospective study of 250 patients who satisfied the criteria for alcohol withdrawal seizures (AWS)—first major generalized convulsion in adult life; recent abstinence from alcohol abuse; no obvious etiology other than alcohol withdrawal—computed tomography (CT) scans disclosed cerebral lesions (mainly traumatic) in 16 patients (6.2 percent). In practically all the alcoholic patients we studied with onset of seizures in adult life, hypomagnesemia and respiratory alkalosis[9] appeared to be important pathogenetic features, but were always a part of alcohol withdrawal.

These observations reinforce a point that has been made repeatedly in writings on alcohol and seizures—namely that alcohol withdrawal, although an important and possibly essential factor in the genesis of seizures, may in itself be an insufficient factor.[8] Such a conclusion seems reasonable because only 10 to 12 percent of alcoholic persons who are hospitalized with neurologic complications of alcoholism develop seizures. Obviously several other factors, some known and others still to be discerned, are operative in the withdrawal period.

This brings us to the most provocative contribution, that of Ng and colleagues,[5] who propose that alcohol withdrawal is not a significant mechanism in the genesis of seizures in alcoholic persons, and that seizures in alcoholic persons are due to the direct toxic effects of alcohol on the brain. I say provocative because these proposals contradict virtually all the pharmacologic, clinical and experimental evidence that has accumulated in the past 40 years. Most of the chapters in this volume are predicated upon the withdrawal theory, and for this reason alone, this study deserves more than passing comment.

In support of their contentions, Ng and colleagues[5] invoke the premise that "alcohol is a known central nervous system toxin and produces other organic brain syndromes," for which reason, they state, "a direct epileptogenic effect of alcohol has been underevaluated." Unfortunately, this statement is supported by neither discussion nor meaningful data. That alcohol is a central nervous system (CNS) toxin hardly needs to be repeated; it is known through commonplace experience. Moreover, experience teaches that the symptoms of intoxication do not generally include seizures. Alcohol is neither a neuronal stimulant nor an excitant, but rather a sedative with all the characteristic pharmacologic effects of the inhalation anesthetics. Like other sedatives, such as barbiturates, alcohol occasionally has a paradoxic effect, inducing excitement and hyperactivity, rather than sedation. But even in such states ("pathological intoxication"), seizures virtually never occur. Occasionally, an alcoholic person insists that a seizure has occurred while he or she was drinking, and cannot identify an element of abstinence; but such instances are rare, and certainly none has ever been documented by measuring blood alcohol levels. In numerous animal experiments, however, it has been shown that without exception, seizures occur not during periods of high, sustained blood alcohol concentrations, but only when the blood alcohol concentration is substantially reduced.

The premises of NG and colleagues aside, what is one to conclude from their data and the conclusions they derive from analyzing these data? On review, it is clear that most seizures occurred during the withdrawal period. First, their definition of abstention time (interval between the last drink and the first seizure) is not inconsistent with the withdrawal phase. Further, only 16% of the seizures in the "alcohol users occurred outside the conventionally defined withdrawal period." This figure is hardly surprising considering the diversity of epileptogenic factors that could have been operative in these patients (notably, idiopathic and symptomatic epilepsy and abuse of drugs other than alcohol). Also, a significant portion of the patients in NG's study were in their teens and early 20s (a common age of onset of idiopathic epilepsy), and some of them had already experienced one or more seizures. It is also noteworthy that the clinical data were obtained entirely from questionnaires filled out by the subjects. Self-reporting allegedly has validity in long-abstinent alcoholic patients, but even in regard to such patients there is no agreement on this point. In a recently completed Veterans Administration Cooperative Study[1] of treatment response in alcoholism, self-report proved *not* to be valid.

Finally, the authors' dismissal of Isbell's classic study is unjustified. Isbell and colleagues[2] were able to control both the precise amount of alcohol ingested by their patients and the periodicity of alcohol ingestion, and to determine accurately the concentrations of blood alcohol, moment of the last drink, diminution of blood alcohol levels, and the relationship of these variables to the occurrence of "rum fits" and other manifestations of alcohol withdrawal. In other words, they were able to eliminate the uncertainty and imprecision that plague open-ward studies. Isbell's conclusions could only be dismissed if replication of the study produced different results. When Mendelson and LaDou[3] and Wolfe and associates[7] replicated the study, however, Isbell's findings (and conclusions) were confirmed.

Simon and colleagues have gone to great lengths to prove that phenytoin is not a useful drug in treating AWS, and their observations, although based on small numbers of patients, certainly support their conclusions. By contrast, phenobarbital and possibly carbamazepine, as demonstrated by Young and Dailey and by Sternebring, are useful in preventing seizures in vulnerable alcoholic patients, that is, early in the withdrawal period. These data vindicate the purely clinical impressions that have long pointed in the same direction.

Concerning the management of AWS, I suggest that assessment and treatment should not be confined to the emergency department, as they were in Young's study. Patients with seizures occurring for the first time in adult life, whatever the presumed cause, should always be admitted to the hospital. In the case of "rum fits," the reasons for hospital admission are obvious. Sixty percent of such patients have more than one seizure, as late as 12 hours after the first seizure. Moreover, about 30% of patients with "rum fits" develop full-blown delirium tremens, a potentially fatal disease.

De Lorenzo's observations on the efficacy and safety of paraldehyde in managing AWS confirm previous clinical observations in all important details. This drug was the therapeutic standby in the 1940s and 1950s, but lost popularity with the advent of benzodiazepine use. Paraldehyde is remarkably effective in modifying early withdrawal symptoms, and dosages many times larger than the average do not harm the patient. There is still no concrete evidence that the benzodiazepines are superior to paraldehyde in controlling alcohol withdrawal symptoms. The packaging of paraldehyde in individual doses negates its major shortcoming, that is, degradation to acetaldehyde. Paraldehyde should be administered only orally or rectally; parenteral use should probably be avoided. Intravenous (IV) use carries a danger of respiratory depression, and intramuscular (IM) injections can damage nerves and create sterile abscesses.

The use of anticonvulsant drugs in treating withdrawal seizures should be discussed further. In most cases of this type, anticonvulsant medication is not necessary. In alcohol withdrawal, the entire convulsive episode may consist of a single seizure, or of a few seizures occurring over a period of a few hours (usually less than 6 hours, sometimes as long as 12 hours). Thus the seizure state has often ended by the time the patient is seen by the physician or by the time certain medications, such as phenytoin, become effective. As was indicated above, there is some evidence that barbiturates and benzodiazepines, given IV in the early stages of alcohol withdrawal, can prevent seizures. Long-term administration of anticonvulsants in patients who have had withdrawal seizures is unnecessary because this type of seizure does not recur if the patient remains abstinent; if the patient resumes drinking, it has been our experience that he or she almost always abandons the prescribed medication.

On the other hand, certain forms of alcoholic epilepsy necessitate treatment with anticonvulsants. Occasionally, seizures in the withdrawal period take the form of *status epilepticus*, that is, repeated seizures in which the patient does not regain consciousness. Such cases should be managed as *status* of other causes. Also, in patients (alcoholic or nonalcoholic) who suffer idiopathic or posttraumatic epilepsy, an episode of even mild alcoholic intoxication may precipitate seizures. Such patients should be cautioned not to use alcohol at all, or in only the smallest amounts, and should, of course, be maintained on their usual anticonvulsant drugs.

Although my task here is to summarize the clinical aspects of alcohol and seizures, this is not where the excitement lies. Certainly the clinicians have defined the problems and posed the appropriate questions about the effects of alcohol on the nervous system, and doubtless they will continue to do so. However, the answers must come from the basic scientists. The fact that the fundamental problems of tolerance and physical dependence are now being addressed at the cellular and even the molecular level, is, from my perspective, the most promising step in our understanding of the relationship between alcohol and seizures.

References

1. Fuller, RK, Lee, KK, and Gordis, E: Validity of self-report in alcoholism research: Results of a Veterans Administration Cooperative Study. Alcoholism: Clin Exp Res 12:201, 1988.
2. Isbell, H, et al: An experimental study of the eti-

ology of "rum fits" and delirium tremens. Quarterly Journal of Studies of Alcohol 16:1, 1955.
3. Lennoy, WG: Alcohol and epilepsy. Quarterly Journal of Studies on Alcohol 2:1, 1941.
4. Mendelson, JH and LaDou, J: Experimentally induced chronic intoxication and withdrawal in alcoholics: II: Psychophysiological findings. Quarterly Journal of Studies on Alcohol 2:14, 1964.
5. Ng, SKC, et al: Alcohol consumption and withdrawal in new-onset seizures. N Engl J Med 319:666, 1988.
6. Victor, M: The pathophysiology of alcoholic epilepsy. Res Publ Assoc Res Nerv Ment Dis 46:431, 1968.
7. Wolfe, SM, et al: Respiratory alkalosis and alcohol withdrawal. Trans Assoc Am Physicians 82:344, 1969.
8. Wolfe, SM and Victor, M: The physiological basis of the alcohol withdrawal syndrome. In Mello, NK and Mendelson, JH (eds): Recent Advances in Studies of Alcoholism. US Government Printing Office, Washington, DC, 1971, p 188.
9. Wolfe, SM and Victor, M: The relationship of hypomagnesemia and alkalosis to alcohol withdrawal symptoms. Ann NY Acad Sci 162:973, 1969.

Index

A page number in *italics* indicates a figure. A "t" following a page number indicates a table.

Absence seizures, epileptic, 6
Absorption, 241
Abstention time, Harlem study, 170–171, *171*, *172*, 172t, *173*, 174–175
Abstinence
 AWS and, 149–150
 EEG patterns and
  animal studies of, 182–184, *183*
  human studies of, 184–190, 187t, 190t, *191–192*, 193
 withdrawal syndrome and, 149–150, 153, *153*
Abuse. *See* Alcoholism
Abuse-associated seizure(s)
 acute, 202–203
 CT scan and, 200–202, 201t, 202t, 203
 first occurrence, 199–202, 200t, 201t
 municipal hospital study of, 198–199, 199t
 studies of, 197–198
Acetaldehyde, biotransformation to, 242–243
Acetylcholine
 AWS treatment and, 273–274
 benzodiazepine actions and, 274
Adaptation
 GABAergic, dependency and, 89–90
 neuronal
  cholesterol and, 46
  lipids and, abnormal, 47–48
  phospholipids and, acidic, 46–47, 47t
Adenosine, 272
Adenosine receptor
 cAMP and
  production of, 26–27, 79–80, *80*
  reduction of, 83t, 83–84, *84*
  signal transduction and, 84–85
 desensitization of, 80–82, 81t, *82*
 studies of, *82*, 82–83
Adenosine triphosphatase, 276
ADH. *See* Alcohol dehydrogenase (ADH) system
Afterhyperpolarization (AHP), 70–71, *71*, 75–76, 77
AHP. *See* Afterhyperpolarization
Alcohol. *See* Ethanol
Alcohol abuse. *See* Alcoholism
Alcohol dehydrogenase (ADH) system
 biotransformation and, 242, 243, 244
 ethanol effect on, acute, 244, 245t
Alcohol dependency. *See* Dependency

Alcohol use. *See also* Alcoholism
 abuse and heavy use of
  age and race in, 15
  definitions of, 13, 14–15
  geographic patterns of, 15–16
  socioeconomic factors in, 16
  time trends in, 16–17
 anti-epileptic drugs and, 241–249, 245t
 chronic use of
  adaptation to, 45–48
  tolerance and, 25–26, 118–120, *121*, 130–131
 dependency and
  calcium channel alterations and, 51–54
  GABA changes in, 87–97
 drinking history and, 206–207
 in epileptic patients, 19–20
 measures of, 12–15
 neurologic complications of, 14, 25–26, 65
 neurophysiologic study of, in nonepileptic patients, 223–229, 235t, *236*, 236t, *237*
 in nonalcoholic patients with epilepsy, 234
 social
  drinking habits in 20th century and, 222–223
  epileptic seizure relationship to, 223
  influence on epilepsy, double-blind study of, 223–228, 225t, 226t, 228t, 229t
  in nonalcoholic patients with epilepsy, 234
  physicians' attitudes toward, in epileptic patients, 228–231, 229t, 230t
  seizure frequency and, 227–228, 228t
Alcohol withdrawal
 animal models and, 265, 266
 central nervous system models of, 265
 drug therapies in, 284t. *See also* Treatment
 neurochemistry of, 266
 neuropharmacology of, benzodiazepine actions and, 267–277
 pathophysiology of, 259
 in randomized, controlled trials, 284t
 single seizure and, 259–260
 status epilepticus in
  diagnosis of, 261
  therapy for, 261–262
Alcohol withdrawal seizures (AWS). *See* Treatment
 binge vs. chronic drinking and, 206–213

333

Alcohol withdrawal seizures (AWS)—*Continued*
   calcium channel activity and, 51–57
   ideal drug therapy for, 285, 285t
   genetics and
      codetermination of, *130, 131,* 131–132,
         135–136
      susceptibility to, *132,* 132–133, *133, 134*
   models of
      animal, 27, 130–136, 265, 266
      cellular, 26–27
      central nervous system and, 265
      tonic-clonic seizures in, 126–127, 127t
Alcohol withdrawal syndrome
   clinical features of
      AWS, 255, 256–257
      delirium tremens, 256
      status epilepticus, 255–256
   concept of
      abstention symptoms in, 149–150
      animal studies of, 151
      delirium tremens and, 148–149, 150, 151
      intoxication versus, 149
      seizures in, 149, 150
   convulsive seizures in alcoholics
      abstention time and, 153, *153*
      alkalosis and, respiratory, *156,* 156–158,
         157, 159, 210
      cerebral trauma-associated, 152–153
      EEG abnormalities in, 153–154
      hypomagnesemia and, 155, *157,* 158
      idiopathic epileptic seizures and, 152
      onset of and drinking cessation, 153
      photomyoclonias and, 154–155, *155, 157,*
         159
   drug therapies in, 284t
   evaluation and differential diagnosis in, 255t,
     256–257
   randomized controlled trials of, 283, 284t
Alcoholic patients
   brains of, calcium channel changes in, 65–66
   cAMP in, 82t, 82–83, *83t, 84*
   epilepsy in, 145, 197, 247–248, 329
   withdrawal seizures in
      abstention time and, 153, *153*
      alkalosis and, *156,* 156–157, *157,* 158, *158,*
         159
      cerebral trauma-associated, 152–153
      EEG abnormalities and, 153–154
      hypomagnesemia and, 155, *157,* 158
      idiopathic epileptic, 152
      photomyoclonus and, 154–155, *155, 157, 159*
Alcoholism
   acute
      SHT current and, 72, *73,* 76
      THT current and, 71, *72, 72,* 75, *75,* 76
   calcium channel blockage and, 65
   cAMP in, 82t, 82–84, *83t*
   chronic, GABA/benzodiazepine receptor
     mediation and, 109–112, *110, 111*
   complications of, medical and neurological,
     255t
   epilepsy in, 145, 197, 247–248, 329
   seizures in
      causes of, 145, 254t
      duration and severity of, 198
      prevalence and incidence of, 18–19
      signs and symptoms of, 255t
   status epilepticus and, 216–220, *218*

Alcohol-related seizure(s). *See also* Alcohol
   withdrawal seizures (AWS)
   acute
      AWS and, 202
      etiology of, 202–203
      head trauma and, 202–203
      laboratory and radiologic findings and, 203
   alcoholism and
      alcohol-induced, 145–146
      causes of, 254t
      cerebral and systemic causes of, 145
      prevalence and incidence of, 18–19
      signs and symptoms of, 255t
      symptomatic epilepsy in, 145
      status epilepticus and, 216–220, *218*
      withdrawal seizures and, 143–145, 144t
   CT scans of, 200–202, 201t, 202t, 203
   epilepsy and
      in alcoholic patient, 146
      nonalcoholic patient and, 147
   first occurence, 199–202, 200t, 201t
   Harlem study of
      abstention time and, 170–171, *171, 173,*
         174–175
      alcohol consumption pattern and, 168t,
         168–169, 169t, 172
      controls in 166, 166t
      demographics of, 168, 168t
      dose-effect of alcohol and, 170t, 170–171,
         172, 172t, 174
      patient selection for, 166–167
      seizure classification in, 167
      seizures in, 170, 172
      withdrawal seizure occurence in, 174–175
   mechanisms of, 163–177
      animal experiments and, 164
      anticonvulsant therapy and, 164
      blood alcohol level and, 163, 164
      chronicity of, 164
      genesis of vs. precipitation of, 162–163
      human experiments and, 164
      observational studies of, 163
   municipal hospital study of, 198–199, 199t
Alkalosis, respiratory, *156,* 156–157, *157, 158, 159,*
   210
Alpha activity
   acute ethanol administration and, 180–181
   early withdrawal and, 185–186
Alpha-adrenergic receptor agonist(s), 322–323
Anticonvulsant therapy. *See* Anti-epileptic drugs;
   Treatment; specific drugs, e.g.
   Benzodiazepine(s)
Anti-epileptic drug(s)
   in alcoholic epileptic patients, 247–248
   alcohol-related seizures and, 164
   in AWS treatment, 331
   blood levels of, alcohol use and, 228, 229t
   enzyme induction by, 244–245
   epileptiform discharges and, 190, 193
   ethanol interactions with
      clinical aspects of, 246–247
      metabolism enhancement and, 245–246
      pharmacodynamics of, 246
   photic stimulation and early withdrawal and,
     189–190, *191–192*
   social alcohol use and, double-blind study of,
     224, 225, 225t, 227, 228, 229, 229t
Antipsychotic drug(s), 258–259

INDEX

Atenolol, 322
Atonic seizure(s), epileptic, 6
Attitude(s), physicians', toward epileptic patient alcohol use, 228–231, 229t, 230t
Automatism(s), 6
AWS. *See* Alcohol withdrawal seizure(s)

Baclofen, GABA and, 325
BAL. *See* Blood alcohol level
Barbiturate(s), 258, 262
Benzodiazepine(s)
  actions of
    acetylcholine and, 274
    adenosine and, 272
    adenosine triphosphatase and, 276
    catecholamine systems and, 271
    cyclic nucleotide system and, 277
    GABA/BZD/chloride ionophore receptor complex and, 269
    glutamate and, 269–270
    hormones and, 277
    opiates and, 276
    serotonin systems and, 272
  in alcohol withdrawal treatment, 257–258
  anticonvulsant effects of, 34–35
  binding sites of
    GABA receptor site and, 36–37, *37*
    micromolar, 37–38, *38*
    nanomolar, 35–37, *36*
  blood levels of, clinical effects and, *40*
  calcium channel inhibition by, 38, *38*
  clinical applications of
    administration and dosage principles in, 286–288
    advantages and disadvantages of, 286, 286t
    in epilepsy, 11, *11*
    as ideal therapy, 285t, 285–286
    pharmacokinetics of, 286, 287t
    placebo versus, 284–285
    in *status epilepticus*, 287t, 287–288
  EEGs and, in later withdrawal, 190, *190*, *191–192*, 193
  ethanol interaction with, 247
  GABA and, 34, 36–37, *37*
  molecular action of, 34
  nanomolar receptors of
    anticonvulsant properties of, 36–37, *37*
    GABA receptor site and, *36*, *37*
  neuronal and nonneuronal tissue and, 35–36
  neuropharmacology of AWS and, 278t
    acetylcholine and, 273–274
    adenosine and, 272
    adenosine triphosphatase and, 276
    calcium metabolism and, 272–273
    catecholamine systems and, 270–271
    cyclic nucleotides system and, 276–277
    GABA systems and, 267–269
    glutamate and, 269–270
    hormones and, 277
    opiates and, 274–276
    serotonin systems and, 271–272
  receptors
    agonists and antagonists of, 106t
    binding sites of, *37*, 37–38, *38*
    GABA receptors site and, 36
    nanomolar, 35–37, *36*
    neuronal excitability regulation and, 34–35

Beta activity, early withdrawal and, 184–185
Beta-adrenergic blockers, 322
Beta-endorphin, AWS treatment and, 275
Binge vs. chronic drinking
  alkalosis and, respiratory, 210
  cerebral seizures and, 210
  diagnoses in, 210–211
  drug use and abuse and, 209–210
  seizures in
    distribution of, gender and time, 207–209, 208t, *209*
    susceptibility to, 212–213
  AWS in
    diagnosis of, 210
    drinking habits and, 211–212
    repeated withdrawals and, 211–212, *212*
Biotransformation, 242–243
Blood alcohol level (BAL)
  epileptiform discharges and, 193
  seizure mechanism and, 163, 164
  withdrawal seizures and, 25–26
BZD. *See* Benzodiazepines

Calcium
  ethanol effect on, 60–61
  flux of
    enhancement of, *63*, 63–64, 65
    inhibition of, 62, *62*, 63, 65
  metabolism of
    alcohol withdrawal treatment and, 272–273
    benzodiazepine actions and, 273
    nervous system and, 30–34, *33*
Calcium channel blocker(s), 52, 325–326
Calcium channel(s)
  activity of
    in alcohol dependency, 51–54
    in AWS, 54, *55*, 56
    depression of, 52–55
    enhancement of, *63*, 63–64, 65
    inhibition of, 62, *62*, 63, 65
  agonists and antagonists of, 55–56
  alcohol-induced alterations in
    cell cultures and, 53–54
    intact animals and, 54–55
  blockade of, 65
  brain studies of, in alcoholic patients, 65–66
  changes in, 60–66
    ethanol effects on, 62, *62*–64, *63*
    neural cell culture studies of, 61–62
  chronic alcoholism effect on, 65–66
  DHP-sensitive, 52, 53
  ethanol effect on
    acute, 62, *62*
    chronic, 65
    depression of, 52–55
    long-term, 62–64, *63*, 65–66
  neuronal excitability and, 31–32
  properties of, ethanol-induced, 64–65
  types of, 31–32, 64–65
  voltage-dependent, 62, *62*, 63, 64
  voltage-gated, 31–32, 64–65
  in withdrawal, 65
Calcium current(s)
  ethanol effect on
    in vitro rat hippocampal neuron study, 69–72, *70*, *71*, *75*, 75

INDEX

Calcium current(s)—*Continued*
    in vivo rat studies, 73–74, *74*
    sedative and anti-epileptic drugs and, 77
    withdrawal and
        in vitro rat studies, *69*, 76
        in vivo rat studies, 73–74, *74*, 76
Calcium signal modulation
    anticonvulsant drugs and, 33
    calmodulin and, 32–33, *33*
    CaM kinase II and, 33–34
    C-kinase and, 34
Calmodulin, calcium signal modulation and, 32–33, *33*
Calmodulin kinase II (CaM kinase II), calcium signal modulation and, 33–34
CaM kinase II. *See* Calmodulin kinase II
cAMP. *See* Cyclic adenosine monophosphate
Carbamazepine
    advantages of, 315–316
    anticonvulsive treatment model of, *317*, 317–318
    in AWS therapy, 315–316
    chemical structure of, *316*
    in epileptic therapy, 8t, 9
    ethanol interaction with, 246
    indications for, 315
    pharmacology of, 316
    prophylactic use of, 315
    treatment problems with, 318–319
    withdrawal seizures following, *317*
Caroverine, 325–326
Catecholamine system(s)
    AWS treatment and
        benzodiazepine actions and, 271
        dopamine and, 270
        norepinephrine in, 270–271
Central nervous system (CNS)
    alcohol effects on, 25–26
    brain, chronic ethanol effect on, 65–66
Cerebral trauma
    alcohol-related seizures and, acute, 202–203
    AWS seizures and, 152–153
Chlordiazepoxide, 87, 88
Chlorpromazine, 321
Cholesterol, chronic ethanol effect on, 46
Chloride (Cl⁻)
    antagonism of, Ro15-4513 and, 108–109
    decrease in
        chronic ethanol and, 109–112, *110*, *111*
        GABA-receptor-mediated, 109–112, *110*, *111*
    GABA-mediated, 51, 57
    inhibition of, Ro15-4513 and, 105–108, *106*, 106t, *107*, 107t
    potentiation of, GABA-receptor-mediated, 103–105, *103*, *104*, *105*
    uptake of, GABA-gated, 94–95
Clonic seizures, epileptic, 6
Clonidine
    naloxone effect on, 323
    withdrawal from, 323
    in withdrawal treatment, 322–323
Coma, 254
Cyclic adenosine monophosphate (cAMP)
    adenosine-receptor-dependence of, 26–27, 79–80, *80*
    in alcoholic patients, 82t, 82–84, 83t, *84*
    production of, 79–80, *80*
    reduction of, 83t, 83–84, *84*
    signal transduction and, 82t, 82–83
Cyclic nucleotide system
    AWS treatment and, 276–277
    benzodiazepine actions and, 277
Cytochrome P450
    biotransformation and, 242–243
    chronic ethanol effect on, 244, 245t

Delirium tremens
    paraldehyde therapy for, 308–309
    in withdrawal, 256
    withdrawal syndrome and, 148–149, 150, 151, 256
Delta activity
    acute ethanol administration and, 180
    early withdrawal and, 185–186
Delta sleep-inducing peptide, 324
Dependency
    adaptation and, GABAergic, 89–90
    calcium channel activity and, 51–54
    enhancement and, GABAergic, *89*, 89
    neuropharmacology of, GABAergic, *96*, 96–97, 98
    postsynaptic
        chloride uptake and, 94–95
        interactions and, 95–96
        receptor ligand binding and, *93*, 93–94
    presynaptic GABA activity and
        release and reuptake of, 90–91
        steady-state concentrations of, *91*, 91
        synthesis of, 90
        turnover of, 91–92
Desialylated transferrin, 207
DHP. *See* 1,4-Dihydropyridine
Diazepam
    in *status epilepticus* treatment, 258, 262, 287t
    in withdrawal treatment, 258
        anti-epileptic drugs and, 258
        antipsychotic drugs and, 258–259
        paraldehyde and, 258
1,4-Dihydropyridine (DHP)
    agonists and antagonists of, 55–56, 57
    binding sites of, 53–54, 325
    Ca^{2+} antagonism and, 52, 53, 57
Disease(s)
    of liver 243–244, 246
    underlying, alcohol-related seizures and, 210–211
Distribution, 241
Dopamine, AWS treatment and, 270, 271
Dose-effect
    EEG activity and
        animal studies of, 179, 181
        human studies of, 180–182
    Harlem study and, 170t, 170–171, 172t
Drinking. *See also* Alcohol use; Social use
    20th century habits of, 222–223
    binge vs. chronic, 206–213, 208t, *209*, *212*
    heavy, 14–17
    patient history of, 206–207
Drug therapy(ies) in alcohol withdrawal treatment. *See* Interactions; Treatment; specific drugs, e.g. Benzodiazepine(s)

Drug use and abuse
    seizures and, binge vs. chronic drinking and, 208–210
    therapy for, 301–302
Drug-effect theory
    contingent tolerance and, 119, 120, *121*
    functional tolerance and, 118–119
Drug-exposure theory
    contingent tolerance and, 119–121, *121*
    functional tolerance and, 118–119
DSIP. *See* Delta sleep-inducing peptide

EAA. *See* Excitatory amino acid receptor(s)
Electroencephalogram (EEG)
    abnormalities in, withdrawal syndrome and, 153–154
    abstinence and
        animal studies and, 182–184, *183*
        human studies and, 184–190, 187t, 190t, *191–192*, 193
    alcohol intake and, 228, 233–234
    anti-epileptic therapy and
        epileptiform discharges and, 190, 193
        photic stimulation and, 189–190, *191–192*
    early abstinence and
        alpha activity and, 185–186
        beta activity and, 184–185
        epileptiform discharges and, 186–188, 187t, *188*
        focal slowing in, 186
        photoconvulsive response and, 188
        photomyogenic response and, 189–190
        photoparoxysmal response and, 188–189, 190, *191–192*
        sleep and, 186–187, 187t
        theta and delta activity and, 185–186
    epileptiform discharges and
        in animal studies, 182–184, *183*
        anti-epileptic therapy and, 190, 193
        BAL and, 193
        early abstinence and, 186–188, 187t, *188*
    ethanol administration and
        acute, 179–181
        chronic, 181–182
    later abstinence and, 190, 193
    usefulness of, in alcohol-related seizures, 193–194
Electrophysiologic recording(s)
    of ethanol effect
        on afterhyperpolarization currents, 70–71, *71*
        on calcium currents, 69–70, *70*, *71*
        on excitatory postsynaptic potentials and, 69–70, *70*
        on inhibitory postsynaptic potentials, 69–70, *70*
    of ethanol–GABA interaction, 95–96
Elimination, 241–242
Enzyme system(s)
    ethanol metabolism and
        alcohol dehydrogenase system in, 242, 243, 244
        microsomal ethanol oxidizing system in, 242–243, 244

Epidemiology
    of alcohol use, 12–17, 18–20
    of epilepsy, 17–18
Epilepsy
    alcohol use and, 19–20, 146
    alcoholism and, concurrent, 197, 329
    definition and classification of, 3–4
    drug therapy for
        benzodiazepines, 11t
        chronic, 8–10, 8t, *9*
        effective plasma levels of, 8t
        fundamentals of, 8
        structure of compounds in, *9*
    epidemiology of, 17–18
    generalized seizures in
        atonic, 6
        clonic, 6
        drug therapy for, 9–10
        myoclonic, 6
        tonic-clonic, 6–7, 7t
    latent, in alcoholic patients, 146
    partial seizures in
        complex, 5–6
        drug therapy for, 8t, 8–9, *9*
        progression of, 5, 5t, 0
        simple, 5
        subgroups of, 4t, 4–5
    seizures in
        generalized, 6–7, 7t
        idiopathic, 152
        latent, 146
        partial, 4t, 4–6, 5t
    syndromes in, 7–8
Epileptic patient(s)
    alcohol use by, physicians' attitudes and, 228–231, 229t, 230t
    alcoholic, therapy of, 247–248
    alcohol-related seizures in, 262–263
    nonalcoholic, neurophysiology of alcohol use by, 233–239, 235t, *236*, 236t 237
    seizures in, 263
    social alcohol use by, 223–228, 225t, 226t, 228t, 229t
Epileptic seizure(s)
    generalized, 6–7, 7t, 9–10
    idiopathic, withdrawal syndrome and, 152
    latent, in alcoholic patients, 146
    partial, 4t, 4–6, 5t
Epileptic syndrome, 7–8
Epileptiform discharge(s)
    blood alcohol level and, 193
    ethanol administration and, 181
    periodic lateralized
        early withdrawal and, 187–188, *188*
        later withdrawal and, 190, 193
    sleep and, early withdrawal and, 186–187, 187t
    in withdrawal, animal studies of, 182–184, *183*
EPSPs. *See* Excitatory postsynaptic potential(s)
Ethanol. *See also* Alcohol
    acute administration of
        calcium currents and, neuronal, 70, 71, 71–72, *72*, *73*
        EEG activity following, 179–181
    adaptation to
        abnormal lipids and, 47–48
        acidic phospholipids and, 46–47, 47t
        cholesterol and fatty acids and, 46

Ethanol—Continued
  anticonvulsant effect of, kindled seizures and, 115–124
  anti-epileptic drug interactions with
    clinical aspects and, 246–247
    concomitant treatment and, 245–246
    mechanism of, 245, 245t
    pharmacodynamics and, 246
    pharmacokinetics and, 246
  calcium and, 60–61
  calcium channels and
    activity of, in dependency, 51–54
    alterations of, in withdrawal, 61–66
  chronic administration of
    calcium currents and, neuronal, 72–73
    EEG patterns in, 181–182
    epileptiform discharges in, 181
  chronopharmacokinetics of, 243
  dependence on
    calcium channels in, 51–57
    GABA changes in, 87–98
  depressant action of, neuronal, 51–53
  drug interactions with
    pentobarbital, 103, 110, 110
    phenobarbital, 245–246
    phenytoin, 246–247
    valproate, 246
  GABA/benzodiazepine receptor complex and, 103–112
    Cl⁻ flux and, 103, 103–105, 104, 105
    Ro15-4513 action on, 105–108, 106, 106t, 107, 107t
  GABAergic changes and
    postsynaptic activity and, 93, 93–96
    presynaptic activity and, 90–92, 91
    withdrawal and, 87, 88, 89, 89–90, 96
  GABAmimetic action and
    neuroanatomic correlates and, 96, 96–97, 98
  metabolism of
    absorption and distribution in, 241
    acetaldehyde and, 243
    biotransformation in, 242–243
    elimination in, 241–242
    factors affecting, 243–244
  neuronal calcium currents and
    acute administration and, 70, 71, 71–72, 72, 73
    chronic administration and, 72–73
    withdrawal and, 73–75, 74, 75
  neuronal depressant action of
    Ca²⁺ channels and, 52–53
    GABAᴬ receptor and Cl⁻ flux and, 51–52
  neuronal effect of, 68, 69
  neuronal membrane lipids interactions with
    biphasic effects and, 44–45
    fluidization and, 44, 46
    neuronal receptor systems and, 45, 45t
    partitioning and, 44
  potentiation of, 244, 245t
  tolerance to anticonvulsant effect of
    contingent dissipation of, 119–122, 120, 121
    development of, 118, 118
    early studies of, 115–116
    in kindled seizures, 118, 118
    kindling model and, 116–118, 117t

Ethosuximide, in epileptic therapy, 8t, 9, 10
Excitability. See Hyperexcitability; Membrane excitability; Neuronal excitability regulation
Excitatory amino acid receptor(s) (EAA), 29–30
Excitatory postsynaptic potential(s) (EPSPs)
  ethanol administration and withdrawal and, 69–70, 70

Fatty acid(s), 46
First seizure(s), 165–166, 199–202, 200t, 201t
Focal slowing, early withdrawal and, 186

GABA. See Gamma-aminobutyric acid
GABAᴬ receptor(s)
  Cl⁻ flux and, 51, 57
  intoxication and, 51–52
GABA/benzodiazepine receptor
  Cl⁻ flux mediation and
    decrease in, chronic alcoholism, 109–112, 110, 111
    ethanol potentiation of, 104–105, 105
    ethanol stimulation of, 103, 103–105, 104
    Ro14-4513 antagonisms of, 108–109
    Ro15-4513 inhibition of, 105–108, 106, 106t, 107, 107t
GABA/BZD/chloride ionophore receptor complex, 267–269
  benzodiazepines and,
    actions of, 269
    receptors of, 268–269
  GABA receptors in, 268
Gamma-aminobutyric acid (GABA)
  baclofen and, 325
  in dependence
    postsynaptic activity of, 92–96, 93
    presynaptic activity of, 90–92, 91
  ethanol relationship and, 324
  GABAergic changes during withdrawal
    adaptation of, 89–90
    enhancement of, by ethanol, 89, 89
    GABAmimetics and withdrawal suppression, 87, 88
  GABA-gated chloride uptake and, 94–95
  interaction of
    postsynaptic, 95–96
    presynaptic, 92
  muscimol and, 324–325
  receptors of
    benzodiazepine receptor sites and, 36–37, 37
    Cl⁻ mediation and, 103–105, 103, 104, 105, 109–112, 110, 111
    depression of, 51–52
    GABAᴬ receptors and, 51–52, 57
    intoxication and, 51–52
    ligand binding in, 93, 93–94
  release and reuptake of, 90–91
  steady-state concentrations of, 91, 91
  synthesis of, 90
  turnover of, 91–92
Gamma-aminobutyric acid (GABA) system(s)
  GABA levels in alcohol withdrawal seizures, 267
  GABA/BZD/chloride ionophore receptor complex, 267–269

benzodiazepine receptors and, 268–269
GABA receptors and, 268
Gamma-glutamyltransferase (GGT), binge drinking and, 207
Generalized tonic-clonic seizure (GTS)
   benzodiazepines and, 34, 37, 39, 40
   classification of, 6–7, 7t
   clonic phase of, 7t
   drug therapy of, 9–10
   tonic phase of, 7t
   withdrawal and, in mice, 126–127, 127t
Genetics
   susceptibility and
      binge vs. chronic drinking and, 212–213
      mouse study of, *130*, 131–133, *131, 132, 133, 134*
   tolerance and, 130–131
GGT. *See* Gamma-glutamyltransferase (GGT)
Glutamate
   benzodiazepine action and, 270
   in withdrawal, 269–270
GTS. *See* Generalized tonic-clonic seizure

5-HT. *See* Serontonin (5-HT) system(s)
Haloperidol, 322
Handling-induced convulsion(s) (HIC)
   genetic mouse model of
      acute withdrawal and, *131*, 131–132
      anticonvulsant treatment sensitivity in, 134–135, *135*
      as AWS sign, 126–127, 127t
      codetermination of withdrawal and, *130, 131*
      differences in, 127–128
      seizure susceptibility and, *132*, 132–134, *133, 134*
      sensitivity and tolerance in, 130–131
      severe- and mild-ethanol withdrawal mice, 135–136
      withdrawal-seizure-prone and resistant mice, *129*, 129–130
Harlem Study
   mechanisms of AWS and
      abstention time in, 179–171, 171t, 172t, *173*, 175
      consumption and, 168t, 168–169, 169t
      demographics in, 168, 168t
      dose-effect in, 170t, 170–171
      first seizure in, 165–166
Head trauma, alcohol-related seizures and, acute, 202–203
HIC. *See* Handling-induced convulsion(s)
Hormone(s)
   AWS treatment and, 277
   benzodiazepine actions and, 277
Hydroxyzine, 322
Hyperexcitability, 51
Hypomagnesemia, 155, 157, 158

Imidazobenzodiazepine, *106*
Inhibition
   of calcium flux, 62, *62, 63*, 65
   of Cl$^-$ flux, GABA/benzodiazepine receptor-mediated, 105–108, *106*, 106t
   GABAergic, 87, *88*, 90

Inhibitory postsynaptic potential(s) (IPSPs), 69–70, *70*, 75, *76*, 77
Interaction(s)
   drug—ethanol
      pentobarbital, *103*, 110, *110*
      phenobarbital, 245–246
      phenytoin, 246–247
      valproate, 246
   phospholipid—membrane proteins, 47, 47t
Intoxication
   acute, 254
   chronic. *See* Alcoholism
   coma in, 254
   GABA$_A$ receptor role in, 51–52
   mechanism of, 51–52
   seizures in, causes of, 254t
Intracranial lesions, alcohol-related seizures and, 199–202, 200t, 201t
IPSPs. *See* Inhibitory postsynaptic potential(s)

Kainic acid, 30
Kindled seizures
   ethanol tolerance and anticonvulsant effect on, 115–118, *118*
   hypothesis of, 211
   kindling model and, 116–118, 117t
   severity of, in rats, 117t

Laboratory markers
   binge drinking and, 207
   blood alcohol level, 25–26, 163, 164, 193
   SGOT, 218
Lipids
   chronic ethanol effect on, 47–48
   neuronal membrane—ethanol interaction and
      biphasic effects and, 44–45
      fluidization and, 44, 46
      receptor systems and, 45, 45t
Liver disease
   ethanol metabolism and, 243–244
   ethanol—anti-epileptic drug pharmacokinetics and, 246
Lofexidine, 323
Lymphocytes, cAMP production in, 83t, 83–84, *84*

Macrocytosis corpuscular volume (MCV), 207
Maximal electric shock (MES), 34, 35
MCV. *See* Macrocytosis corpuscular volume
Mechanism(s)
   of chronic alcohol effect, 65
   Harlem study of
      abstention time in, 170–171, *171*, 172t, *173*, 175
      consumption in, 168t, 168–169, 169t, 172t
      demographics in, 168, 168t
      dose-effect in, 170t, 170–171
      first seizure in, 165–166
      seizure classification in, 167
   of intoxication, 51
   past studies of, 163–165
Membrane excitability
   benzodiazepine receptors and, 34–35, *35*
      binding sites of, 37, 37–38, *38*
      GABA receptor side and, 36

Membrane excitability—*Continued*
    micromolar receptors and, 37–38, *38*
    nanomolar receptors and, 35–37, *36*
MEOS. *See* Microsomal ethanol oxidizing system
Meprobamate, 322
MES. *See* Maximal electric shock
Mesoridazine, 322
Metabolism
    of acetaldehyde, 243
    of calcium, 272–273
    of ethanol
        absorption and distribution in, 241
        biotransformation in, 242–243
        elimination in, 242–242
        factors affecting, 242–244
    of paraldehyde, 306
Methionine-enkephalin
    AWS treatment and, 275
    in withdrawal treatment, 323–324
Microsomal ethanol oxidizing system (MEOS)
    acute ethanol effect on, 244
    biotransformation and, 242–243, 244
Muscimol
    Cl^- uptake stimulation, ethanol and, *105*, 111, *111*
    GABA and, in withdrawal syndrome, 324–325
    withdrawal suppression and, 87, 88, 89
Myoclonia(s), epileptic, 6

Naloxone
    clonidine and, 323
    delta sleep-inducing peptide and, 324
    in ethanol-induced seizures, 324
Neural cells
    cAMP production in
        adenosine-receptor-dependent, 79–80, *80*
        PGE_1-receptor dependent, 80–81, 81t
    ethanol effect on
        cAMP signal transduction in, 79, 82t, 82–85
        culture studies of, 61–62
        receptor systems of, 45, 45t
Neuronal excitability regulation
    benzodiazepine receptors and, 34–35, *35*
        binding sites of, 37, 37–38, *38*
        GABA receptor site and, 36
        micromolar receptors, 37–38, *38*
        nanomolar benzodiazepine receptors and, 35–37, *36*
    calcium regulation and
        calcium channels and, 31
        calcium signal modulation and, 32–34, 33
        voltage-gated calcium channels and, 31–32
    EAA receptors and, 29–30
    sustained repetitive firing and
        anticonvulsant action and, 39
        benzodiazepines and, 39–41
        drug and second messenger modulation of, 39–41, *40*
    withdrawal and, 29–41
Neuropharmacology, 278t
    acetylcholine and, 273–274
    adenosine and, 272
    adenosine triphosphatase and, 276
    calcium metabolism and, 272–273
    catecholamine systems and, 270–271
    cyclic nucleotide system and, 276–277
    GABA systems and, 267–269
    GABAergic, 96, *96*–97, *98*
    glutamate and, 269–270
    hormones and, 277
    opiates and, 274–276
    serotonin systems and, 271–272
Neurophysiology study(ies)
    of alcohol intake in nonalcoholic epileptic patients
        clinical effects of, 233, 234–235, 235t, 236t
        EEG effects of, 233, *236*, 236–237, *237*, 238–239
        seizure exacerbation and, 235–236, 235t, 236t, 238, 239
        seizure occurrence and, 223–224, 238
Neuroreceptor system(s)
    in AWS
        adenosine receptors and, 26–27, 79–83, 81t, *82*, 83t, *84*
        benzodiazepine receptor complex, 27, 35–38, *36*, 37, *38*, 106t
        GABA/benzodiazepine/chloride ionophore complex, 27, 268–269 complex, 27
        opiate, 323–324
Neurotransmission
    GABAergic
        drugs and, 87, 88
        ethanol and, 89–90
Norepinephrine, AWS treatment and, 270–271

Opiate receptor(s), agonists and antagonists of, 323–324
Opiate(s)
    AWS treatment and, 275–276
    benzodiazepine action and, 276
    endogenous, 323–324
Opioid peptide(s)
    antagonists of, 275
    beta-endorphin, 275
    methionine-enkephalin, 275

Paraldehyde
    administration of
        intramuscular, 310–311
        intravenous, 311–312
        oral, 309–310
        rectal, 310–311
    in agitated and delirious patients, 305
    in AWS treatment, 331
    clinical pharmacology and action of, 306–307
    diazepam and, 258
    dosages of, recommended, 310t
    historical uses of
        as pre-anesthetic and analgesic agent, 305
        as sedative and hypnotic agent, 304
    metabolism of, 306
    precautions with, 313
    protocol for, recommended, 312t, 312–313
    side effects of, 305–306, 310t

therapeutic usage of
    in delirium tremens, 308–309
    in *status epilepticus*, 311
    in withdrawal treatment, 258, 262, 308
Partial epileptic seizure(s)
  complex, 5–6
  progression of, 5, 5t
  simple, 5
  subgroups of, 4t, 4–5
PC12 cell line culture(s)
  ethanol effect on, 62, 63, 64, 65
PCR. *See* Photoconvulsive response
Pentobarbital, ethanol interaction with, *103*, 110, *110*
Pentylentetrazol (PTZ), benzodiazepines and, 34, 36, 37
Phenobarbital
  in alcoholic epileptic patients, 248
  in convulsion management, 302
  in epileptic therapy, 8t, 9, *9*
  ethanol interaction with, 245–246
  intravenous
    dosage—blood level relationship, 301
    prospective uncontrolled trial of, 298–301, 299t
  rationale for use of, 298
  sedative withdrawal treatment with, 301–302
  in *status epilepticus* therapy, 262, 301, 302
  versus benzodiazepines, 298
Phenytoin
  in AWS, 258, 262, 330
  in epileptic therapy, 8–9, 8t, *9*
  ethanol interaction with, 246–247
  rationale for
    animal studies and, 291t, 291–292
    cross-tolerance with alcohol, 290–291
    human trials, 292
    San Francisco General Hospital study
      patient population in, 293–295, 294t, 295t
      results of, 295
  in *status epilepticus*, loading dosage of, 217t, 220, 221
Phosphatidylcholine, chronic ethanol effect on, 46
Phosphatidylethanol, abnormal lipids and, 47
Phosphatidylserine, neuronal function and, 47, 47t
Phospholipid(s)
  chronic ethanol effect on
    administration mode and, 47
    concentrations of, 46
    interactions with membrane proteins, 47, 47t
Photic stimulation
  early withdrawal and
    anti-epileptic therapy and, 189–190, *191–192*
    photoconvulsive response and, 188
    photomyogenic response and, 189–190
    photoparoxysmal response and, 188–189, 190, *191–192*
    sensitivity to, 190t
  photomyoclonus and, 154–155, *155*, *157*, 159
Photoconvulsive response (PCR), 188
Photomyoclonus, alcohol withdrawal syndrome and, 154–155, *155*, *157*, 159
Photomyogenic response (PMR), 189–190

Photoparoxysmal response (PPR), 188–189, 190, *191—192*
Physician(s)
  attitudes of, alcohol use by epileptic patients and, 228–231, 229t, 230t
PMR. *See* Photomyogenic response
Postassium current(s)
  neuronal effects of, 68–79. *See also* Calcium current(s)
Potentiation, concomitant drug use and, 244, 244t
PPR. *See* Photoparoxysmal response
Primodone, in epileptic therapy, 8t, 9, *9*
Propranolol, 322
Protein kinase C (C-kinase)
  abnormal lipids and, 47
  calcium signal modulation and, 34
PTZ. *See* Pentylentetrazol

Ro15-4513
  antagonism of ethanol-induced behaviors and, 108–109
  GABA/benzodiazepine receptor complex and, 105–109, *106*, 106t, *107*, 107t
  inhibition of GABA-mediated Cl⁻ flux by, 105–108, *106*, 106t, *107*, 107t

Sedative withdrawal, phenobarbital therapy in, 301–302
Seizure(s). *See also* Alcohol-related seizures; Alcohol withdrawal seizure(s) (AWS); *Status epilepticus*
  alcohol abuse-associated, etiologies of, 197–203
  in alcoholic patients
    epileptogenic factors and, 330
    genesis of, 329–330
  alcoholism and
    epidemiology of, 12, 17–19
    withdrawal seizures in, 143–146, 144t
  alcohol-related
    alcoholism and, 143–146, 144t
    EEGs in, 179–194
    etiologies of, 197–203
    mechanisms of, 162–176
  epileptic, 144t
    alcohol use and, 19–20, 146
    alcohol-induced, 145–146
    classification of, 4t, 4–7, 5t, 7t
    drug therapy for, 8t, 8–11, *9*, 11t
    exacerbation of, chlorpromazine and, 321
    generalized, 6–7, 7t
    incidence and prevalence of, 17–18
    neurophysiologic study of, 228–231, 229t, 230t, 234–239, 235t, *236*, *237*
    partial, 4t, 4–6, 5t
    patients with chronic alcoholism and, 18–20
    provocation of, 230t, 230–231
    social alcohol use and, 223–229, 225t, 226t, 228t, 229t
  kindled, 115–118
  MES-induced, benzodiazepines and, 34, 35, 37, 40, 41
  pentylenetetrazol-induced, benzodiazepines and, 34, 36, 37, 40, 41
  serial, *status epilepticus* and, 217t

Seizure(s)—*Continued*
  single, 259–260
  susceptibility to, genetic, *132*, 132–133, *133*
  withdrawal
    binge vs. chronic drinking and, 206–213
    genetic models of, mouse, 126–137
    models for, 26–27
Serotonin (5-HT) system(s)
  AWS treatment and, 271–272
  benzodiazepine actions and, 272
Sex steroid hormone(s), ethanol metabolism and, 243
SGOT, in *status epilepticus* and, *218*
SHT. *See* Sustained high threshold (SHT) current
Sleep
  epileptiform discharges in, 186–187, 187t
  ethanol effect on, 243
Social uses of alcohol
  20th century drinking habits and, 222–223
  in epileptic patients, 223–228, 225t, 226t, 228t
  physicians' attitudes toward, in epileptic patients, 228–231, 229t, 230t
SRF. *See* Sustained repetitive firing
St. Paul Ramsey study, 216–220
Status epilepticus
  clinical features of, 255–256
  diagnosis of, 261
  St. Paul Ramsey Study
    alcohol use and related seizures in, *218*
    etiology analysis in, 217–219
    frequency of, 220
    mortality and, 219t
    phenytoin loading and, 217t, 220, 221
    seizure classification in, 217t
    serial seizures and, 217t
    subjects in, 219t
    SGOT values and, *218*
  therapy for
    benzodiazepines in, 287t, 287–288
    diazepam in, 287t
    general, 9, 10
    paraldehyde in, 311
    phenobarbital in, 262, 301, 302
    phenytoin in, 8–9, 217t, 220, 221
  tonic-clonic seizures in, 261–262
Susceptibility
  in binge vs. chronic drinking, 212–213
  genetic, mouse study, *130*, 131–133, *131*, *132*, *133*, *134*
Sustained high threshold (SHT) current
  acute alcoholism and, *72*, *73*, *76*
Sustained repetitive firing (SRF)
  anticonvulsant drugs and, 39–41
  benzodiazepine receptors and, 39–41, *40*
  drug and second messenger modulation of, 39–41, *40*
  neuronal excitability and, 38–39

Theta activity
  acute ethanol administration and, *180*, *181*
  early withdrawal and, 185–186
THT. *See* Transient high threshold (THT) current
Tolerance
  acute, 25
  chronic, 26
  in chronic alcoholism, 254

contingent
  dissipation of, 122–123, *123*
  drug-effect theory and, 119, 120, *120*
  drug-exposure theory and, 119–121, *121*
  generality of, 124
cross-tolerance with phenytoin, 290–291
functional, drug-exposure and drug-effect theories of, 118–119
genetics and, mouse studies, 130–131
Tonic-clonic seizures
  classification of, 6–7, 7t
  clonic phase of, 7t
  drug therapy for, 9–10
  in *status epilepticus*, 261–262
  tonic phase of, 7t
  withdrawal and, mouse study, 126–127, 127t
Transient high threshold (THT) current
  acute alcoholism and, *71*, *72*, *72*, *75*, *75*, *76*
Treatment
  alpha-adrenergic receptor agonists in, 322–3
  anti-epileptic drugs and, 244–247, 258, 331
  antipsychotic drugs in, 258–259
  baclofen in, 325
  barbiturates in, 258, 262
  benzodiazepines in
    clinical applications of, 283–289
    general, 257–258
    neuropharmacology of withdrawal and, 267–277
  beta-adrenergic blockers in, 322
  beta-endorphin and, 275, 323–324
  calcium channel blockers in, 325–326
  carbamazepine in, 315–316, *316*, *317*, 317–9
  chlorpromazine in, 321
  clonidine in, 322–323
  delta sleep-inducing peptide in, 324
  diazepam in, 258, 262
  GABA and, 324
  general principles of, 257–259, 262
  haloperidol in, 322
  lofexidine in, 323
  methionine-enkephalin and, 295, 323–324
  muscimol and, 324–325
  naloxone and, 324
  neuroleptics in, 321–322
  paraldehyde in, 258, 262, 304–313
  phenobarbital in, 262, 299–301
  phenytoin in, 262
    rationale for, 291t, 291–292
    San Franciso General Hospital study of, 293–295, 294t, 295t
  valproate in, 315, 316, *316*, 318, 319
Trimethadione, in epileptic therapy, 9, 10

Valproate
  anticonvulsive treatment model of, 318
  chemical structure of, *316*
  in epileptic therapy, 8t, 10
  ethanol interaction with, 246
  hepatotoxicity of, 319
  indications for, 315
  literature on, 315
  pharmacology of, 316
  treatment problems with, 319

Withdrawal. *See* Alcohol withdrawal